# Computational Biophysics of the Skin

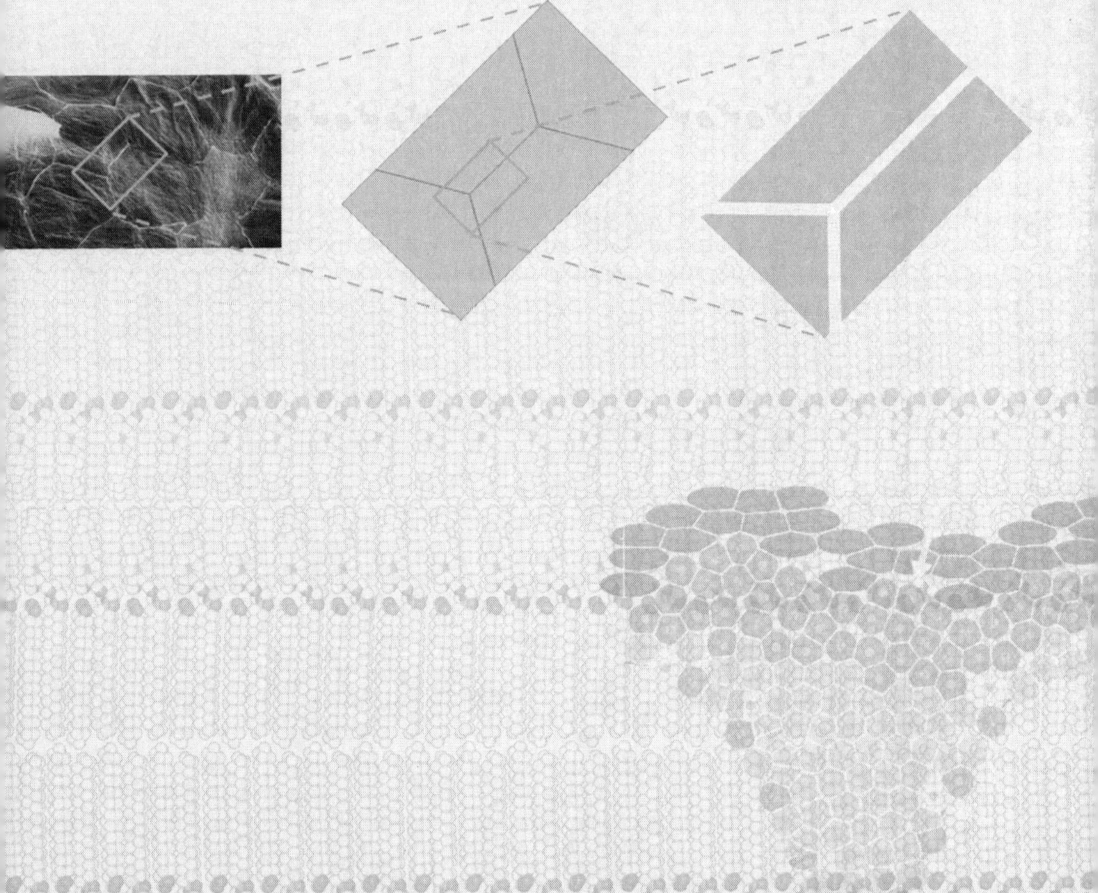

# Computational Biophysics of the Skin

edited by
**Bernard Querleux**

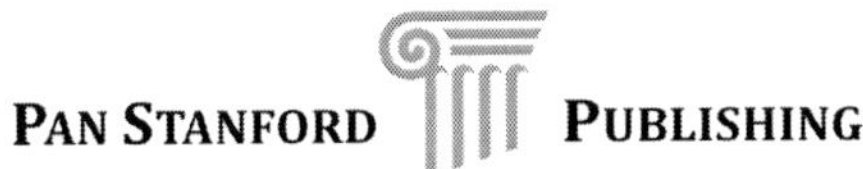

PAN STANFORD PUBLISHING

*Published by*

Pan Stanford Publishing Pte. Ltd.
Penthouse Level, Suntec Tower 3
8 Temasek Boulevard
Singapore 038988

Email: editorial@panstanford.com
Web: www.panstanford.com


**British Library Cataloguing-in-Publication Data**
A catalogue record for this book is available from the British Library.

**Computational Biophysics of the Skin**



ISBN 978-981-4463-84-3 (Hardcover)
ISBN 978-981-4463-85-0 (eBook)

Printed in the USA

*To my wife, Sylvie*
*To my sons, Simon, Samuel, and Elie*

Look at the invisible skin to understand
the visible skin

—*Inspired by* The Picture of Dorian Gray,
*Oscar Wilde, 1891*
*"The true mystery of the world is the visible,
not the invisible"*

# Contents

## PART 3: SKIN BARRIER

**12. Accurate Multiscale Skin Model Suitable for Determining the Sensitivity and Specificity of Changes of Skin Components**    **353**

*Jürg Fröhlich, Sonja Huclova, Christian Beyer, and Daniel Erni*

# Foreword

We have learned much about skin. Starting in the 19th century, the observations can truly be described as enlightenment. Traditionally, this term is used for our basic knowledge in physics and chemistry; however, it represents what occurred in skin knowledge. The basics of anatomy, dissection, histology, cellular anatomy, the cell, and the power of special stains propelled us to what became possible in the 20th century.

The 20th century saw a rapid expansion, as the decades went along, from a handful of laboratories to dozens of strong basic and clinical science laboratories that took advantage of the start of the 19th century knowledge. Special stains rapidly gained prominence, followed by biochemistry, electron microscopy, and eventually molecular biology.

By the end of the 20th century, the critical mass had been reached that made this textbook possible.

The 21st century will see modeling become a main line part of cutaneous science and many other areas of investigation.

In this textbook, Bernard Querleux has amassed a monumental amount of information that had been widely dispersed and not previously readily available to the passive and active scholar.

By dividing the book in broad sweeps, it becomes readily absorbed. Scientists interested in color, mechanics, the inordinate complexity of the many skin barriers, the numerous fluids, and that all-encompassing area known as homeostasis will find well-disciplined packages that make for easy reading.

The limitation of this book's scholar relates not to the power of the computer or the programming but to the limitations of high-quality biological observations that are currently available.

Whether at the subcellular, cellular, anatomic, functional (physiology), pathologic, or pathology levels, the human brain, programming, and the computer can do more than what is available in terms of hard high-quality scientific observations.

Much of this is in the realm of so-called big science obtaining cooperative study groups to provide the data that is necessary to predict with the power of the computer.

This volume will serve as the standard textbook for undergraduates, masters, and PhD students wishing to utilize the computer and programs to understand the complexity of human cutaneous biology.

It will likely be the source of dozens of masters and PhD theses in the decades to come.

Because we are now at the critical mass and we have this superb concise overview, we predict that the next decades will be highly fruitful and will benefit many areas of science, in addition to skin.

**Howard I. Maibach, M.D.**
The University of California School of Medicine
Department of Dermatology
San Francisco, California 94143-0989, USA
May 2014

# Preface

For a long time, skin properties have been considered easy to explore, as the skin is accessible to palpation and visual control. If clinical exam remains the reference approach for individual diagnosis, it has also shown its limits in reproducibility and accuracy for quantifying skin properties, for instance, in clinical studies aiming at characterizing chronological and photoaging, skin specificity related to ethnic origins, and the evaluation of the efficacy and safety of dermatological and cosmetic products.

Taking advantage of the accessibility of the skin in vivo, non-invasive methods were developed for about 40 years, which nowadays offer accurate measurements of the skin color through optical methods, firmness and elasticity measurements through biomechanical devices, and even direct measurements of some skin functions such as excretion, transepidermal water loss, perfusion, and the barrier function. In vivo skin imaging has also appeared in the past decades and gives us much information on the skin structures from the microscopic to macroscopic levels.

However, we should admit that at the dawn of the 21st century, the mechanisms involved in these properties are still partly understood owing to the multidomain (biological, biochemical, and biophysical domains) and multiscale dimension (cellular and below to tissular and beyond) of the mechanisms. In many domains, including biomedical engineering, numerical modeling is nowadays recognized as a complementary key actor for improving our knowledge.

This book presents for the first time the contributions that focus on scientific computing and numerical modeling and simulations to offer a deeper understanding of mechanisms involved in some skin functions. The book is structured around some skin properties and functions, with—for each of them—several chapters describing either biological or physical models at different scales.

Part 1 is dedicated to skin optics. From skin color simulation to the biology of skin pigmentation, these three chapters offer key issues to modulate skin appearance.

Part 2 deals with the biomechanical properties of the skin, which are analyzed from the tissular scale toward the cellular scale. These chapters bring new insights on the relative impact of the main skin components on its non-linear biomechanical properties.

One major function of the skin is to work as a protective barrier against the penetration of external substances, allergens, and microorganisms. Part 3 considers this function at different scales and represents the state of the art in the understanding of skin permeation.

Part 4 is focused on skin fluids, whose impact on the skin physiology is very important but surprisingly have not been studied much. Water behavior and state in the different skin layers and a deeper description about skin microcirculation through numerical simulation allow a better knowledge of some dynamic properties of the skin physiology.

The last part of the book is more prospective and gathers two chapters that introduce new modeling approaches based on the "systems biology" approach. Aiming at integrating a large quantity of data, the chapters discuss mathematical and non-mathematical modeling of skin homeostasis.

I would like to thank all the authors for providing outstanding contribution to this book and also for their support to this idea that computational biophysics is a key approach to foster our understanding of the physiology of organs such as the skin.

I am personally deeply grateful to Stanford Chong, from Pan Stanford Publishing, who first suggested that I edit this book and helped me broaden the covered topics. I don't forget to thank Sarabjeet Garcha and Arvind Kanswal from Pan Stanford Publishing, not only for their great job concerning the publishing but also for their permanent kindness to solve all the problems.

I hope this book will help all the readers, from master students to confirmed researchers, coming from many disciplines such as dermatology, cosmetic science, biology, chemistry, physics, and computer science, in developing their own research of this fascinating but complex organ, which is the human skin.

**Bernard Querleux**
May 2014

# PART 1

## SKIN COLOR

# Chapter 1

# Multilayer Modeling of Skin Color and Translucency


Gladimir V. G. Baranoski,[a] Tenn F. Chen,[a] and Aravind Krishnaswamy[b]

[a]*University of Waterloo,*
*200 University Ave. West, Waterloo, Ontario, N2L 3G1, Canada*
[b]*Google Inc.,*
*1600 Amphitheatre Parkway, Mountain View, CA 94043, USA*
gvgbaran@curumin.cs.uwaterloo.ca


## 1.1 Introduction

The computer modeling of skin appearance has a wide range of applications, from the generation of realistic images for educational and entertainment purposes to the screening of medical conditions and the assessment of the efficacy of sunscreens and cosmetics. Skin appearance attributes, such as color and translucency, result from complex light interaction processes. In order to simulate these processes and obtain reliable predictions about skin appearance attributes, it is necessary to take into account the biophysical properties of the different skin tissues such as thickness, refractive index, and the presence of light absorbers and scatterers. Although the main skin tissues are normally represented by layers during light transport simulations, the number of skin layers and


*Computational Biophysics of the Skin*

Edited by Bernard Querleux

Copyright © 2014 Pan Stanford Publishing Pte. Ltd.

ISBN 978-981-4463-84-3 (Hardcover), 978-981-4463-85-0 (eBook)

www.panstanford.com

the level of detail employed to characterize them may vary among the different skin multilayer models available in the literature.

In this chapter, we concisely address these modeling efforts from a practical perspective. We start with an outline of relevant radiometric concepts related to the measurement of appearance of skin specimens, followed by an overview of the different approaches normally used to simulate light propagation and absorption within skin multilayer modeling frameworks. We then discuss predictability and reproducibility guidelines that should be followed so that skin appearance models can be effectively employed in interdisciplinary investigations and applications that involve the high fidelity simulation of skin color and translucency. During this discussion, we briefly examine a biophysically based spectral model of light interaction with human skin (BioSpec [1]) that has been employed in different application domains, from realistic image synthesis [2] to biomedical optics [3] and pattern recognition [4]. This particular case study is used to illustrate issues related to model development and evaluation procedures, as well as current trends involving the reproducibility of model predictions and code transparency. We close the chapter with an outlook on open research avenues that can lead to future advances in the predictive modeling of skin appearance attributes.

## 1.2  Measurement of Skin Appearance

The group of measurements necessary to characterize the appearance of a given material is called its measurement of appearance [5]. These measurements involve the spectral and the spatial energy distribution of the light propagated by the material. The variations in the spectral distribution of the propagated light are responsible for appearance attributes such as hue, lightness, and saturation, while changes in the spatial distribution of the propagated light affect appearance characteristics such as glossiness and translucency.

The spectral energy distribution of the propagated light is usually measured in terms of reflectance and transmittance. There are nine different representations of reflectance and transmittance. These representations depend on the incident and propagated (collected) light geometries, which are designated as directional, conical, and hemispherical [6].

The spatial patterns of light distribution are represented by the bidirectional scattering-surface distribution function (BSSDF) [6]. The BSSDF is considered to be a difficult function to measure, store and compute due to its dependency on four parameters: the incidence direction, the propagation direction, the wavelength of the incident light, and the position on the target surface [6]. Hence, for practical purposes, the bidirectional scattering distribution function (BSDF, or simply BDF) is often employed to describe the light scattering behavior of complex biological materials such as human skin.

The BDF assumes that the point of light incidence and the point of light propagation by the material are separated by a negligible distance. This function can be further decomposed into two components: the bidirectional reflectance distribution function (BRDF) and the bidirectional transmittance distribution function (BTDF).

Although the spectral and spatial distributions of light propagated by human skin can be measured separately, they work together to give us the different visual impressions of this biological surface. More specifically, incident light interacts with a skin specimen characterized by a BSSDF, and it may be directionally propagated toward our eyes. Upon reaching our visual system, the incoming light is translated to appearance attributes such as color, glossiness, and translucency. Hence, the appearance of human skin depends on spectral and spatial light distributions, which, in turn, are controlled by the optical properties of biological structures (e.g., cells, organelles, and fibers) present in the cutaneous tissues. These structures are directly associated with the processes of light absorption and scattering within the skin layers, whose histological and optical complexity determine the wide range of spectral signatures and scattering profiles found in the human population.

## 1.3  Light Transport Simulation Approaches

A large number of multilayered models have been developed for the simulation of light interactions with human skin. Although these models employ the same intuitive concept of layers to represent the cutaneous tissues, their formulation is usually tailored to their target applications. Typically, models developed for biomedical applications provide as output the spectral power distribution of skin tissues, while models developed for image synthesis applications provide as output spatial power distribution quantities [2]. In order to obtain these modeled quantities, different light transport simulation approaches can be applied, and no single approach is superior in all the cases. The selection of a given approach is usually determined by the requirements of the application at hand. In this section, we outline the two major groups of simulation approaches, namely deterministic and stochastic, employed in the modeling of skin appearance attributes. Combinations of elements of these two groups may be classified as belonging to a third group of hybrid approaches. Although the following presentation is supported by selected key examples, the reader interested in a broader review of light transport simulations approaches used in this area is referred to comprehensive texts on this topic [2,7,8].

### 1.3.1 Deterministic Simulations

The deterministic simulation approaches used in the modeling of skin appearance attributes rely on the explicit solution of light transport equations through standard numerical techniques. For example, within the Kubelka–Munk theory framework [9], differential equations are used to describe light transport in a medium using as parameters its scattering and absorption coefficients. In skin optics, the Kubelka–Munk theory was initially applied to specific skin tissues. For example, Anderson and Parish [10] developed a model that employed the Kubelka–Munk theory to compute absorption and scattering coefficients for the dermis tissues. Wan et al. [11] extended this model to compute the absorption and scattering coefficients for the epidermis tissues, taking into account both collimated and diffuse incident irradiance. Later on, Doi and Tominaga [12] presented a model that considers the skin composed of two layers representing the epidermis and dermis tissues. They applied the Kubelka–Munk theory to both layers. More recently, the Kubelka–Munk theory has been employed in the modeling of skin appearance attributes for image synthesis applications [13]. Although models based on the Kubelka–Munk theory cannot be considered comprehensive models of optical radiation transfer since they lack a more detailed analysis of the structure and optical properties of the different skin tissues, their relative simplicity makes them competitive candidates for model inversion procedures used to derive tissue optical parameters from reflectance and transmittance measurements.

Photon propagation in optically turbid media, such as skin tissues, can be described by the time and energy independent equation of radiative transport known as the Boltzmann photon transport equation [14]. The diffusion theory can be seen as an approximate solution to this equation [15]. For example, Farrell and Patterson [16] proposed a model based on the diffusion theory to be used in the noninvasive determination of the absorption and scattering properties of mammalian tissues. Their model incorporates a photon dipole source approximation in order to satisfy the tissue boundary conditions, namely light being propagated from a tissue from a point different from the incidence point, and the presence of thin layers of dirt, blood or other fluids on the surface of the tissue under investigation. Models based on the diffusion theory [17] are amenable to analytic manipulation and relatively easy to use. However, it has been stated that when the absorption coefficient of a turbid medium is not significantly smaller than the scattering coefficient, the diffusion theory provides a poor approximation for the photon transport equation [18–20]. Accordingly, it can be successfully applied only when scattering events are more probable than absorption events. In the case of mammalian tissues, this condition is observed in the red and near infrared regions of the light spectrum [21]. For this reason, in the biomedical field, models based on the diffusion theory are usually employed to support investigations involving red lasers [15,22]. Nonetheless, in the computer graphics field, the diffusion theory has been employed to render believable images of human skin [23,24].

When more reliable solutions to the radiative light transport equation in biological tissues are required, more robust methods, such as the adding-doubling method and the discrete ordinate method, can be used. The adding-doubling method [7,25] requires that the reflectance and transmittance of two identical homogeneous thin layers to be known. They are used to compute the reflectance and transmittance of another layer formed by the juxtaposition of these two individual layers. Once the transmittance and reflectance of this paired layer are known, the reflectance and transmittance of a target layer can be computed by repeating this process, i.e., doubling the ensemble of paired layers, until the thickness of the resulting multilayered structure matches the thickness of the target layer.

The discrete ordinate method divides the radiative transport equation into $n$ discrete fluxes to obtain $n$ equations with $n$ unknowns. These equations are then solved using numerical techniques. For example, Nielsen et al. [26] have proposed a skin model composed of five epidermal layers of equal thickness, a dermal layer, and a subcutaneous layer. The subdivision of the epidermis into five layers allowed Nielsen et al. [26] to simulate different contents and size distributions of the melanin-containing organelles (melanosomes). The radiative light transport equation associated with this layered model is then solved using the discrete ordinate algorithm proposed by Stamnes et al. [27] for the simulation of radiative transfer in layered media. This approach is feasible when the phase function (used to describe the bulk scattering of the material under investigation) can be expressed as a sum of Legendre polynomials [28]. For highly asymmetric phase functions, it is necessary to consider a large number of fluxes, which may result in a numerically ill-conditioned system of equations [7].

### 1.3.2 Stochastic Simulations

Models based on stochastic simulation approaches rely on Monte Carlo methods [29] to account for the different optical phenomena affecting light transport within the skin tissues. These methods are usually applied in conjunction with ray optics techniques. More specifically, the light transport processes are simulated as random walks in which the photon (ray) histories are recorded as they are scattered and absorbed within a given skin layer.

Monte Carlo models are extensively used in skin related applications in image synthesis, biomedicine, colorimetry, and pattern recognition, either online (e.g., to determine skin optical properties and other biophysical attributes through inversion procedures) or offline (e.g., to evaluate the effectiveness of modeling frameworks based on deterministic approaches). For example, Shimada et al. [30] proposed a regression analysis algorithm to determine melanin and blood concentration in human skin. In their investigation, they applied the modified Beer–Lambert law [2] and considered three-layered (epidermis, dermis and subcutaneous tissue) skin phantoms. To assess the accuracy of their predictions, they employed a general-purpose Monte Carlo algorithm for light transport in multilayered tissues (Monte Carlo modeling of light transport in multi-layered tissues, or simply MCML) developed by Wang et al. [31]. The same algorithm was employed by Nishidate et al. [32] in their regression analysis investigation aimed at the estimation of melanin and blood concentration in the human skin. However, Nishidate et al. [32] considered two-layered (epidermis and dermis) skin phantoms, and employed the MCML model not only to verify the fidelity of their predictions, but also to derive input data from a number of MCML simulated absorption spectra.

Monte Carlo methods can provide flexible and yet rigorous solutions to light transport within skin tissues [31]. However, many trials (sample rays) are required to determine the overall local light transport behavior of a given skin specimen. For this reason, Monte Carlo models are often employed offline to generate data or to assess the accuracy of predictions provided by other models (e.g., [21,33]). Although most Monte Carlo models share a similar mathematical formulation, key aspects distinguish one model from another and affect the overall accuracy of their predictions. These aspects include the level of abstraction used to represent the skin tissues (e.g., number of layers) and their parameter space. In addition, the correctness of their simulation algorithms is bound by the use of proper representations for the mechanisms of scattering and absorption of photons (rays) as well as the reliability of their input data. Hence, the use of a Monte Carlo model to generate input or evaluation data to another model is scientifically sound only if the predictions provided by the reference Monte Carlo model have been properly evaluated in the first place. It is worth noting that this information is often omitted in related publications.

## 1.4 Practical Guidelines

Multilayered skin models are usually developed for specific applications. For example, they can be designed to simulate variations in the reflectance of skin specimens as responses to physiological changes caused by pathological conditions, or to add glossiness effects on the face of a virtual character. However, it is possible to develop models that can be used in different fields as long as a set of practical guidelines is taken into account. Ideally, such models should enable the computation of spectral and spatial readings for the light propagated by a given skin specimen. More importantly, these models need to be predictive, i.e., their simulation algorithms need to be controlled by biophysically meaningful parameters, and their predictions should be quantitatively and qualitatively evaluated through comparisons with actual measured data. Furthermore, the results provided by such models should be fully reproducible, which requires the complete disclosure of the data and computer code used in the simulations. After all, the reproduction of research findings is one of the fundamental criteria employed to assess scientific contributions.

To date, only a handful of light transport models fulfill these guidelines [3]. A noteworthy exception to this trend is the biophysically based spectral model of light interaction with human skin (BioSpec [1]), which has been used not only in realistic image synthesis applications [2], but also in biomedical applications [3,4]. In the remainder of this section, we provide an overview of BioSpec, and use this model as a case study to illustrate the feasibility of the practical guidelines mentioned above.

## 1.4.1 BioSpec Model Overview

The BioSpec model employs Monte Carlo techniques to simulate light interactions with human skin. Within the BioSpec framework, this organ is considered to be composed of four main layers, namely stratum corneum, epidermis, papillary dermis, and reticular dermis (Fig. 1.1). Accordingly, the BioSpec parameter space includes the refractive index and thickness of each of these layers as well as the specific absorption coefficient, concentration and volume fraction of their main pigments (eumelanin, pheomelanin, oxyhemoglobin, deoxyhemoglobin, methemoglobin, sulfhemoglobin, carboxihemoglobin, β-carotene, and bilirubin). In addition, the aspect ratio of the skin surface folds is also included in the model parameter space along with the refractive index and the diameter of the collagen fibers present in the dermal layers.

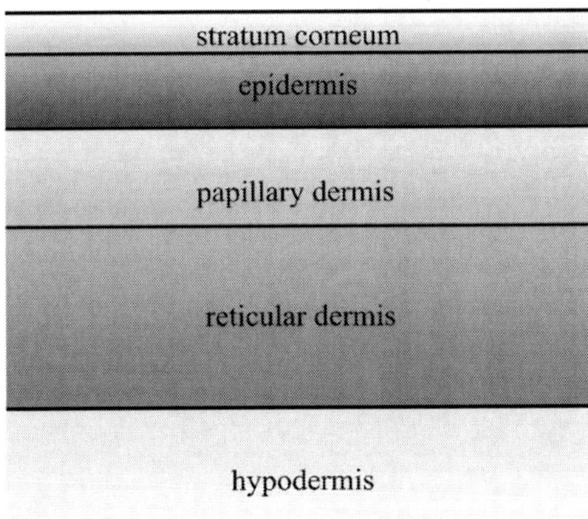


**Figure 1.1** Diagram depicting the skin layers considered by the BioSpec model.

The propagation of light within the skin layers is simulated by the BioSpec model as a random walk process (that relies on the generation of random numbers $\xi_j$, for $j = 1, 2, ..., 9$, uniformly distributed in the interval [0, 1]) using ray optics. In this random walk process, the transition probabilities are associated with Fresnel coefficients computed at each interface between the layers, and the termination probabilities are determined by the ray free path length.

Once a ray impinges on the skin surface, it can be reflected back to the environment or transmitted into its internal tissues. In the former case, the distribution of the reflected light is computed taking into account the aspect ratio, denoted by $\sigma$, of the skin surface folds. As the surface folds become flatter (lower $\sigma$), the reflected light becomes more specular. In order to account for this change in the light reflection behavior, the reflected rays are perturbed using angular displacements obtained from the surface-structure function proposed by Trowbridge and Reitz [34], which represents rough air–material interfaces using microareas randomly curved. These displacements are given in terms of a polar perturbation angle:

$$\theta_s = \cos^{-1}\left[\left(\left(\frac{\sigma^2}{\sqrt{\sigma^4 - \sigma^4 \xi_1 + \xi_1}} - 1\right)b\right)^{1/2}\right], \tag{1.1}$$

where $b$ corresponds to $1/(\sigma^2 - 1)$. The corresponding azimuthal perturbation angle $\phi_s$ is given by $2\pi\xi_2$.

If the ray is transmitted into the skin, then it can be reflected and refracted multiple times within the skin layers before it is either absorbed or propagated back to the environment through the air/stratum corneum interface. In the stratum corneum and epidermis, the scattering of the propagated ray is simulated using angular displacements measured by Bruls and van der Leun [35].

Every ray transmitted into one of the dermal layers is initially tested for Rayleigh scattering [36]. If the test fails or the ray has already been bounced off one of the dermal interfaces, then the ray is randomized around the normal direction using a warping function based on a cosine distribution in which the polar perturbation angle, $\alpha_c$, and the azimuthal perturbation angle, $\beta_c$, are given by

$$(\alpha_c, \beta_c) = (\cos^{-1}((1-\xi_3)^{1/2}), 2\pi\xi_4). \tag{1.2}$$

In order to perform the Rayleigh scattering test, the spectral Rayleigh scattering amount, $S(\lambda)$, is computed using the appropriate expression for Rayleigh scattering involving particles [36]. Next, a random number $\xi_5$ is generated. If $\xi_5 < 1 - e^{-S(\lambda)}$, then the ray is scattered using an azimuthal perturbation angle, $\beta_R$, given by $2\pi\xi_6$, and a polar perturbation angle, $\alpha_R$, obtained using the following rejection sampling algorithm based on the Rayleigh phase function [36]:

```
do        αR = πξ7

          χ = 3ξ8/2

while  (χ > 3√6(1 + cos²αR)sinαR/8)
```

Since the subcutaneous tissue is a highly reflective medium, it is assumed that light impinging on the reticular dermis/hypodermis interface is reflected toward the upper layers.

Once a ray has been scattered in a given layer, it is probabilistically tested for absorption. This test consists in estimating the ray free path length using a formulation based on the Beer–Lambert law [2]. Accordingly, the ray free path length, $p(\lambda)$, is computed using the following expression:

$$p(\lambda) = -\frac{1}{\mu_i(\lambda)}\ln(\xi_7)\cos\theta, \tag{1.3}$$

where $\theta$ corresponds to the angle between the ray and the specimen's normal, and $\mu_i(\lambda)$ represents the total absorption coefficient of a given layer $i$. If $p(\lambda)$ is greater than the thickness of the layer, then the ray is propagated. Otherwise, it is absorbed.

The total absorption coefficient, $\mu_i(\lambda)$, of a given layer $i$ accounts for the specific absorption coefficient (s.a.c.) and the concentration of the pigments present in this layer such as the eumelanin and pheomelanin found in the epidermis. These specific absorption coefficients may be incorporated into the model directly if their values are available. Otherwise, they are calculated using the spectral molar extinction coefficients, $\varepsilon$, and molar weights, $\omega$, of the organic absorbers. The expression used to compute the s.a.c. of an absorber $j$ is given by

$$s_j(\lambda) = \frac{\varepsilon_j(\lambda)}{\omega_j}\ln 10. \tag{1.4}$$

Note that the factor of $\ln 10$ in Eq. 1.4 is needed to convert from an absorbance value (molar extinction) to a specific absorption coefficient.

## 1.4.2 Predictability

The BioSpec design is based on a first-principles strategy in which the simulations are controlled by the fundamental properties of a given skin specimen such as the contents of individual absorbers. The default values assigned for these biophysically meaningful parameters are selected within valid ranges reported in the literature. Accordingly, the radiometric predictions provided by the BioSpec model are amenable to evaluation through comparisons with actual measured data [2]. For example, modeled spectral curves can be obtained using a virtual spectrophotometer [37], and compared with measured ones. This procedure is illustrated in Fig. 1.2, which depicts comparisons of modeled and measured reflectance curves for two skin specimens with different levels of pigmentation, namely a lightly pigmented (LP) and a moderately pigmented (MP) specimen. In these comparisons, the measured curves correspond to measurements provided by Vrhel et al. [38]. These measurements were made available in a spectra database at the North Carolina State University (NCSU spectral files 113 and 82, respectively). The pigmentation parameters used to generate the modeled curves (Table 1.1) were selected based on the skin type description of the actual specimens provided in the NCSU spectra database and the corresponding ranges for these parameters available in the literature [39]. The values assigned for the remaining BioSpec parameters employed in the computation of the modeled curves were gathered from related scientific publications (Table 1.2). Both sets of modeled and measured curves were obtained considering the same angle of incidence (45°).

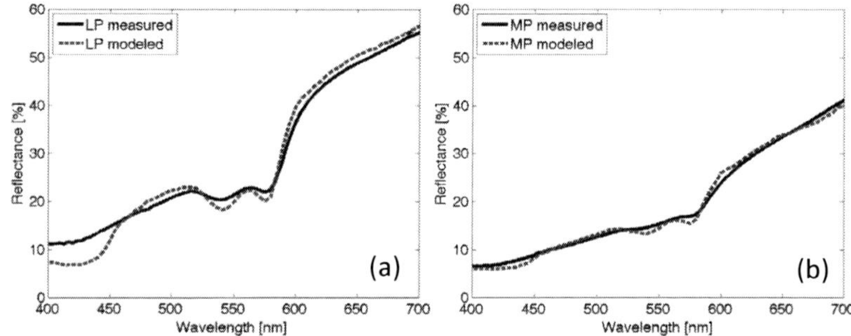


**Figure 1.2**  Comparisons of modeled directional-hemispherical reflectance curves (obtained using the BioSpec model [1] and considering specimens characterized by the parameters provided in Tables 1.1 and 1.2) with measured directional-hemispherical reflectance curves provided by Vrhel et al. [38]. All modeled and measured curves were obtained considering an angle of incidence equal to 45°. (a) Lightly pigmented (LP) specimen. (b) Moderately pigmented (MP) specimen.

**Table 1.1**  Skin pigmentation–related parameters employed by BioSpec model to characterize a lightly pigmented (LP) specimen and a moderately pigmented (MP) specimen

| Parameter | LP | MP |
|---|---|---|
| Percentage of epidermis occupied by melanosomes | 1.6% | 3.6% |
| Percentage of papillary dermis occupied by blood | 0.8% | 0.6% |
| Percentage of reticular dermis occupied by blood | 0.8% | 0.6% |

**Table 1.2**  Biophysical parameters used by the BioSpec model to characterize skin specimens under normal conditions

| Parameter | Value | Reference |
|---|---|---|
| Aspect ratio of skin surface folds | 0.75 | [41,42] |
| Thickness of stratum corneum | 0.001 cm | [43] |
| Thickness of epidermis | 0.01 cm | [43] |
| Thickness of papillary dermis | 0.01 cm | [44] |
| Thickness of reticular dermis | 0.1 cm | [44] |
| Radius of collagen fibers | 25 nm | [45] |
| Concentration of eumelanin in the melanosomes | 80 g/L | [39,46] |
| Concentration of pheomelanin in the melanosomes | 5.2 g/L | [47] |
| Concentration of $\beta$-carotene in the stratum corneum | 2.1e-4 g/L | [48] |
| Concentration of $\beta$-carotene in the epidermis | 2.1e-4 g/L | [48] |
| Concentration of $\beta$-carotene in the blood | 7.0e-5 g/L | [48] |
| Concentration of bilirubin in the blood | 0.05 g/L | [49] |
| Concentration of oxy/in the blood | 147 g/L | [50] |
| Ratio of oxy/deoxyhemoglobin | 75% | [51] |
| Concentration of methemoglobin in the blood | 1.5 g/L | [52] |
| Concentration of carboxyhemoglobin in the blood | 1.5 g/L | [53] |
| Concentration of sulfhemoglobin in the blood | 0 g/L | [54] |
| Refractive index of stratum | 1.55 | [55] |
| Refractive index of epidermis | 1.4 | [8] |
| Refractive index of papillary dermis | 1.36 | [56] |
| Refractive index of reticular dermis | 1.38 | [56] |
| Refractive index of collagen | 1.5 | [39] |

Besides quantifying the spectral distribution of the light impinging on a skin specimen in terms of reflectance and transmittance, BioSpec also accounts for the spatial distribution of light interacting with the cutaneous tissues, which is quantified in terms of BDF. For example, Fig. 1.3 presents modeled BRDF curves obtained using BioSpec to illustrate variations in skin glossiness associated with different values assigned to the aspect ratio ($\sigma$) of the skin surface folds, as well as the angular dependency of light reflected on the skin surface. Modeled BDF curves, in turn, can also be used in quantitative and qualitative comparisons with actual measured BDF data, thus strengthening the evaluation of the model's predictive capabilities.

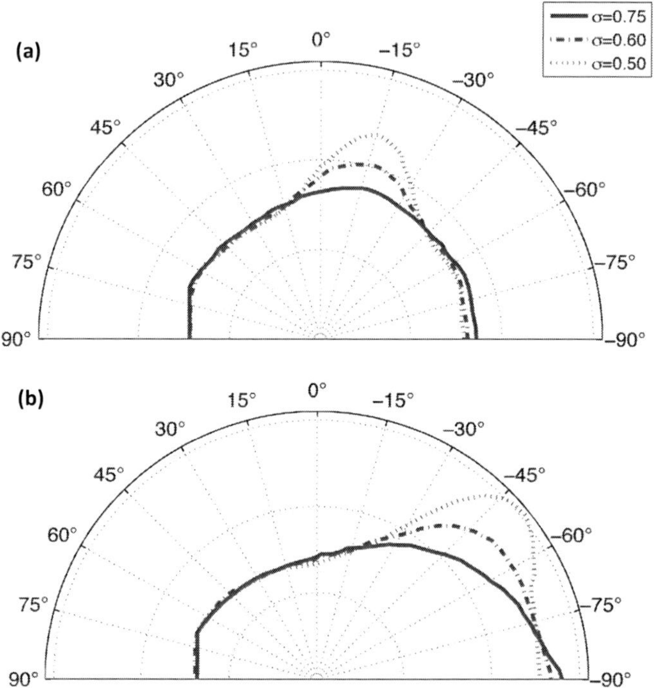


**Figure 1.3**  Modeled BRDF curves provided by the BioSpec model [1] depicting glossiness variations associated with different values assigned to the aspect ratio ($\sigma$) of the surface folds, and considering two angles ($\theta_i$) of incidence. (a) $\theta_i = 15°$, (b) $\theta_i = 45°$.

It is worth remarking that although BioSpec provides as output bidirectional readings, one can obtain directional-hemispherical quantities by integrating the propagated light (rays) with respect to the propagation (collection) hemisphere [37]. Similarly, bihemispherical quantities can be calculated by integrating bidirectional values with respect to incident and collection hemispheres [40].

These aspects in conjunction with its algorithmic nature, make the incorporation of the BioSpec multilayered skin model into existing rendering systems straightforward. Accordingly, it can be effectively employed to generate realistic images depicting the appearance attributes of human skin (Fig. 1.4).

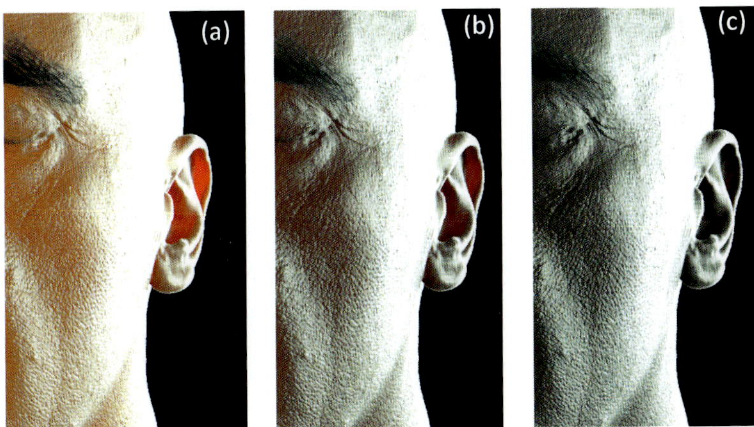


**Figure 1.4** Computer-generated images illustrating color and translucency variations resulting from different levels of melanin pigmentation associated with distinct percentages of melanosomes ($\vartheta_m$) present in the epidermis tissue. (a) $\vartheta_m$ = 3.6%, (b) $\vartheta_m$ = 10%, (c) $\vartheta_m$ = 20%. These images were rendered using a path-tracer algorithm [2] and skin spectral predictions provided by the BioSpec model (Head polygonal mesh courtesy of XYZ RGB Inc.).

### 1.4.3 Reproducibility

The BioSpec source code and supporting simulation data (e.g., molar extinction coefficients for pigments) were made available for download [57] to ensure code transparency and the full reproducibility of the BioSpec predictions. In addition, BioSpec can be run online via a model distribution framework (Natural Phenomena Simulation Group Distributed, or simply NPSGD) [58]. Accordingly, researchers can access its web interface (Fig. 1.5), manipulate simulation parameters associated with experimental conditions (e.g., angle of incidence and spectral range) and skin characterization data (e.g., percentage of epidermis occupied by melanosomes), and receive customized simulation results (e.g., spectral directional-hemispherical reflectance curves). It is worth mentioning that the BioSpec source code available for download corresponds to an updated "fresh" implementation. This reimplementation of the model allowed the filtering of "bugs" and the improvement of its running performance through the use of more efficient software and hardware features.

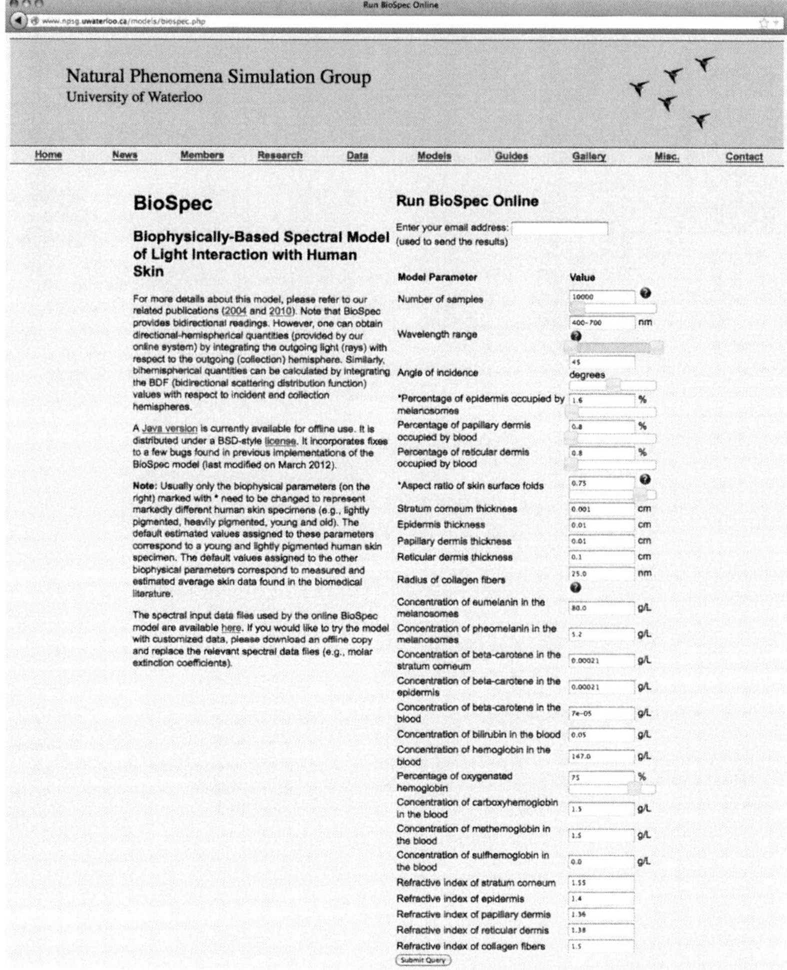

**Figure 1.5**   The Web interface for the BioSpec model available through the Natural Phenomena Simulation Group Distributed (NPSGD) framework [58]. Accessing this interface, researchers can configure biophysical parameters, execute light transport simulations involving different skin specimens, and receive customized results.

## 1.5  Future Prospects

In recent years, a substantial amount of work has been devoted to the multilayer modeling of skin appearance attributes. However, these efforts are often limited by the scarcity of measured data to characterize the optical properties of different skin specimens. Furthermore, in order to be used in a predictive manner, computer models need to be properly evaluated, which, in turn, requires comparisons of modeled data with actual measured data. Besides being also scarce, these datasets rarely include characterization data (e.g., thickness, refractive indexes, ...) for the specimens employed in the measurements. The absence of this information further impairs the proper evaluation of modeled predictions. Clearly, to overcome these hurdles, it is essential to enhance quantitatively and qualitatively the measurement and dissemination of fundamental biophysical skin data.

From a scientific point of view, the modeling of skin appearance attributes is far from being a solved problem. In fact, there are a number of relevant topics that remain largely unexplored by the skin research community. For example, most current models work on the visible domain. However, there is a wide range of applications outside this domain. Noteworthy examples include the accurate modeling of appearance changes due excessive light exposure, such as tanning and photoaging, which involve predictive simulations of light and skin interactions in the ultraviolet and infrared domains, respectively. Furthermore, the biophysical characteristics of important tissue constituents, such as the size, shape, orientation, and distribution of melanosomes, are rarely taken into account in current simulation frameworks.

Finally, we believe that interdisciplinary collaborations supported by accessible data resources and code transparency can lead to significant advances in this area. After all, a well-designed model is of little use without reliable data, and code disclosure is instrumental not only for the reproduction of research results but also for the refinement of the corresponding simulation algorithms.

## References


1. Krishnaswamy A and Baranoski G (2004). A biophysically-based spectral model of light interaction with human skin, *Comput Graph Forum,* **23**(3), 331–340.

2. Baranoski G and Krishnaswamy A (eds) (2010). *Light and Skin Interactions Simulations for Computer Graphics Applications*, Morgan Kaufmann, Amsterdam.

3. Baranoski G, Chen T, Kimmel B, Miranda E, and Yim D (2012). On the noninvasive optical monitoring and differentiation of methemoglobinemia and sulfhemoglobinemia, *J Biomed Opt,* **17**(9), 097005-1–097005-14.

4. Cavalcanti P, Scharcanski J, and Baranoski G (2013). A two-stage approach for discriminating melanocytic skin lesions using standard cameras, *Expert Syst Appl,* **40**(10), 4054–4064.

5. Hunter R and Harold R (eds) (1987). *The Measurement of Appearance*, 2nd ed., Wiley-Interscience, New York.

6. Nicodemus FE, Richmond JC, Hsia JJ, Ginsberg IW, and Limperis T (1992). Geometrical considerations and nomenclature for reflectance, in *Physics-Based Vision Principles and Practice: Radiometry* (Wolf LB, Shafer SA, and Healey GE, eds), Jones and Bartlett Publishers, Sudbury, pp. 94–145.

7. Prahl S (1988). *Light Transport in Tissue*, Ph.D. thesis, The University of Texas at Austin, TX, USA.

8. Tuchin V (ed) (2007). *Tissue Optics: Light Scattering Methods and Instruments for Medical Diagnosis*, SPIE PM (SPIE/International Society for Optical Engineering).

9. Kubelka P and Munk F (1931). Ein beitrag zur optik der farbanstriche, *Zurich Tech Phys,* **12**, 593–601.

10. Anderson R and Parrish J (1981). The optics of human skin, *J Invest Dermatol,* **77**(1), 13–19.

11. Wan S, Anderson R, and Parrish J (1981). Analytical modeling for the optical properties of the skin with in vitro and in vivo applications, *Photochem Photobiol,* **34**, 493–499.

12. Doi M and Tominaga S (2003). Spectral estimation of human skin color using the Kubelka–Munk theory, in *SPIE/IS&T Electronic Imaging* (SPIE, vol 5008), pp. 221–228.

13. Donner C and Jensen H (2005). Light diffusion in multi-layered translucent materials, *ACM T Graphic,* **24**(3), 1032–1039.

14. Ishimaru A (ed) (1978). *Wave Propagation and Scattering in Random Media*, vol 1, 2nd ed., IEEE Press, New York.

15. van Gemert M, Welch A, Star W, Motamedi M, and Cheong W (1987). Tissue optics for a slab geometry in diffusion approximation, *Laser Med Sci,* **2**, 295–302.

16. Farell T, Patterson M, and Wilson B (1992). A diffusion theory model of spatially resolved, steady-state diffuse reflectance for the noninvasive determination of tissue optical properties in vivo, *Med Phys,* **19**, 879–888.

17. Hielscher A, Alcouffe R, and Barbour R (1998). Comparison of finite-difference transport and diffusion calculations for photon migration in homogeneous tissues, *Phys Med Biol,* **43**, 1285–1302.

18. Chen B, Stamnes K, and Stamnes J (2001). Validity of the diffusion approximation in bio-optical imaging, *Appl Opt,* **40**(34), 6356–6336.

19. Sardar D and Levy L (1998). Optical properties of whole blood, *Laser Med Sci,* **13**, 106–111.

20. Steinke J and Shepherd A (1988). Diffusion model of the optical absorbance of whole blood, *J Opt Soc Am,* **5**(6), 813–822.

21. Flock S, Patterson M, Wilson B, and Wyman D (1989). Monte Carlo modeling of light propagation in highly scattering tissues—I: model predictions and comparison with diffusion theory, *IEEE T Biomed Eng,* **36**(12), 1162–1168.

22. Yoon G, Prahl S, and Welch A (1989). Accuracies of the diffusion approximation and its similarity relations for laser irradiated biological media, *Appl Opt,* **28**(12), 2250–2255.

23. Donner C and Jensen H (2006). A spectral BSSRDF for shading human skin, in *Rendering Techniques 2006: 17th Eurographics Workshop on Rendering*, pp. 409–418.

24. Donner C, Weyrich T, d'Eon E, Ramamoorthi R, and Rusinkiewicz S (2008). A layered, heterogeneous reflectance model for acquiring and rendering human skin, *ACM T Graphic,* **27**(5), 140:1–140:12.

25. Prahl S, van Gemert M, and Welch A (1993). Determining the optical properties of turbid media using the adding-doubling method, *Appl Opt,* **32**(4), 559–568.

26. Nielsen K, Zhao L, Stamnes J, Stamnes K, and Moan J (2004). Reflectance spectra of pigmented and nonpigmented skin in the UV spectral region, *Photochem Photobiol,* **80**, 450–455.

27. Stamnes K, Tsay S-C, Wiscombe W, and Jayaweera K (1988). Numerically stable algorithm for discrete-ordinate-method radiative transfer in multiple scattering and emitting layered media, *Appl Opt,* **27**(12), 2502–2509.

28. Chandrasekhar S (ed) (1960). *Radiative Transfer,* Dover Publications Inc., New York.

29. Hammerley J and Handscomb D (eds) (1964). *Monte Carlo Methods,* Wiley, New York.

30. Shimada M, Yamada Y, Itoh M, and Yatagai T (2001). Melanin and blood concentration in human skin studied by multiple regression analysis: assessment by Monte Carlo simulation, *Phys Med Biol,* **46**, 2397–2406.

31. Wang L, Jacques S, and Zheng L (1995). MCML–Monte Carlo modeling of light transport in multi-layered tissues, *Comput Meth Prog Bio,* **47**, 131–146.

32. Nishidate I, Aizu Y, and Mishina H (2004). Estimation of melanin and hemoglobin in skin tissue using multiple regression analysis aided by Monte Carlo simulation, *J Biomed Opt,* **9**(4), 700–710.

33. Prahl S, Keijzer M, Jacques S, and Welch A (1989). A Monte Carlo model of light propagation in tissue, in *SPIE Proceedings of Dosimetry of Laser Radiation in Medicine and Biology*, vol IS 5 (Müller G and Sliney D, eds), pp. 102–111.

34. Trowbridge T and Reitz K (1975). Average irregularity representation of a rough surface for ray reflection, *J Opt Soc Am,* **65**(5), 531–536.

35. Bruls W and van der Leun J (1984). Forward scattering properties of human epidermal layers, *Photochem Photobiol,* **40**, 231–242.

36. McCartney E (ed) (1976). *Optics of the Atmosphere: Scattering by Molecules and Particles,* John Wiley & Sons Inc., New York.

37. Baranoski G, Rokne J, and Xu G (2001). Virtual spectrophotometric measurements for biologically and physically-based rendering, *Visual Comput,* **17**(8), 506–518.

38. Vrhel M, Gershon R, and Iwan L (1994). The measurement and analysis of object reflectance spectra, *Color Res Appl,* **19**(1), 4–9.

39. Jacques S (1996). Origins of tissue optical properties in the UVA, visible, and NIR regions, in *OSA TOPS on Advances in Optical Imaging and Photon Migration* (Alfano RR, and Fujimoto JG, eds), vol 2, pp. 364–369.

40. Krishnaswamy A, Baranoski G, and Rokne J (2004). Improving the reliability/cost ratio of goniophotometric measurements, *J Graph Tool,* **9**(3), 31–51.

41. Magnenat-Thalmann N, Kalra P, Lévêque J-L, Bazin R, Batisse D, and Querleux B (2002). A computational skin model: fold and wrinkle formation, *IEEE T Inf Technol B,* **6**(4), 317–323.

42. Talreja P, Kasting G, Kleene N, Pickens W, and Wang T-F (2001). Visualization of the lipid barrier and measurement of lipid pathlength in human stratum corneum, *AAPS Pharmsci,* **3**(2), 48–56.

43. Gambichler T, Boms S, Stücker M, Kreuter A, Moussa G, Sand M, Altmeyer P, and Hoffmann K (2006). Epidermal thickness assessed by optical coherence tomography and routine histology: preliminary results of method comparison, *J Eur Acad Dermatol,* **20**(7), 791–795.

44. Agache P (2004). Main skin physical constants, in *Measuring the Skin* (Agache P and Humbert P, eds), Springer-Verlag, Berlin, pp. 747–757.

45. Li S (2003). Biologic biomaterials: tissue-derived biomaterials (collagen), in *Biomaterials Principles and Applications* (Park J and Bronzano J, eds), CRC Press, Boca Raton, pp. 117–139.

46. Kollias N and Baqer A (1986). On the assessment of melanin in human skin in vivo, *Photochem Photobiol,* **43**(1), 49–54.

47. Hennessy A, Oh C, Diffely B, Wakamatsu K, Ito S, and Rees J (2005). Eumelanin and pheomelanin concentrations in human epidermis before and after UVB irradiation, *Pigm Cell Res,* **18**(3), 220–223.

48. Lee R, Mathews-Roth M, Pathak M, and Parrish J (1975). The detection of carotenoid pigments in human skin, *J Invest Dermatol,* **64**(3), 175–177.

49. Martin C and Cloherty J (2008). Neonatal hyperbilirubinemia, in *Manual of Neonatal Care* (Cloherty J, Eichenwald E, and Stark A, eds), Wolters Kluwer, Philadelphia, pp. 181–212.

50. Yaroslavsky A, Priezzhev A, Rodriquez J, Yaroslavsky I, and Battarbee H (2002). Optics of blood, in *Handbook of Optical Biomedical Diagnostics* (Tuchin V, ed), SPIE-Press, pp. 169–216.

51. Öberg P (2003). Optical sensors in medical care, *Sens Update,* **13**(1), 201–232.

52. Haymond S, Cariappa R, Eby C, and Scott M (2005). Laboratory assessment of oxygenation in methemoglobinemia, *Clin Chem,* **51**(2), 434–444.

53. Cunnington A, Kendrick S, Wamola B, Lowe B, and Newton C (2004). Carboxyhemoglobin levels in Kenyan children with plasmodium falciparum malaria, *Am J Trop Med Hyg,* **71**(1), 43–47.

54. Yarynovska IH and Bilyi AI (2006). Absorption spectra of sulfhemoglobin derivatives of human blood, in *Optical Diagnostics and Sensing VI* (Cote G and Priezzhev A, eds), SPIE, pp. 1–6.

55. Diffey B (1983). A mathematical model for ultraviolet optics in skin, *Phys Med Biol,* **28**(6), 647–657.

56. Jacques S, Alter C, and Prahl S (1987). Angular dependence of HeNe laser light scattering by human dermis, *Laser Life Sci,* **1**, 309–333.

57. NPSG (2011). Run BioSpec Online, School of Computer Science, University of Waterloo, http://www.npsg.uwaterloo.ca/models/biospec.php.

58. Baranoski G, Dimson T, Chen T, Kimmel B, Yim D, and Miranda E (2012). Rapid dissemination of light transport models on the web, *IEEE Comput Graph,* **32**, 10–15.

# Chapter 2

# Dermal Component–Based Optical Modeling of Skin Translucency: Impact on Skin Color

Igor Meglinski,[a,b] Alexander Doronin,[b] Alexey N. Bashkatov,[a] Elina A. Genina,[a] and Valery V. Tuchin[a,c,d]

[a]*Research-Educational Institute of Optics and Biophotonics,*
*Saratov State University, 83 Astrakhanskaya, Saratov, 410012 Russia*
[b]*The Jack Dodd Centre for Quantum Technology,*
*Department of Physics, University of Otago,*
*P.O. Box 56, Dunedin, 9054 New Zealand*
[c]*Laboratory of Laser Diagnostics of Technical and Living Systems,*
*Institute of Precise Mechanics and Control of the Russian Academy of Sciences,*
*24 Rabochaya, Saratov, 410028 Russia*
[d]*Optoelectronics and Measurement Techniques Laboratory, University of Oulu,*
*P.O. Box 4500, Oulu, FIN-90014 Finland*

tuchinvv@mail.ru

Computational modeling of skin color and/or skin reflectance spectra opens up new ways to investigate functional properties of human skin. Modeling of skin color and its variations associated with the physiological changes in human skin, such as blood oxy- and deoxygenation, melanin content, etc., is frequently required in various medical and biomedical applications. We present an open-access computational tool for online simulation of skin color and/or skin reflectance and transmittance spectra in real time. Human

*Computational Biophysics of the Skin*
Edited by Bernard Querleux
Copyright © 2014 Pan Stanford Publishing Pte. Ltd.
ISBN 978-981-4463-84-3 (Hardcover), 978-981-4463-85-0 (eBook)
www.panstanford.com

skin is presented as multi-layered medium. The variations in spatial distribution of blood, pheomelanin, eumelanin, index of blood oxygen saturation, hematocrit, and volume fraction of water are taken into account. The developed Monte Carlo (MC)-based calculator of spectra and color of human skin is supported by Compute Unified Device Architecture (CUDA), introduced by NVIDIA Corporation, that provides acceleration of modeling up to $10^3$ times, allowing produce the results of simulation within seconds. The calculator is based on the object-oriented programming (OOP) paradigm and available online at www.biophotonics.ac.nz.

Examples of MC modeling of skin optical properties optimal for removal the tattoo or any other localized absorbing abnormality by laser thermolysis are also presented. This optimization is based on the laser wavelength selection and application of immersion optical clearing for enhancement of laser light selective absorption.

## 2.1   Introduction

In vivo measurements of human skin spectra serve as an important supplement to standard non-invasive optical techniques for diagnosing various skin diseases [1], such as venous ulcers, skin necrosis, and interstitial edema. However, the quantified analysis of the reflectance spectra is complicated by the fact that skin has a complex multilayered non-homogeneous structure with a spatially varying absorption coefficient, mainly determined by melanin pigmentation, oxygen saturation of cutaneous blood, index of erythema, contents of bilirubin, $\beta$-carotene, and other chromophores. Various approaches targeting the modeling of human skin reflectance spectrum and associated colors exist, but in our current work we apply the recently developed multipurpose graphics-processing unit (GPU)-accelerated MC tool for the needs of biophotonics and biomedical optics [2–4].

The description of optical radiation propagation within random media is based on the radiative transfer theory [5] that forms a basis of MC modeling of photons migration in biological tissues [6]. Originally introduced in biomedical optics for the counting of fluence rate distribution in biological tissues for the purpose of estimation laser radiation dose [7], in the last decades the MC approach has become a primary tool for a number of needs in biomedical optics. Incorporated with the computational model of human skin [8] MC technique has been used for simulation of skin visual and near-infrared reflectance spectra [9,10], analysis of skin fluorescence excitation [11–13], simulation of optical coherence tomography (OCT) images of human skin [14,15], analysis of scattering orders, and OCT image formation [16–18]. The MC approach has been generalized for simulation of coherent effects of multiple scattering, such as enhancement of coherent back-scattering (CBS) and changes of temporal intensity correlation function depending on the dynamics of scattering particles [19,20]. Based on these developments a new approach of handling polarization has been introduced and some effects such as a helicity flip of circular polarization has been observed [21,22]. The obtained modeling results have been comprehensively validated by comparison with the known exact solution by Milne [23,24] and with the results of experimental studies of image transfer through the water solution of spherical microparticles of known size and density [25,26]. Meanwhile, a number of other MC algorithms has been developed in the past, see for example [27–30].

In this chapter, we discuss an MC approach specially designed for imitation of reflectance spectra and associated colors of human skin. The developed skin spectrum/color calculator utilizes seven-layered skin model corresponding to *Stratum corneum*, living epidermis, papillary dermis, upper blood net dermis, reticular dermis, deep blood net dermis, and subcutaneous fat. In the framework of the calculator, different modeling parameters can be independently varied, including concentration of blood, hematocrit, oxygen saturation, volume fraction of hemoglobin in erythrocytes, concentration of water, and thickness of the layers. Some examples of MC modeling of skin optical properties for practical use, such as tattoo and other absorbing abnormalities imaging and selective ablation by laser thermolysis, will be discussed in the framework of tissue optical clearing concept.

## 2.2 Skin Color Calculator

### 2.2.1 Online Object-Oriented Graphics-Processing Unit—Accelerated Monte Carlo Tool

Due to a number of practical applications in skin optics, the MC model undergoes continuous modifications and changes dedicated to the inclusion of diverse properties of incident optical/laser radiation, configuration of the sources and detectors, structure of the medium and the conditions of light detection [8–30]. Past attempts to unify the MC codes [31] are mainly based on the use of structured programming. While structured programming is known for years, it limits the ability to handle a large code without decreasing its functionality and manageability [32]. In practice, the increasing diversity of the MC applications results to a substantial growth of the model's source code and leads to the development of a set of separate MC codes dedicated each for a particular purpose.

To generalize and unify the code for a multi-purpose use in various biomedical optics applications we apply the OOP concept. Object-oriented programming is widely used in mainstream application development and has been found extremely effective in design of complex multi-parametric systems, providing highly intuitive approach of programming [33]. The key features of OOP allow for the MC to be separated into logical components, described by objects.

Thus, the OOP approach significantly increases the efficiency of the model manageability and provides superior opportunities to generalize MC to combine previously developed MC models in a way to imitate a particular skin optics experiment taking into account various features of optical radiation and light-tissue interaction.

### 2.2.2  Graphics-Processing Unit Acceleration of MC

Launching of a large number ($\sim 10^8$–$10^9$) of photon packets and computing their interaction with medium and with the probe is a highly intensive computational process. Owing to a required computational performance, processing time has always been a significant issue in stochastic modeling, taking hours or even a few days to complete on a standard central processing unit (CPU). To achieve the supreme performance of simulation, a number programming approaches and optimizations of algorithms have been used in the past, including parallel and cluster computing [34,35].

We use recently introduced by NVIDIA Corporation parallel computing framework, known as Compute Unified Device Architecture (CUDA) technology, which provides an unlimited access to computational resources of graphic card: processor cores, different types of memory (of various capacity and speed) making

GPU a massive co-processor in parallel computations [34,35]. The graphic chip is capable of executing executes up to 30,000 threads simultaneously, without context switch performance losses and has a very fast (up to 4 Gbit/s) on-chip GDDR5 memory. Graphics-processing unit's shared memory has been used to store the intermediate results; constant memory is applied for data input, whereas the global memory is used to store parameters of photon objects (e.g., path-length, state of polarization, outlet angles, etc.).

The OOP MC model has been developed using CUDA 4.0 C/C++ and supports multiple GPUs. The hardware is presented by a MPICH2 cluster of four Tesla M2090/GeForce GTX 480 graphic cards with NVIDIA CUDA computing capability 2.0 totally having up to 5 Tflops of computational power on board. This cutting-edge graphic technology also incorporates a powerful set of instruments applied for optimized simulation of objects motion, rotation, reflection, ray-tracing, etc. The NVIDIA CUDA provides GPU-accelerated mathematical libraries, such as CULA, CUBLAS—Linear Algebra, CUFFT—Fast Fourier Transform, and CURAND—Random Number Generators [36]. Their incorporation into MC allows for speeding up the simulation of each photon packet up to $10^3$ times.

### 2.2.3  Online Solution

With the rapid growth of the Internet, rich, browser-based applications have become more and more popular. Solutions such as Google Apps, Google Docs, online video sharing, and gaming portals have become a large part of our everyday life. In comparison with traditional desktop applications, they are much easier to deploy and update, as a capable Web-browser is the only requirement [37]. Leveraging modern, Web-based technology, we have created a free online MC computational tool for researchers in the area of biophotonics and biomedical optics [2,3]. On the server side, the tool is accelerated by CUDA GPUs. On the client side, a lightweight, user-friendly Web interface allows multiple clients to set up optical system parameters, perform modeling, and download results in a typical journal paper format. We have combined powerful GPU technology with a modern Web application development approach, allowing researchers to use, check, and validate our MC model using our group's GPU computing facilities [38].

A conceptual design of the online solution is schematically presented in Fig. 2.1.

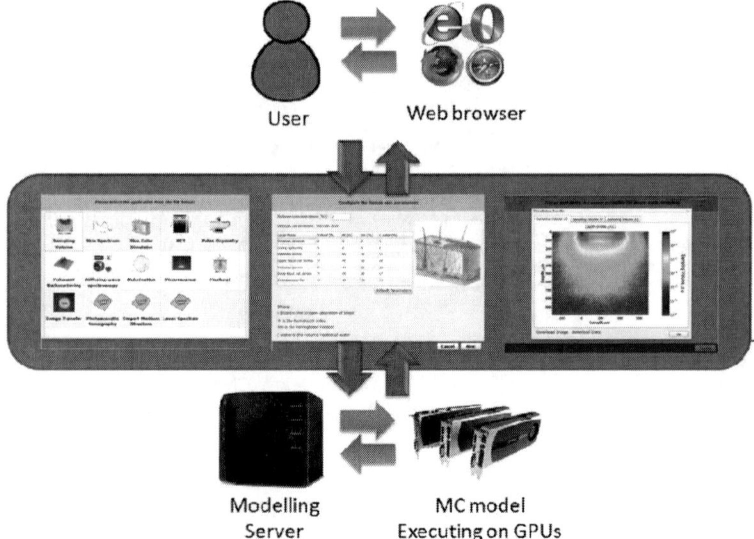


**Figure 2.1** Schematic presentation of the online MC tool. The server hosts a Web frontend, which accepts the user's simulation requests and displays the obtained results. The developed components provide interoperability between the interactive user interface and GPUs, executing all heavy-duty MC-related tasks.

Integrating CUDA acceleration with the modern Web technologies, such as Microsoft Silverlight and ASP.NET Framework, the Online Object Oriented MC (O3MC) computational tool was developed [39]. The key idea behind O3MC development is the creation a universal computational tool to simulate the results of real experiments typically used in major applications in biomedical optics and related areas that could provide researchers with practical results nearly in real time.

Object-oriented programming and GPU implementations enable speeds up the procedure of MC simulation up to $10^3$ times [39]. However, due to the multi-user architecture of the online solution, concurrent simulations by multiple clients significantly degrade performance of O3MC. For example, if one user accessing the O3MC can get the results in 4.3 seconds on TESLA M2090 GPU, 100 users accessing O3MC at the same time can be stacked in a queue and wait for 10–15 min.

Therefore, in framework of further development of O3MC to deal with the multi-user access we apply a peer-to-peer (P2P) network [39]. The proposed P2P network consists of a set of computers, called nodes or peers, which communicate and share their GPUs (Fig. 2.2). The peers in P2P network are equal among each other, acting as both clients and servers. P2P approach has gained a lot of popularity in the recent years, especially in terms of multimedia content delivery and communication (e.g., BitTorrent, Skype).

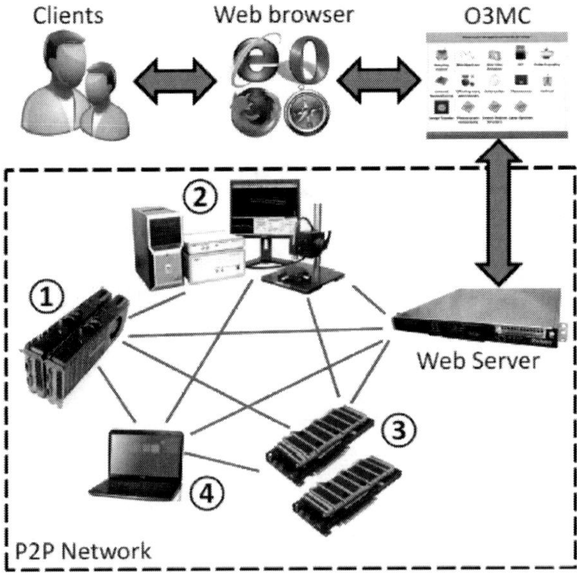


**Figure 2.2** **Schematic presentation of P2P O3MC implementation.** Clients interact with the O3MC Web interface via a preferred Web browser. The server accepts O3MC simulation requests and keeps track of the participating peers. The P2P network consists of different computers equipped with the CUDA-supporting GPUs: (1) a workstation with two GeForce GTX 480 GPUs each 480 CUDA cores, 1540 Gigaflops of the peak single precision FPP/85 Gigaflops double precision FPP, 1536 GB of GDDR5 memory; (2) Thorlabs OCT imaging system workstation with Quadro FX580 featuring 32 CUDA cores, 512 MB GDDR3 memory; (3) computational server equipped with two Tesla M2090 GPUs each 512 CUDA cores, 1331 Gigaflops of the peak single precision floating point performance (FPP)/665 Gigaflops double precision FPP, 6 GB of GDDR5 memory; (4) Dell laptop with GeForce GT555M featuring 144 CUDA cores, 3072 GB GDDR3 memory. Adapted with permission from [39].

Web server hosts the online MC tool user interface, accepts O3MC simulation requests from clients, and keeps track of the other nodes (see Fig. 2.2). The nodes are responsible for sharing the information about currently queuing MC simulations, processing them on GPUs, uploading, downloading and hosting the outcomes (presented in a typical journal-paper format) among themselves without the need of the central server [39].

Figure 2.3 shows the welcome screen of the online O3MC tool available at http://www.biophotonics.ac.nz. This is a starting point providing access to a number of MC applications, including sampling volume, fluence rate distribution, skin spectra and skin color modeling, and other.

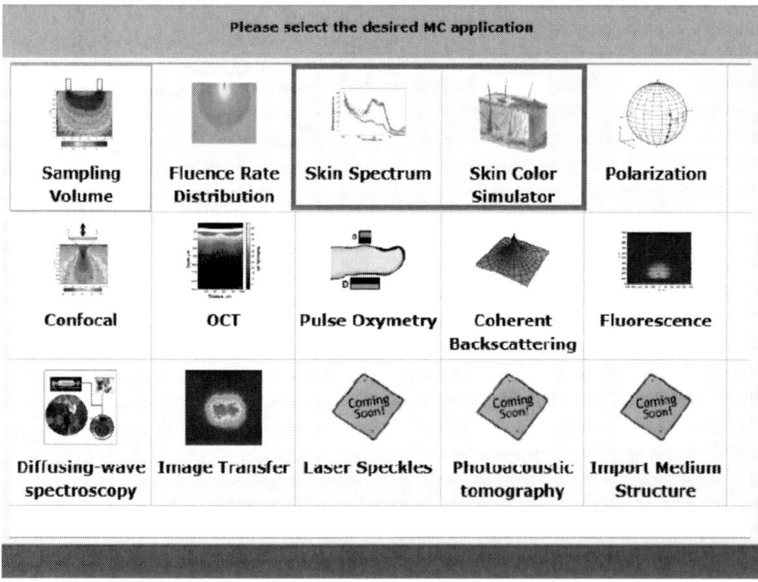


**Figure 2.3**   Front screen of the online O3MC tool. Each icon represents a different application. Skin color and skin spectra calculators are highlighted by frame. The application can be started by clicking the corresponding icon.

To use "skin spectrum" or "skin color simulator" applications a user should select the corresponding icon. Once the icon is clicked, the user will be taken to the page where he can either set up the detailed parameters of human skin model (Fig. 2.4) of the MC simulation or start the simulation using default parameters.

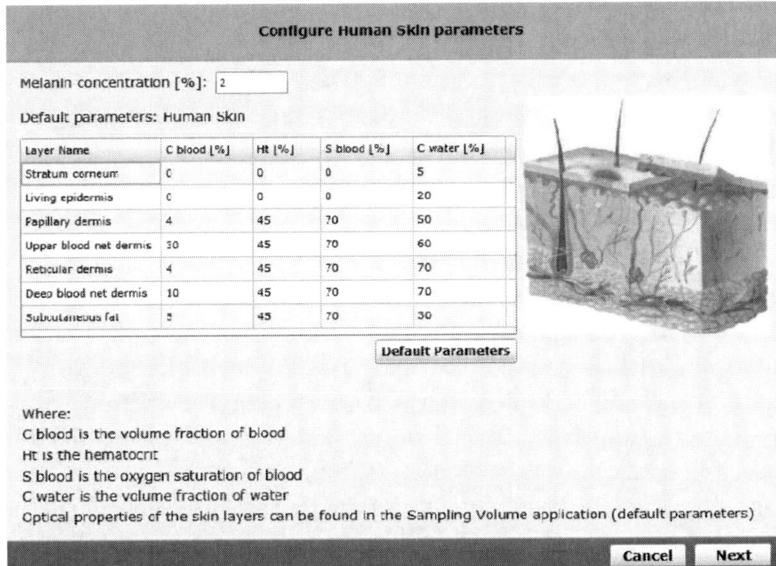


**Figure 2.4**    Configuring parameters of the seven layer human skin model, including blood concentration (C blood), hematocrit (Ht), the oxygen saturation of blood (S), fraction of water (C water).

When the parameters are configured, the server will perform a MC simulation and provide the user with the results in a typical journal paper format (see Section 2.3), which can be downloaded and further used.

## 2.3    Skin Spectra and Skin Color Simulation

### 2.3.1    Basics of MC

The MC is based on the consequent simulation of the photon packet trajectories as they travel through scattering medium [8,9]. The simulation of the photon trajectories consists of the following key stages: injection of a photon packet in medium, generation of photon path-lengths, generation of scattering events, definition of reflection/refraction at the medium boundary and detection. The random path length $l$ a photon packet goes for a step $i$ is given by

$$l = -\frac{\ln\xi}{\mu_s},$$

(2.1)

where $\xi$ is the computer-generated random number, uniformly distributed in the interval $[0,1]$, $\mu_s$ is the scattering coefficient.

Internal reflections on medium boundary are taken into account by splitting the photon packet into reflected and transmitted parts. The weights of these parts are attenuated according to the Fresnel reflection coefficients [40]:

$$W = W_0 \left[1 - R_0(\alpha)\right] \cdot \prod_{p=1}^{M} R_p(\alpha) \tag{2.2}$$

Here, $W_0$ is the initial weight of the photon packet, $M$ is the number of times the photon packet experiences a partial reflection on medium boundary, $R_p(\alpha)$ is the Fresnel reflection coefficient for the $p$-th photon-boundary interaction, $R_0(\alpha)$ is the Fresnel reflection coefficient for the initial photon-boundary interaction, where the photon packet enters the medium, $\alpha$ is the angle of incidence on the medium boundary [8]. The details of the reflection and refraction at the medium layers boundaries are given in detail in Refs. [8–12]. The simulation of the photon tracing within the medium is stopped when a photon packet has been scattered more than $10^4$ times and does not depend on absorption. The counting of normalized skin spectra $I(\lambda)$ is based on the microscopic Beer–Lambert law and defined as follows [9,10]:

$$I(\lambda) = \frac{1}{N_{\text{ph}} W_0} \sum_{j=1}^{N_{\text{ph}}} W_j \exp\left\{ -\sum_{i=1}^{K_j} \mu_{\text{ai}}(\lambda) l_i \right\}, \tag{2.3}$$

where $W_j$ is the final weight of the $j$-th photon packet defined by Eq. (2.3), $K_j$ is the total number of scattering events for the $j$-th photon packet, $\lambda$ is the wavelength, $\mu_{\text{ai}}$ and $l_i$ are the medium-local absorption coefficient and the path length of photon packet at $i$-th step, respectively [8]. The total number of the photon packets $N_{\text{ph}}$ typically used in spectra simulation is $\sim 10^8$–$10^9$.

## 2.3.2 Skin Model and Skin Tissues Optical Properties

To simulate the reflectance spectra of human skin, we adopted the seven layers skin model developed in Ref. [9,10]. The absorption of main skin chromophores [41] and skin layers are summarized in Fig. 2.5.

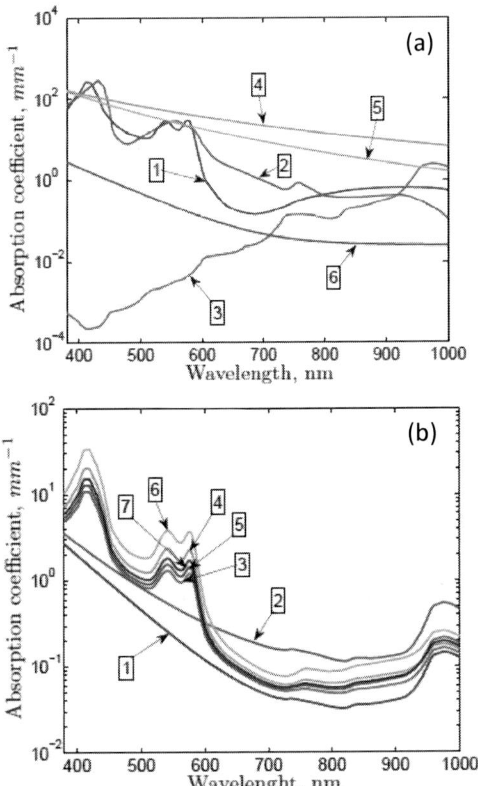

**Figure 2.5**  Absorption properties of skin tissues used in the simulation. (a) Absorption coefficients of major skin tissues chromophores: (1) oxy-hemoglobin, (2) deoxy-hemoglobin, (3) water, (4) eumelanin, (5) pheomelanin, and (6) baseline. (b) Absorption coefficients of the human skin layers counted by Eqs. 2.4–2.6. Adapted with permission from [44].

The absorption of skin layers takes into account concentration of blood ($C_{\text{blood}}$) in various vascular beds, oxygen saturation ($S$), water content ($C_{\text{H}_2\text{O}}$), melanin fraction ($C_{\text{mel}}$), and defined as [9,10]

$$\mu_a^{\text{Strat.corneum}}(\lambda) = (1 - C_{\text{H}_2\text{O}})\mu_a^{\text{baseline}}(\lambda) + C_{\text{H}_2\text{O}}\mu_a^{\text{water}}(\lambda) \tag{2.4}$$

$$\mu_a^{\text{Living epidermis}}(\lambda) = (1 - C_{\text{H}_2\text{O}})\{C_{\text{mel}}[B_{\text{mel}}\mu_a^{\text{mel}}(\lambda) + (1 - B_{\text{mel}})\mu_a^{\text{ph.mel}}(\lambda)] +$$
$$(1 - C_{\text{mel}})\mu_a^{\text{baseline}}(\lambda)\} + C_{\text{H}_2\text{O}}\mu_a^{\text{water}}(\lambda) \tag{2.5}$$

$$\mu_a^{\text{Dermis}}(\lambda) = C_{\text{blood}}\{F_{\text{Hb}}F_{\text{RBC}}\text{Ht}[S\mu_a^{\text{oxy}}(\lambda) + (1-S)\mu_a^{\text{deoxy}}(\lambda)] + (1-\text{Ht})\mu_a^{\text{water}}(\lambda)\}$$
$$+ (1-C_{\text{blood}})(1-C_{\text{H}_2\text{O}})\mu_a^{\text{baseline}}(\lambda) + (1-C_{\text{blood}})C_{\text{H}_2\text{O}}\mu_a^{\text{water}}(\lambda)$$

$$(2.6)$$

Here $\mu_a^{\text{mel}}(\lambda)$ is the absorption coefficient of eumelanin, $\mu_a^{\text{ph.mel}}(\lambda)$ is the absorption coefficient of pheomelanin, $B_{\text{mel}}$ is the volume fraction of the blend between two melanin types, $\mu_a^{\text{oxy}}(\lambda)$ is the absorption coefficient of oxy-hemoglobin, $\mu_a^{\text{deoxy}}(\lambda)$ is the absorption coefficient of deoxy-hemoglobin, $\mu_a^{\text{baseline}}(\lambda)$ is the absorption coefficient of other water-free tissue components, Ht is the hematocrit, $F_{\text{Hb}}$ is the volume fraction of hemoglobin in a single erythrocyte, and $F_{\text{RBC}}$ is the volume fraction of erythrocytes. The actual values of these parameters are presented in Table 2.1. $C_{\text{mel}}$ varies within the ranges 0–45%.

**Table 2.1**    Parameters of skin layers, used in the simulation [9,10]

| Layer | $d$ (μm)$^*$ | Ht | $F_{\text{Hb}}$ | $F_{\text{RBC}}$ | $C_{\text{H}_2\text{O}}$ | $C_{\text{blood}}$ |
|---|---|---|---|---|---|---|
| *Stratum corneum* | 20 | 0 | 0 | 0 | 0.05 | 0 |
| Living epidermis | 150 | 0 | 0 | 0 | 0.2 | 0 |
| Papillary dermis | 250 | 0.4 | 0.99 | 0.25 | 0.3 | 0.04 |
| Upper blood net dermis | 330 | 0.45 | 0.99 | 0.25 | 0.4 | 0.3 |
| Reticular dermis | 1830 | 0.45 | 0.99 | 0.25 | 0.5 | 0.04 |
| Deep blood net dermis | 1910 | 0.5 | 0.99 | 0.25 | 0.5 | 0.1 |
| Subcutaneous fat | 8000 | 0.45 | 0.99 | 0.25 | 0.6 | 0.05 |

$^*d$ is the thickness of the layer.

The scattering coefficients of skin layers (Fig. 2.6) are approximated basing on combination of Mie and Rayleigh scattering suggested in Ref. [42], as

$$\mu_s^{\text{Rayleigh}}(\lambda) = 2.2 \times 10^{11} \times \lambda^{-4}, \tag{2.7}$$

$$\mu_s^{\text{Mie}}(\lambda) = 11.74 \times \lambda^{-0.22}, \tag{2.8}$$

$$\mu_s^{\text{Layer}}(\lambda) = N[\mu_s^{\text{Rayleigh}}(\lambda) + \mu_s^{\text{Mie}}(\lambda)], \tag{2.9}$$

where $N$ is the coefficient representing the fraction of scattering centers in the skin tissue, varying in a range 1 to 10.

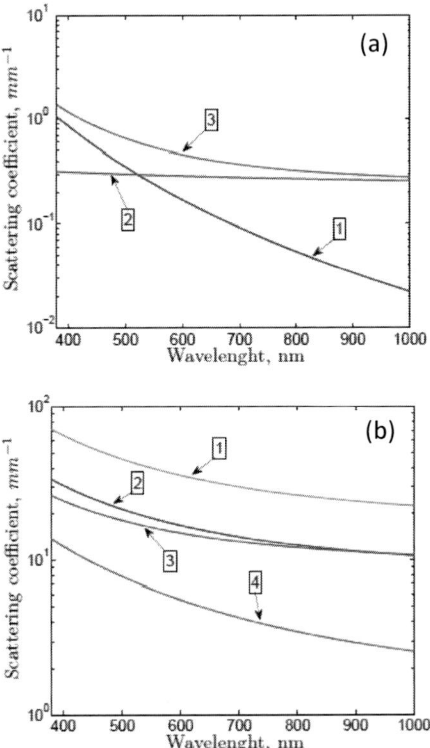

**Figure 2.6**  Scattering properties of tissues used in the simulation. (a) Reduced scattering coefficients: (1) Rayleigh scattering by Eq. 2.7, (2) Mie scattering by collagen fibers by Eq. 2.8, (3) the combined Rayleigh and Mie scattering by Eq. 2.9. (b) Scattering properties of human skin layers: (1) *stratum corneum*; (2) epidermis; (3) dermis; (4) subcutaneous fat. Adapted with permission from [44].

The skin reflection spectrum is modeled assuming that absorption and scattering coefficients of the layers of human skin are changed over the wavelength range (380–1000 nm) as presented in Fig. 2.6. This approach significantly enhances the modeling and allowed one to improve the overall quality of the outcomes.

Converting the spectral power distribution $I(\lambda)$ to the CIE XYZ coordinates and then to the actual RGB-gamut color images is done using the standard CIE 2° observer/tristimulus values utilizing D65 illuminant. The resulting images have been textured using a human skin surface BRDF mask [42].

## 2.4 Modeling Results

The online GPU-accelerated MC approach, presented above, has been used for both skin spectra and associated skin color simulations. Figure 2.7 presents the results of the modeling of human skin spectra and associated skin colors with various blood concentration and melanin content. The obtained results of skin spectra modeling are well agreed with the results of experimental measurements, e.g., by using the standard Ocean Optics spectrophotometer (Fig. 2.8).

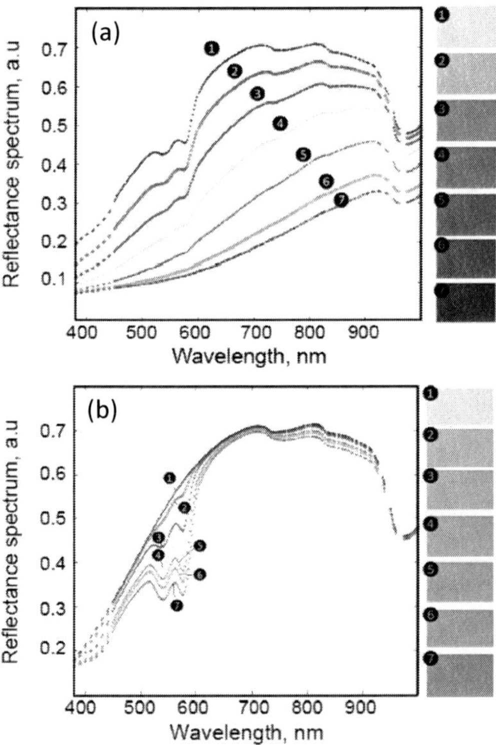

**Figure 2.7**  The results of MC simulation of human skin spectra (left) and corresponding colors (right) while varying the melanin content in living epidermis (a)—(1): 0%, (2): 2%, (3): 5%, (4): 10%, (5): 20%, (6): 35%, (7): 45%—and (b) while varying the blood concentration in the layers from papillary dermis to subcutaneous tissue: (1) 0%, (2) 2%, (3) 5%, (4) 10%, (5) 20%, (6) 35%, (7) 45%, respectively. The melanin concentration is 2% and fraction between eumelanin and pheomelanin is 1:3. Adapted with permission from [44].

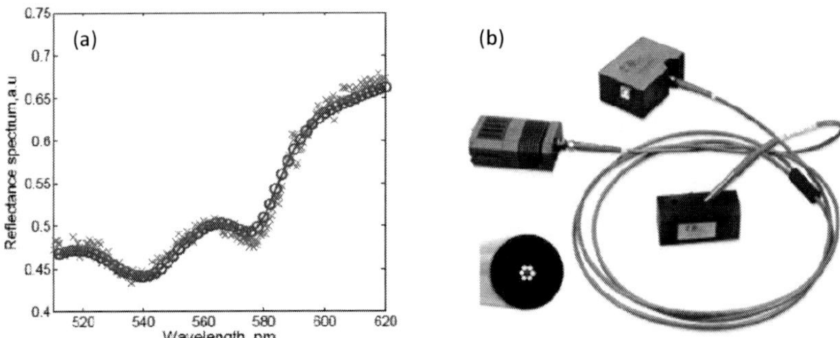

**Figure 2.8**  (a) Human skin reflectance spectrum simulated by the developed MC model (circles) compared with the results (crosses) obtained in vivo by a High-Resolution spectrometer (Ocean Optics USB4000). (b) Standard Ocean Optics USB4000 spectrometer and QR400-7-VIS-NIR probe (adapted from the manufacturer's Web site). Adapted with permission from [44].

Figure 2.9 displays the experimental results [43] for different parts of a human body in chromaticity coordinates plotted in the CIE 1931 color space in comparison with the results of MC simulation. It is clear that the experimental results and computational results are in a good agreement with each other.

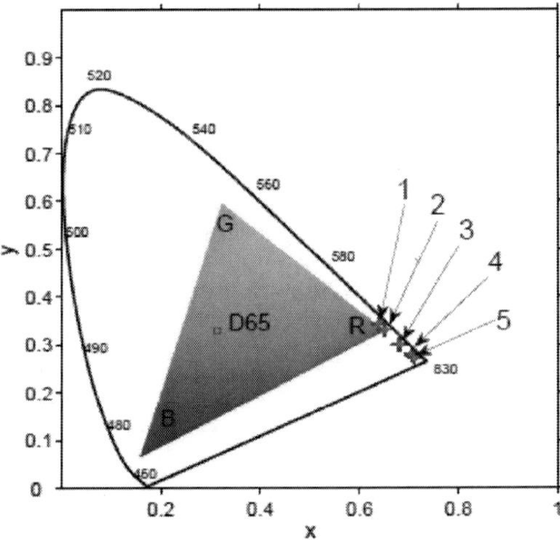

**Figure 2.9**  Chromaticity coordinates for fingernail (1), finger (2), palm (3), wrist (4) and forearm (5): crosses display experimental data and circles—the results of computer O3MC simulations. Adapted with permission from [44].

The design of the CIE 1931 color space splits the concept of color into brightness and chromaticity. The black contour in Fig. 2.9 is the spectral locus with the corresponding wavelengths. D65 is the standard daylight illuminant used in the O3MC model. The triangle represents a color gamut that can be reproduced by a standard computer monitor. As one can see the modeled tissue colors outside the gamut cannot be displayed properly on a standard color reproduction device and require a conversion procedure. Moreover, the diagram does not allow displaying of the actual brightness (luminance) of the colors. However, the actual colors are observed by a naked eye during the experiment.

To make the luminance visible, we converted the modeled CIE chromaticity coordinates into the Lab color space. Figure 2.10 shows experimentally observed and computer simulated near-IR transmission colors of different parts of a human arm, presented in CIE 1976 L*a*b* color space. The simulation is done for the actual experimental geometry and the fiber probe position used to collect the data. The simulated CIE 1976 L*,a*,b* coordinates in the color space, plotted in Fig. 2.10, are presented in Table 2.2 with the converted sRGB colors.

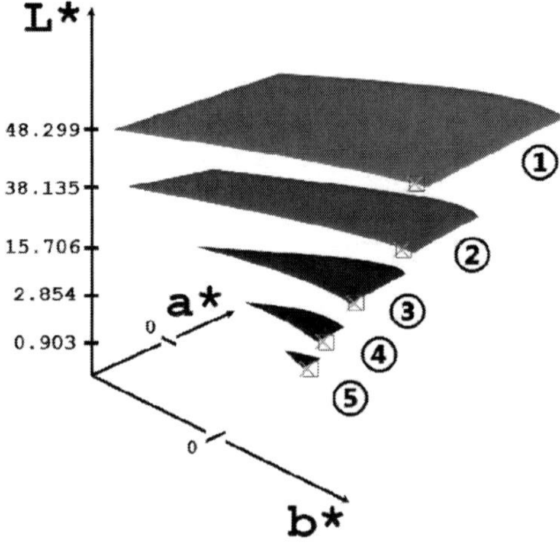


**Figure 2.10**  The changes of human skin color presented in CIE 1976 L*a*b* color space simulated by the developed MC model (crosses) compared with the results of measurements/observations in vivo (squares) for near-IR light transmitted through the various parts of human body: (1) fingernail, (2) finger, (3) palm, (4) wrist, (5) forearm. Adapted with permission from [44].

**Table 2.2**   The results of the MC simulation of skin color CIE coordinates in L*,a*,b* color space

| Sample | L* | a* | b* | Standard deviation | sRGB Color |
|---|---|---|---|---|---|
| Fingernail | 48.299 | 67.372 | 68.396 | 0.001 | |
| Finger | 38.135 | 62.883 | 54.705 | 0.001 | |
| Palm | 15.706 | 44.938 | 24.774 | 0.001 | |
| Wrist | 2.854 | 19.824 | 4.601 | 0.001 | |
| Forearm | 0.930 | 7.024 | 1.532 | 0.001 | |

*Note:* The standard deviation is calculated between the experimental data and the modeling output. CIE XYY coordinates converted to sRGB values are presented the resulting color in sRGB column.

Observing the effect of the changes of tissues color due to, for example, changes of blood and/or melanin content, and variations in blood oxygenation, is of a potential use for the practical diagnostic purpose and bioengineering applications. These changes can be quantified and characterized with the developed MC model.

## 2.5 Simulation of Skin Tattoo: Toward Its Effective Removal

### 2.5.1 Introductory Remarks

In this section, we present one of the examples of modeling of skin optical properties for some practical use: to optimize tattoo removal by laser thermolysis [47–50]. This optimization is based on the laser wavelength selection and application of immersion optical clearing [51–54] for enhancement of laser light absorption by tattoo pigments or any other localized absorbing substance (for example, malignant neoplasm) lying at some depth in the skin.

Nano-sized pigmented ink particles used for tattoo are located within dermis fibroblasts and mast cells, predominantly in a perivascular region. Red and NIR laser radiation penetrates deeply into skin and it is absorbed more or less strongly by blue, green, and black tattoo pigments included in the composition of the most tattoos [47]. Although, short-wavelength radiation is well absorbed by tattoo pigments, the use of visible lasers is limited by a strong light scattering in skin and hemoglobin absorption.

The immersion optical clearing (IOC) based on the impregnation of tissue by an optical clearing agent (OCA) can improve laser tattoo removal due to reduction of light scattering of the upper tissue layers and correspondingly due to more effective laser beam delivery to the embedded ink particles [47–50]. The major mechanisms of IOC are well discussed in literature (see, for example, Refs. [51–54]) and can be explained in terms of refractive index matching concept because exogenous OCAs having a high index of refraction as penetrating into tissue and dissolving by interstitial fluid (ICF), match the refractive indices of scattering centers (collagen and elastin fibers) and ICF. Most of the OCAs are hyperosmotic liquids and thus intensively dehydrate tissue and therefore provide its temporal and reversible shrinkage, which also lead to better optical homogeneity of tissue and its lesser thickness. All these phenomena give the better penetration for light beams at their transportation in tissues, in particular in skin.

A number of laser diagnostic, surgery, and therapy technologies may have a significant benefit at a reversible skin optical clearing. However, slow diffusion of OCAs, such as glucose or glycerol water solutions, through human skin barrier makes practical application of IOC difficult. To overcome barrier function of skin epidermis a number of different chemical and physical methods such as skin stripping, microdermabrasion, laser fractional ablation of skin surface, iontophoresis, ultrasound, laser induced photomechanical waves, and needle-free injection were proposed [51–54].

In our work we use two different types of skin fractional ablation using lamp and laser (fractional laser microablation (FLMA)) techniques. The fractional ablation of SC can be done using a variety of light sources and delivery optics, including application of lenslet arrays, phase masks, and matrices of exogenous point-wise absorbers. The lamp technique is based on creation of the lattice of damaged micro-zones of stratum corneum (SC) by multi-dot intensive lamp heating of skin surface via transparent appliqué with many black dots, which absorb light and locally heat SC [55,56]. For the optimized procedure, a long-term effect of such damage is only the transient deterioration of skin barrier function, because no any damage to viable tissue can be provided. That leads to the local increase of OCA's permeability via SC.

FLMA technique is one of the relatively safe and minimally invasive methods used to administer not only OCAs and drugs, but also micro and nanoparticles into the skin at sufficiently large depth in comparison with surface ablation and mechanical treatments because of the low area of skin damage and, therefore, reduced risk of infection [57].

Figure 2.11 illustrates how fractional ablation combined with IOC works for in vitro testing of human skin sample with the modeled black ink tattoo at fractional ablation of SC and glycerol application during 24 hours [49]. Tattoo is poorly recognized on the right image and clearly seen on the right image and dot areas of ablated skin via which glycerol penetrates are also well seen. Evidently, that this demonstration is valid for imaging of any in-depth absorbing pathology of the skin.

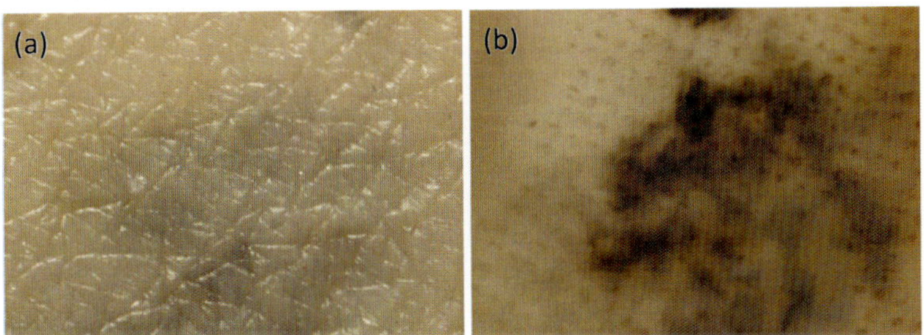


**Figure 2.11**   In vitro images of skin sample surface with black ink tattoo model: before processing (a) and after skin fractional ablation (lamp/transparent appliqué with many black dots) and glycerol application during 24 h (b) [49]. Tattoo is clearly seen on the right image (b) and dot areas of ablated skin are also well seen. Image (b) is done with polarization filtering.

Figure 2.12 illustrates the possibility of in vivo enhancement of tattoo imaging using skin surface preprocessing by the cyanoacrylate glue-stripping technique allowed for rapid and complete SC removal and glycerol delivery under pressure. There are shown unadjusted pre- (a) and post-glycerol (b) photographs of the treated skin region. Figures 2.12c,d are close-ups of the areas indicated in Figs. 2.12a,b, respectively. Enhanced visualization of the vasculature of the skin is also well seen.

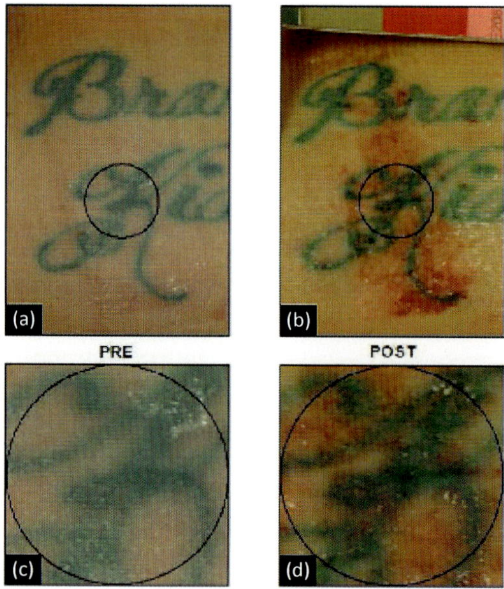


**Figure 2.12** In vivo raw images pre (a and c) and post (b and d) glycerol application for a patient with the preprocessed skin by cyanoacrylate glue-stripping technique allowed for rapid and complete SC removal. A 100%-glycerol was used as an OCA, which was delivered into skin under pressure. The fluid pressure was maintained through continuous addition of glycerol from a dispenser using regulated compressed air over a separate glycerol in order to maintain a pressure of 30–70 mmHg for 30–60 min. After the bandage was drained through the fluid access port and removed, any remaining glycerol was wiped away with a paper towel. The intensification of the ink vision and the ability to visualize vasculature is seen in the post glycerol treatment (b and d) [48].

## 2.5.2  Skin Model and MC Simulation

The efficiency of laser radiation delivery to the skin sites where tattoo pigment is localized can be evaluated on the basis of MC simulations for variable optical properties of skin layers due to tissue clearing potency. We will consider that the absorption properties of skin are mainly determined by the absorption of melanin, water, and blood hemoglobin; as well as scattering is determined by the tissue structure components, such as collagen/elastin fibrils of dermis, mitochondria, and nuclei of epidermal cells.

In accordance with the optical and the structural-morphological properties of skin, the six-layer skin model was used [49,50] with the main parameters presented in Table 2.3 [58].

**Table 2.3**     Parameters of skin layers used in the MC simulations [58]

| Skin layer | Thickness ($\mu$m) | Refractive index | Water content (%) | Blood content (%) | Scattering coefficient of a bloodless tissue at 577 nm cm$^{-1}$ | Mean vessel diameter ($\mu$m) |
|---|---|---|---|---|---|---|
| Epidermis & SC | 100 | 1.45 | 60 | 0 | 300 | — |
| Basal membrane | 15 | 1.40 | 60 | 0 | 300 | — |
| Dermis & upper blood plexus | 200 | 1.38 | 75 | 1.7 | 120 | 6 |
| Reticular dermis | 1500 | 1.35 | 75 | 1.4 | 120 | 15 |
| Dermis & lower blood plexus | 200 | 1.38 | 75 | 1.7 | 120 | 6 |
| Subcutaneous adipose tissue | 3000 | 1.44 | 5 | 0 | 130 | — |

In the visible and NIR spectral ranges the absorption coefficient of each skin layer is defined as

$$\mu_{\text{a}k} = B_k C_k \mu_{\text{a}}^{\text{bl}}(\lambda) + \left(1 - B_k - W_k\right)\mu_{\text{a}}^{\text{bg}} + M_k \mu_{\text{a}}^{\text{mel}}(\lambda)$$
$$+ W_k \mu_{\text{a}}^{\text{w}}(\lambda), \tag{2.10}$$

where $k = 1, \ldots, 6$ is a layer number, $B_k$ and $W_k$ are the volume fractions of blood and water in the each layer; for the melanin containing layers (epidermis and basal membrane) $M_k = 1$, for the other skin layers $M_k = 0$; $\mu_{\text{a}}^{\text{bl}}$, $\mu_{\text{a}}^{\text{mel}}$, $\mu_{\text{a}}^{\text{w}}$, and $\mu_{\text{a}}^{\text{bg}}$ are the absorption coefficients of blood, melanin, water and background matter (collagen) of tissue, respectively (in the framework of the model $\mu_{\text{a}}^{\text{bg}}$ is assumed to be wavelength independent and equal to 0.15 cm$^{-1}$ [58]); $C_k$ is a dimensionless correction factor. The correction factor is a number from 0 to 1 and taking into account the fact that blood is localized in vessels rather than distributed homogeneously in the skin dermis. If the blood vessel diameter is large enough, and light does not penetrate to the inner part of the vessel, then hemoglobin of the interior part has not to be taken into account as an absorber; and in this case, the correction factor will be considerably smaller than unity. Otherwise, for thin vessels the correction factor is close to unity. Taking into account that the correction factor depends on the vessel diameter, we used in the model the following empirical expression [49,50]:

$$C_k = \frac{1}{1 + a\left(0.5\mu_a^{bl} d_k^{ves}\right)^b},$$

(2.11)

where $d_k^{ves}$ is the blood vessel diameter in centimeters and $\mu_a^{bl}$ should be expressed in inverse centimeters. If blood vessels lying in parallel to the skin surface are illuminated by a collimated light beam $a = 1.007$ and $b = 1.228$, while for the diffuse illumination of the vessels $a = 1.482$ and $b = 1.151$. The blood optical properties (i.e., anisotropy factor and both absorption and scattering coefficients) were calculated on the basis of algorithm described in detail in Ref. [59]. In the framework of the modeling, it was assumed that degree of hemoglobin oxygenation is 0.8 (oxygenation for arterial blood is 0.9 and that for venous blood is 0.7) and value of blood hematocrit is of 0.4.

The scattering coefficient of skin layers is defined as

$$\mu_{sk}(\lambda) = B_k C_k \mu_s^{bl}(\lambda) + (1 - B_k)\mu_{sk}^{bg}(\lambda)$$

(2.12)

Here

$$\mu_{sk}^{bg}(\lambda) = \mu_{sk}^0 \left(\frac{577}{\lambda}\right)$$

is the scattering coefficient of bloodless tissue [58]; $\mu_{sk}^0$ is the scattering coefficient of bloodless tissue at the wavelength 577 nm (see Table 2.3); $\lambda$ is expressed in nanometers.

The anisotropy scattering factor is expressed in the following form:

$$g_k(\lambda) = \frac{B_k C_k \mu_s^{bl}(\lambda) g^{bl} + (1 - B_k)\mu_{sk}^{bg}(\lambda) g^{bg}(\lambda)}{\mu_{sk}(\lambda)},\qquad(2.13)$$

where

$$g^{bg}(\lambda) = 0.7645 + 0.2355\left[1 - \exp\left(-\frac{\lambda - 500}{729.1}\right)\right]$$

is the scattering anisotropy factor of bloodless tissue [58]. The absorption coefficient of melanin is described by the following empirical expression [58]:

$$\mu_a^{mel}(\lambda) = A\exp\left(-\frac{\lambda - 800}{182}\right),\qquad(2.14)$$

where $A$ is the ratio of the optical density of pigmented skin layer (epidermis and basal membrane) to their thickness. In the model $A$ was taken as 0.87 cm$^{-1}$ for epidermis and 13.5 cm$^{-1}$ for basal membrane [58].

### 2.5.3 Skin Immersion Optical Clearing and Tattoo Modeling

The optical clearing of different skin layers was simulated using Mie scattering theory [60], which requires the knowledge of the refractive indices of skin scatterers and surrounding interstitial fluid (ICF), and also sizes of the scatterers. Calculations for epidermis and basal membrane have been performed using the model of spherical particles, since cell mitochondria are the main scatterers for epithelial tissues, while for dermis the model of cylindrical particles was used, because of fibrous structure of dermis [61]. As the particle size distribution and the corresponding packing factor of the scatterers are unknown, monodisperse, so-called Mie-equivalent particles, were used for the simulation.

The scattering coefficient of the epithelial skin layers was calculated in the following form [60]:

$$\mu_s(\lambda) = \frac{3}{4}\frac{\varphi}{\pi a_{sph}^3}\pi a_{sph}^3 Q_s(a_{sph}, n_s, n_l)F(\lambda),\qquad(2.15)$$

where $a_{\mathrm{sph}}$ is the radius of spherical particle; $Q_{\mathrm{s}}(a_{\mathrm{sph}}, n_{\mathrm{S}}, n_{\mathrm{I}})$ is the scattering efficiency factor; $F(\lambda)$ is the packing factor of the particles; $n_{\mathrm{s}}$ is the refractive index of the particles; $n_{\mathrm{I}}$ is the refractive index of the ISF; $\varphi$ is the volume fraction of particles for each layer. For dermal layers the scattering coefficient was calculated as [60]:

$$\mu_{\mathrm{s}}(\lambda) = \frac{\varphi}{\pi \alpha_{\mathrm{c}}^2} 2a_{\mathrm{c}} Q_{\mathrm{s}}(a_{\mathrm{c}}, n_{\mathrm{s}}, n_{\mathrm{I}}) F(\lambda), \tag{2.16}$$

where $a_{\mathrm{c}}$ is the radius of cylindrical particles. Both the effective size of the particles and their packing factor were calculated by the minimization of the target function

$$\mathrm{TF}(a(\lambda), F(\lambda)) = (\mu_{\mathrm{s}}^{\mathrm{mod}} - \mu_{\mathrm{s}}^{\mathrm{Mie}})^2 + (g^{\mathrm{mod}} - g^{\mathrm{Mie}})^2, \tag{2.17}$$

where $\mu_{\mathrm{s}}^{\mathrm{mod}}$ and $g^{\mathrm{mod}}$ correspond to the data calculated according to Eqs. 2.12 and 2.13 for each layer; $\mu_{\mathrm{s}}^{\mathrm{Mie}}$ and $g^{\mathrm{Mie}}$ are the scattering coefficient (Eqs. 2.15 and 2.16) and the anisotropy factor calculated for each layer on the basis of Mie theory. To minimize the target function the Nelder and Mead simplex method described in detail in Ref. [62] has been used.

The influence of clearing agent on the skin optical properties was simply modeled by increasing of ISF index of refraction up to 1.45. It was assumed that effective size, packing factor, and index of refraction of the scatterers have not being changed at the immersion optical clearing.

For modeling of tattoo, an absorbing layer in the form of cross with thickness 50 μm and size $1 \times 1$ cm$^2$ was added to the skin model. Total area of the modeled skin sample was $3 \times 3$ cm$^2$. Absorption coefficient of the cross was equal to absorption coefficient of ink, i.e., 11770, 10776, 8673, 7872, 6150, and 5253 cm$^{-1}$ at wavelengths 470, 532, 650, 694, 850, and 1064 nm, respectively. Scattering properties of this layer was taken as similar to the scattering properties of reticular dermis. The depth of ink location in the model was chosen as 0.5 or 1 mm.

The MC simulation has been performed on the basis of the algorithm presented in Ref. [7]. For the calculation of the photon fraction absorbed in tattoo area the following procedure was used: When a photon trajectory passed through the tattoo area, parameter $A_{\mathrm{t}}$ (the photon fraction absorbed in tattoo area) increased on $w\mu_a/(\mu_a + \mu_s)$ at the each act of interaction [7], where $w$ is the current weight of photon packet, and $\mu_a$ and $\mu_s$ are the coefficients of absorption and scattering in the given point, respectively. After the detection of all photon packets, the value $A_t$ was summed over all packets and normalized to the total weigh of the packets, which were used for the simulation. A new propagation direction of the scattered photon packet was determined according to the Henyey–Greenstein scattering phase function:

$$f_{HG}(\theta) = \frac{1}{4\pi} \frac{1-g^2}{(1+g^2-2g\cos\theta)^{3/2}}, \tag{2.18}$$

where $\theta$ is the polar scattering angle. The distribution over the azimuthal scattering angle was assumed as uniform.

For the simulation of skin images with tattoo $25 \times 10^6$ photon packets was used. Photons normally incident on the skin surface were uniformly distributed over the area $3 \times 3$ cm$^2$. For the detection of backscattered photons, this area ($3 \times 3$ cm$^2$) was separated on the grid with area of the grid cells of $0.01$ mm$^2$. When backscattered photon went out, its weigh was recorded to the array cell, which corresponded to the coordinates of the point of going out, then was summed over all packets. After the finishing of the simulation it was normalized to the average weight of the incident packets upon corresponding area.

The thicknesses and refractive indices of skin layers used in the MC simulations are presented in Table 2.3. Without optical clearing for each wavelength and each skin layer, absorption coefficient, scattering coefficient, and anisotropy factor were calculated using Eqs. 2.10, 2.12, and 2.13, respectively. At the immersion skin optical clearing, scattering coefficient and anisotropy factor of each skin layer were calculated using Eqs. 2.15 and 2.16.

### 2.5.4   Results of MC Modeling and Discussion

Monte Carlo simulations of reflectance spectra and images of the human skin with black tattoo localized in reticular dermis at the depth of 0.5 and 1.0 mm are presented in Figs. 2.13 and 2.14 [49,50]. In Fig. 2.13, the reflection spectra are shown: for the intact skin without tattoo (curves 1); for the skin with tattoo located at the depth of 0.5 mm (a) and 1.0 mm (b) (curves 2); with skin layers over or under tattoo are immersed (curves 3 and 4, respectively); and totally immersed skin without/with tattoo (curves 5 and 6, respectively). In all cases the subcutaneous adipose tissue layer was not immersed. The shape of the intact skin reflectance spectrum is determined by light scattering of tissue components and absorption of melanin, blood hemoglobin with bands at 416, 542, and 575 nm, and water

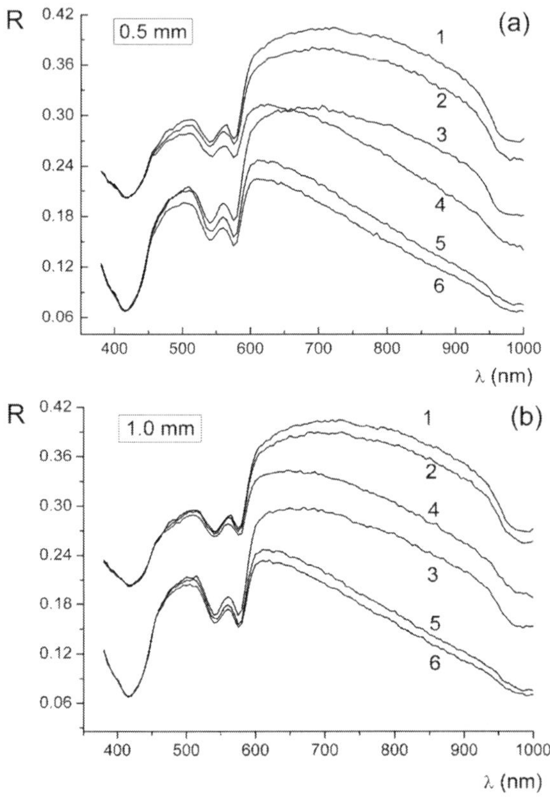


**Figure 2.13** MC simulated human skin reflectance spectra with a black color tattoo at a depth of 0.5 (a) and 1.0 mm (b): (1) normal skin; (2) skin with tattoo; (3) skin layers above tattoo are immersed by an OCA (model of topical OCA administration); (4) skin layers under tattoo (between tattoo and subcutaneous adipose tissue) are immersed by an OCA (model of intradermal injection of an OCA); (5) and (6) all skin layers from the surface up to subcutaneous adipose tissue are immersed by an OCA (model of combined OCA administration—topical and via injection): (5) normal skin, (6) skin with tattoo [49].

at 980 nm. The presence of tattoo reduces the skin reflectance due to light absorption by the ink pigment. For smaller pigment location depth, the skin reflectance decreases more significantly. The modeling demonstrates well that optical clearing of different skin layers, upper and lower tattoo location, allows for control of skin reflectivity in a rather wide range within the visible and NIR wavelengths. However, to use IOC effects in practice to image and/ or ablate absorbing inhomogeneity like tattoo or tumor, we are able to introduce and calculate two more parameters, such as image contrast $K$ and fraction of light absorbed by this inhomogeneity $A$ [49,50].

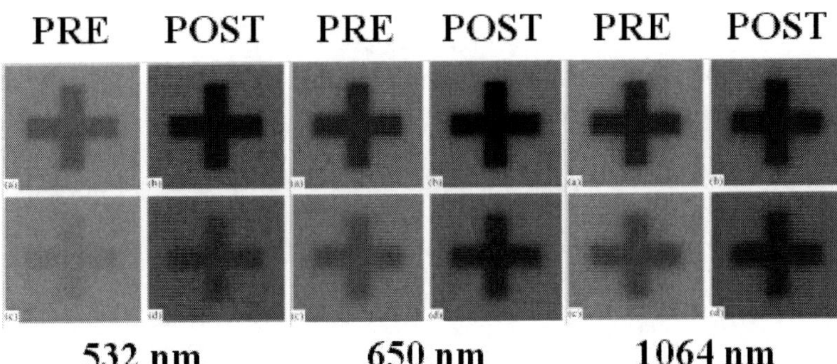


**Figure 2.14** Three sets of MC simulated skin tattoo images at the wavelengths 532, 650, and 1064 nm: (a, b) the depth of the tattoo is 0.5 mm and (c, d) 1.0 mm; the size of the tattoo is $1 \times 1$ cm$^2$; (a, c) no clearing; (b, d) skin layers above the tattoo are optically cleared (model of topically applied immersion agent) [50].

The images, presented in Fig. 2.14, were simulated using optical properties of skin at $\lambda = 532$ nm, 650 nm, and 1064 nm. The left images of each set correspond to the skin with tattoo, as the right images correspond to the same skin but with optically cleared skin layers above the tattoo in accordance with the model of topically administered immersion agent [50]. The tattoo image boundaries without IOC look rather blurred due to high light scattering by the upper tissue layers. The simulation of photon migration in skin has shown that the immersion of the upper skin layers is more efficient for image contrast improvement and increasing of the number of photons absorbed by the tattoo.

As it follows from Fig. 2.14, the optical clearing of the upper skin layers significantly enhances the image contrast, which improves the tattoo localization and imaging. The image contrast can be estimated as:

$$K = \frac{\left(R_1 - R_2\right)}{\left(R_1 + R_2\right)}, \tag{2.19}$$

where $R_1$ and $R_2$ are the skin reflectance outside the tattoo area and inside it, respectively.

Results of tattoo image contrast calculations for normal and optically cleared skin are also presented in Table 2.4 and Fig. 2.15. It is well seen that contrast of the tattoo images increases with the wavelength of illuminating light with some saturation in the NIR spectral range. At the same time, clearing efficiency expressed as a ratio of the contrast images of tattoo in immersed skin to the contrast images of tattoo in native skin, somewhat decreases with the wavelength. However, the efficiency is still very high, especially for deeper tattoo localization, and less dependent on the wavelength in the range above 700 nm (Fig. 2.15).

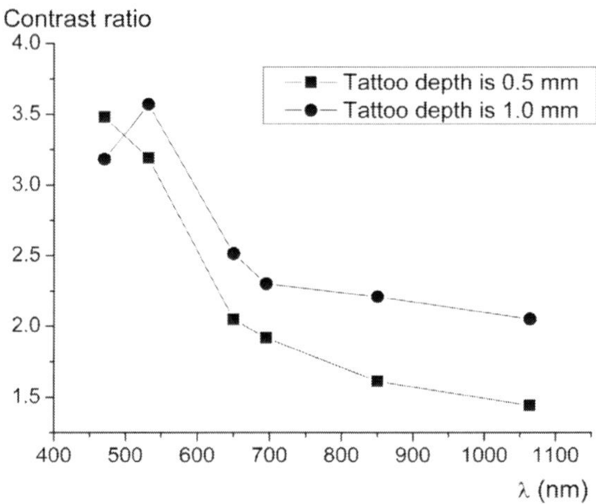


**Figure 2.15** The wavelength dependences of contrast ration $K_{\text{POST}}/K_{\text{PRE}}$ for tattoo images (POST and PRE are after and before optical clearing (model of OCA topical application), respectively) [50].

**Table 2.4**  Result of MC simulation of image contrast of 1 mm-depth skin tattoo pre- and post-OCA topical application [50]

| Wavelength (nm) | Immersed skin, $K_{POST}$ | Native skin, $K_{PRE}$ | $K_{POST}/K_{PRE}$ |
|---|---|---|---|
| 470 | 0.070 | 0.022 | 3.182 |
| 532 | 0.100 | 0.028 | 3.571 |
| 650 | 0.284 | 0.113 | 2.513 |
| 694 | 0.382 | 0.166 | 2.301 |
| 850 | 0.380 | 0.172 | 2.209 |
| 1064 | 0.371 | 0.181 | 2.050 |

Figure 2.16 presents the spectral dependences of the fraction of photons absorbed by the skin layer with tattoo $A$ at depths of 0.5 and 1 mm. Curves 1 and 5, which describing intact and totally immersed skin without tattoo, are very similar to each other and close to zero due to small absorption of native skin in this range and this particular localization—this is a base line for modeling of absorbed fraction by tattoo. The presence of tattoo changes

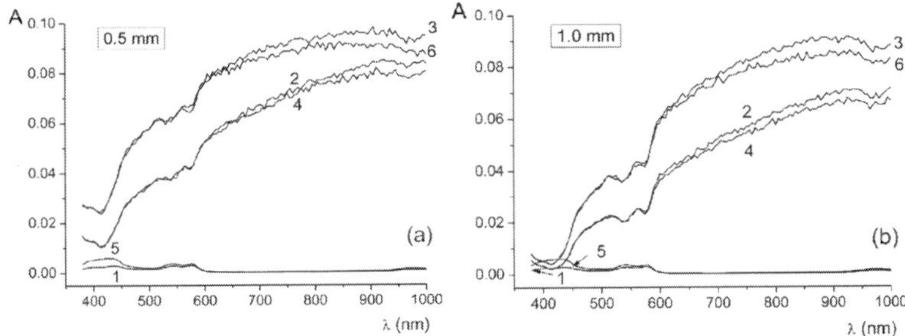


**Figure 2.16**  Result of MC simulation of absorbed photon fraction in the black tattoo area of skin at a depth of 0.5 (a) or 1.0 mm (b) under the different conditions: (1) normal skin; (2) skin with tattoo; (3) skin layers above tattoo are immersed by an OCA (model of topical OCA administration); (4) skin layers under tattoo (between tattoo and subcutaneous adipose tissue) are immersed by an OCA (model of intradermal injection of an OCA); (5) and (6) all skin layers from the surface up to subcutaneous adipose tissue are immersed by an OCA (model of combined OCA administration—topical and via injection): (5) normal skin, (6) skin with tattoo [49].

the spectral dependence of the fraction of absorbed photons in accordance with the absorption spectrum of the used ink or dye. The immersion of layers under tattoo reduces the number of photons absorbed in the given area, which is well seen in Fig. 2.16, curves 4. At the same time, if only upper layers over the tattoo are cleared, a significant number of photons propagate through the upper layers almost without scattering and are absorbed in the tattoo area. Photons that have passed through the absorbing layer to down skin layers, which are not cleared, can be effectively backscattered and also absorbed by the tattoo. The fraction of photons absorbed in the wavelength range from 600 to 1000 nm increases upon clearing of upper skin layers on average by 30% and 40% for tattoos at depths of 0.5 and 1 mm, respectively. Thus, for deeply located tattoo this method of clearing is more efficient.

Table 2.5 summarizes data of IOC efficiency for a 1 mm-depth location of tattoo. It is seen that the absorbed fraction increases with the increase of the wavelength similar to the image contrast behavior (see Table 2.4), and the ratio of the light fraction absorbed in tattoo embedded in immersed skin to the fraction for tattoo embedded in the native skin decreases with the wavelength (see Fig. 2.17). The ratio decreases from 1.588 ($\lambda$ = 470 nm) to 1.197 ($\lambda$ = 1064 nm) for tattoo located at the depth of 1.0 mm and from 1.633 ($\lambda$ = 470 nm) to 1.082 ($\lambda$ = 1064 nm) for tattoo located at the depth of 0.5 mm. That is related to general decrease of skin scattering for the longer wavelengths; so less overall photons circulate within absorbing layer and are absorbed by tattoo.

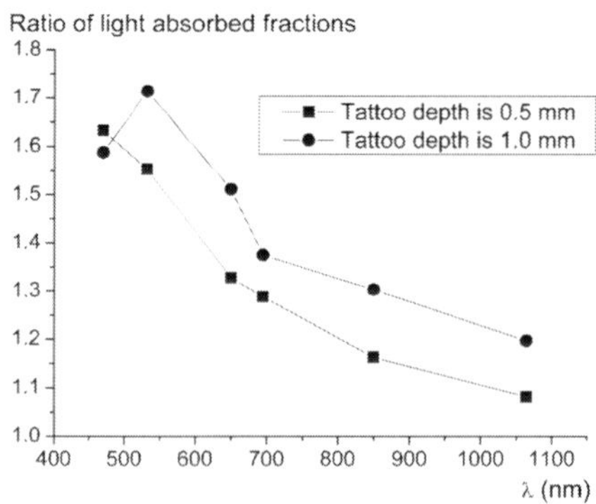


**Figure 2.17** The wavelength dependences of the ratio of light absorbed fractions by tattoo $A_{\mathrm{POST}}/A_{\mathrm{PRE}}$ (POST and PRE are after and before optical clearing, respectively) [50].

However, the efficiency of IOC is still good to provide laser thermolysis of tattoo or other skin absorbing abnormality for a number of wavelengths. Basing on literature data for different laser systems it was estimated [50] that to achieve the similar tattoo damage, which can be obtained without skin optical clearing, at optical clearing the density of laser energy can be reduced in dependence on the tattoo localization depth up to 50–60% for the blue-green spectral range, 30–40% for the red, and 10–20% for the NIR.

**Table 2.5**  MC simulation of light absorbed fraction $A$ by tattoo located at 1.0 mm depth

| Wavelength, nm | $A_{\mathrm{PRE}}$ | $A_{\mathrm{POST}}$ | $A_{\mathrm{POST}}/A_{\mathrm{PRE}}$ |
|---|---|---|---|
| 470 | 0.017 | 0.027 | 1.588 |
| 532 | 0.021 | 0.036 | 1.714 |
| 650 | 0.045 | 0.068 | 1.511 |
| 694 | 0.056 | 0.077 | 1.375 |
| 850 | 0.066 | 0.086 | 1.303 |
| 1064 | 0.071 | 0.085 | 1.197 |

*Note*: $A_{\mathrm{PRE}}$ is for normal skin; $A_{\mathrm{POST}}$ is for upper skin layers immersed by an OCA [50].

## 2.6  Summary

Facing the problem of combining properties of optical radiation and the ability to cope with the parameters of biological tissues, which are anticipated to vary spatially and temporally, as well as individually, the MC technique becomes a primary tool in biophotonics and biomedical optics. The developed O3MC tool can be used for direct on-line real-time simulation of human skin spectra and colors depending on the blood, water, melanin content. The geometry of particular probes is taken into account for skin spectra simulation as well as controllable and selective immersion optical clearing of skin layers. With the further development of the technique additional parameters such as spatial distribution of blood vessels, tissue shrinkage and swelling, red blood cells aggregation and their velocity will be included. In addition, by applying recently developed approach of handling polarization [45,46] the MC can be used for direct simulations of sampling volume for various probe geometry, skin reflectance spectra for non-, co- and cross- polarized light, fluorescence spectra modeling, and other. We believe with the new developments the MC technique will find a number of new straightforward applications related to the non-invasive optical based skin studies.

## Acknowledgments

This study was supported in part by the Ministry of Business, Innovations, and Employment of New Zealand; by the University of Oulu, Finland, project FiDiPro TEKES 40111/11; as well as by a Grant of the President of the Russian Federation no. NSh-1177.2012.2 and by state contracts of the Russian Federation nos. 14.V37.21.0728 and 14.V37.21.0563.

## References

1. Tuchin VV (ed.) (2010). *Handbook of Photonics for Biomedical Science*, CRC Press, Taylor & Francis Group, London.

2. Doronin AV and Meglinski IV (2011). Online object oriented Monte Carlo computational tool for the needs of biomedical optics, *Biomed Opt Express*, **9**, 2461–2469.

3. Doronin AV and Meglinski IV (2011). Monte Carlo simulation of photon migration in turbid random media based on the object-oriented programming paradigm, in *Biomedical Applications of Light Scattering V* (Wax AP and Backman V, eds), Proc. SPIE, 7907, 790709.

4. Doronin AV and Meglinski IV (2010). GPU-accelerated Object-Oriented Monte Carlo modeling of photon migration in turbid media, in *Optical Technologies in Biophysics and Medicine* XII (Tuchin VV and Genina EA, eds), *Proc. SPIE*, 7999, 79990K.

5. Dolin LS (2009). Development of radiative transfer theory as applied to instrumental imaging in turbid media, *Phys-Usp*, **52**, 519–526.

6. Martelli F, Del Bianco S, Ismaelli A, and Zaccanti G (eds) (2009). *Light Propagation through Biological Tissue and Other Diffusive Media: Theory, Solutions, and Software*, SPIE Press.

7. Wang LH, Jacques SL, and Zheng LQ (1995). MCML—Monte Carlo modeling of photon transport in multilayered tissues, *Comput Meth Prog Bio*, **47**, 131–146.

8. Meglinski IV and Matcher SJ (2001). Modeling the sampling volume for the skin blood oxygenation measurements, *Med Biol Eng Comput*, **39**, 44–50.

9. Meglinski IV (2001). Modeling the reflectance spectra of the optical radiation for random inhomogeneous multi-layered highly scattering and absorbing media by the Monte Carlo technique, *Quantum Electron*, **31**, 1101–1107.

10. Meglinski IV and Matcher SJ (2003). Computer simulation of the skin reflectance spectra, *Comput Meth Prog Bio*, **70**, 179–186.

11. Churmakov DY, Meglinski IV, and Greenhalgh DA (2004). Amending of fluorescence sensor signal localization in human skin by matching of the refractive index, *J Biomed Opt*, **9**, 339–346.

12. Churmakov DY, Meglinski IV, Greenhalgh DA, and Piletsky SA (2003). Analysis of skin tissues spatial fluorescence distribution by the Monte Carlo simulation, *J Phys D: Appl Phys*, **36**, 1722–1728.

13. Meglinski IV and Churmakov DY (2004). Spatial localization of biosensor fluorescence signals in human skin under the effect of equalization of the refractive Index of the surrounding medium, *Opt Spectrosc*, **96**, 946–951.

14. Meglinski IV, Kirillin M, Kuzmin VL, and Myllyla R (2008). Simulation of polarization-sensitive optical coherence tomography images by a Monte Carlo method, *Opt Lett*, **33**, 1581–1583.

15. Kirillin M, Meglinski I, Sergeeva E, Kuzmin VL, and Myllyla R (2010). Simulation of optical coherence tomography images by Monte Carlo modeling based on polarization vector approach, *Opt Express*, **18**, 21714–21724.

16. Kirillin MY, Priezzhev AV, and Meglinski IV (2006). Effect of photons of different scattering orders on the formation of a signal in optical low-coherence tomography of highly scattering media, *Quantum Electron*, **36**, 247–252.

17. Romanov VP, Churmakov DY, Berrocal E, and Meglinski IV (2004). Low-order light scattering in multiple scattering disperse media, *Opt Spectrosc*, **97**, 796–802.

18. Meglinski IV, Romanov VP, Churmakov DY, Berrocal E, Jermy MC, and Greenhalgh DA (2004). Low and high orders light scattering in particulate media, *Laser Phys Lett*, **1**, 387–390.

19. Kuzmin VL and Meglinski IV (2004). Coherent multiple scattering effects and Monte Carlo method, *JETP Lett*, **79**, 109–112.

20. Meglinski IV, Kuzmin VL, Churmakov DY, and Greenhalgh DA (2005). Monte Carlo simulation of coherent effects in multiple scattering, *Proc Roy Soc A*, **461**, 43–53.

21. Kuzmin VL and Meglinski IV (2010). Anomalous polarization phenomena of light scattered in random media, *J Exp Theor Phys*, **137**, 742–753.

22. Kuzmin VL and Meglinski IV (eds) (2010). *Helicity Flip of Backscattered Circularly Polarized Light, Proc. SPIE*, 7573, 75730Z.

23. Kuzmin VL and Meglinski IV (2007). Coherent effects of multiple scattering for scalar and electromagnetic fields: Monte-Carlo simulation and Milne-like solutions, *Opt Commun*, **273**, 307–310.

24. Kuzmin VL, Meglinski IV, and Churmakov DY (2005). Stochastic modeling of coherent phenomena in strongly inhomogeneous media, *J Exp Theor Phys*, **101**, 22–32.

25. Berrocal E, Meglinski IV, Greenhalgh DA, and Linne MA (2006). Image transfer through the complex scattering turbid media, *Laser Phys Lett*, **3**, 464–468.

26. Berrocal E, Sedarsky D, Paciaroni M, Meglinski IV, and Linne MA (2007). Imaging through the turbid scattering media: part I: experimental and simulated results for the spatial intensity distribution, *Opt Express*, **15**, 10649–10665.

27. Boas DA, Culver JP, Stott JJ, and Dunn AK (2002). Three dimensional Monte Carlo code for photon migration through complex heterogeneous media including the adult human head, *Opt Express*, **10**, 159–170.

28. Ramella-Roman J, Prahl S, and Jacques S (2005). Three Monte Carlo programs of polarized light transport into scattering media: part I, *Opt Express*, **13**, 4420–4438.

29. Fang Q (2010). Mesh-based Monte Carlo method using fast ray-tracing in Plücker coordinates, *Biomed Opt Express*, **1**, 165–175.

30. Shen H and Wang G (2011). A study on tetrahedron-based inhomogeneous Monte Carlo optical simulation, *Biomed Opt Express*, **2**, 44–57.

31. Meglinski IV, Kirillin M, and Kuzmin VL (2008). The concept of a unified modelling of optical radiation propagation in complex turbid media, *Proc. SPIE*, 7142, 714204.

32. Schach S (ed) (2006). *Object-Oriented and Classical Software Engineering*, Seventh Ed., McGraw-Hill, New York.

33. McConnell S (ed) (2004). *Code Complete*, 2nd ed., Microsoft Press, Redmond.

34. Kirk DB, Hwu WW (eds) (2010). *Programming Massively Parallel Processors: A Hands-on Approach*, Morgan Kaufmann Publishers, Burlington.

35. Sanders J and Kandrot E (ed) (2010). *CUDA by Example: An Introduction to General-Purpose GPU Programming*, Addison-Wesley, Boston.

36. CUDA Programming Guide 4.0; CUBLAS Library; CUFFT Library; CURAND Library (2011). NVIDIA Corporation.

37. Shklar L and Rosen R (eds) (2009). *Web Application Architecture: Principles, Protocols and Practices*, John Wiley & Sons Ltd, Chichester.

38. Doronin AV (2011). GPU-Accelerated Biophotonics & Biomedical Optics, NVIDIA Corporation, interview, Aug. 28.

39. Doronin A and Meglinski I (2012). Peer-to-Peer Monte Carlo simulation of photon migration in topical applications of biomedical optics, *J Biomed Opt*, **17**, 090504.

40. Churmakov DY, Meglinski I, and Greenhalgh DA (2002). Influence of refractive index matching on the photon diffuse reflectance, *Phys Med Biol*, **47**, 4271–4285.

41. Jacques S (2013). Optical properties of biological tissues: a review, *Phys Med Biol*, **58**, R37–R61.

42. Saidi I, Jacques S, and Tittel F (1995). Mie and Rayleigh modeling of visible-light scattering in neonatal skin, *Appl Opt*, **34**, 7410–7418.

43. Donner G and Jensen HW (2006). A spectral BSSRDF for shading human skin, in: *Rendering Techniques 2006: 17th Eurographics Workshop on Rendering*, pp 409–418.

44. Petrov GI, Doronin A, Whelan HT, Meglinski I, and Yakovlev VV (2012). Human tissue colour as viewed in high dynamic range optical spectral transmission measurements, *Biomed Opt Express*, **3**, 2154–2161.

45. Churmakov DY, Kuzmin VL, and Meglinski IV (2006). Application of the vector Monte Carlo method in polarization optical coherence tomography, *Quantum Electron*, **36**, 1009–1015.

46. Kuzmin VL and Meglinski IV (2009). Backscattering of linearly and circularly polarized light in randomly inhomogeneous media, *Opt Spectrosc*, **106**, 257–267.

47. McNichols RJ, Fox MA, Gowda A, Tuya S, Bell B, and Motamedi M (2005). Temporary dermal scatter reduction: quantitative assessment and implications for improved laser tattoo removal, *Lasers Surg Med*, **36**, 289–296.

48. Fox AM, Diven, DG, Sra K, Boretsky A, Poonawalla T, Readinger A, Motamedi M, and McNichols RJ (2009). Dermal scatter reduction in human skin: a method using controlled application of glycerol, *Lasers Surg Med*, **41**, 251–255.

49. Genina EA, Bashkatov AN, Tuchin VV, Altshuler GB, and Yaroslavski IV (2008). Possibility of increasing the efficiency of laser-induced tattoo removal by optical skin clearing, *Quant Electron*, **38**(6), 580–587.

50. Bashkatov AN, Genina EA, Tuchin VV, and Altshuler GB (2009). Skin optical clearing for improvement of laser tattoo removal, *Laser Phys*, **19**(6), 1312–1322.

51. Tuchin VV (ed) (2006). *Optical Clearing of Tissues and Blood*, PM154, SPIE Press, Bellingham.

52. Genina EA, Bashkatov AN, and Tuchin VV (2010). Tissue optical immersion clearing, *Expert Rev Med Devices*, **7**(6), 825–842.

53. Larin KV, Ghosn MG, Bashkatov AN, Genina EA, Trunina NA, and Tuchin VV (2012). Optical clearing for OCT image enhancement and in-depth monitoring of molecular diffusion, *IEEE J Select Tops Quant Electron*, **18**(3), 1244–1259.

54. Zhu D, Larin KV, Luo Q, and Tuchin VV (2013). Recent progress in tissue optical clearing, *Laser Photonics Rev*, 1–26.

55. Tuchin VV, Altshuler GB, Gavrilova AA, Pravdin AB, Tabatadze D, Childs J, and Yaroslavsky IV (2006). Optical clearing of skin using flashlamp-induced enhancement of epidermal permeability, *Lasers Surg Med*, **38**(9), 824–836.

56. Genina EA, Bashkatov AN, Korobko AA, Zubkova EA, Tuchin VV, Yaroslavsky I, and Altshuler GB (2008). Optical clearing of human skin: comparative study of permeability and dehydration of intact and photothermally perforated skin, *J Biomed Opt*, **13**(2), 021102-1–8.

57. Genina EA, Bashkatov AN, Dolotov LE, Maslyakova GN, Kochubey VI, Yaroslavsky IV, Altshuler GB, and Tuchin VV (2013). Transcutaneous delivery of micro- and nanoparticles with laser microporation, *J Biomed Opt*, **18**(11), 111406-1–9.

58. Altshuler G, Smirnov M, and Yaroslavsky I (2005). Lattice of optical islets: a novel treatment modality in photomedicine, *J Phys D: Appl Phys*, **38**, 2732–2747.

59. Bashkatov AN, Zhestkov DM, Genina EA, and Tuchin VV (2005). Immersion optical clearing of human blood in the visible and near infrared spectral range, *Opt Spectrosc*, **98**(4), 638–646.

60. Bohren CF and Huffman DR (eds) (1983). *Absorption and Scattering of Light by Small Particles*, Wiley, New York.

61. Tuchin VV (ed) (2007). *Tissue Optics: Light Scattering Methods and Instruments for Medical Diagnosis*, PM 166, SPIE Press, Bellingham.

62. Bunday B (ed) (1984). *Basis Optimization Methods*, Edward Arnold, London.

# Chapter 3

# Mathematics and Biological Process of Skin Pigmentation

Josef Thingnes,[a] Leiv Øyehaug,[b] and Eivind Hovig[a,c,d]

[a]*Department of Tumor Biology, Institute for Cancer Research,*
*The Norwegian Radium Hospital, Part of Oslo University Hospital, Oslo, Norway*
[b]*Norwegian Defence Research Establishment,*
*Land and Air Systems Division, P. O. Box 25, 2027 Kjeller, Norway*
[c]*Institute of Medical Informatics, University of Oslo,*
*Oslo University, Hospital, Oslo, Norway*
[d]*Biomedical Research Group, Department of Informatics,*
*Faculty of Mathematics and Natural Sciences, University of Oslo,*
*Oslo, Norway*

joseft@ifi.uio.no

Human skin pigmentation is facilitated by melanocytes that synthesize the pigment melanin. The melanocytes reside in the basal layer of epidermis. Melanin is produced by specialized organelles within the melanocytes, called melanosomes. In healthy skin, melanocytes are distributed in a characteristic regularly dispersed pattern. Sun tanning results from a UV-induced increase in the production and release of melanin to the neighbouring keratinocytes, as well as a redistribution of melanin among these cells. The regulatory mechanisms of pigmentation and the tanning

*Computational Biophysics of the Skin*
Edited by Bernard Querleux
Copyright © 2014 Pan Stanford Publishing Pte. Ltd.
ISBN  978-981-4463-84-3 (Hardcover),  978-981-4463-85-0 (eBook)
www.panstanford.com

response encompass cell self-organization, UV-sensing, auto- and paracrine signalling, melanocyte dendrite formation, as well as melanogenesis and melanosome transfer.

In this chapter, we give a detailed presentation of the biological process of the skin pigmentation. Further, we review the mathematical models that have been deployed up until now in the field. We also present one of our own models more deeply. This is an ODE model describing the distribution of melanin in the layers of epidermis in response to UV irradiation.

## 3.1 Background

Around 1 million years ago, a tanning response evolved in our hominid ancestors in which the accumulation of melanin granules in skin cells provided physical protection against the DNA-damaging effects of sunlight [1]. Today, the tanning response is exploited by millions of people each year for cosmetic reasons. Because of the increased risks for melanoma and squamous cell carcinoma following overexposure to sunlight [2], the molecular biology of the tanning response has been given substantial biomedical attention over the last decades from dermatologists and oncologists (reviewed by [3–7]), as well as from those seeking ways to achieve tanning independent of sunlight [8].

### 3.1.1 The Tanning Response

The tanning response is the additional production and distribution of melanin, exceeding the constitutive level, following UV stimulation. The UV signal is transduced from the primary recipient to the melanocyte, where the photoprotective pigment melanin is produced and distributed. In addition to the optical shielding effects, melanin and its precursors and intermediates act as free-radical scavengers, as well as signalling molecules [9–11]. The tanning response thus encompasses UV sensing, signal transduction, melanogenesis, melanosome mobilization and transfer to keratinocytes, as well as the further distribution through the epidermis via keratinocyte migration.

## 3.1.2   Photobiology of the UV Radiation

UV radiation is electromagnetic radiation with wavelengths just below visual light (100–400 nm). The biologically most relevant wavelength segments are UVA (320–400 nm) and UVB (290–320 nm). UVB represents the most bio-reactive part of the spectrum both as inducer of erythema and tanning. Our current conception is that UV radiation causes basal cell skin cancers, such as basal cell carcinoma and malignant melanoma, through its mutagenic effect on basal layer cells. Melanin has a remarkable capacity to absorb UV radiation and to reflect it at the shortest wavelengths (<300 nm) [13] (Fig. 3.1).

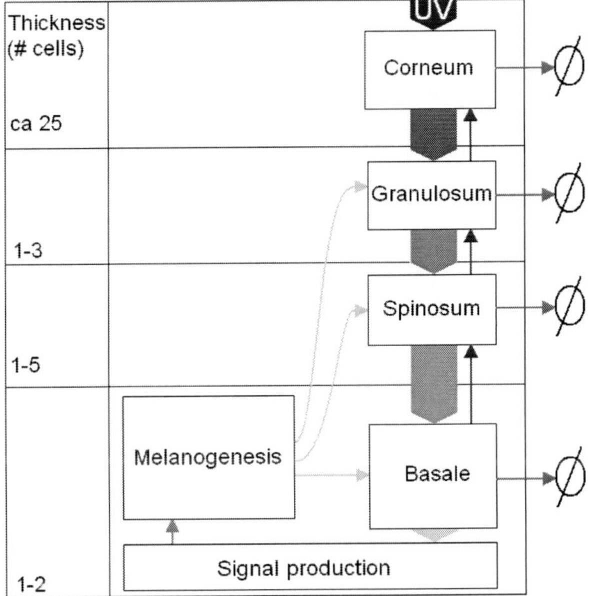


**Figure 3.1**   Melanin production and distribution as response to UV radiation. Outline of the melanin unit. The melanin content of each layer is a function of melanin delivered from the melanocyte, melanin degradation and the melanin in the cells moving upwards. The distributed melanin absorbs UV radiation (described by decreasing darkness of the arrows with increasing depth). Increase of the UV radiation reaching the basal layer triggers signal substance production. In turn, the signal substances stimulate melanogenesis and dendrite growth in the melanocyte. Reprinted from [12].

### 3.1.3  Signal Transduction

UV radiation is the major inducer of the tanning response. Both keratinocytes and melanocytes produce various substances that stimulate melanogenesis upon UV irradiation [14–16]. These comprise the elements controlling the activity of the hypothalamus–pituitary–adrenal axis which are expressed in the skin, including corticotropin releasing hormone (CRH), urocortin, and proopiomelanocortin (POMC), with its products adrenocorticotropic hormone (ACTH), β- and γ-lipotropic hormone (LPH), corticotropin-like intermediate lobe peptide (CLIP), α- and β-melanocyte-stimulating hormone (MSH), and β-endorphin [17–19]. The skin is therefore conceived to possess a complete stress handling system of which the tanning response is an important part [20]. The hormone α-MSH and its receptor MC1R are important mediators of UV induced tanning [16,21–23]. It has been proposed that the increased POMC transcription in keratinocytes following UV exposure is p53 dependent [24]. Even though the POMC derivatives do not seem to be crucial in constitutive melanin production in mouse [25,26], genetic variants of their receptor, MC1R, are deemed to be the main determinant of constitutive melanin levels, and also of the tanning ability in human [21,27,28]. This enigmatic situation substantiates the challenges involved in understanding the intercellular signalling network of the skin.

Also, some contradictive clues have emerged over the last decade regarding the cellular origin of the regulatory signals for constitutive as well as UV-induced melanin production. On the one hand, it has been reported that, following UV irradiation in mice, p53 activation stimulates transcription from the POMC promoter in keratinocytes, thereby increasing the release of POMC-derived α-MSH [29]. Keratinocyte-derived α-MSH then stimulates the receptor MC1R on melanocytes, resulting in increased production of eumelanin [24]. On the other hand, the suggested dominant role of the keratinocyte in the p53-mediated a-MSH stimulation in human tanning has been challenged [30] and is inconsistent with the strong p53-mediated melanogenic response to UV irradiation by human melanocytes and melanoma cells in vitro in the absence of keratinocytes [31].

Yoshida et al. have conducted some fascinating experiments that shed light on the roles played by melanocytes and keratinocytes in regulating melanogenesis [32,33]. By grafting mixtures of cultured keratinocytes, melanocytes and fibroblasts into chambers inserted onto the back skin of severe combined immunedeficient mice, they constructed human skin substitutes (HSS) from a combination of donor skin types. They show that even if the constitutive pigmentation level is mostly governed by the melanocyte, the keratinocyte makes a significant contribution. Further, they found that HSS constructed from dark skin–derived keratinocytes (KD) had the same number of melanosomes compared to HSS constructed with light skin–derived keratinocytes (KL) and that the observed difference in pigmentation is due to the melanosomes being more mature and individually distributed in the former.

### 3.1.4 Melanogenesis

Melanogenesis, which occurs within discrete cytoplasmic organelles of the melanocyte, called melanosomes, is a process where the amino acid tyrosine is converted into melanin pigment. Tyrosinase is regarded as the rate-limiting enzyme in this process. The transcriptional regulation and the posttranslational activation of tyrosinase are the key regulation points for the melanogenesis. Microphthalmia-associated transcription factor (MITF) is a central protein in the transcriptional regulation of tyrosinase and thereby melanogenesis, as demonstrated by its role in Waardenburg syndrome type 2 and Tietz syndrome [34]. The architecture of the MITF promoter region suggests that several transcription factors (like SOX10, PAX3, LEF1/TCF, CREB and ONECUT2) are involved in melanogenesis and the tanning response [3,5,35]. LEF1/TCF and CREB are responsible for the immensity of MITF promoter responsiveness to UV radiation via MC1R/cAMP/PKA and the WNT/β-catenin pathways [3,5,36–38]. MITF is therefore proposed to act as a self-regulating switchboard for diverse pathways originating in the cell membrane or the intracellular environment and regulating the activity of the melanogenic apparatus [5]. Other transcription factors can also activate melanin production, like the ubiquitous basic helix-loop-helix-leucine zipper transcription factor USF1, which is reported to be essential for the tanning response, and indeed MITF and USF1 share binding site specificity [39].

Both p38, ERK1/2 and other MAP kinases are involved in MITF signalling and regulation [3,5,40]. The MAP kinase pathway is in turn activated by several ligands such as KITLG, FGF2 and EGF. The MAPK pathway may also activate CREB via RSK1, illustrating the complexity of the structure in these networks. The key second messenger cAMP appears to be another point of cross talk between the αMSH-MC1R pathway and the MAP kinase pathway [41]. See [3–5,42] for comprehensive reviews of the molecular biology of melanogenesis.

### 3.1.5 Melanin is Delivered to Nearby Keratinocytes through Dendrites

An additional effect of UV irradiation and the subsequent release of CRH, the POMC derivatives and even endothelins and nitric oxide is the stimulation of melanocyte dendrite growth and melanosome delivery to keratinocytes [5,23,41,43–45]. Each melanocyte attached to the epidermal basement membrane exports mature melanosomes to nearby keratinocytes through its dendrites. The uptake of melanosomes by the keratinocytes is an active process involving regulatory processes in the dendrites as well as in the keratinocytes [9,19,32,46,47].

### 3.1.6 Further Distribution through Keratinocyte Movement

Ninety-five percent of the cells in the epidermis are keratinocytes and a fraction of the keratinocytes in the basal layer is "stem" keratinocytes, which produce new keratinocytes continuously through cell division. From being attached to the epidermal basement membrane initially, these "non-stem" keratinocytes move progressively toward the skin surface. In a cross section of the epidermis, the keratinocytes form four distinguishable layers named *stratum basale, stratum spinosum, stratum granulosum* and *stratum corneum* [48]. The thicknesses of the viable parts of the epidermis (*basale, spinosum, granulosum*) and of *stratum corneum* vary between individuals and are correlated with a number of factors like age, body site, gender, UV exposure, smoking habit, and physical tiredness [49].

## 3.2 Mathematical Modelling of Pigment Production and Distribution

To our knowledge, a few mathematical models are made with the goal to describe and understand the pigmentation process. The oldest one is by Stolnitz et al. in 2001 [50] and is a signal transduction model of melanogenesis relevant pathways in melanocytes. This model takes into account α-MSH binding to the MC1R, adenylate cyclase activation by G-protein, increase of the intracellular cAMP concentration, PKA activation by cAMP, CREB phosphorylation by PKA, MITF gene expression, MITF binding to the TYR gene promoter, and increase of tyrosinase synthesis. Positive and negative feedback loops of this system are analyzed. Though for its time a comprehensive model, it lacks important concepts like MITF and TYR activation by phosphorylation. The phosphorylation of MITF seems important to include in such a model, both because MITF is a central protein in the melanocytes and melanomas [3,34,51] and because the phosphorylation changes the stability of the MITF protein [52,53], the MITF protein ability to act as a transcription factor, and the affinity of MITF to inhibiting proteins like PIAS3 [54–57] and 14-3-3 [58].

In 2002, Øyehaug et al. developed a mathematical model of the switching between eumelanin and pheomelanin production (melanogenic switching) depending on the extracellular signalling context [59]. Different explanatory hypotheses of the observed switching were tested against available data. The results suggest that melanogenic switching may be due to a jump between two stable production pattern states when the tyrosinase activity varies between two bifurcation levels. This implies that small changes in the levels of external regulatory factors may cause an accentuated change in the proportion of the produced colour pigments and may explain the fact that mammalian coat patterns often exhibit sharply delimited patches of either black or reddish colour. Even if some signalling is included in this model, it is mostly a metabolic network model describing the two chemical pathways in the synthesis of eumelanin and pheomelanin from the amino acid tyrosine, and the switching between them in accordance with cues in the extracellular environment. As a model that primarily explores mammalian coat coloration, its relevance for understanding the melanocyte in human epidermis comes from the fact that the same two forms of melanin exist in humans, and that hair follicle melanocytes and epidermal melanocytes have a lot in common. On the other hand, the switching is not relevant for humans in the way that we do not express patterns of differently coloured hair (like a zebra, tiger or Dalmatian dog).

Stolnitz et al. proposed a mathematical model of melanosome transport along filaments in intact and UV-irradiated melanocytes in 2004 [60]. They considered processes at three levels: Dynamics of the single motor, transport of melanosome by an ensemble of motors, and melanosomes distribution along microtubules. A single motor is considered as a stochastic ratchet; modelled by transitions between internal states described by chemical kinetics equations, thus permitting determination of "force-velocity" dependence for the motor. The ensemble of motors is described by a system of equations for average motor velocities, and transported melano-somes move with average velocity, which in turn is determined by the sum of forces generated by each elastically coupled motor. The distribution of melanosomes along a microtubule is described by a system of equations for bidirectional motion of each attached melanosome and free diffusion of unattached melanosomes. The effect of UV radiation is modelled as a change in the number of each type of motor simultaneously linked to one melanosome. It induces redistribution of melanosomes between centre and periphery of the melanocytes.

In 2009 we proposed a dynamic model of the distribution of melanin between the layers of epidermis in response to UV irradiation [12]. This model was designed to assemble current knowledge of the tanning response and was calibrated to resemble available data. The model describes the melanin level in each layer, considering UV exposure, cell signalling, melanogenesis, dendrite growth, and keratinocyte movement. The ODE model is solved analytically and the results indicate that the implemented concepts were not sufficient to explain the data. This model is presented in further detail below, as an example.

Another part of the epidermal homeostasis and pigmentation apparatus is the distribution of melanocytes in the basal layer. We have deployed an agent-based model to describe this distribution [61]. The model describes cells as incompressible spheres capable of progressing through the cell cycle, of migration, and able to differentiate as well as sending and sensing paracrine signals. The environment in which these cells are modelled is a virtual dish measuring 400 μm × 400 μm. The cells are dividing or differentiating according to their cell cycle status and the signal sensed in the immediate surroundings. The migration is stochastic, but biased by the gradients of the paracrine signals.

On a higher level of resolution, several modelling efforts that investigate signalling networks or gene regulatory networks are relevant for melanocyte biology, without focusing directly on melanogenesis. Melanocyte relevant pathways that are investigated by mathematical models include (but are not limited to) the MAP kinase pathway (e.g., [62–69]), the TGFβ receptor trafficking [70], the SMAD nucleocytoplasmic shuttling [71], the combination of TGFβ receptor trafficking and SMAD nucleocytoplasmic shuttling [72], the IL-6 signal transduction [73] and the MITF–PIAS3–STAT3 interaction [57].

## 3.3　Mathematics of Tanning

This chapter presents and discusses a dynamic model previously published in [12] aimed at providing a mathematical conceptualization of our current knowledge of the tanning response. The resolution level of the model was tuned to available data, and its primary focus was to describe the tanning response following UV exposure.

The model appears capable of accounting for some, but not all of the available experimental data on the tanning response. The data set consists of measured melanin levels in the different layers of epidermis from nine individuals of different constitutive pigmentation level, before and seven days after UV irradiation [74]. The dynamic model of pigment production and distribution presented here provides a framework in which to interpret such data, which hopefully will lead to a deeper and more quantitative understanding of the tanning phenomenon.

The model is presented in detail in the Methods section, but here we state its most important premises. The model is designed to describe the dynamics associated with what is called a melanin unit, which consists of one melanocyte and the keratinocytes with which it maintains functional contact. In one melanin unit there are around 36 keratinocytes distributed between the three viable layers [48].

The model describes the melanin content $M_j$ in layer $j$, $j \in \{c,g,s,b\}$ (layers are referred to by their initial letter), the signal substance concentration $s$ and the dendrite length relative to the length from mid-melanocyte to *stratum corneum*, $x$. In the constitutive condition, i.e., in the absence of UV radiation, the melanin produced in the melanocyte is assumed delivered only to the basal layer. The melanin is then distributed outwards by the continuous movement of keratinocytes towards the skin surface. The constitutive level of melanin production and delivery is in equilibrium with the melanin degradation and the loss of melanin through keratinocytes shed from the skin surface. Exposure to UV radiation triggers signal substance production, which, in turn, leads to enhanced melanogenic activity. Due to the resolution level of our model, the complex signal processing is condensed into one signal concentration value $s$, which alters the ratio of the number of ligand-bound receptors to the total number of receptors on the melanocyte membrane. While this is a severe simplification of a complex phenomenon, we are still able to capture the systemic behaviour on the current level of resolution. Dendrite growth and melanin production are both assumed to depend on this ratio. Consistent with how biological compounds are normally degraded and in accordance with common modelling practice, degradation of melanin and signal substance are assumed to be linear.

The dendritic growth following UV exposure may show a quite complex geometry, and in the model this growth process has been very much simplified. To derive the functions which describe how melanin is distributed into the epidermal layers, we assume a uniform growth process and that all keratinocytes that can be reached from one melanocyte with a dendrite of a given length will receive the same amount of melanin.

### 3.3.1   Available Data

Even though a considerable amount of empirical data has been used as a basis for model construction, the amount of available relevant validation data is very modest. To the best of our knowledge, there is currently only one experimental study reported where human skin exposed to UV radiation is subsequently biopsied to analyse the melanin content in the different epidermal layers [74,75]. In this work, Tadokoro et al. exposed nine individuals to a single 1 minimal erythema dose (MED) of UVA/UVB radiation.

Biopsies were taken before and seven days after the exposure. Using the Fontana–Masson method, they established the melanin content in the *basale*, *spinosum* and *granulosum* layers of epidermis on these two time points. These data points are reported as single measurements, i.e., no standard errors or standard deviations are given. The amount of melanin is given in a not scaled unit and with no measurement of volume. The thicknesses of the different epidermal layers are varying a great deal and it is therefore difficult to establish good concentration measures from these data.

## 3.3.2 Results

### 3.3.2.1 Reproduction of empirical data

The model was parameterized to fit available data on the distribution of melanin in the different epidermal layers and how different skin types respond to UV radiation. Consistent with Tadokoro et al.'s [74] experiments, the model was exposed to a UV pulse. The eight free parameters of the model where optimized to fit nine different data sets representing nine different individuals (S5, S30, S21, S27, S47, S35, S37, S19, S26, using the denotation of Tadekoro et al.). For six of the individuals (S21, S47, S35, S37, S19, S26), the model successfully describes the observed melanin distributions and can be calibrated to mimic individual differences (Table 3.1 and Fig. 3.2, lower panels). The model is not able to describe data corresponding to the three remaining individuals (S5, S30 and S27, see Section 3.3.3). Results for these individuals are therefore not shown in the table or the figure.

**Table 3.1**  Goodness of fit

| Layer | Day | S21 | S47 | S35 | S37 | S19 | S26 |
|---|---|---|---|---|---|---|---|
| Granulosum | 0 | 0.001 | 0.000 | 0.001 | 0.003 | 0.231 | 0.006 |
| Spinosum | 0 | 0.005 | 0.000 | 0.000 | 0.001 | 0.007 | 0.004 |
| Basal | 0 | 0.000 | 0.004 | 0.003 | 0.018 | 0.000 | 0.002 |
| Granulosum | 7 | 0.002 | 0.000 | 0.000 | 0.000 | 0.048 | 0.002 |
| Spinosum | 7 | 0.000 | 0.001 | 0.001 | 0.008 | 0.003 | 0.001 |
| Basal | 7 | 0.007 | 0.003 | 0.001 | 0.006 | 0.000 | 0.001 |
| Sum | — | 0.016 | 0.008 | 0.006 | 0.037 | 0.290 | 0.015 |

*Note*: The goodness-of-fit $((M_{\mathrm{data}} - M_{\mathrm{model}})/M_{\mathrm{data}})^2$, where $M_{\mathrm{data}}$ and $M_{\mathrm{model}}$ are the measured data and model prediction, respectively, for each individual whose data can be successfully described by the model in the three epidermal layers at times $t = 0$ d and $t = 7$ d.

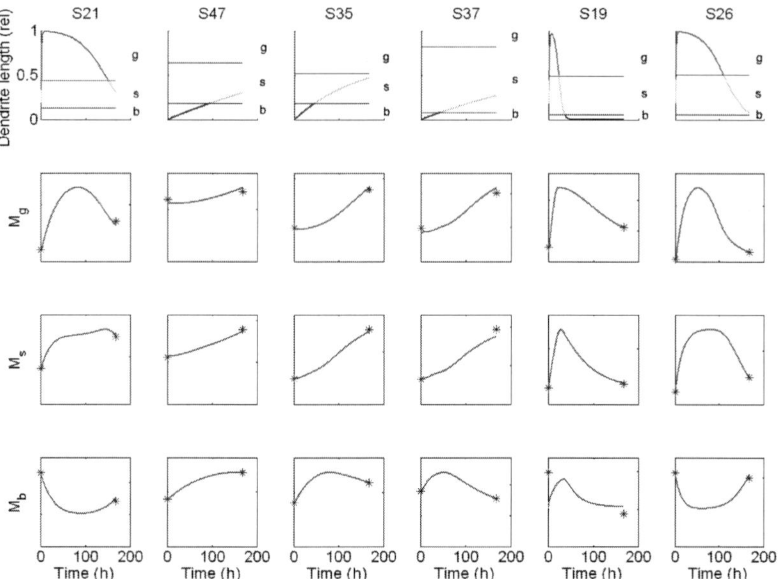

**Figure 3.2**   Temporal evolution of dendrite length and melanin levels in epidermal layers after a pulse of UV radiation. Each column corresponds to individuals whose melanin data can be described by our model. Top panels: Length of the dendrites relative to total layer thickness. The horizontal lines define the boundaries between the layers, which are indicated by a letter on the right hand side (b; *basale*, s; *spinosum*, g; *granulosum*). Lower panels: Temporal evolution of the melanin level in each layer, stars indicate observed data. In both the experiment and the model, the UV-pulse was given immediately after the first measurement. In plots displaying melanin levels, scaling is omitted to highlight the fitting of the model to data. Reprinted from [12].

### 3.3.2.2   Dendricity

After the UV pulse, the dendrites first grow and then retract (Fig. 3.2, top panels). The dendrite extension into the layers of epidermis differs substantially between individuals in both length and duration. Individuals S47, S35 and S37 are described by the model with intermediate dendrite lengths lasting longer than the one-week simulation time, while S21, S19 and S26 exhibit longer dendrites over a shorter period of time.

### 3.3.3  Discussion

Due to the paucity of relevant experimental data, the model is intentionally very simple. Despite this, it is capable of making quite strong predictions concerning the relationship between observed temporal development of melanin production and distribution following UV exposure and the thicknesses of the epidermal layers as well as the degree of dendricity.

The resolution level of the model is a trade-off between the benefits and disadvantages of simple models compared to complex models containing a large amount of molecular detail. In this work we do not explicitly model different signal substances, different receptors (and their genetic variants or their refractory periods), different second messengers and all the actors in the different pathways leading to melanogenesis and dendrification as well as the biochemical regulatory effects of melanin. This does not mean that the model is in conflict with the available information concerning these processes. Given more spatiotemporal experimental data on the tanning response as suggested by the current work, we think the stage will be set for the making of more high-resolution models.

Tadokoro et al. [74] provide measurements of three additional individuals for which the model is not capable of achieving consistency with the empirical data. The reason for this is that the melanin levels in the *granulosum* or *spinosum* layers in these three individuals are lower 7 days after than before UV exposure, and the model does not include mechanisms that can produce such behaviour. A possible explanation can be that the UV exposure causes alteration of the thicknesses of the epidermal layers. A thinner *spinosum* or *granulosum* 7 days after UV radiation can, even with a higher relative melanin density, result in a decrease in measured melanin levels with the methods applied by Tadokoro et al. [74]. It should be stressed that such a mechanism can easily be implemented so that the model can account for all nine individuals, but no insight is gained by this exercise before more empirical data become available. In fact, the above discrepancy between model results and empirical data clearly documents the need for including specific measurements of the thickness of epidermal layers in experimental set-ups like that of Tadokoro et al. [74].

The model does not take into account the possibility that DNA damage due to UV exposure causes the production of signals stimulating melanogenesis long after the cessation of UV exposure (reviewed in [76]). Neither does it take into account that the thickness of stratum corneum may change with UV exposure [77] and that this may influence the UV absorbance [13]. Since, so far, the data on how DNA damage might enhance and prolong signal substance production is so scarce, we find it premature to include this effect in our model. Moreover, the time window of UV radiation in the experiments used to validate our model is probably not long enough for the thickening of *stratum corneum* to take place and give an effect. Thus, we do not have data to assess whether or not the UV-induced thickening of *stratum corneum* plays an important role in the tanning process. This does not mean that the above phenomena are not interesting, but that, in the lack of quantitative data, not much would be gained by including them in the model.

This model can be viewed as an implementation of current knowledge. The part of the model that is most abstracted and least based on observations is the melanin delivery equations. The combination of the observation that dendrites grow longer on melanocytes, given the same stimuli that they receive in skin after UV exposure [44,78], with the fact that melanosomes are delivered through the dendrites (reviewed in [47]), formed the basis for the derivation of these equations. Even if this part of the model may be somewhat speculative, it still represents an implementation of the current understanding of this complex phenomenon.

The view of the model as an implementation of current knowledge of the melanogenesis and melanosome transfer mechanisms has the implication that a possible failure of the model reflects that our basic understanding of the mechanisms involved contain wrong assumptions. However, due to the lacking thickness dimension in the data currently available, there is not enough support for rejection of the model. A program that sets out to uncover these mechanisms should, in addition to generating more and better data, propose mechanisms that can explain all the observations.

The goal of any mathematical modelling effort should be to gain biological insights about the system under study. A further development of this model is one possible such effort. Another possibility is to combine individual based modelling techniques with individual cell measurements of melanin level. Individual based computational models have been extensively deployed in the study of epidermal cell organisation, e.g., [61,79–84]. Yoshida et al. [32,33] provide interesting data motivating further effort along these lines.

## 3.3.4 Methods

The aim of the model is to describe the temporal distribution of melanin in the epidermal layers following an UV pulse. Whenever b, s, g or c is used as subscripts below, they refer to the epidermal layers stratum *basale, stratum spinosum, stratum granulosum*, and *stratum corneum*, respectively. See Table 3.2 for an overview of parameters and their dimensions.

**Table 3.2**     Parameters of the model with approximate magnitudes, references, descriptions and units

| Parameter | Approximate value | Reference | Description | Unit |
|---|---|---|---|---|
| $\gamma_s$ | $10^{-1}$ | Optimized | Signal substance degradation rate | 1/h |
| $f_{min}$ | $10^3$ | Optimized | Constitutive melanin production | tau/h |
| $f_{ind}$ | $10^3$ | Optimized | Tanning ability | tau/h |
| $a$ | $10^0$ | Optimized | Dendrites growth rate | cd/h |
| $\gamma_M$ | $10^{-2}$ | Optimized | Melanin degradation rate | 1/h |
| $w$ | $10^{-1}$ | [48] | Cell movement rate | cell/h |
| $T_c$ | 25 | [48] | Thickness, corneum | cd |
| $T_g$ | 2 | [48] | Thickness, granulosum | cd |
| $T_s$ | 4 | [48] | Thickness, spinosum | cd |
| $T_b$ | 1 | [48] | Thickness, basale | cd |
| Area | 5 | [48,74,85] | Area of melanin unit | cd*cd |

*Note*: The unit of volume is the number of cells and unit of length is cell diameter (cd). Melanin amount is measured in the arbitrary unit of [74] (tau). Estimated values are related to each other and the rest of the model. Their absolute values are not regarded as predictions.

### 3.3.4.1 UV intensity and signal substance dynamics

The spatial intensity of the UV pulse is assumed to decrease exponentially with depth and absorbance down through the epidermis. As increased melanin content enhances UV absorption, the net signal substance production rate relative to baseline conditions as a function of UV intensity $I$ and melanin content $M$ may be expressed as

$$p(I, M) = a_1 \frac{I^2}{I^2 + \Theta^2} e^{-a_2 \frac{M}{M_0}}. \tag{3.1}$$

We assume that there is a maximal production rate $a_1$ and that the actual production is a sigmoidal function of $I$ with threshold parameter $\Theta$ (i.e., the production rate is half of its maximum when $I$ equals $\Theta$). In the exponential term, $M_0$ is the constitutive melanin level and $M$ is the current total melanin level in all layers; $M = \Sigma_{j=c,g,s,b} M_j$. In the simulations, since the melanin amount in the epidermis does not change significantly during the first hour, and the model is exposed to UV radiation only during this period, the exponential term can be regarded as a constant. Furthermore, the UV intensity is assumed constant during the 1 h of exposure and therefore the fraction term can be regarded as a constant as well. In the simulations, the production rate can thus be regarded to be constant: $p(I, M) = \tilde{p}$.

The concentration of free signal substance is determined by the balance between its production and degradation, described by

$$\dot{s} = p(I, M) - \gamma_s s, \tag{3.2}$$

where we assume a linear degradation rate $\gamma_s$ and that the pulse of signal substance production (with magnitude $\tilde{p}$) endures for only 1 h, i.e., the ODE to be solved is

$$\dot{s} = \begin{cases} \tilde{p} - \gamma_s s, & 0 \leq t \leq 1\,\text{h}, \\ -\gamma_s s, & 1\,\text{h} \leq t. \end{cases} \tag{3.3}$$

The analytical solution of Eq. 3.3 is

$$s(t) = \begin{cases} \dfrac{\tilde{p}}{\gamma_s}(1 - \exp(-\gamma_s t)), & 0 \leq t \leq 1\,\text{h}, \\[2ex] \dfrac{\tilde{p}}{\gamma_s}(\exp(\gamma_s) - 1)\exp(-\gamma_s t), & 1\,\text{h} < t. \end{cases} \tag{3.4}$$

Let $R$ stand for the fractional occupancy of melanocyte receptors binding signal substance. Then the rate of change of $R$ is given by $k_+s(1 - R) - k_-R$, where $k_+s$ and $k_-$ are coupling and decoupling relative rates, respectively. We assume that equilibrium between binding and release of signal molecules from the melanocyte surface is set up so fast relative to the time scale of the model that the rate of change can be set equal to zero, giving $R$ in terms of signal substance concentration, i.e.

$$R = \frac{s}{s + K}, \tag{3.5}$$

where $K = k_-/k_+$. Thus, we are able to express $R(t)$ as a function of the signal substance production, $\tilde{p}$, degradation rate, $\gamma_s$, and the relation between the coupling and decoupling constants, $K$:

$$R(t) = \frac{s(t)}{s(t) + K},$$

$$= \begin{cases} \dfrac{(\exp(\gamma_s t)-1)/(\exp(\gamma_s)-1)}{(\exp(\gamma_s t)-1)/(\exp(\gamma_s)-1) + A\exp(\gamma_s t)} & 0 \le t \le 1\,\mathrm{h}, \\[2em] \dfrac{1}{1 + A\exp(\gamma_s t)} & 1\,\mathrm{h} < t. \end{cases} \tag{3.6}$$

where $A = (K\gamma_s/(\tilde{p}(\exp(\gamma_s)-1)))$.

### 3.3.5 Melanin Production

Melanocytes have a constitutive melanin production as well as the ability to increase melanin production as a response to receptor mediated signals. The melanin synthesis rate can thus be expressed as

$$f(R) = f_{\min} + f_{\mathrm{ind}}R. \tag{3.7}$$

In the absence of UV radiation the net signal substance level (not including base line levels) and hence the net fractional occupancy, $R$, is zero, such that $f_{\min}$ expresses the constitutive melanin production.

### 3.3.5.1 Dynamics of dendrite length

We assume that all the melanin is delivered to nearby keratinocytes. The melanin delivered to one particular layer is described as the production $f(R)$ times a function $d_j$ for each layer $j$, where the $d_j$'s are functions of the dendrite length relative to the maximum dendrite length, here denoted $x$. The dendrites grow when the melanocyte is stimulated by signal substances [5,41]. Therefore, we assume that $x$ is governed by

$$\dot{x} = a(R(T) - x), \tag{3.8}$$

where the parameter $a$ is the time constant of dendrite growth and retraction. Assuming that the dendrite is of zero extension initially, Eq. 3.8 can be analytically solved to give

$$x(t) = a \int_0^t R(\tau) \exp(-a(t - \tau)) d\tau. \tag{3.9}$$

### 3.3.5.2 Distribution of melanin as function of dendrite length

Assume a sphere with the melanocyte in the middle and radius equal to the dendrite length $x$ (Fig. 3.3a). The proportion of this sphere that resides in each layer of the epidermis is equated with the proportion of melanin delivered to this layer. As the radius of the sphere grows, the proportion of the volume residing in each layer changes. We use these proportions as guidelines for distributing the melanin produced. The proportion functions below (Eq. 3.10) derived from the formula for volume of a sphere and the thickness of the different layers are plotted in Fig. 3.3b. We define all dendrite tips to be in the basal layer provided that the relative dendrite length $x$ is below $h_{bs}$, where $h_{bs} = \frac{1}{2}T_b / (\frac{1}{2}T_b + T_s + T_g)$ ($T_j$ denotes thickness of layer $j$) is the distance from the centre of the melanocyte to the border between *stratum basale* and *stratum spinosum* relative to the maximal dendrite length which equals $h_{gc} = \frac{1}{2}T_b + T_s + T_g$. The dendrite tips extend to the *spinosum* layer when $h_{bs} \leq x \leq h_{sg}$ and to the *granulosum* layer when $x > h_{sg}$, where $h_{sg} = (h_{bs} + T_s)/(\frac{1}{2}T_b + T_s + T_g)$ is the distance from the centre of the melanocyte to the border between *stratum spinosum* and *stratum granulosum* relative to $h_{gc} = \frac{1}{2}T_b + T_s + T_g$. We then obtain the functions $d_j, j = b, s, g$, describing the melanin delivery distributions,

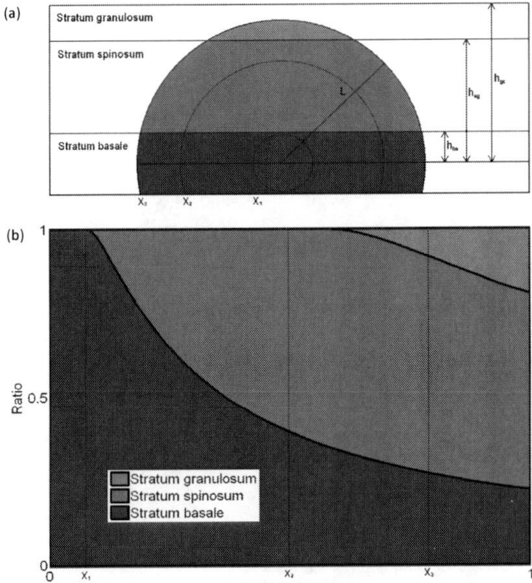


**Figure 3.3** Melanin distribution ratios between the different layers as a function of the dendrite length. As the length of the dendrite, $x$, grows, the ratio of reached volume in each layer changes (a). In (b) these ratios are plotted versus the dendrite length. With short dendrites ($x_1$) all melanin is delivered to the basal layer. As the dendrite is growing, more is delivered to *stratum spinosum* ($x_2$), and when they are long enough, they also distribute melanin to the *stratum granulosum* ($x_3$). Reprinted from [12].

$$
d_g(x) = \begin{cases} x < h_{sg}: & 0 \\[2ex] x \geq h_{sg}: & \dfrac{\frac{2}{3}x^3 - x^2 h_{sg} + \frac{1}{3}h_{sg}^3}{\frac{2}{3}x^3 + x^2 h_{bs} - \frac{1}{3}h_{bs}^3} \end{cases}
$$

$$
d_s(x) = \begin{cases} x < h_{bs}: & 0 \\[2ex] h_{bs} \leq x < h_{sg}: & \dfrac{\frac{2}{3}x^3 - x^2 h_{bs} + \frac{1}{3}h_{bs}^3}{\frac{2}{3}x^3 + x^2 h_{bs} - \frac{1}{3}h_{bs}^3} \\[3ex] x \geq h_{sg}: & \dfrac{x^2 h_{sg} - \frac{1}{3}h_{sg}^3 - x^2 h_{bs} + \frac{1}{3}h_{bs}^3}{\frac{2}{3}x^3 + x^2 h_{bs} - \frac{1}{3}h_{bs}^3} \end{cases}
$$

$$d_{\mathrm{b}}(x) = \begin{cases} x < h_{\mathrm{bs}}: & 1 \\[2ex] x \geq h_{\mathrm{bs}}: & \dfrac{2\left(x^2 h_{\mathrm{bs}} - \dfrac{1}{3} h_{\mathrm{bs}}^3\right)}{\dfrac{2}{3}x^3 + x^2 h_{\mathrm{bs}} - \dfrac{1}{3} h_{\mathrm{bs}}^3} \end{cases} \qquad (3.10)$$

It should be noted that $d_{\mathrm{g}}(x) + d_{\mathrm{s}}(x) + d_{\mathrm{b}}(x) = 1$ holds for all $x$.

### 3.3.5.3  Melanin dynamics within keratinocytes

The data obtained by Tadokoro et al. [74] are given in an absolute but not scaled unit of the amount of melanin in each layer. Using the same unit, we model the melanin content in each layer by the following set of differential equations, where $M_j$ denotes melanin content in layer $j$,

$$\begin{aligned} \dot{M}_{\mathrm{c}} &= -\gamma_{\mathrm{M}} M_{\mathrm{c}} + \omega_{\mathrm{g}} M_{\mathrm{g}} - \omega_{\mathrm{c}} M_{\mathrm{c}}, \\ \dot{M}_{\mathrm{g}} &= d_{\mathrm{g}}(x)f(R) - \gamma_{\mathrm{M}} M_{\mathrm{g}} + \omega_{\mathrm{s}} M_{\mathrm{s}} - \omega_{\mathrm{g}} M_{\mathrm{g}}, \\ \dot{M}_{\mathrm{s}} &= d_{\mathrm{s}}(x)f(R) - \gamma_{\mathrm{M}} M_{\mathrm{s}} + \omega_{\mathrm{b}} M_{\mathrm{b}} - \omega_{\mathrm{s}} M_{\mathrm{s}}, \\ \dot{M}_{\mathrm{b}} &= d_{\mathrm{b}}(x)f(R) - \gamma_{\mathrm{M}} M_{\mathrm{b}} - \omega_{\mathrm{b}} M_{\mathrm{b}}, \end{aligned} \qquad (3.11)$$

where the terms $d_j(x)\, f(R)$, $j = $ b, s, g represent melanin delivery rates from melanocytic dendrites into keratinocytes of layer $j$ and $\omega_j = w/V_j$, $j = $ b, s, g, c ($w$ and $V_j$ are described below). We assume that melanin has a degradation rate $\gamma_{\mathrm{M}}$ (with unit h$^{-1}$) and that $w$ (unit: cell h$^{-1}$) describes the speed by which keratinocytes move towards the surface. The scope of this model is the melanin unit (defined in Background and not to be confused with a unit of measurement) which we assume to have the same area throughout the epidermis (described by the parameter *area*). The volume of each layer is then $V_j = T_j \times$ area.

With the above definition of $\omega_j$, $j = $ b, s, g, the quantities $h_{\mathrm{bs}}$ and $h_{\mathrm{sg}}$ can be defined in terms of the model parameters as follows:

$$\begin{aligned} h_{\mathrm{bs}} &= \frac{T_{\mathrm{b}}/2}{T_{\mathrm{b}}/2 + T_{\mathrm{s}} + T_{\mathrm{g}}} = \frac{\omega_{\mathrm{b}}^{-1}/2}{\omega_{\mathrm{b}}^{-1}/2 + \omega_{\mathrm{s}}^{-1} + \omega_{\mathrm{g}}^{-1}}, \\[2ex] h_{\mathrm{sg}} &= \frac{T_{\mathrm{b}}/2 + T_{\mathrm{s}}}{T_{\mathrm{b}}/2 + T_{\mathrm{s}} + T_{\mathrm{g}}} = \frac{\omega_{\mathrm{b}}^{-1}/2 + \omega_{\mathrm{s}}^{-1}}{\omega_{\mathrm{b}}^{-1}/2 + \omega_{\mathrm{s}}^{-1} + \omega_{\mathrm{g}}^{-1}}. \end{aligned} \qquad (3.12)$$

The sum of the inverses of the $\omega_j$'s, $j$ = b, s, g, equals $(T_b/2 + T_s + T_g) \times area/w$, which is approximately 400 (Table 3.2). Thus, if $\omega_b$ and $\omega_g$ are given, $\omega_s$ follows by a simple calculation.

### 3.3.5.4 Estimates of parameter ranges

The parameters of the model and their values are presented in Table 3.2. In the following, we describe the derivations of parameter value ranges.

The volume of each layer is given as the number of cells in one melanin unit. In the simulations we have divided the volume into thickness $T_j$, $j$ = c, g, s, b and *area*. In this model the melanin unit has a fixed area throughout the epidermis, hence only the thickness varies between the layers. The layer thicknesses, presented in Table 3.2, are obtained from [48]. The melanocyte density, and thus the area of one melanin unit, does not vary between different skin colours but it does vary with body location [48]. Melanocyte density is measured in different ways, but from [48,74,85] we have derived an average of the area of the melanin unit on the actual body site (lower back) to be 4–6 cells.

The parameter $w$ (with unit cell per hour) describes the movement of keratinocytes upwards from layer to layer. The epidermal turnover time $t_{\text{turnover}}$; the time from a cell is born in the basal layer until it is shred off the *corneum* layer, is 52–75 days in normal skin [48]. The parameter $w$ can then be estimated from the relation

$$w = \frac{T}{t_{\text{turnover}}}, \tag{3.13}$$

where $T$ is the total thickness of all four layers.

## 3.4 Conclusions

In this chapter, we have discussed current knowledge of the biological processes involved in skin pigmentation, presented the mathematical models currently available on these processes, and finally portrayed one of our models in the field.

Generally, the field is not thoroughly explored by mathematical modelers and could benefit from increased application of systems biology methods and approaches. The nature of the pigmentation apparatus and the tanning response expose some challenges on the choice of modelling paradigm. On a tissue level, the cell self-organization properties of the epidermis are probably best modelled with individual based models. However, how one best represents the complex shape of the melanocyte with its dendrites in such a model, is a challenging task. An individual based model of melanosome maturation and distribution in the epidermis would be a useful tool for understanding the melanocyte-keratinocyte transfer process, and eventually the keratinocyte-keratinocyte transfer mechanism.

On the cellular level, the ODE-paradigm is the standard for signalling network and gene regulatory network models. One challenge for modelling, which is general for all multicellular eukaryotes, is choosing the number of compartments. In the case of pigmentation, one has to consider the melanosome in addition to the nucleus, the cytoplasm, the membrane and the extracellular space. The challenge is to tune the level of abstraction to the available data and the task at hand.

## References


1. Jablonski NG (2004). The evolution of human skin and skin color, *Annu Rev Anthropol*, **33**(1) 585–623.

2. Rigel DS (2008). Cutaneous ultraviolet exposure and its relationship to the development of skin cancer, *J Am Acad Dermatol*, **58**(5 Suppl 2), S129–S132.

3. Steingrimsson E, Copeland NG, and Jenkins NA (2004). Melanocytes and the microphthalmia transcription factor network, *Annu Rev Genet*, **38,** 365–411.

4. Lin JY and Fisher DE (2007). Melanocyte biology and skin pigmentation, *Nature*, **445**(7130), 843–850.

5. Slominski A, Tobin DJ, Shibahara S, and Wortsman J (2004). Melanin pigmentation in mammalian skin and its hormonal regulation, *Physiol Rev*, **84**(4), 1155–1228.

6. Kondo T and Hearing VJ (2011). Update on the regulation of mammalian melanocyte function and skin pigmentation, *Expert Rev Dermatol*, **6**(1), 97–108.

7. Schiaffino MV (2010). Signaling pathways in melanosome biogenesis and pathology, *Int J Biochem Cell Biol*, **42**(7), 1094–1104.

8. Dorr RT, Ertl G, Levine N, Brooks C, Bangert JL, Powell MB, Humphrey S, and Alberts DS (2004). Effects of a superpotent melanotropic peptide in combination with solar UV radiation on tanning of the skin in human volunteers, *Arch Dermatol*, **140**(7), 827–835.

9. Slominski A and Paus R (1994). Towards defining receptors for L-tyrosine and L-dopa, *Mol Cell Endocrinol*, **99**(2), C7–C11.

10. Slominski A, Paus R, and Schadendorf D (1993). Melanocytes as "sensory" and regulatory cells in the epidermis, *J Theor Biol*, **164**(1), 103–120.

11. Slominski A and Paus R (1990). Are L-tyrosine and L-dopa hormone-like bioregulators? *J Theor Biol*, **143**(1), 123–138.

12. Thingnes J, Oyehaug L, Hovig E, and Omholt SW (2009). The mathematics of tanning, *BMC Syst Biol*, **3**, 60.

13. Nielsen KP, Lu Z, Juzenas P, Stamnes JJ, Stamnes K, and Moan J (2004). Reflectance spectra of pigmented and nonpigmented skin in the UV spectral region, *Photochem Photobiol*, **80**(3), 450–455.

14. Sturm RA (1998). Human pigmentation genes and their response to solar UV radiation, *Mutat Res*, **422**(1), 69–76.

15. Costin GE and Hearing VJ (2007). Human skin pigmentation: melanocytes modulate skin color in response to stress. *FASEB J*, **21**(4), 976–994.

16. Slominski A and Pawelek J (1998). Animals under the sun: effects of ultraviolet radiation on mammalian skin. *Clin Dermatol*, **16**(4), 503–515.

17. Hoogduijn MJ, Ancans J, Suzuki I, Estdale S, and Thody AJ (2002). Melanin-concentrating hormone and its receptor are expressed and functional in human skin, *Biochem Biophys Res Commun*, **296**(3), 698–701.

18. Slominski A, Roloff B, Curry J, Dahiya M, Szczesniewski A, and Wortsman J (2000). The skin produces urocortin, *J Clin Endocrinol Metab*, **85**(2), 815–823.

19. Slominski A and Wortsman J (2000). Neuroendocrinology of the skin, *Endocr Rev*, **21**(5), 457–487.

20. Slominski A, Wortsman J, Luger T, Paus R, and Solomon S (2000). Corticotropin releasing hormone and proopiomelanocortin involvement in the cutaneous response to stress, *Physiol Rev*, **80**(3), 979–1020.

21. Abdel-Malek ZA, Knittel J, Kadekaro AL, Swope VB, and Starner R (2008). The melanocortin 1 receptor and the UV response of human melanocytes—a shift in paradigm, *Photochem Photobiol*, **84**(2), 501–508.

22. Chakraborty AK, Funasaka Y, Slominski A, Ermak G, Hwang J, Pawelek JM, and Ichihashi M (1996). Production and release of proopiomelano-cortin (POMC) derived peptides by human melanocytes and kerati-nocytes in culture: regulation by ultraviolet B, *Biochim Biophys Acta*, **1313**(2), 130–138.

23. Im S, Moro O, Peng F, Medrano EE, Cornelius J, Babcock G, Nordlund JJ, and Abdel-Malek ZA (1998). Activation of the cyclic AMP pathway by alpha-melanotropin mediates the response of human melanocytes to ultraviolet B radiation, *Cancer Res*, **58**(1), 47–54.

24. Cui R, Widlund HR, Feige E, Lin JY, Wilensky DL, Igras VE, D'Orazio J, Fung CY, Schanbacher CF, Granter SR, and Fisher DE (2007). Central role of p53 in the suntan response and pathologic hyperpigmentation, *Cell*, **128**(5), 853–864.

25. Slominski A, Plonka PM, Pisarchik A, Smart JL, Tolle V, Wortsman J, and Low MJ (2005). Preservation of eumelanin hair pigmentation in proopiomelanocortin-deficient mice on a nonagouti (a/a) genetic background, *Endocrinology*, **146**(3), 1245–1253.

26. Smart JL and Low MJ (2003). Lack of proopiomelanocortin peptides results in obesity and defective adrenal function but normal melanocyte pigmentation in the murine C57BL/6 genetic background, *Ann N Y Acad Sci*, **994,** 202–210.

27. Rana BK, Hewett-Emmett D, Jin L, Chang BH, Sambuughin N, Lin M, Watkins S, Bamshad M, Jorde LB, Ramsay M, Jenkins T, and Li WH (1999). High polymorphism at the human melanocortin 1 receptor locus. *Genetics*, **151**(4), 1547–1557.

28. Rouzaud F, Costin GE, Yamaguchi Y, Valencia JC, Berens WF, Chen KG, Hoashi T, Böhm M, Abdel-Malek ZA, and Hearing VJ (2006). Regulation of constitutive and UVR-induced skin pigmentation by melanocortin 1 receptor isoforms, *FASEB J*, **20**(11), 1927–1929.

29. Nylander K, Bourdon JC, Bray SE, Gibbs NK, Kay R, Hart I, and Hall PA (2000). Transcriptional activation of tyrosinase and TRP-1 by p53 links UV irradiation to the protective tanning response, *J Pathol*, **190**(1), 39–46.

30. Slominski A, Tobin DJ, and Paus R (2007). Does p53 regulate skin pigmentation by controlling proopiomelanocortin gene transcription? *Pigment Cell Res*, **20**(4), 307–308; author reply 309–310.

31. Friedmann PS and Gilchrest BA (1987). Ultraviolet radiation directly induces pigment production by cultured human melanocytes, *J Cell Physiol*, **133**(1), 88–94.

32. Yoshida Y, Hachiya A, Sriwiriyanont P, Ohuchi A, Kitahara T, Takema Y, Visscher MO, and Boissy RE (2007). Functional analysis of keratinocytes in skin color using a human skin substitute model composed of cells derived from different skin pigmentation types, *FASEB J*, **21**(11), 2829–2839.

33. Yoshida-Amano Y, Hachiya A, Ohuchi A, Kobinger GP, Kitahara T, Takema Y, and Fukuda M (2012). Essential role of RAB27A in determining constitutive human skin color, *PLoS One*, **7**(7), e41160.

34. Tachibana M (2000). MITF: a stream flowing for pigment cells, *Pigment Cell Res*, **13**(4), 230–240.

35. Jacquemin P, Lannoy VJ, O'Sullivan J, Read A, Lemaigre FP, and Rousseau GG (2001). The transcription factor onecut-2 controls the microphthalmia-associated transcription factor gene, *Biochem Biophys Res Commun*, **285**(5), 1200–1205.

36. Bellei B, Flori E, Izzo E, Maresca V, and Picardo M (2008). GSK3beta inhibition promotes melanogenesis in mouse B16 melanoma cells and normal human melanocytes, *Cell Signal*, **20**(10), 1750–1761.

37. Miller AJ and Mihm MC Jr (2005). Melanoma, *N Engl J Med*, **355**(1), 51–65.

38. Shibahara S, Takeda K, Yasumoto K, Udono T, Watanabe K, Saito H, and Takahashi K (2001). Microphthalmia-associated transcription factor (MITF): multiplicity in structure, function, and regulation, *J Invest Dermatol Symp Proc*, **6**(1), 99–104.

39. Galibert MD, Carreira S, and Goding CR (2001). The Usf-1 transcription factor is a novel target for the stress-responsive p38 kinase and mediates UV-induced Tyrosinase expression, *EMBO J*, **20**(17), 5022–5031.

40. Saha B, Singh SK, Sarkar C, Bera R, Ratha J, Tobin DJ, and Bhadra R (2006). Activation of the Mitf promoter by lipid-stimulated activation of p38-stress signalling to CREB, *Pigment Cell Res*, **19**(6), 595–605.

41. Busca R and Ballotti R (2000). Cyclic AMP a key messenger in the regulation of skin pigmentation, *Pigment Cell Res*, **13**(2), 60–69.

42. Park HY, Kosmadaki M, Yaar M, and Gilchrest BA (2009). Cellular mechanisms regulating human melanogenesis, *Cell Mol Life Sci*, **66**(9), 1493–1506.

43. Huber WE, Price ER, Widlund HR, Du J, Davis IJ, Wegner M, and Fisher DE (2003). A tissue-restricted cAMP transcriptional response: SOX10 modulates alpha-melanocyte-stimulating hormone-triggered expression of microphthalmia-associated transcription factor in melanocytes, *J Biol Chem*, **278**(46), 45224–45230.

44. Hara M, Yaar M, and Gilchrest BA (1995). Endothelin-1 of keratinocyte origin is a mediator of melanocyte dendricity, *J Invest Dermatol*, **105**(6), 744–748.

45. Romero-Graillet C, Aberdam E, Clément M, Ortonne JP, and Ballotti R (1997). Nitric oxide produced by ultraviolet-irradiated keratinocytes stimulates melanogenesis, *J Clin Invest*, **99**(4), 635–642.

46. Seiberg M (2001). Keratinocyte-Melanocyte Interactions During Melanosome Transfer, *Pigment Cell Res*, **14**(4), 236–242.

47. Hearing VJ (2007). Regulating melanosome transfer: who's driving the bus? *Pigment Cell Res*, **20**(5), 334–335.

48. Burns TF and Rook A (2004). *Rook's Textbook of Dermatology*, 7th ed., Blackwell Science, Malden.

49. Sandby-Moller J, Poulsen T, and Wulf HC (2003). Epidermal thickness at different body sites: relationship to age, gender, pigmentation, blood content, skin type and smoking habits, *Acta Derm Venereol*, **83**(6), 410–413.

50. Stolnitz MM and Peshkova AY (2001). Mathematical model of cAMP-dependent signaling pathway in constitutive and UV-induced melanogenesis, in *Optical Technologies in Biophysics and Medicine* (Tuchin VV, ed), **4707**, pp. 375–383.

51. Strub T, Giuliano S, Ye T, Bonet C, Keime C, Kobi D, Le Gras S, Cormont M, Ballotti R, Bertolotto C, and Davidson I (2011). Essential role of microphthalmia transcription factor for DNA replication, mitosis and genomic stability in melanoma, *Oncogene*, **30**(20), 2319–2332.

52. Liu F, Singh A, Yang Z, Garcia A, Kong Y, and Meyskens FL Jr (2010). MiTF links Erk1/2 kinase and p21 CIP1/WAF1 activation after UVC radiation in normal human melanocytes and melanoma cells, *Mol Cancer*, **9**, 214.

53. Wu M, Hemesath TJ, Takemoto CM, Horstmann MA, Wells AG, Price ER, Fisher DZ, and Fisher DE (2000). c-Kit triggers dual phosphorylations, which couple activation and degradation of the essential melanocyte factor Mi, *Genes Dev*, **14**(3), 301–312.

54. Levy C, Nechushtan H, and Razin E (2002). A new role for the STAT3 inhibitor, PIAS3: a repressor of microphthalmia transcription factor, *J Biol Chem*, **277**(3), 1962–1966.

55. Levy C, Sonnenblick A, and Razin E (2003). Role played by microphthalmia transcription factor phosphorylation and its Zip domain in its transcriptional inhibition by PIAS3, *Mol Cell Biol*, **23**(24), 9073–9080.

56. Sonnenblick A, Levy C, and Razin E (2004). Interplay between MITF, PIAS3, and STAT3 in mast cells and melanocytes, *Mol Cell Biol*, **24**(24), 10584–10592.

57. Thingnes J, Lavelle TJ, Gjuvsland AB, Omholt SW, and Hovig E (2012). Towards a quantitative understanding of the MITF-PIAS3-STAT3 connection, *BMC Syst Biol*, **6**, 11.

58. Bronisz A, Sharma SM, Hu R, Godlewski J, Tzivion G, Mansky KC, and Ostrowski MC (2006). Microphthalmia-associated transcription factor interactions with 14-3-3 modulate differentiation of committed myeloid precursors, *Mol Biol Cell*, **17**(9), 3897–3906.

59. Oyehaug L, Plahte E, Vage DI, and Omholt SW (2002). The regulatory basis of melanogenic switching. *J Theor Biol*, **215**(4), 449–468.

60. Stolnitz MM and Udryashov AA (2004). Interaction of motor proteins of various types at melanosomes redistribution in melanocytes under action of UV-radiation, in *Complex Dynamics, Fluctuations, Chaos, and Fractals in Biomedical Photonics* (Tuchin VV, ed), **5**(19), pp. 185–193.

61. Thingnes J, Lavelle TJ, Hovig E, and Omholt SW (2012). Understanding the melanocyte distribution in human epidermis: an agent-based computational model approach, *PLoS One*, **7**(7), e40377.

62. Hirashima T (2012). A kinetic model of ERK cyclic pathway on substrate control, *Math Biosci*, **239**(2), 207–212.

63. Posta F and Chou T (2010). A mathematical model of intercellular signaling during epithelial wound healing, *J Theor Biol*, **266**(1), 70–78.

64. Sarma U and Ghosh I (2012). Different designs of kinase-phosphatase interactions and phosphatase sequestration shapes the robustness and signal flow in the MAPK cascade, *BMC Syst Biol*, **6,** 82.

65. Bluthgen N and Legewie S (2008). Systems analysis of MAPK signal transduction, *Essays Biochem*, **45,** 95–107.

66. Brightman FA and Fell DA (2000). Differential feedback regulation of the MAPK cascade underlies the quantitative differences in EGF and NGF signalling in PC12 cells, *FEBS Lett*, **482**(3), 169–174.

67. Muller M, Obeyesekere M, Mills GB, and Ram PT (2008). Network topology determines dynamics of the mammalian MAPK1,2 signaling

network: bifan motif regulation of C-Raf and B-Raf isoforms by FGFR and MC1R, *Faseb J*, **22**(5), 1393–1403.

68. Walker DC, Georgopoulos NT, and Southgate J (2008). From pathway to population—a multiscale model of juxtacrine EGFR-MAPK signalling, *BMC Syst Biol*, **2**, 102.

69. Shvartsman SY, Coppey M, and Berezhkovskii AM (2009). MAPK signaling in equations and embryos, *Fly (Austin)*, **3**(1), 62–67.

70. Vilar JM, Jansen R, and Sander C (2006). Signal processing in the TGF-beta superfamily ligand-receptor network, *PLoS Comput Biol*, **2**(1), e3.

71. Schmierer B, Tournier AL, Bates PA, and Hill CS (2008). Mathematical modeling identifies Smad nucleocytoplasmic shuttling as a dynamic signal-interpreting system, *Proc Natl Acad Sci USA*, **105**(18), 6608–6613.

72. Zi Z and Klipp E (2007). Constraint-based modeling and kinetic analysis of the Smad dependent TGF-beta signaling pathway, *PLoS One*, **2**(9), e936.

73. Singh A, Jayaraman A, and Hahn J (2006). Modeling regulatory mechanisms in IL-6 signal transduction in hepatocytes, *Biotechnol Bioeng*, **95**(5), 850–862.

74. Tadokoro T, Yamaguchi Y, Batzer J, Coelho SG, Zmudzka BZ, Miller SA, Wolber R, Beer JZ, and Hearing VJ (2005)? Mechanisms of skin tanning in different racial/ethnic groups in response to ultraviolet radiation, *J Invest Dermatol*, **124**(6), 1326–1332.

75. Tadokoro T, Kobayashi N, Zmudzka BZ, Ito S, Wakamatsu K, Yamaguchi Y, Korossy KS, Miller SA, Beer JZ, and Hearing VJ (2003). UV-induced DNA damage and melanin content in human skin differing in racial/ethnic origin, *Faseb J*, **17**(9), 1177–1179.

76. Agar N and Young AR (2005). Melanogenesis: a photoprotective response to DNA damage? *Mutat Res*, **571**(1–2), 121–132.

77. Wulf HC, Sandby-Møller J, Kobayasi T, and Gniadecki R (2004). Skin aging and natural photoprotection, *Micron*, **35**(3), 185–191.

78. Hara M, Yaar M, Tang A, Eller MS, Reenstra W, and Gilchrest BA (1994). Role of integrins in melanocyte attachment and dendricity, *J Cell Sci*, **107**(Pt 10), 2739–2748.

79. Adra S, Sun T, MacNeil S, Holcombe M, and Smallwood R (2010). Development of a three dimensional multiscale computational model of the human epidermis, *PLoS One*, **5**(1), e8511.

80. Smallwood R (2011). Cell-centred modeling of tissue behaviour, in *Understanding the Dynamics of Biological Systems* (Dubitzky W, Fuß H, and Southgate J, eds), Springer, London, pp. 175–194.

81. Sun T, Adra S, Smallwood R, Holcombe M, and MacNeil S (2009). Exploring hypotheses of the actions of TGF-beta1 in epidermal wound healing using a 3D computational multiscale model of the human epidermis, *PLoS One*, **4**(12), e8515.

82. Sun T, McMinn P, Coakley S, Holcombe M, Smallwood R, and Macneil S (2007). An integrated systems biology approach to understanding the rules of keratinocyte colony formation, *J R Soc Interface*, **4**(17), 1077–1092.

83. Walker D, Sun T, MacNeil S, and Smallwood R (2006). Modeling the effect of exogenous calcium on keratinocyte and HaCat cell proliferation and differentiation using an agent-based computational paradigm, *Tissue Eng*, **12**(8), 2301–2309.

84. Walker D, Wood S, Southgate J, Holcombe M, and Smallwood R (2006). An integrated agent-mathematical model of the effect of intercellular signalling via the epidermal growth factor receptor on cell proliferation, *J Theor Biol*, **242**(3), 774–789.

85. Whiteman DC, Parsons PG, and Green AC (1999). Determinants of melanocyte density in adult human skin, *Arch Dermatol Res*, **291**(9), 511–516.

# PART 2

# SKIN BIOMECHANICS

# Chapter 4

# State-of-the-Art Constitutive Models of Skin Biomechanics

**Georges Limbert**

*National Centre for Advanced Tribology,*
*Faculty of Engineering and the Environment,*
*University of Southampton, University Road,*
*Southampton, SO17 1BJ, United Kingdom*

g.limbert@soton.ac.uk

This chapter provides a review of what are considered state-of-the-art of constitutive models used to describe and predict the biomechanics of skin. The focus is on the mathematical constitutive formulations that, ultimately, have also to be implemented into computational codes so that practical problems featuring complex geometries and boundary conditions can be solved via appropriate numerical techniques (e.g., the finite element method (FEM)). Structurally and phenomenologically based constitutive modeling approaches, together with a combination of those two are presented. Models featuring elastic and inelastic responses (e.g., viscoelasticity, viscoplasticity) are reviewed. Mechanobiological models, going beyond the traditional realm of continuum mechanics by incorporating coupling between mechanics and

*Computational Biophysics of the Skin*

Edited by Bernard Querleux

Copyright © 2014 Pan Stanford Publishing Pte. Ltd.

ISBN 978-981-4463-84-3 (Hardcover), 978-981-4463-85-0 (eBook)

www.panstanford.com

biology are also discussed in the context of growth. For sake of completeness, a brief on non-linear continuum mechanics is also provided in this review. Finally, as an illustration, a practical application of the computational modeling of skin (wrinkles) is presented.

## 4.1 Introduction

The skin, the largest organ of the human body [1], is a multi-functional biophysical interface to the external environment. It ensures cohesion and protection of the internal body structures from thermo-mechanical loads, is a dynamic barrier against chemical, bacterial, and radiological agents, provides a network of sensory receptors, and plays a major role in the synthesis of various biochemical compounds such as vitamin D [2].

Nowadays, computational techniques such as finite element methods (FEM) and computational fluid dynamics (CFD) numerical procedures are routinely used in a wide range of industrial and academic sectors. As far as skin biomechanics is concerned, the domains of application have expanded well beyond medicine and civil/military safety to reach other fields such as consumer products, cosmetics [3], sport equipment, and computer graphics. Experimentally characterizing and mathematically describing the mechanical behavior of skin is an essential requirement for conducting computational experiments using the numerical techniques mentioned previously (e.g., FEM and CFD). It is therefore critical to develop constitutive models (i.e., a set of mathematical equations characterizing the explicit dependency between strains and mechanical stresses in the material) that can capture particular mechanical features operating at specific length scales so that these models are adapted for their intended applications.

Besides its living nature, as a macroscopic biological structure, the skin possesses strong anisotropic, inhomogeneous, and non-linear mechanical properties that vary according to body site, gender, individuals, age, ethnicity and exposure to specific environmental conditions [1]. In skin, like in other biological tissues, there is an intimate relationship between structure and function [4]. Given the multiple functions of skin it is not surprising that skin features a complex multi-scale hierarchical structure [2,5]. At the meso-macroscopic level, skin is generally considered as a multi-layer assembly made up of three main distinct structures: the epidermis, dermis, and hypodermis. The epidermis—which is avascular—can be further divided into the *stratum corneum* and living epidermis (also called viable epidermis), which contains living basal cells— mainly corneocytes—which undergo mitosis and continuously migrate from the *stratum basale* in the living epidermis to the *stratum corneum* [5].

The dermis is mainly made of a dense array of collagen fibers with preferred directions embedded into a soft compliant matrix of proteoglycans [1].

Moreover, in vivo, skin is in a state of complex heterogeneous tension patterns that depend on individuals, their age and body location [6]. This presents a number of challenges for the experimental characterization of the mechanical properties of skin (as a material or as a multi-component structure) as well as their mathematical and computational realization.

A variety of methods can be used to measure the mechanical properties of skin: e.g., uniaxial and biaxial tensile tests [7], multiaxial tests [8,9], application of torsion loads [10], indentation [11], suction [12,13], and bulge testing [14]. Recent techniques have focused on the experimental characterization of the mechanical properties of the epidermis [15–17] that are particularly relevant for cosmetic and pharmaceutical applications.

It is often assumed that the dermis is the main load-bearing component of skin because of its high collagen content under the form of stiff fibers (when uncrimped). Depending on the nature of loads, this is not necessarily the case (e.g., hydrostatic pressure) and certain loading situations will only solicit the upper layers of skin. Nonetheless, if one wants to develop realistic constitutive models of skin as a multi-layer structure or constitutive models of the dermis (see Chapter 5 of this book), it is essential to consider the anisotropic mechanical characteristics introduced by the collagenous microstructure (either implicitly or explicitly as will be described in the subsequent sections of this chapter). Here, it is relevant to point out that the anisotropic properties of skin measured in vivo also arise from the inhomogeneous residual tension lines—the so-called Langer lines—present all over most of the body.

Based on these considerations and on the nonlinear nature of skin mechanics, and with very few exceptions, only nonlinear anisotropic constitutive models of skin will be presented in this review. Particular emphasis will be placed on nonlinear elastic models as they can serve as a basis for extension to any type of inelastic models. These nonlinear dissipative models are also reviewed.

## 4.2  Modeling Approaches for Skin Biomechanics

The formulation of any constitutive model relies on a number of assumptions that must be considered in view of the intended application of the model. For example, the chemo-mechanical interplay between the *stratum corneum*, living epidermis, and dermis is critical for understanding the appearance of skin in a cosmetical context but less so if one is interested in simulating skin failure as a result of military blast loading. Spatial and temporal scales are also important elements to consider. Constitutive models of skin can be classified into three main categories: phenomenological, structural, and structurally based phenomenological models.

The first type of models assumes that the skin is a homogeneous material where the geometrically and mechanically explicit accounting of the various structural elements of the tissue (e.g., corneocytes, collagen fibers) is ignored. These phenomenological models aim to capture the overall—generally macroscopic—behavior of the tissue without accounting for the individual behavior of the different sub-structures and their mutual interactions [18]. Typically, if one considers mechanical behavior only, a phenomenological model is a set of mathematical relations that describe the evolution of stress as a function of strain [4]. It is generally always possible to fit[1] such a constitutive law to a set of experimental data. However, the main drawback is that the resulting constitutive parameters often do not have a direct physical interpretation.

Structural models of skin consider the tissue as a composite material made of key microstructural elements (e.g., collagen fiber bundles with a certain degree of dispersion, proteoglycans). The way these structural elements interact can also be specified by

---

[1]Fitting a mathematical model to set of experimental data consists in calculating the optimal parameters that minimize the difference between the model and the experimentally measured data (typically the stress–strain response).

developing appropriate equations (e.g., fiber–fiber or matrix–fiber interactions). In this approach, not only the mechanical properties of the individual basic structures need to be determined or known but also the way they are geometrically arranged to form the macroscopic tissue. The overall properties of the tissue is the result of this—generally nonlinear—coupling between geometry and mechanics.

Structural models require an explicit description of the different microstructures and it is easy to realize that, in a computational finite element context, this can lead to computationally prohibitively expensive analyses, particularly if one considers several spatial scales. The advantage of this class of models is that constitutive parameters are directly related to the mechanical properties and geometric characteristics of the microstructures. Structural models can be viewed as homogenized geometric assemblies of phenomenological models. For example, a structural model of skin could consider a phenomenological law to represent the behavior of individual collagen fibers (e.g., Hooke's law). For this reason, one could argue that strictly structural models do not exist and it is matter of spatial scale. Structural models ultimately rely on phenomenological equations. Only when models will be built ab initio from first principles of quantum chemistry could we talk about structural models.

Finally, the third class of models is represented by a combination of the characteristics found in phenomenological and structural models. Nano-, meso-, microstructurally based features such as particular geometric arrangements or deformation mechanisms can be incorporated into macroscopic constitutive laws. Nowadays, these models represent the dominant trend and their level of sophistication is ever increasing.

In the last decade, there has been a tremendous drive in skin biophysics research, which has resulted in the development of innovative experimental techniques and advanced mathematical and computational models of skin. Some of these constitutive models have gone beyond single-physics (e.g., mechanics) by introducing equations coupling mechanics and biological adaptation (i.e., growth). Constitutive models featuring thermo-mechanical coupling are out of the scope of the present review and the interested reader is advised to consult the recent excellent monograph on this subject by Xu and Lu [19]. Similarly, constitutive models related to skin wound healing [20] are not treated here.

## 4.3 A Brief on Continuum Mechanics

Because current state-of-the-art constitutive models of skin mechanobiology rely on finite deformation continuum mechanics [21,22] it is relevant to provide a brief on the kinematic description of a continuum in the general case (arbitrarily large deformations) as well as how constitutive equations are derived (expression of stress and elasticity tensors) for the simple case of hyperelasticity.

The traditional approach to formulate constitutive laws for biological soft tissues, including skin, has been mainly based on invariant formulations that postulate the existence of a strain energy function depending on a set of tensorial invariants of a given deformation or strain measure [22–25]. The key element in these procedures is to select a set of tensor invariants that characterize the particular deformation modes the tissue is known to be subjected to and that have also a physical interpretation so that constitutive parameters can be directly related to experimental measurements. For collagen fiber-rich tissues, a classic assumption is to consider the tissue as a *continuum* composite material made of one or several families of (oriented) collagen fibers embedded in a highly compliant isotropic solid matrix composed mainly of proteoglycans. The preferred fiber alignment is defined by the introduction of a so-called structural tensor that appears as an argument of the strain energy function [23,25]. These concepts are explained below.

### 4.3.1 Kinematics of a Continuum

Following standard usage in continuum mechanics one defines the (potentially time-dependent) deformation gradient $\mathbf{F}$ as:

$$\mathbf{F}(\mathbf{X}) = \frac{\partial \varphi(\mathbf{X})}{\partial \mathbf{X}} = \sum_{i,I=1}^{3} \frac{\partial \varphi_i}{\partial X_I} \mathbf{e}_i \otimes \mathbf{E}_I \tag{4.1}$$

$\mathbf{X}$ is the position of the material point in the *Lagrangian*—or *reference*—configuration while $\mathbf{x} = \varphi(\mathbf{X})$ is the material placement in the *Eulerian*—or *current*—configuration. $\{\mathbf{E}_I\}_{I=1,2,3}$ and $\{\mathbf{e}_i\}_{i=1,2,3}$ are fixed orthonormal bases in the *Lagrangian* and *Eulerian* configurations, respectively. $\otimes$ and "T" denote the tensor outer product and transpose operators.

The right Cauchy–Green deformation tensors is defined as

$$\mathbf{C} = \mathbf{F}^{\mathrm{T}} \cdot \mathbf{F} \tag{4.2}$$

This tensor only contains change of length and therefore excludes rigid body rotations so is appropriate to define valid constitutive equations. For future developments, one also defines **1** as the second-order identity tensor. The classical three principal deformation invariants of **C** that define the isotropic (or non-directional response) response of a given material are defined as follows [21,22,24]:

$$I_1 = \mathrm{trace}\,(\mathbf{C}), \quad I_2 = \frac{1}{2}[I_1 - \mathrm{trace}\,(\mathbf{C}^2)], \quad I_3 = \det(\mathbf{C}) \tag{4.3}$$

To characterize a general orthotropic symmetry one can introduce three unit vectors associated, respectively, with the principal material directions *i* in the reference configuration. Because these material directions are *signed* directional properties, it is convenient to introduce the concept of structural tensors [22–25], which are even functions of these unit vectors:

$$\mathbf{L}_0^i = \mathbf{n}_0^i \otimes \mathbf{n}_0^i \{i = 1,2,3\} \tag{4.4}$$

For the material *isotropy* case all material directions are equivalent and

$$\mathbf{L}_0^1 = \mathbf{L}_0^2 = \mathbf{L}_0^3 = \mathbf{n}_0^1 \otimes \mathbf{n}_0^1 = \mathbf{n}_0^2 \otimes \mathbf{n}_0^2 = \mathbf{n}_0^3 \otimes \mathbf{n}_0^3 = \mathbf{1} \otimes \mathbf{1} \tag{4.5}$$

For *transverse isotropy*, if the preferred material direction is given by $\mathbf{n}_0^3$,

$$\mathbf{L}_0^3 = \mathbf{n}_0^3 \otimes \mathbf{n}_0^3, \qquad \mathbf{L}_0^1 = \mathbf{L}_0^2 = \frac{1}{2}(\mathbf{1} - \mathbf{L}_0^3) \tag{4.6}$$

In the context of soft tissue mechanics, a single unit vector $\mathbf{n}_0^i$ can represent the local orientation of a single collagen fiber bundle or family of fibers. This gives rise to a *transverse isotropy* symmetry if one assumes that these fibers are embedded in an isotropic matrix.

Two additional tensorial invariants characteristic of the transverse isotropy symmetry can be defined [22,23,25]:

$$I_4^i = \mathbf{C} : \mathbf{L}_0^i, \quad I_4^i = \mathbf{C}^2 : \mathbf{L}_0^i \tag{4.7}$$

## 4.3.2 Constitutive Equations

From the set of five invariants $\{I_1, I_2, I_3, I_4^i, I_5^i\}^{i=1}$, it is now possible to fully characterize the transversely isotropic hyperelastic behavior of a fibrous material by defining a strain energy form that is a scalar-valued isotropic function of its five scalar invariants:

$$\psi^1 = \psi(I_1, I_2, I_3, I_4^1, I_5^1) \tag{4.8}$$

If one considers a second family of fibers and assume that the two families of fibers do not interact [22,24,26], one can postulate the existence of a strain energy function

$$\psi^{1,2} = \psi(I_1, I_2, I_3, I_4^1, I_5^1, I_4^2, I_5^2) \tag{4.9}$$

The Lagrangian stress tensor, **S**, known as the second Piola–Kirchhoff stress tensor, is readily obtained by differentiation of the strain energy density function with respect to the right Cauchy–Green deformation tensor while applying the chain rule of differentiation for the deformation $n$ invariants $I_i$:

$$\mathbf{S} = 2 \sum_{i=1}^{n\,\text{invariants}} \left( \frac{\partial \psi}{\partial I_i} \frac{\partial I_i}{\partial \mathbf{C}} \right) \tag{4.10}$$

The Cauchy stress tensor, often referred as *true* stress tensor, is obtained by push-forward operation of the second Piola–Kirchhoff stress tensor **S** from the reference to the current configuration [22]:

$$\sigma = \frac{1}{J}(\varphi_* \mathbf{S}) = \frac{1}{J}\mathbf{F}\cdot\mathbf{S}\cdot\mathbf{F}^\mathrm{T} = \frac{2}{J}\mathbf{F}\cdot\left(\frac{\partial \psi}{\partial \mathbf{C}}\right)\cdot\mathbf{F}^\mathrm{T} \tag{4.11}$$

The elasticity tensors that characterize the stiffness of the material can be defined in the Lagrangian and Eulerian configurations, respectively, as

$$\mathbf{C} = 2\frac{\partial \mathbf{S}}{\partial \mathbf{C}} = 4\frac{\partial^2 \psi}{\partial \mathbf{C} \otimes \partial \mathbf{C}} \quad \text{and} \quad \mathbf{c} = \frac{1}{J}(\mathbf{F} \otimes \mathbf{F}^{\mathrm{T}}):\frac{\partial^2 \psi}{\partial \mathbf{C}\partial \mathbf{C}}:(\mathbf{F}^{\mathrm{T}} \otimes \mathbf{F})$$

$$(4.12)$$

These elasticity tensors are generally not constant and depend on the deformations [22,24].

They are essential in the implementation of constitutive models into non-linear implicit-based finite element codes as they are used to calculate the numerical tangent stiffness and therefore condition the rate of convergence of the system of non-linear equations [27].

## 4.4 Nonlinear Elastic Models of Skin

This section presents a selection of current state-of-the-art models of skin that make the assumption of elastic behavior. Chapter 5 of this book covers the fiber-matrix models of the dermis in details with special emphasis on models accounting for fiber dispersion via appropriate continuous and discrete statistical distributions.

### 4.4.1 Models Based on the Gasser–Ogden–Holzapfel Anisotropic Hyperelastic Formulation

The Gasser–Ogden–Holzapfel (GOH) constitutive formulation [28] was designed to capture the orthotropic hyperelastic behavior of arterial tissues while accounting for statistical distributions of fiber along their two main directions (see Section 5.3.2 of this book). Introducing $\mathbf{H}_i$ as structural tensors accounting for fiber dispersion, the strain energy function was defined as ($\mu$, $k_{i1}$, $k_{ki2}$) are material parameters)

$$\psi = \frac{\mu}{2}(I_1 - 3) + \mu \sum_{i=1}^{2} \frac{k_{i1}}{k_{ki2}}(\exp\{k_{ki2}[\text{trace}(\mathbf{H}_i \cdot \mathbf{C}) - 1]^2\} - 1) \quad (4.13)$$

Ní Annaidh et al. conducted a series of physical uniaxial tensile tests to failure using digital image correlation to measure stress–strain characteristics [29] and mean collagen fiber distribution [30] in cadaveric human skin specimens at various body locations and along several orientations (defined with respect to Langer lines). The

GOH model was fitted to the experimental tensile stress–strain curves and implemented into the finite element environment of ABAQUS (Simulia, Dassault Systèmes, Providence, RI, USA). The physical experiments were replicated by means of finite element analysis and demonstrated the very good performance of the numerical model.

In a recent study, Tonge et al. [14] determined the in-plane anisotropic mechanical properties of post-mortem human skin using cyclic full-field bulge tests with 3D digital image correlation techniques. Two main directions of anisotropy were considered and a series of full skin samples (located on the back torso) obtained from six male and female donors (43, 44, 59, 61, 62, and 83 years old) were used. The effect of preconditioning and humidity of the sample on the stress–strain response was investigated and was shown to be negligible. Age of the donors had a significant effect on the stiffness and directional properties of the skin. Specimens for older donors exhibited a stiffer and more isotropic response compared to those of younger donors. The authors also found that the bulge test method was limited by its inability to accurately determine stress and material parameters due to significant bending effects. In a companion paper, Tonge et al. [31] analyzed the results of their bulge tests [14] using an analytical method based on thin shell theory, which considered the effects of bending stiffness of skin. The method accounts for through-the-thickness linear strain gradients. Their experimental data were fitted to the GOH model and to a similar anisotropic model featuring a fully integrated fiber distribution. Two cases were considered for the GOH model—2D and 3D fiber distributions—while the fully integrated fiber model was restricted to 2D planar fiber orientation. It was found that both the 2D and 3D GOH model were unable to capture the anisotropic mechanics of skin from bulge tests unlike the 2D fully integrated fiber model, which was shown to capture it very well. Tonge et al. [31] attributed the differences between their results and those of Ní Annaidh et al. [29,30] mainly to the younger age of their donors, lower strain level considered in their tests and their assumption in terms of fiber orientation. Tonge et al. [31] considered only one fiber family aligned with the principal stretch direction while Ní Annaidh et al. [29,30] assumed that skin was made of two fiber families symmetric about the loading axis.

## 4.4.2 Models Based on the Weiss's Transversely Isotropic Hyperelastic Formulation

Weiss et al. [32] developed a transversely isotropic hyperelastic formulation to model the mechanics of the ligaments of the knee joint. The constitutive equations did not account for fiber dispersion.

Recently, Weiss's model was applied to model the anisotropic mechanics of skin by Groves et al. [33]. The strain energy function was defined as the sum of a Veronda–Westmann (VW) potential $\psi^{\mathrm{VW}}$ [18] and three tri-valued anisotropic fiber functions $\psi_i^{\mathrm{fiber}}$ [32] to model the isotropic and anisotropic responses, respectively:

$$\psi(I_1, I_2, I_4^1, I_4^2, I_4^3) = \psi^{\mathrm{VW}}(I_1, I_2) + \sum_{i=1}^{3} \psi_i^{\mathrm{fiber}}(I_4^i), \tag{4.14}$$

where

$$\psi^{\mathrm{VW}} = c_1(\exp\{c_2(I_1 - 3)\} - 1) - \frac{c_1 c_2}{2}(I_2 - 3), \quad \text{and} \tag{4.15}$$

$$\sqrt{I_4^i}\,\frac{\partial \psi_i^{\mathrm{fiber}}(I_4^i)}{\partial \sqrt{I_4^i}} = \begin{cases} 0 & \text{if } \sqrt{I_4^i} \leq 1 \\ c_3(\exp\{c_4(\sqrt{I_4^i} - 1)\} - 1) & \text{if } 1 < \sqrt{I_4^i} < \sqrt{\overline{I_4^i}} \\ c_5\sqrt{I_4^i} + c_6 & \text{if } \sqrt{I_4^i} \geq \sqrt{\overline{I_4^i}} \end{cases}$$

$$\tag{4.16}$$

Here, $\sqrt{\overline{I_4^i}}$ represents the stretch at which the (collagen) fibers are assumed to be fully taut. $c_1$ is a shear-like modulus while $c_2$ is a dimensionless parameter that scales the response connected to the second invariant. $c_3$ is an elastic modulus-like parameter scaling the exponential response, $c_4$ controls the rate of un-crimping of the fibers, $c_5$ is the elastic modulus of the taut fibers while $c_6$ is a correcting factor to ensure continuity of the stiffness response at $I_4 = \overline{I_4^i}$.

In their experimental procedure, Groves et al. [33] used 8 human discoid skin samples from two female donors (aged 56 and 68) following mastectomy and 14 post-mortem murine skin samples obtained from eight mice (aged 18–24 months). For each sample, tensile tests were simultaneously conducted along three axes ($0°$, $45°$, and $90°$). Using an inverse analysis based on finite element simulations of the testing procedures, constitutive parameters were determined. For each sample, three sets of four parameters ($c_3, c_4, \sqrt{\overline{I}_4^i}$ and an additional parameter characterizing the deviation from the assumed fiber orientation) for each fiber energy function were obtained in addition to the two parameters of the VW function.

Although Groves et al. [33] demonstrated a good fit between their three-fiber family model and their experimental data, they also acknowledged the limitations of using a simplex optimization algorithm for their inverse analysis, which could only capture *local* minima of their cost function.

### 4.4.3 Models Based on the Bischoff–Arruda–Grosh's Formulation

Bischoff et al. [34] extended the eight-chain model of Arruda and Boyce [35] to orthotropy by considering distinct dimensions for the three characteristic dimensions of the original cuboid unit cell defined by Arruda and Boyce. This model and the isotropic Arruda-Boyce model applied to human skin by Bischoff et al. [36] are not detailed here (see Section 5.3.3 of Chapter 5 in this book). Flynn et al. have developed a series of skin models based on the Bischoff–Arruda–Grosh (BAG)'s formulation [37–39].

Kuhl et al. [40] later particularized the BAG's model to the case of transverse isotropy by setting two of the unit cell dimensions equal. The model was shown to capture very well the anisotropic response of rabbit skin [41] and was further extended to model collagen fiber reorientation in response to a strain-driven stimulus such that the fiber direction progressively aligns with the first principal direction of the Cauchy–Green deformation tensor.

### 4.4.4 Models Based on the Flynn–Rubin–Nielsen's Formulation

The general constitutive model developed by Flynn et al. [42] to model the anisotropic response of biological soft tissues is described in details in Section 5.3.4 of this book. A notable feature of the constitutive formulation is the use of a discrete fiber distribution kernel that does not rely on computationally expensive integration and leads to an attractive closed-form solution for the constitutive equations. This model was notably applied to model the biaxial response of rabbit skin [41] and uniaxial tensile response of pig skin [43]. The model was later extended by Flynn and Rubin [44] to address shortcomings linked to the relation between fiber weight and anisotropic response.

## 4.4.5 Model Based on the Limbert–Middleton/ Itskov–Aksel's Formulation

A *polyconvex*[2] anisotropic strain energy function for soft tissues was developed by Limbert and Middleton [45] and independently formulated by Itskov et al. [46] shortly after. The constitutive framework was based on the generalized structural tensor invariant formulation developed by Itskov and Aksel [47]. Limbert and Middleton applied the constitutive formulation to model rabbit skin biaxial tensile test data from Lanir and Fung [41] and showed the adequacy of their formulation to capture the data accurately using a three-term series as detailed below. The starting point of the formulation that features novel invariants (compared to those described in Section 4.3) is the definition of a generalized structural tensor as the weighted sum of three mutually orthogonal structural tensors [46]:

$$\mathbf{L}_{0[k]} = \sum_{i=1}^{3} \omega_k^i \mathbf{L}_0^i = \omega_k^1 \mathbf{L}_0^1 + \omega_k^2 \mathbf{L}_0^2 + \omega_k^3 \mathbf{L}_0^3, \quad \{k = 1,2,...,n\}, \tag{4.17}$$

where $\omega_k^i (i = 1, 2, 3; k = 1, 2, ..., n)$ are non-negative scalars dependent on the principal directions. The generalized structural tensors must satisfy the normalization condition so that

$$\text{trace}(\mathbf{L}_{0[k]}) = 1 \ \text{ if } \ \sum_{i=1}^{3} \omega_k^i = 1 \tag{4.18}$$

Itskov and Aksel [47] proposed the following two sets of invariants to describe the generalized orthotropic behavior of hyperelastic materials:

$$I_{[k]} = \omega_1^k \text{ trace}(\mathbf{CL}_1) + \omega_2^k \text{ trace}(\mathbf{CL}_2) + \omega_3^k \text{ trace}(\mathbf{CL}_3) \tag{4.19}$$

---

[2]Polyconvexity is a mathematical requirement that ensures the existence of a global minimizer of the energy of the system under consideration.

$$J_{[k]} = I_3 [\omega_1^k \operatorname{trace}(\mathbf{C}^{-1}\mathbf{L}_1) + \omega_2^k \operatorname{trace}(\mathbf{C}^{-1}\mathbf{L}_2) + \omega_3^k \operatorname{trace}(\mathbf{C}^{-1}\mathbf{L}_3)]$$

$$(4.20)$$

The original strain energy function sproposed by Itskov and Aksel [47] was designed to model the mechanics of transversely isotropic calendered rubber sheets at high strains, which it did very well:

$$\psi = \frac{1}{4}\sum_{k=1}^{n} \mu_k \left[ \frac{1}{\alpha_k}(I_{[k]}^{\alpha_k} - 1) + \frac{1}{\beta_k}(J_{[k]}^{\beta_k} - 1) + \frac{1}{\chi_k}(I_3^{-\chi_k} - 1) \right] \qquad (4.21)$$

This function was subsequently modified by Limbert and Middleton [45] to capture the typical exponential behavior of the toe region of the stress–strain curve of biological soft tissues.

$$\psi = \frac{1}{4}\sum_{k=1}^{n} \mu_k \left[ \frac{1}{\alpha_k}(e^{(I_{[k]}-1)^{\alpha_k}} - 1) + \frac{1}{\beta_k}(J_{[k]}^{\beta_k} - 1) + \frac{1}{\chi_k}(I_3^{-\chi_k} - 1) \right] \qquad (4.22)$$

For both strain energy functions $\psi$, the polyconvexity condition is fulfilled if the material coefficients $\mu_k$, $\alpha_k \cdot \beta_k$ and $\chi_k$ satisfy the following inequalities:

$$\mu_k \geq 0, \quad \alpha_k \geq 1, \quad \beta_k \geq 1, \quad \chi_k \geq -\frac{1}{2} \quad \{k = 1, 2, ..., n\} \qquad (4.23)$$

Although the function developed by Limbert and Middleton was able to fit very well the data from Lanir and Fung [41], it featured 12 parameters with no direct physical interpretation.

### 4.4.6 Model Based on the Limbert's Formulation

Recently, Limbert [26] developed a novel invariant-based multi-scale constitutive framework to characterize the transversely isotropic and orthotropic elastic responses of biological soft tissues. The constitutive equations were particularized to model skin. The model was not only capable to accurately reproduce the experimental multi-axial behavior of rabbit skin, as in [48] but could also a posteriori predict stiffness values of individual tropocollagen molecules in agreement with physical and molecular-dynamics-based computational experiments [26].

A key aspect of the formulation is that the constitutive parameters can be directly extracted from physical measurements by segregating the orthogonal deformation modes of its constituents.

Of particular significance is the ability to capture *explicit* fiber–fiber and matrix–fiber interactions unlike all the models described in this section. The network models based on the BAG's formulation captures only *implicitly* and *globally* these interactions. Another desirable feature of the constitutive equations is that the response is based on physical geometrical/structural parameters that can be measured experimentally or determined ab initio from molecular dynamic simulations.

Limbert's formulation is based on the constitutive framework of Lu and Zhang [49] for transversely isotropic materials, which make use of four invariants that characterize decoupled deformations modes solely related to purely volumetric ($J$), deviatoric stretch in the fiber direction ($\bar{\lambda}$), cross-fiber shear ($\alpha_1^i$) and fiber-to-fiber/ matrix-to-fiber shear ($\alpha_2^i$) stress responses. Orthotropic symmetry is accounted for by introducing a second family of fibers. The index $i$ = 1, 2 identifies each fiber family:

$$J = \sqrt{I_3}; \quad \bar{\lambda}_i = I_3^{-\frac{1}{6}}\sqrt{I_4^i}; \quad \alpha_1^i = \frac{I_1 I_4^i - I_5^i}{\sqrt{I_3 I_4^i}}; \quad \alpha_2^i = \frac{I_5^i}{(I_4^i)^2} \tag{4.24}$$

Limbert proposed the following strain energy function:

$$\psi = \psi^v(J) + \sum_{i=1}^{2}[\psi_i^{\bar{\lambda}}(\bar{\lambda}_i) + \hat{\psi}_i^1(\alpha_1^i) + \tilde{\psi}_i^2(\alpha_2^i, \bar{\lambda}_i)] \tag{4.25}$$

$\psi^v$, $\psi_i^{\bar{\lambda}}$, $\hat{\psi}_i^1$, and $\tilde{\psi}_i^2$ are, respectively, the volumetric, deviatoric fiber, cross-fiber shear and fiber-to-fiber/fiber-to-matrix shear energies. The functional forms of the energies and the constitutive parameters are detailed below.

$$\hat{\psi}_i^1(\alpha_1^i) = \frac{1}{2}\mu_1^i(\alpha_1^i - 2) \tag{4.26}$$

$$\tilde{\psi}_i^2(\alpha_2^i, \bar{\lambda}_i) = \frac{1}{2}\mu_2^i(\alpha_2^i - 1)^2 \; \underbrace{\frac{1}{1 + a_i\, e^{-b_i(\bar{\lambda}_i - \bar{\lambda}_i^c)}}}_{\text{Sigmoid coupling function}} \tag{4.27}$$

The novelty of the present approach is that the collagen fibers and the matrix are allowed to interact via explicit decoupled shear interactions while the collagen fibers behave like a worm-like chain model [40,50].

$$\psi_i^{\bar{\lambda}}(\bar{\lambda}_i) = \begin{cases} \aleph_i \mu_0^i \left( \bar{\lambda}_i^2 + \dfrac{2}{\bar{\lambda}_i} - 3 \right) + \xi_0^i \aleph_i \ln(\bar{\lambda}_i^{r_{0i}^2}) & \text{if } \bar{\lambda}_i \leq 1 \\[2em] \aleph_i \mathcal{K}\theta \dfrac{L_i}{4L_p^i} \left( 2\dfrac{\bar{\lambda}_i^2 r_{0\beta}^2}{L_i^2} + \dfrac{1}{\left(1 - \dfrac{\bar{\lambda}_i r_{0i}}{L_i}\right)} - \dfrac{\bar{\lambda}_i r_{0i}}{L_i} \right) \\[1em] \quad + \xi_0^i \aleph_i \ln(\bar{\lambda}_i^{r_{0\beta}^2}) & \text{if } \bar{\lambda}_i > 1 \end{cases}$$

$$(4.28)$$

The constitutive model resulted in a set of 23 constitutive parameters $\mathbf{p} = \mathbf{p}^1 \cup \mathbf{p}^2 = \{\mathcal{K}, \theta, \kappa, \mu_0^i, \mu_1^i, \mu_2^i, \aleph_i, L_i, L_p^i, r_i, a_i, b_i, \bar{\lambda}_i^c\}_{i=1,2}$. A notable feature of this multi-scale formulation is that all the parameters have a direct physical interpretation. Limbert [26] determined the parameter set $\mathbf{p}^2$ using a numerical global optimization algorithm while the parameter set $\mathbf{p}^1$ was assumed a priori based on existing data [40] and data obtained via visual inspection of the biaxial stress–strain curves [48]. The parameters are listed below while their physical meaning is provided in Table 4.1.

$$\mathbf{p}^1 = \{\mathcal{K}, \theta, \kappa, \mu_0, \alpha_{n_0}, b_{n_0}, a_{m_0}, b_{n_0}, \aleph_{n_0}, \aleph_{m_0}, \bar{\lambda}_{n_0}^c, \bar{\lambda}_{m_0}^c\};$$

$$\mathbf{p}^2 = \{\mu_1, \mu_2, L_{n_0}, L_p^{n_0}, r_{n_0}, \aleph_{m_0}, L_{m_0}, L_p^{m_0}, r_{m_0}\}$$

$$(4.29)$$

Although the model slightly under-predicts the response of rabbit skin along the head-tail direction at low stretch (<1.35), an excellent fit was obtained (Fig. 4.1). Limbert implemented the non-linear constitutive model as tri-linear hexahedral finite element using an enhanced strain formulation [51], which has been proven to be superior to a standard displacement-based formulation, particularly for shear-dominated problems and nearly incompressible materials. Moreover, analytically exact direct sensitivity analyses subroutines were also implemented to assess the sensitivity of the shear response of the model to its constitutive parameters during a simulated indentation test [26].

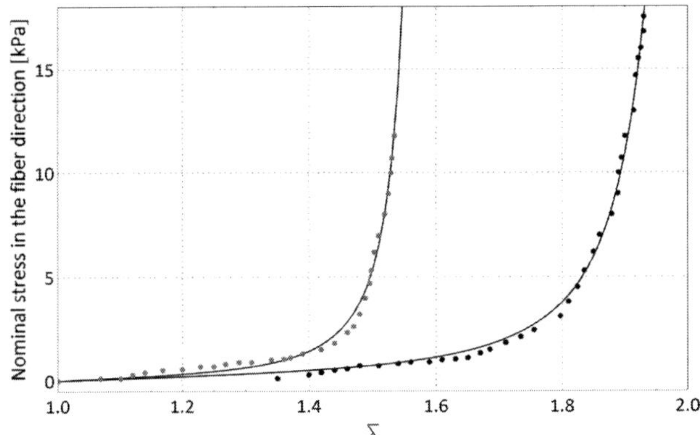

**Figure 4.1**     Experimental data from uniaxial tensile tests on rabbit skin from Lanir and Fung [41] and the corresponding theoretical values (continuous lines) calculated after identification of the constitutive parameters (gray: head-to-tail fiber direction, $r^2 = 0.997$; black: perpendicular to head-to-tail direction, $r^2 = 0.998$).

**Table 4.1**     Constitutive parameters of the rabbit skin model [26]

| | **Measured or estimated constitutive parameters** |
|---|---|
| $\mathcal{R}$ | Boltzmann constant |
| $\theta$ | Absolute temperature |
| $\kappa$ | Bulk modulus of the matrix |
| $\mu_0$ | Shear modulus of collagen fibers |
| $a_{n_0}, a_{m_0}$ | First shape parameter for sigmoid coupling function (families 1 and 2) |
| $b_{n_0}, b_{m_0}$ | Second shape parameter for sigmoid coupling function (families 1 and 2) |
| $\overline{\lambda}^c_{n_0}, \overline{\lambda}^c_{m_0}$ | Critical stretch for sigmoid coupling function (families 1 and 2) |
| $\aleph_{n_0}, \aleph_{m_0}$ | Density of collagen fibers (families 1 and 2) |
| | **Constitutive parameters determined by numerical optimization** |
| $\mu_1$ | Matrix shear modulus |
| $\mu_2$ | Maximum fiber–fiber/matrix–fiber shear modulus |
| $L_{n_0}, L_{m_0}$ | Contour length of a tropocollagen molecule (families 1 and 2) |
| $L_p^{n_0}, L_p^{m_0}$ | Persistence length of a tropocollagen molecule (families 1 and 2) |
| $r_{n_0}, r_{m_0}$ | Initial length of a crimpled collagen molecule (families 1 and 2) |

From the persistence lengths of tropocollagen molecules determined from the optimization procedure (22 and 65 nm for fiber families 1 and 2) Limbert [26] calculated equivalent Young's moduli of, respectively, 293 and 865 MPa. These values lie within one order of magnitude less of what has been determined experimentally and obtained trough computational modeling studies (see, for example, Gautieri et al. [52]). However, using the same equation used by Limbert to calculate the Young's modulus, Sun et al. [53] estimated the Young's modulus of collagen molecules to range between 350 MPa and 12 GPa.

## 4.5 Nonlinear Viscoelastic Models of Skin

Key aspects of viscoelasticity are represented by stress relaxation, creep, possible rate-dependency of stress and hysteresis [4]. A large number of researchers have characterized the viscoelastic properties of skin under various testing conditions [54–61]. To date, there are only very few nonlinear viscoelastic anisotropic constitutive models of skin [62,63]. This is mainly due to the considerable challenges of experimentally characterizing the behavior of skin, particularly in vivo. The literature on general viscoelastic constitutive models is rich and, here, only a brief account of the most common approaches to model biological soft tissues (following the classification of Ehret [64]) is reported. State-of-the-art nonlinear viscoelastic models of skin are presented.

### 4.5.1 Quasi-Linear Viscoelasticity and Its Derivatives

The application of quasi-linear viscoelasticity (QLV) theory to soft tissue mechanics has been particularly popularized by the work of Fung and co-workers [4,65]. The idea behind QLV is to assume that the time-dependent stress response $\sigma(t)$ in response to a uniaxial loading can be expressed as a convolution integral of the form:

$$\sigma(t) = \int_{-\infty}^{t} G(t-\tau)\frac{\partial \sigma_e(\tau)}{\partial t}d\tau, \tag{4.30}$$

where $\sigma_e$ is the instantaneous elastic stress and $G$ the reduced relaxation function. This function controls how the current stress response is affected by past loading history.

The notion of quasi-linearity stems from the linear relation of the integrand terms and the analogy with rate equations of linear viscoelasticity. The uniaxial relationship can be extended to a full 3D representation by introducing second-order and fourth-order tensors describing, respectively, the stress and reduced relaxation function [4]. This represents a flexible framework where anisotropic properties and decoupling between deviatoric and volumetric responses can be captured by appropriate constitutive equations.

Bischoff [66] applied QLV to model porcine skin by developing an anisotropic microstructurally motivated constitutive model including the viscoelastic properties of collagen and fiber dispersion. A notable feature of the model is the ability to capture a fiber-level viscoelastic orthotropic response with only seven parameters. However, the authors recognized the need for additional experiments to fully characterize the mechanical response.

### 4.5.2 Explicitly Rate-Dependent Models

By design, these types of model—also called viscoelastic models of the *differential* type—are capturing strain-rate sensitivity and viscous effects in the close time vicinity of the application of load [67]. They are based on differential rather than integral equations like for QLV and are therefore inappropriate to capture long-term memory viscoelastic effects such as relaxation. Coleman and Noll [68] formulated the principle of fading memory, which states that the deformations that occurred in the recent time history have greater influence on the actual stresses than those which occurred in a more distant past history. Explicitly rate-dependent models of soft tissues are particularly well suited to high strain rate situations such as those occurring during car crash, sport activities, impact and blast [67,69–71].

These models generally postulate the existence of a viscous potential $\psi^v$ from which the viscous dissipative effects D arise by differentiation with respect to the rate of the Cauchy–Green deformation tensor $\dot{\mathbf{C}} = \partial \mathbf{C}/\partial t$ (see Section 4.1.3.1):

$$\mathbf{D} = \frac{\partial \psi^{\mathrm{v}}}{\partial \dot{\mathbf{C}}} : \dot{\mathbf{C}} \qquad (4.31)$$

The total second Piola–Kirchhoff stress tensor, which includes purely elastic effects through a potential $\psi^{\mathrm{e}}$ and purely viscous effects through $\psi^{\mathrm{v}}$, is obtained by differentiation of the total potential $\psi$ assuming that $\dot{\mathbf{C}}$ is a parameter or internal variable:

$$\mathbf{S} = 2 \left( \frac{\partial \psi^{\mathrm{e}}}{\partial \mathbf{C}} + \frac{\partial \psi^{\mathrm{v}}}{\partial \dot{\mathbf{C}}} \right) \qquad (4.32)$$

The framework proposed by Pioletti et al. [67] for modeling the rate-dependent isotropic viscohyperelastic behavior of ligaments and tendons was later extended by Limbert and Middleton [70] to transverse isotropy using a tensor formalism. This model was subsequently combined with damage equations to model the failure of human skin in response to puncturing biting loads [69] (see Fig. 4.2).

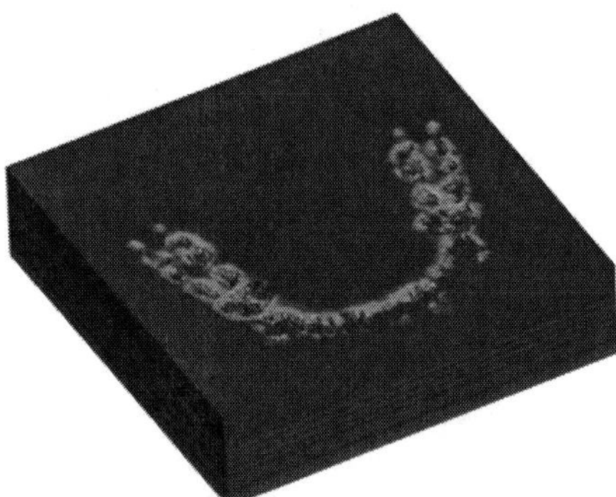

**Figure 4.2**    Simulation of skin damage as a result of human bite. The constitutive model is based on an anisotropic viscohyperelastic formulation [70] combined to a damage model implemented in a commercial explicit finite element code [69] (published data not in the public domain).

### 4.5.3  Internal Variables Based on Strain Decomposition

Unidimensional (small-strain) rheological models based on combinations of spring and dashpot elements are very useful to conceptualize particular viscoelastic behaviors [22]. The arrangement of a dashpot and a spring in series constitutes a Maxwell element with viscosity $\eta$ and elastic modulus $E$. The total strain $\varepsilon$ in the element can be decomposed into elastic and inelastic strains as $\varepsilon = \varepsilon_e + \varepsilon_i$ and the total strain rate is

$$\frac{\partial \varepsilon}{\partial t} = \frac{1}{E}\frac{\sigma}{\eta} + \frac{\partial \sigma}{\partial t} \qquad (4.33)$$

Borrowing this concept of linear strain decomposition and applying it to the 3D finite strain regime, on can establish a multiplicative decomposition of the deformation gradient into an elastic and inelastic parts as $\mathbf{F} = \mathbf{F}^e \cdot \mathbf{F}^i$ [72]. From this definition on can define the *elastic* and *inelastic* right Cauchy–Green deformation tensors as

$$\mathbf{C}^e = \mathbf{F}^{eT} \cdot \mathbf{F}^e; \qquad \mathbf{C}^i = \mathbf{F}^{iT} \cdot \mathbf{F}^i \qquad (4.34)$$

One can postulate the existence of a free energy $\psi(\mathbf{C}, \mathbf{C}^i)$ decomposed into equilibrium and non-equilibrium terms where $\mathbf{C}^i$ is treated as an internal variable [72]:

$$\psi(\mathbf{C}, \mathbf{C}^i) = \psi^{\text{equilibrium}}(\mathbf{C}) + \psi^{n.\text{equilibrium}}(\mathbf{C}^i) \qquad (4.35)$$

Naturally, one can generalize this concept to $n$ Maxwell elements so that one introduces $n$ internal (tensor) variables $\mathbf{C}^i_k$:

$$\psi(\mathbf{C}, \mathbf{C}^i_k) = \psi^{\text{equilibrium}}(\mathbf{C}) + \sum_{k=1}^{n} \psi^{n.\text{equilibrium}}_k(\mathbf{C}^i_k) \qquad (4.36)$$

The second Piola–Kirchhoff stress is then obtained as the sum of equilibrium and non-equilibrium terms as

$$\mathbf{S} = \mathbf{S}^{\text{equilibrium}} + \sum_{k=1}^{n} \mathbf{S}^{n.\text{equilibrium}}_k \qquad (4.37)$$

Bischoff et al. [73] combined this type of formulation with their previous orthotropic eight-chain model [34] to model the viscoelastic behavior of soft tissues. The model was fitted to the experimental data on rabbit skin [41]. Vassoler et al. [74] recently proposed a variational framework making use of the multiplicative decomposition of the deformation gradient into elastic and inelastic parts to represent the mechanics of fiber-reinforced biological composites and this would be appropriate for skin.

### 4.5.4  Internal Variables Based on Stress Decomposition

If one considers a set of non-measurable strain-like internal variables $\mathbf{E}_k$ in the reference configuration, the free energy of a viscoelastic material can be defined as follows [22]:

$$\psi(\mathbf{C},\mathbf{E}_k) = \psi^{\text{equilibrium}}(\mathbf{C}) + \sum_{k=1}^{n} \psi_k^{n.\text{equilibrium}}(\mathbf{C},\mathbf{E}_k), \tag{4.38}$$

where, in analogy with Eq. 4.36, the free energy (and stress) can be split into equilibrium and non-equilibrium contributions associated, respectively, with elastic and viscous deformation mechanisms:

$$\mathbf{S} = \mathbf{S}^{\text{equilibrium}} + \sum_{k=1}^{n} \mathbf{Q}_k^{n.\text{equilibrium}} \tag{4.39}$$

The over-stress $\mathbf{Q}_k^{n.\,\text{equilibrium}}$ are work-conjugate to $\mathbf{E}_k$. Drawing a parallel with rheological elements of linear viscoelasticity, and instead of formulating evolution equations fort the strain-like variables $\mathbf{E}_k$, one can formulate rate equations in terms of the stress-like internal variables $\mathbf{Q}_k^{n.\,\text{equilibrium}}$. These equations can be solved by means of convolution integrals [72,75]. Using a multi-modal Maxwell element rheological analogy, this type of formulation was applied by Holzapfel and Gasser [75] to model the viscoelastic orthotropic behavior of arteries. Peña et al. [76,77] developed a similar approach to model the ligaments of the knee but conceptually used a combination of Kelvin-Voigt elements. Ehret et al. [78] recently proposed a microstructurally motivated finite strain viscoelastic model for soft tissues, which is very relevant for skin mechanics.

The non-equilibrium energy in Eq. 4.38 could have been equivalently defined in terms of internal stress-like variables $\mathbf{Q}_k^{n.\,\text{equilibrium}}$ as proposed by Simo [79]. Only in special cases, the approach based on the multiplicative decomposition of the deformation gradient is consistent with the one based on convolution integrals [79].


## 4.6  Other Inelastic Models of Skin

### 4.6.1  Softening and Damage

Preconditioning effects are often associated with viscoelasticity [4]. They are linked to short-term rearrangement of the tissue microstructure and, in some instances, permanent damage of the microstructure. For example, Muñoz et al. [80] observed a typical softening effect—well known as the Mullins effect in the context of filled rubber mechanics—during cyclic uniaxial testing of murine skin at large deformations. A similar effect was reported by Edsberg et al. [81] for human skin under cyclic pressures.

Ehret and Itskov [82] developed a constitutive framework to capture the Mullins effects observed in biological soft tissues and fitted it to the experimental data of Muñoz et al. [80] demonstrating an excellent agreement. Ehret et al. [83] later applied their constitutive model to porcine dermis.

## 4.6.2 Plasticity

Mazza et al. [84,85] developed a non-linear elasto-visco-plastic model to simulate ageing of the human face [84,85]. It is based on the constitutive model of Rubin and Bodner [86] to model the dissipative response of soft tissues. In this study, the dissipative effects were a combination of elastic and visco-plastic mechanisms. Rubin and Bodner [86] demonstrated the relevance of their model by capturing very well the cyclic dissipative response of superficial musculoaponeurotic system tissue. The constitutive equations were implemented as a user subroutine in the commercial finite element code ABAQUS (Simulia, Dassault Systèmes, Providence, RI, USA) to simulate gravimetric descent of facial tissue [84]. Mazza et al. [84,85] extended the model of Rubin and Bodner [86] by including an aging parameter equipped with its own time evolution equation. This parameter controlled the stiffness degradation of aging tissues. A four-layer model of facial skin combined with a face-like geometric base was developed and showed the great potential of this kind of computational models to study the effects of skin aging on facial appearance.

## 4.6.3 Growth

In the context of tissue expansion procedures [87], Socci et al. [88] developed an axisymmetric computational model of skin growth. Motivated by the same medical application, Tepole et al. [89] proposed a 3D constitutive model for skin growth embedded into a rigorous theoretical framework based on the thermodynamics of opens systems [90] where the rate of variation of the material density $\rho_0$ is balanced by mass in- and out-fluxes $\nabla_x \cdot \mathbf{R}$ and mass sources/sinks $R_0$:

$$\frac{d\rho_0}{dt} = \nabla_x \cdot \mathbf{R} + R_0 \tag{4.40}$$

The general point of departure of growth theories consists in multiplicatively splitting the deformation gradient $\mathbf{F}$ into a growth part (inelastic) $\mathbf{F}^g$ and an elastic deformation gradient $\mathbf{F}^e$ [91]:

$$\mathbf{F} = \mathbf{F}^e \cdot \mathbf{F}^g \tag{4.41}$$

This effectively assumes that there exists an intermediate virtual configuration between the reference and current configurations in which individual *material particles* have their volume changed. However, the growth (positive or negative) of each material particle renders them geometrically incompatible with their neighbors [92,93]. The elastic deformations characterized by $\mathbf{F}^e$ bring back compatibility and, by doing so, introduce residual stress [94].

Rather than describing volumetric growth, Tepole et al. [89] considered in-plane skin growth driven by a strain-based stimulus: growth occurs when a critical in-plane stretch is reached. The growth factor is described by a temporal evolution equation. The skin was modeled as a neo-Hookean material.

3D tissue expansions were simulated by considering a series of expanders with different shapes and showed the promising potential of the computational model of skin growth.

Tepole et al. [95] later extended this model by considering skin as a eight-chain transversely isotropic material [40]. Computational relaxation and creep tests were conducted to study the evolution of in-plane area stretch. Skin growth due to the application of circular-, square-, rectangular-, and crescent-shaped tissue expanders was also simulated and confirmed the usefulness of the approach to simulate complex surgical procedures where predictive tools are very attractive. Several iterations of the original Tepole et al.'s model [89] were done by the same group, mostly focusing on refining the computational procedures for simulating the inflation of the tissue expander [96–98].

## 4.7  A State-of-the-Art Application: Skin Wrinkles

As humans age, the chemo-mechano-biology of their skin undergoes a series of alterations that occur in combination with the effects of external environmental factors such as solar radiations or chemical pollution. These biophysical changes lead to modifications of the skin appearance that can be translated into the appearance or accentuation of wrinkles. Skin wrinkles have been the subject of much attention because of their societal importance in relation to age and beauty but also, in the case of expression wrinkles, because of their role in conveying emotions and thus as a vehicle for communication. Understanding and predicting the biophysics of the skin, particularly in relation to wrinkles, is essential for developing novel solutions for a wide range of industries such as biomedical, pharmaceutical, toiletry and cosmetic products, sport equipment among many others. For example, wet shaving products (razors) do not interact in the same way with the wrinkled skin of an 85-year-old man and the skin of a 15-year-old teenager. It is therefore essential to take these facts into consideration when developing products that interact with the skin surface.

From a general physical and geometrical view point, wrinkles are the result of a complex interplay between material and structural properties, boundary and loading conditions, the exact nature of which remains to be elucidated [99]. Wrinkling, ubiquitous in nature, is also a multi-scale spatial phenomenon that spans over eight orders of magnitude [100].

There is no consensus on the classification and terminology used to describe the various types of skin wrinkles [101,102]. Piérard et al. [102] established a classification of skin wrinkles based on the following four types: atrophic (Type I), elastotic (Type II), gravitational (Type III), and expressional (Type IV). Each of these four wrinkle types is characterized by specific micro-anatomical alterations occurring each at distinct body locations. One might want to distinguish between *skin microrelief*—characterized by characteristic intersecting lines and regularly splayed follicular and eccrine duct openings—and *skin wrinkles* (or skin folds) [102] generally associated with ageing and *dynamic wrinkles* associated with skin movement. The characteristics of skin microrelief can be further classified according to the orientation and depth of featured lines [103–105] into *primary, secondary, tertiary* and *quaternary* lines [105].

The study of skin wrinkles has received much attention in the dermatology and cosmetics communities [102]—and references therein—but only few studies can be found in the biomechanics and biophysics research arenas [3,37–39,106–112] although this is rapidly changing [3,113,114]. Research into visually realistic computational models of skin wrinkling has been mainly driven by the computer graphics community [111]. Despite a growing trend of physics-based animations, these models have not considered the underlying structural properties of skin together with advanced constitutive models valid for arbitrary kinematics.

Magnenat-Thalmann et al. [110] developed a 2D model featuring the *stratum corneum* and the dermis only that demonstrated that the geometry of the interface between the *stratum corneum* and the dermis was essential in producing realistic wrinkle patterns and that, as opposed to a two-layer, a three-layer model corroborated clinical observations. Flynn and McCormack [109] developed a computational model of skin wrinkling. The three-layer model features the *stratum corneum*, the dermis, and the hypodermis, respectively, modeled as a neo-Hookean, orthotropic viscohyperelastic, and a Yeoh material. The model, implemented in the finite element code ABAQUS/Explicit (Simulia, Dassault Systèmes, Providence, RI, USA), was validated against in vivo 3D experimental measurements on the forearm of a series of volunteers. This model provided a valuable insight into the influence of the number of layers and pre-stress on wrinkle formation.

The living epidermis was not included in the model and the coupled effects of structural dimensions, mechanical properties and loading conditions were not investigated.

This was recently addressed by Limbert [3], who developed a three-layer model of skin to simulate compression wrinkles in the finite element code ABAQUS/Standard in order to explore the relative influence of geometry, mechanical properties, boundary and loading conditions on wrinkle formation via a design of computer experiment. The computational procedure was based on a perturbation technique combining buckling and post-buckling analyses. The initial geometry of the skin composite was made of three perfectly bonded *planar* cuboid geometries (Fig. 4.3). The probabilistic finite element analyses revealed the strong interplay between the geometry and mechanical properties of each layer and also highlighted the current limitation of traditional Lagrange interpolation-based finite element techniques in simulating highly non-linear phenomena such as wrinkling and folding, which need to accurately capture changes in surface curvature. The development of alternative techniques to simulate different types of skin wrinkles is under way in the author's research group.

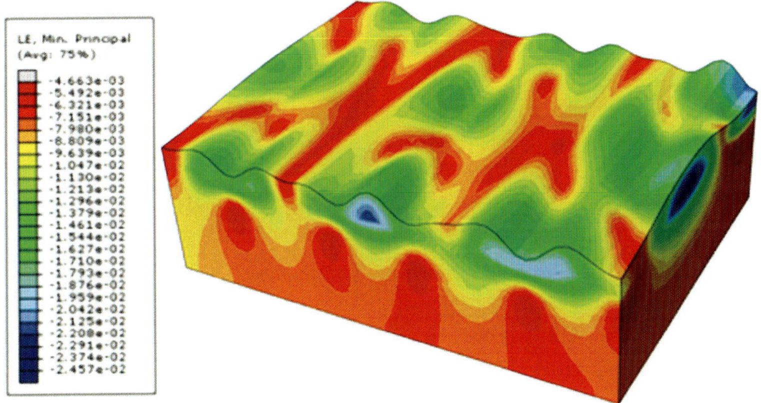


**Figure 4.3**    Post-buckling finite element analysis of compression wrinkle on a three-layer model of human skin. The color plot represents the distribution of third principal strains in the skin composite [3,114].

## 4.8   Conclusion

This chapter has presented a selection of non-linear constitutive formulations to represent the biomechanics of skin. Every model has its own advantages and drawbacks as well as its (restricted) domain of validity. As George P. E. Box (professor emeritus of statistics at the University of Wisconsin, USA) rightly said, *"All models are wrong, but some are useful."* It is the present author's opinion that it is in this spirit that models should be conceived, developed, validated, used, extended, and discarded.

As stated in the introduction, computational models of skin offer a vast potential as practical tools to assist research and development in a wide range of research areas, and so, industrial sectors. A clinically and experimentally validated computational model of skin (or a series of models addressing specific modeling objectives) can be an invaluable numerical assay to perform hypothesis driven research and unravel some of the complex non-linear mechanisms associated with the natural (or otherwise) physiological processes occurring in skin.

Before reaching the point where mathematical and computational models of skin have a sufficient predictive power such that physical experiments can be significantly reduced, it is essential to develop simple models with constitutive parameters that can be *directly* linked to physical measurements. Developing advanced mathematical and computational models of biological tissues is relatively "easy"; the main difficulty lies in the physical measurement of biophysical properties (either in vitro or in vivo) to feed and validate these models. Mathematical models of skin should be developed in conjunction with physical experimental techniques so that their relevance could be directly put to the test. Mathematical and computational models have also an important role to play in guiding the design of physical experiments.

It is believed that the evolution of skin imaging techniques will also be instrumental in answering the challenges that make the experimental characterization of skin so difficult. Image-based modeling techniques [115,116] will also lead to more and more accurate micromechanical models where, for example, the geometry of individual collagen fibers could be captured explicitly.

Probabilistic finite element techniques [3,114,117] are worth mentioning as they offer an attractive solution to account for the variability in biological systems and experimental techniques.

Computational multi-scale methods combining atomistic, molecular and continuum techniques are bound to play an increasing role in the modeling of skin biophysics [118–122].

From this review, one can appreciate that skin provides an exciting research "playground" to develop and apply new theories, computational and experimental techniques so that clinicians, biologists, mathematicians, chemists, physicists, and engineers can embrace a truly multi-disciplinary approach. There is much to be done before we could even contemplate replacing *physical* tests on skin by fully validated in silico analyses. This is likely to keep us busy for many decades. In the meantime, let's enjoy the work!

# References


1. Lanir Y (1987). Skin mechanics, in *Handbook of Bioengineering* (Skalak R, Chien S, eds), McGraw-Hill, New York, pp. 11.11–11.25.

2. Burns T, Breathnach S, Cox N, and Griffiths C (eds) (2004). *Rook's Textbook of Dermatology*, 7th ed., Blackwell Science, Oxford.

3. Limbert G (2009). A stochastic finite element study of the wrinkling behaviour of skin, in *Third International Conference on Mechanics of Biomaterials and Tissues*, Elsevier, Clearwater.

4. Fung YC (ed) (1981). *Biomechanics: Mechanical Properties of Living Tissues*, Springer-Verlag, New York.

5. Shimizu H (ed) (2007). *Shimizu's Textbook of Dermatology*, Hokkaido University Press—Nakayama Shoten Publishers.

6. Alexander H and Cook TH (1977). Accounting for natural tension in the mechanical testing of human skin, *J Invest Dermatol*, **69**, 310–314.

7. Wan Abas WAB (1994). Biaxial tension test of human skin in vivo, *Biomed Mater Eng*, **4**, 473–486.

8. Kvistedal YA and Nielsen PMF (2004). Investigating stress–strain properties of in-vivo human skin using multiaxial loading experiments and finite element modeling, in *Proceedings of the 26th Annual International Conference of the IEEE Engineering in Medicine and Biology Society, Vols 1–7*, **26**, pp. 5096–5099.

9. Kvistedal YA and Nielsen PMF (2009). Estimating material parameters of human skin in vivo, *Biomech Model Mechanobiol*, **8**, 1–8.

10. Batisse D, Bazin R, Baldeweck T, Querleux B, and Lévêque J-L (2002). Influence of age on the wrinkling capacities of skin, *Skin Res Technol*, **8**, 148–154.

11. Delalleau A, Josse G, Lagarde J-M, Zahouani H, and Bergheau J-M (2006). Characterization of the mechanical properties of skin by inverse analysis combined with the indentation test, *J Biomech*, **39**, 1603–1610.

12. Diridollou S, Patat F, Gens F, Vaillant L, Black D, Lagarde J-M, Gall Y, and Berson M (2000). In vivo model of the mechanical properties of the human skin under suction, *Skin Res Technol*, **6**, 214–221.

13. Hendriks FM, Brokken D, Oomens CWJ, Bader DL, and Baaijens FPT (2006). The relative contributions of different skin layers to the mechanical behavior of human skin in vivo using suction experiments, *Med Eng Phys*, **28**, 259–266.

14. Tonge TK, Atlan LS, Voo LM, and Nguyen TD (2013). Full-field bulge test for planar anisotropic tissues: Part I—Experimental methods applied to human skin tissue, *Acta Biomater*, **9**, 5913–5925.

15. Geerligs M, Oomens CWJ, Ackermans PAJ, Baaijens FPT, and Peters GWM (2011). Linear shear response of the upper skin layers. *Biorheology*, **48**(3–4), 229–245.

16. Geerligs M, van Breemen LCA, Peters GWM, Ackermans PAJ, Baaijens FPT, and Oomens CWJ (2011). In vitro indentation to determine the mechanical properties of epidermis, *J Biomech*, **44**, 1176–1181.

17. Lamers E, van Kempen THS, Baaijens FPT, Peters GWM, and Oomens CWJ (2013). Large amplitude oscillatory shear properties of human skin, *J Mech Behav Biomed Mater*, S1751–6161(13)00039-8.

18. Veronda DR and Westmann R (1970). Mechanical characterization of skin—finite deformations, *J Biomech*, **3**, 111–124.

19. Xu F and Lu T (2011). *Introduction to Skin Biothermomechanics and Thermal Pain*, Springer, Heidelberg Dordrecht London New York.

20. Vermolen FJ, Gefen A, and Dunlop JWC (2012). In vitro "Wound" healing: experimentally based phenomenological modeling, *Adv Eng Mater*, **14**, B76–B88.

21. Marsden JE and Hughes TJR (eds) (1994). *Mathematical Foundations of Elasticity*, Dover Publ, New-York.

22. Holzapfel, G. A. (ed) (2000). *Nonlinear Solid Mechanics. A Continuum Approach for Engineering*, John Wiley & Sons, Chichester.

23. Boehler JP (1978). Lois de comportement anisotrope des milieux continus. *J de Mécanique*, **17**, 153–190.

24. Limbert G and Taylor M (2002). On the constitutive modeling of biological soft connective tissues. A general theoretical framework and tensors of elasticity for strongly anisotropic fiber-reinforced composites at finite strain, *Int J Solids Struct*, **39**, 2343–2358.

25. Spencer AJM (ed) (1992). *Continuum Theory of the Mechanics of Fibre-Reinforced Composites*, Springer-Verlag, New York.

26. Limbert G (2011). A mesostructurally-based anisotropic continuum model for biological soft tissues—Decoupled invariant formulation, *J Mech Behav Biomed Mater*, **4**, 1637–1657.

27. Belytschko T, Liu WK, and Moran B (eds) (2000). *Nonlinear Finite Elements for Continua and Structures*, Wiley, Oxford.

28. Gasser TC, Ogden RW, and Holzapfel GA (2006). Hyperelastic modelling of arterial layers with distributed collagen fibre orientations, *J Roy Soc Int*, **3**, 15–35.

29. Ní Annaidh A, Bruyère K, Destrade M, Gilchrist MD, and Otténio M (2011). Characterization of the anisotropic mechanical properties of excised human skin, *J Mech Behav Biomed Mater*, **5**, 139–148.

30. Ní Annaidh A, Bruyère K, Destrade M, Gilchrist MD, Maurini C, Otténio M, and Saccomandi G (2012). Automated estimation of collagen fibre dispersion in the dermis and its contribution to the anisotropic behaviour of skin, *Ann Biomed Eng*, **40**, 1666–1678.

31. Tonge TK, Voo LM, and Nguyen TD (2013). Full-field bulge test for planar anisotropic tissues: Part II—A thin shell method for determining material parameters and comparison of two distributed fiber modeling approaches, *Acta Biomater*, **9**, 5926–5942.

32. Weiss JA, Maker BN, and Govindjee S (1996). Finite element implementation of incompressible transversely isotropic hyperelasticity, *Comput Meth Appl Mech Eng*, **135**, 107–128.

33. Groves RB, Coulman SA, Birchall JC, and Evans SL (2013). An anisotropic, hyperelastic model for skin: experimental measurements, finite element modelling and identification of parameters for human and murine skin, *J Mech Behav Biomed Mater*, **18**, 167–180.

34. Bischoff JE, Arruda EA, and Grosh K (2002). A microstructurally based orthotropic hyperelastic constitutive law, *J Appl Mech*, **69**, 570–579.

35. Arruda EM and Boyce MC (1993). A three-dimensional constitutive model for the large stretch behavior of rubber elastic-materials, *J Mech Phys Solids*, **41**, 389–412.

36. Bischoff JE, Arruda EM, and Grosh K (2000). Finite element modeling of human skin using an isotropic, nonlinear elastic constitutive model, *J Biomech*, **33**, 645–652.

37. Flynn C and McCormack BAO (2008). Finite element modelling of forearm skin wrinkling, *Skin Res Technol*, **14**, 261–269.

38. Flynn C and McCormack BAO (2008). A simplified model of scar contraction, *J Biomech*, **41**, 1582–1589.

39. Flynn CO and McCormack BAO. (2010). Simulating the wrinkling and aging of skin with a multi-layer finite element model, *J Biomech*, **43**, 442–448.

40. Kuhl E, Garikipati K, Arruda E, and Grosh K (2005). Remodeling of biological tissue: mechanically induced reorientation of a transversely isotropic chain network, *J Mech Phys Solids*, **53**, 1552–1573.

41. Lanir Y and Fung YC (1972). Two-dimensional mechanical properties of rabbit skin—II: experimental results, *J Biomech*, **7**, 171–182.

42. Flynn C, Rubin MB, and Nielsen P (2011). A model for the anisotropic response of fibrous soft tissues using six discrete fibre bundles, *Int J Numer Meth Bio*, **27**, 1793–1811.

43. Ankersen J, Birkbeck AE, Thomson RD, and Vanezis P (1999). Puncture resistance and tensile strength of skin simulants, in *Proceedings of the Institution of Mechanical Engineers Part H-Journal of Engineering in Medicine*, **213**, pp. 493–501.

44. Flynn C and Rubin MB (2012). An anisotropic discrete fibre model based on a generalised strain invariant with application to soft biological tissues, *Int J Eng Sci*, **60**, 66–76.

45. Limbert G and Middleton J (2005). A polyconvex anisotropic strain energy function. Application to soft tissue mechanics, in *ASME Summer Bioengineering Conference*, Vail.

46. Itskov M, Ehret AE, and Mavrilas D (2006). A polyconvex anisotropic strain-energy function for soft collagenous tissues, *Biomech Model Mechanobiol*, **5**, 17–26.

47. Itskov M and Aksel N (2004). A class of orthotropic and transversely isotropic hyperelastic constitutive models based on a polyconvex strain energy function, *Int J Solids Struct*, **41**, 3833–3848.

48. Bischoff JE, Arruda EM, and Grosh K (2002). Finite element simulations of orthotropic hyperelasticity, *Finite Elem Anal Des*, **38**, 983–998.

49. Lu J and Zhang L (2005). Physically motivated invariant formulation for transversely isotropic hyperelasticity, *Int J Solids Struct*, **42**, 6015–6031.

50. Kratky O and Porod G (1949). Röntgenuntersuchungen gelöster Fadenmoleküle, *Recueil des Travaux Chimiques des Pays-Bas et de la Belgique*, **68**, 1106–1122.

51. Korelc J, Šolinc U, and Wriggers P. (2010). An improved EAS brick element for finite deformation, *Comput Mech*, **46**, 641–659.

52. Gautieri A, Vesentini S, Redaelli A, and Buehler MJ (2011). Hierarchical structure and nanomechanics of collagen microfibrils from the atomic scale up, *Nano Lett*, **11**, 757–766.

53. Sun YL, Luo ZP, Fertala A, and An KN (2002). Direct quantification of the flexibility of type I collagen monomer, *Biochem Biophys Res Commun*, **295**, 382–386.

54. Barbenel JC and Evans JH (1973). The time-dependent mechanical properties of skin, *J Invest Dermatol*, **69**, 165–172.

55. Pereira JM, Mansour JM, and Davis BR (1990). Analysis of shear-wave propagation in skin—application to an experimental procedure, *J Biomech*, **23**, 745–751.

56. Pereira JM, Mansour JM, and Davis BR (1991). Dynamic measurement of the viscoelastic properties of skin, *J Biomech*, **24**, 157–162.

57. Lanir Y (1979). The rheological behavior of the skin: experimental results and a structural model, *Biorheology*, **16**, 191–202.

58. Wu JZ, Cutlip RG, Welcome D, and Dong RG (2006). Estimation of the viscous properties of skin and subcutaneous tissue in uniaxial stress relaxation tests, *Bio-Med Mater Eng*, **16**, 53–66.

59. Khatyr F, Imberdis C, Vescovo P, Varchon D, and Lagarde J-M (2004). Model of the viscoelastic behaviour of skin in vivo and study of anisotropy, *Skin Res Technol*, **10**, 96–103.

60. Boyer G, Laquieze L, Le Bot A, Laquieze S, and Zahouani H (2009). Dynamic indentation on human skin in vivo: ageing effects, *Skin Res Technol*, **15**, 55–67.

61. Boyer G, Zahouani H, Le BA, and Laquieze L (2007). In vivo characterization of viscoelastic properties of human skin using dynamic micro-indentation, in *Annual International Conference of the IEEE Engineering in Medicine and Biology Society, Vols 1–16*, pp. 4584–4587.

62. Lokshin O and Lanir Y (2009). Viscoelasticity and preconditioning of rat skin under uniaxial stretch: microstructural constitutive characterization, *J Biomech Eng*, **131**, 031009–031010.

63. Lokshin O and Lanir Y (2009). Micro and macro rheology of planar tissues, *Biomaterials*, **30**, 3118–3127.

64. Ehret A (2011). Generalised concepts for constitutive modelling of soft biological tissues, *PhD Thesis RWTH Aachen University*, pp. 1–230.

65. Fung YC (1973). Biorheology of soft tissues, *Biorheology*, **10**, 139–155.

66. Bischoff J (2006). Reduced parameter formulation for incorporating fiber level viscoelasticity into tissue level biomechanical models, *Ann Biomed Eng*, **34**, 1164–1172.

67. Pioletti DP, Rakotomanana LR, Benvenuti JF, and Leyvraz PF (1998). Viscoelastic constitutive law in large deformations: application to human knee ligaments and tendons, *J Biomech*, **31**, 753–757.

68. Coleman BD and Noll W (1961). Foundations of linear viscoelasticity, *Rev Mod Phys*, **3**, 239–249.

69. Limbert G (2004). Development of an advanced computational model for the simulation of damage to human skin, in *Cardiff: Welsh Development Agency (Technology and Innovation Division)—FIRST Numerics Ltd.*, pp. 1–95.

70. Limbert G and Middleton J (2004). A transversely isotropic viscohyperelastic material: application to the modelling of biological soft connective tissues, *Int J Solids Struct*, **41**, 4237–4260.

71. Limbert G and Middleton J (2005). An anisotropic viscohyperelastic constitutive model of the posterior cruciate ligament suitable for high loading-rate situations, in *IUTAM Symposium on Impact Biomechanics: from Fundamental Insights to Applications*, Dublin, pp. 1–8.

72. Reese S and Govindjee S (1998). A theory of finite viscoelasticity and numerical aspects, *Int J Solids Struct*, **35**, 3455–3482.

73. Bischoff JE, Arruda EM, and Grosh K (2004). A rheological network model for the continuum anisotropic and viscoelastic behavior of soft tissue, *Biomech Model Mechanobiol*, **3**, 56–65.

74. Vassoler JM, Reips L, and Fancello EA (2012). A variational framework for fiber-reinforced viscoelastic soft tissues, *Int J Numer Meth Eng*, **89**, 1691–1706.

75. Holzapfel GA and Gasser TC (2001). A viscoelastic model for fiber-reinforced composites at finite strains: continuum basis, computational aspects and applications, *Comput Meth Appl Mech Eng*, **190**, 4379–4403.

76. Pena E, Calvo B, Martinez MA, and Doblare M (2007). An anisotropic visco-hyperelastic model for ligaments at finite strains. Formulation and computational aspects, *Int J Solids Struct*, **44**, 760–778.

77. Pena E, Calvo B, Martinez MA, and Doblare M (2008). On finite-strain damage of viscoelastic-fibred materials. Application to soft biological tissues, *Int J Numer Meth Eng*, **74**, 1198–1218.

78. Ehret AE, Itskov M, and Weinhold GW (2009). A micromechanically motivated model for the viscoelastic behaviour of soft biological tissues at large strains, *Nuovo Cimento C*, **32**, 73–80.

79. Simo JC (1987). On a fully three-dimensional finite-strain viscoelastic damage model: formulation and computational aspects, *Comput Meth Appl Mech Eng*, **60**, 153–173.

80. Muñoz MJ, Bea JA, Rodríguez JF, Ochoa I, Grasa J, Pérez del Palomar A, Zaragoza P, Osta R, and Doblaré M (2008). An experimental study of the mouse skin behaviour: damage and inelastic aspects, *J Biomech*, **41**, 93–99.

81. Edsberg LE, Mates RE, Baier RE, and Lauren M (1999). Mechanical characteristics of human skin subjected to static versus cyclic normal presures, *J Rehabil Res Dev*, **36**, 133–141.

82. Ehret AE and Itskov M (2009). Modeling of anisotropic softening phenomena: application to soft biological tissues, *Int J Plast*, **25**, 901–919.

83. Ehret AE, Hollenstein M, Mazza E, and Itskov M (2011). Porcine dermis in uniaxial cyclic loading: sample preparation, experimental results and modeling, *J Mech Mater Struct*, **6**, 1125–1135.

84. Mazza E, Papes O, Rubin MB, Bodner SR, and Binur NS (2005). Nonlinear elastic-viscoplastic constitutive equations for aging facial tissues, *Biomech Model Mechanobiol*, **4**, 178–189.

85. Mazza E, Papes O, Rubin MB, Bodner SR, and Binur NS (2007). Simulation of the aging face, *J Biomech Eng*, **129**, 619–623.

86. Rubin MB and Bodner SR (2002). A three-dimensional nonlinear model for dissipative response of soft tissue, *Int J Solids Struct*, **39**, 5081–5099.

87. Neumann CG. (1959). The expansion of an arrea of skin by progressive distension of a subcutaneous balloon; us eo fthe method for securing skin for subtotal reconstruction of the ear, *Plast Reconstr Surg*, **19**, 124–130.

88. Socci L, Pennati G, Gervaso F, and Vena P (2007). An axisymmetric computational model of skin expansion and growth, *Biomech Model Mechanobiol*, **6**, 177–188.

89. Tepole AB, Ploch CJ, Wong J, Gosain AK, and Kuhl E (2011). Growing skin: a computational model for skin expansion in reconstructive surgery, *J Mech Phys Solids*, **59**, 2177–2190.

90. Kuhl E and Steinmann P (2003). Theory and numerics of geometrically non-linear open system mechanics, *Int J Numer Meth Eng*, **58**, 1593–1615.

91. Rodriguez EK, Hoger A, and McCulloch AD (1994). Stress-dependent finite growth in soft elastic tissues, *J Biomech*, **27**, 455–467.

92. Lubarda VA and Hoger A (2002). On the mechanics of solids with a growing mass, *Int J Solids Struct*, **39**, 4627–4664.

93. Taber LA (1995). Biomechanics of growth, remodeling and morphogenesis, *Appl Mech Rev*, **48**, 487–545.

94. Menzel A and Kuhl E (2012). Frontiers in growth and remodeling, *Mech Res Commun*, **42**, 1–14.

95. Tepole AB, Gosain AK, and Kuhl E (2012). Stretching skin: the physiological limit and beyond, *Int J Non-Linear Mech*, **47**, 938–949.

96. Zollner A, Tepole AB, Gosain AK, and Kuhl E (2012). Growing skin: tissue expansion in pediatric forehead reconstruction, *Biomech Model Mechanobiol*, **11**, 855–867.

97. Zöllner AM, Holland MA, Honda KS, Gosain AK, and Kuhl E (2013). Growth on demand: reviewing the mechanobiology of stretched skin, *J Mech Behav Biomed Mater*, **28**, 495–509.

98. Zollner AM, Tepole AB, and Kuhl E (2012). On the biomechanics and mechanobiology of growing skin, *J Theor Biol*, **297**, 166–175.

99. Zöllner AM, Holland MA, Honda KS, Gosain AK, and Kuhl E (2013). Growth on demand: Reviewing the mechanobiology of stretched skin. *J Mech Behav Biomed Mater*, **28**, 495–509.

100. GenzerJ and Groenewold J (2006). Soft matter with hard skin: From skin wrinkles to templating and material characterization, *Soft Matter*, **2**, 310–323.

101. Hatzis, J. (2004). The wrinkle and its measurement—a skin surface profilometric method, *Micron*, **35**, 201–219.

102. Piérard GE, Uhoda I, and Piérard-Franchimont C (2004). From skin microrelief to wrinkles. An area ripe for investigation, *J Cosm Derm*, **2**, 21–28.

103. Piérard-Franchimont C, and Piérard GE (1987). Assessment of aging and actinic damages by cyanocrylate skin surface strippings, *Am J Dermopathol*, **9**, 500–509.

104. Lévêque J-L (1999). EEMCO guidance for the assessment of skin topography, *J Eur Acad Derm Vener*, **12**, 103–114.

105. Piérard GE, Hermanns JF, and Lapière CH (1974). Stéréologie de l'interface dermo-épidermique, *Dermatologica*, **149**, 266–273.

106. Cavicchi A, Gambarotta L, and Massabo R (2009). Computational modeling of reconstructive surgery: the effects of the natural tension on skin wrinkling, *Finite Elem Anal Des*, **45**, 519–529.

107. Cerda E (2005). Mechanics of scars, *J Biomech*, **38**, 1598–1603.

108. Evans SL (2009). On the implementation of a wrinkling, hyperelastic membrane model for skin and other materials, *Comput Meth Biomech Biomed Eng*, **12**, 319–332.

109. FlynnCO and McCormack BAO (2009). A three-layer model of skin and its application in simulating wrinkling, *Comput Meth Biomech Biomed Eng*, **12**, 125–134.

110. Magnenat-ThalmannN, Kalra P, Lévêque J-L, Bazin R, Batisse D, and Querleux B (2002). A computational skin model: fold and wrinkle formation, *IEEE Trans Inf Technol Biomed*, **6**, 317–323.

111. Wu Y, Kalra P, Moccozet L, and Magnenat-Thalmann N (1999). Simulating wrinkles and skin aging, *Visual Comp*, **15**, 183–198.

112. Sopher R and Gefen A (2011). Effects of skin wrinkles, age and wetness on mechanical loads in the stratum corneum as related to skin lesions, *Med Biol Eng Comput*, **49**, 97–105.

113. Lévêque J-L and Audoly B (2013). Influence of Stratum Corneum on the entire skin mechanical properties, as predicted by a computational skin model, *Skin Res Technol*, **19**, 42–46.

114. LimbertG (2010). Dynamic skin wrinkles: geometry or mechanics? A probabilistic finite element approach, in *STLE/ASME 2010 International Joint Tribology Conference*, San Francisco.

115. LimbertG, Bryan R, Cotton R, Young P, Hall-Stoodley L, Kathju S, and Stoodley P (2013). On the mechanics of bacterial biofilms on non-dissolvable surgical sutures: a laser scanning confocal microscopy-based finite element study, *Acta Biomater*, **9**, 6641–6652.

116. YoungPG, Beresford-West TBH, Coward SRL, Notarberardino B, Walker B, and Abdul-Aziz A (2008). An efficient approach to converting three-dimensional image data into highly accurate computational models, *Philos T R Soc A*, **366**, 3155–3173.

117. Forrester A, Sobester A, and Keane A (eds) (2008). *Engineering Design via Surrogate Modelling: A Practical Guide*, John Wiley & Sons, Chichester, UK.

118. Buehler MJ (2006). Large-scale hierarchical molecular modeling of nanostructured biological materials, *J Comput Theor Nanos*, **3**, 603–623.

119. Rim JE, Pinsky PM, and van Osdol WW. (2005). Finite element modeling of coupled diffusion with partitioning in transdermal drug delivery, *Ann Biomed Eng*, **33**, 1422–1438.

120. RimJE, Pinsky PM, and van Osdol WW (2007). Using the method of homogenization to calculate the effective diffusivity of the stratum corneum, *J Membr Sci*, **293**, 174–182.

121. RimJE, Pinsky PM, and van Osdol WW (2008). Using the method of homogenization to calculate the effective diffusivity of the stratum corneum with permeable corneocytes, *J Biomech*, **41**, 788–796.

122. RimJE, Pinsky PM, and van Osdol WW (2009). Multiscale Modeling Framework of Transdermal Drug Delivery, *Ann Biomed Eng*, **37**, 1217–1229.

# Chapter 5

# Fiber-Matrix Models of the Dermis

**Cormac Flynn**

*The Centre for Engineering and Industrial Design,*
*Waikato Institute of Technology, Hamilton 3240, New Zealand*

Cormac.Flynn@wintec.ac.nz

This chapter presents a review of fiber-matrix models that have been used to simulate the mechanical response of the dermis. It summarizes the physical and mechanical properties of the dermis. Different categories of fiber-matrix models are presented. These include structurally based models that represent the orientation and undulation of collagen fibers using probability density functions; models that represent the collagen fiber undulation in a phenomenological sense using exponential functions; eight-chain non-Gaussian network models; and, more recently, discrete-fiber icosahedral models. The ability of each model type to simulate experimental data is discussed, as well as the strengths and weaknesses of each approach. The chapter concludes with a discussion on the experimental protocols that are needed to validate and further develop physical fiber-matrix models of the dermis.

## 5.1  Introduction

Computational models of the dermis are being increasingly used to further knowledge in a broad range of disciplines. These include

*Computational Biophysics of the Skin*
Edited by Bernard Querleux
Copyright © 2014 Pan Stanford Publishing Pte. Ltd.
ISBN 978-981-4463-84-3 (Hardcover), 978-981-4463-85-0 (eBook)
www.panstanford.com

improving the design of consumer personal care products [1], the design of transdermal drug delivery devices [2], and improving the design of surgical incisions for better wound healing [3,4].

Constitutive models of the dermis can be broadly divided into two categories. The first category consists of phenomenological models, which are based on observed behavior only and have no direct physical connection with the underlying mechanism responsible for that behavior. Some phenomenological models are mathematically simple and therefore straightforward to implement [5,6]. However the parameters of these models tend to have little physical meaning. The form of the model can also change depending on the type of test and the material being tested and so phenomenological models may not accurately represent the material in reality under all conditions such as a uniaxial model by Ridge and Wright [7].

The other category consists of physical models, which attempt to establish a connection between the microstructure of the dermis and its mechanical behavior. The material parameters in a physical model are more easily identifiable and many can be measured in the laboratory [8]. The realistic basis for such models also results in better predictive capabilities than phenomenological models [9]. Therefore, physical models can be used to predict changes in the mechanical response of the dermis due to aging or disease by altering the constituent properties.

This chapter is concerned with physically-based fiber-matrix constitutive models of the dermis. Firstly, a description of the physical and mechanical properties of the dermis will be presented. Secondly, a detailed overview will be given of different fiber-matrix models used to simulate the mechanical response of the dermis or whole skin. The chapter will conclude with a discussion of the experimental data needed to further develop the models.

## 5.2 Characteristics of the Dermis

### 5.2.1 Physical Components

The dermis is a dense network of collagen, reticulin, and elastin fibers imbedded in a semi-gel matrix of ground substance. Approximately 75% of the dry weight of dermal tissue consists of strong, stiff collagen fibers, while the rubber-like elastin make up 4% of the dry-weight and the semi-fluid ground substance makes up 20% of the dry-weight [10]. Only trace amounts of reticulin (about 0.4% of the dry-weight) are found in adult skin [11]. In addition, there are blood and lymph vessels, nerve endings, hair follicles, and glands within the layer. Collagen fibers are arranged in bundles ranging in diameter from 1 to 40 $\mu$m. These in turn are composed of fibrils whose mean diameter is on the order of 100 nm. Elastin fibers form a delicate scattered network lying between the collagen [12]. Unlike collagen fibers, they do not have a fibrillar substructure and range in diameter from 0.5 to 8 $\mu$m. The semi-fluid ground substance is an amorphous mass of proteoglycans and water. The water molecules are not free and are bonded by hygroscopic hyaluronic acid, which is a component of the proteoglycans [11].

The dermis is usually subdivided into two layers: the papillary dermis and the reticular dermis. The papillary dermis is thinner and lies adjacent to the epidermis. It contains a less dense distribution of elastin and collagen fibers and proportionally more of ground substance [13].

The dermis varies in thickness from 0.5 mm in the eyelid and inguinal regions to 2.0 mm in the back region [14].

## 5.2.2 Mechanical Properties

The highly non-linear stress–strain behavior of skin can be attributed in large part to the structure of the dermal layer. The non-linear behavior can be divided into three phases. The first phase is characterized by low-stiffness (Fig. 5.1). In this phase the collagen network is undulated and unaligned and does not contribute significantly to the mechanical properties. The initial low stiffness response of skin can be attributed to the elastin network [15]. In the second phase, the collagen fibers begin to align and straighten in the direction of the applied load. As a result, the stiffness of the skin increases. In the third phase, the collagen network is hypothetically aligned and straightened. Further extension of the skin requires extension of the collagen fibers. The high stiffness of the skin in this region is similar to that of pure collagen [11]. The elastic behavior of skin is facilitated by the elastin network, which provides a return spring mechanism for the collagen [15]. This property varies with age [16].

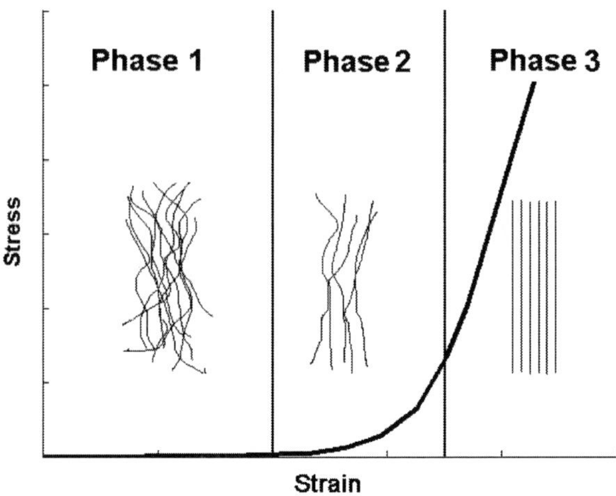



**Figure 5.1** Typical stress–strain response of dermis. Phase 1: The collagen fibers are not carrying load. Phase 2: Some fibers are straight and are starting to carry load. Phase 3: Most of the fibers are straight and are carrying the load.

The dermis in general is an anisotropic material—its behavior is direction-dependent. Dupuytren [17] first investigated the directional effects in skin. Langer [18] punctured the skin of cadavers with conically pointed instruments and found elliptical splits were produced. The lines of the major axes of these slits are known as Langer Lines. The skin's mechanical anisotropy follows the same pattern of Langer Lines and stretches the least in the direction of the lines. It has been concluded that the collagen and elastin fibers form an irregular multidirectional system in which there is a preferential orientation in the lines' direction [10,19]. When a sample is stretched in the direction of minimum extensibility the fiber networks align along the load axis at lower strains [11].

The mechanical properties of the dermis are time-dependent. Lanir and Fung [20] have shown the viscoelastic nature of skin with significant hysteresis loops in stress–strain relations. Flynn et al. [21,22] and Wan Abas [23] demonstrated significant in vivo viscoelastic characteristics in human forearm and facial skin. Viscoelastic effects in skin are very noticeable for strains corresponding to the region when collagen fibers are carrying part of the load [15] although Pereira et al. [24] report that viscoelastic effects are also present in the large strain–low stress region.

Individual collagen fibrils also exhibit viscoelasticity through the unwinding of collagen fibril and collagen molecules sliding relative to each other [25]. However, the relaxation times of these mechanisms are much shorter than for whole dermis or skin so other mechanisms at the tissue level must dominate [25,26]. The viscoelastic response of skin has been attributed in part to the relative movement between the alignable collagen network and the ground substance in the dermis [11].

It is known that soft tissues subject to successive cyclic tests yield different results over the first few cycles, but the results converge as the number of cycles increase. This phenomenon is known as preconditioning and several experimental studies have shown this behavior in skin [20,21,23,27]. Preconditioning in skin can be attributable to the collagen fibers in the dermis orientating and changing their gage length in response to the cyclical load. Also, the stiffness of the elastin fibers decreases [8]. Eventually, after a number of cycles, a steady state is reached where no further changes take place unless the upper or lower limits of the cycling are changed [28].

## 5.2.3   In vivo Tension

The skin on the human body is normally in a state of tension. Langer's experiments [18] mentioned in Section 5.2.2 demonstrate the existence of an anisotropic tension field in the skin. The tension field results in a good fit of the skin on the human body with appropriate wrinkling occurring to allow free movement of the joints. The magnitude of the tension field is dependent on many factors including site, body position, and age of the individual [10]. Estimates of the in vivo tension range widely from 1.7 N/m to 138 N/m [29], [22,30–32]. According to Silver et al. [33], the level of in vivo tension varies from region to region in order to regulate extracellular matrix metabolism through mechanochemical transduction.

Whatever the reasons and causes of the in vivo tension in skin, knowledge of its level is important as it allows us to determine the stress-free configuration of the soft tissue [34]. Inclusion of this quantity is essential when determining the material parameters of constitutive models from in vivo skin deformation data [22,32,35,36].

## 5.3  Computational Fiber-Matrix Dermis Models

What follows are descriptions of constitutive models that have been used to simulate the mechanical response of the dermis. Many of the models were developed for simulating other fibrous soft tissues but were subsequently used to model the dermis. Most of the models were tested by fitting them to various experimental tensile testing data of whole skin. It has been assumed that the dermis dominates the tensile response of skin and that the contribution of the epidermis is negligible [7]. The models are sorted into different subsections according to their principal characteristics. A selection of the models is summarized in Table 5.1.

**Table 5.1**    Selection of fiber-matrix models of the dermis

| Model | Characteristics modeled | Comments |
|---|---|---|
| Lanir [38] | Non-linear elasticity, anisotropy, viscoelasticity | Dermis response is the sum of its constituent responses; Fibers are thin and perfectly flexible; Only straightened undulated collagen fibers resist load; Simulated forearm and porcine skin [39,40]; Computationally intensive |
| Shoemaker et al. [43] | Non-linear elasticity, orthotropy, viscoelasticity | Similar to [38]; Stress due to sum of compliant and stiff fibrous parts; Linear viscoelastic law; Stretching of human skin; Phenomenological parameters |
| Lokshin and Lanir [8] | Non-linear elasticity, anisotropy, viscoelasticity, pre-conditioning (PC) | Similar to [38]; Collagen fiber PC due to increase in reference gage length; Elastin fiber PC due to Mullins effect; Biaxial stretching of rabbit skin; 31 parameters |
| Gasser et al. [9] | Non-linear elasticity, anisotropy | Collagen fibers dispersed about two preferred orientations; Collagen fibers represented by exponential functions; Simulated stretching of human skin [19] |

| Model | Characteristics modeled | Comments |
| --- | --- | --- |
| Arruda and Boyce [50] | Non-linear elasticity, isotropy | Unit cubic cell with eight collagen fibers; Strain energy of fiber based on non-Gaussian statistics; Simulated in vivo and in vitro skin tests [35] |
| Bischoff et al. [53] | Non-linear elasticity, orthotropy | Similar to [50] but with orthotropic unit cell; Simulated stretching of rabbit skin |
| Bischoff et al. [54] | Non-linear, anisotropy, viscoelasticity | As [53] but with two cells in parallel and one viscoelastic component; Viscoelasticity modeled using reptation dynamics theory; 14 material parameters |
| Bischoff et al. [60] | Non-linear, orthotropic, viscoelastic | One cell as in [53]; Viscoelasticity modeled at the fiber level using QLV; Simulated stress relaxation of porcine skin; 7 material parameters |
| Limbert [63] | Non-linear elasticity, orthotropy | Worm-like chain model represents collagen; Multi-scale model; Decoupled shear interactions; 23 parameters |
| Flynn et al. [68] | Non-linear, anisotropic | 6 weighted fibers oriented within a regular icosahedron; Analytical distribution functions simulate undulated fibers; Simulated stretching of rabbit and pig skin; 11 material parameters; Undesirable anisotropy |
| Flynn and Rubin [70] | Non-linear elasticity, anisotropy | Discrete fiber model based on generalized strain invariant Unambiguous interpretation of anisotropy |

## 5.3.1 Statistical Distribution Models

One of the earliest structural models of skin was proposed by Lanir [37,38]. The model considers skin as a collection of collagen and elastin fibers embedded in a ground matrix. The fiber orientations within the matrix are represented by a distribution function $R_k(\theta)$ ($k$ indicates fiber type), which typically takes the form of a Von Mises distribution [39].

The collagen fibers are assumed to be undulated and can only resist loads when fully straightened and they buckle under compressive loads. The undulations of the collagen fibers oriented in the direction $\theta$ are not equal. The distribution of undulations is assumed to follow a Gaussian profile $D(x)$, where $x$ is the stretch required to straighten an undulated fiber. The Cauchy stress–strain relation for the fiber and matrix composite is given by

$$\sigma = J^{-1} \sum_k V_k \int_0^\pi \left( R_k(\theta) f_k^*(\lambda) \mathbf{F} \frac{\partial \lambda}{\partial \mathbf{E}} \mathbf{F}^\mathrm{T} \right) d\theta - p\mathbf{I}, \tag{5.1}$$

where $\mathbf{F}$ is the deformation gradient, $J = \det(\mathbf{F})$ is the ratio of deformed to undeformed volume, $V_k$ is the volume fraction of fiber type $k$, $f_k^*(\lambda)$ is the force per unit undeformed cross sectional area of an individual fiber at stretch $\lambda$, $\mathbf{E} = \frac{1}{2}(\mathbf{F}^\mathrm{T}\mathbf{F} - \mathbf{I})$ is the Green strain tensor, and $p$ is a hydrostatic pressure representing the response of the ground matrix. For collagen fibers, $f_c^*(\lambda)$ accounts for the undulations

$$f_c^*(\lambda) = \int_1^\lambda D(x) f_c\left(\frac{\lambda}{x}\right) dx, \tag{5.2}$$

where $f_k(\lambda)$ is the force per unit undeformed cross sectional area of an individual fiber. The fibers are generally considered linear elastic with the force given by

$$f_k(\lambda) = K_k(\lambda - 1), \quad \lambda \geq 1$$
$$f_k(\lambda) = 0, \quad \text{otherwise} \tag{5.3}$$

where $K_k$ is the fiber stiffness. The elastin fibers do not have any undulation so $f_e^*(\lambda) = f_e(\lambda)$.

Lanir [37,38] did not evaluate the model by testing its ability to simulate soft tissue deformations. Meijer et al. [40] characterized the in-plane mechanical properties of human forearm skin using a combined numerical-experimental approach. The skin was represented by the Lanir [38] constitutive model. By measuring the force on extensometer tabs and the displacement field of the area of interest, they estimated some of the Lanir [38] material parameters that best fit the numerical model to the experimental results. The parameters estimated were the collagen fiber stiffness, the mean undulation of the collagen fibers, and two parameters that describe the distribution of the collagen fibers. Other parameters were fixed at values specified in the literature. The estimated parameters were within the range of previously reported values. They conclude that the applied strains in the experiments were not high enough to engage a sufficient portion of the collagen fibers. Therefore, the calculated collagen fiber stiffness (ranging from 51 MPa to 86 MPa) was not as accurate as other calculated parameters.

Jor et al. [39] used the Lanir [38] model within a finite element framework to characterize porcine skin samples under equi-biaxial tension. Using non-linear optimization techniques, a sub-set of the material parameters that best fit the model to experimental results was determined. The ground matrix stiffness ranged from 5 kPa to 32 kPa, the collagen fiber stiffness ranged from 48 MPa to 366 MPa, and the mean orientation of the fibers was from 2° to 13° from the torso mid-line, which are consistent to experimental measurements. The authors commented on the difficulty of optimizing the material parameters. Multiple parameter-sets with similar error levels were determined demonstrating that the experimental data was not sufficient to determine unique parameter-sets. A priori knowledge of the orientation of the collagen fibers would help greatly in parameter identification as the optimization procedure was most sensitive to this parameter.

Belkof and Haut [41] used some aspects of the Lanir [38] model to simulate the mechanical response of rat skin. The proposed uniaxial model assumes the collagen fibers are all arranged in the same direction. A similar fiber undulation model as Lanir [38] is used. The model is limited to uniaxial deformations. They determined the collagen fiber stiffnesses, and means and standard deviations of the fiber undulation of rat skin of different ages and orientations under uniaxial extension.

Manschot and Brakkee [42] took a similar simplified approach and developed a uniaxial model, which assumed all the collagen fibers were aligned. Unlike Lanir [38], they assumed that the more undulated a collagen fiber is the more stress is needed to straighten it. The undulated collagen fibers are also assumed to have a sinusoidal waveform. The three parameters of the model represented the collagen fiber stiffness, fibril corrugation, and a strain value at which the fiber becomes straight. Values for these parameters were determined that best-fit the model to in vivo uniaxial extensometer tests of human calf skin.

A structural model similar to Lanir [38] was proposed by Shoemaker et al. [43]. It was assumed that the stress in the soft tissue was due to the sum of compliant and stiff fibrous components in the tissue. The compliant component was assumed to depend on strain rate components. Both the compliant and stiff fibrous components were characterized with a linear viscoelastic law, which was specified by a relaxation function. The distribution function describing the orientation of the stiff fibers was simplified as a constant. While the foundations of the model are structural, the nine material parameters cannot be directly related to physical properties of the dermis and so are phenomenological in nature. Experimental biaxial tests on human skin were fitted to the model with limited success. One deficiency was that the model tended to predict a more abrupt change in slope at the "elbow" region of the stress–strain curve compared with the experimental data.

Lokshin and Lanir [8] developed a micro-structural model that encompassed the non-linear, anisotropic, viscoelastic, and pre-conditioning characteristics of skin. The model is similar to Lanir's earlier model [38] in that it assumes the skin is a collection of fibers arranged in a ground matrix and the tissue response is the sum of the responses of its constituent parts. The response of the tissue at low strains is dominated by the elastin, while both the elastin and collagen networks contribute at higher strains. Both networks are also assumed to be quasi-linear viscoelastic with each characterized by a normalized bi-exponential relaxation function. Preconditioning is represented in the elastin and collagen fiber networks using two different mechanisms. For the collagen fibers, their gage length increases under repeated cycling, while for the elastin fibers, preconditioning is due to a reduction in the elastic stiffness (known as the Mullins effect).

There are 31 material parameters in total for the model, which is obviously a major challenge to determine for a particular skin sample. The descriptive and predictive power of the model was evaluated using a series of biaxial rabbit skin tests [20]. A good model-to-data-fit was obtained using a single set of parameters and the entire test protocol. There was a relatively low variance in the parameter values for different skin samples—a feature that is characteristic of structural models according to Lokshin and Lanir [8]. A parsimony analysis determined that most of the material parameters were significant. In particular, the collagen non-linear elasticity, viscoelasticity, undulation, and pre-conditioning characteristics were the most significant of parameters. The least significant parameter was the non-linear elasticity of the elastin.

### 5.3.2  Structural Models with Phenomenological Uncrimping Representations

Representing the uncrimping of the collagen fibers with statistical distribution functions as done in Section 5.3.1 can be computationally expensive. An alternative phenomenological approach captures the unfolding of the collagen fibers using exponential laws. This makes it more efficient to implement into a finite element framework.

The Holzapfel and Gasser [44] model was developed to simulate the response of arterial layers. It considers the soft tissue to consist of collagen fibers with two preferred orientations embedded in an isotropic ground matrix. Vasoler et al. [45] used this model within a viscoelastic variational framework to simulate the uniaxial extension of mouse skin.

Gasser et al. [9] generalized these earlier models [44,46] by including the dispersion of collagen fibers about the preferred directions. The resulting strain energy density function is a superposition of the ground matrix strain energy and the collagen fiber network strain energy:

$$W = \frac{\mu}{2}(I_1 - 3) + \mu \sum_{i=1}^{2} \frac{k_{i1}}{2k_{i2}} \{\exp(k_{i2}[tr(\mathbf{H}_i\mathbf{C}) - 1]^2) - 1\}, \qquad (5.4)$$

where $\mu$ is a material parameter related to the shear modulus of the ground matrix. $k_{i1}$ and $k_{i2}$ are dimensionless material constants related to the collagen fiber stiffness in the low strain and high strain regimes, respectively. $I_1 = tr(C)$ is the first strain invariant, and $\mathbf{H}_1$ and $\mathbf{H}_2$ are structural tensors that depend on the two preferred directions of the fibers and their dispersion about those directions.

Ní Annaidh et al. [19] characterized human cadaveric skin samples using Eq. 5.4. They performed histological analyses of different skin samples taken from human cadavers to determine the preferred fiber directions and their dispersions assuming a Von Mises distribution. Performing uniaxial tension tests on some of the samples, optimized values for $\mu$, $k_{i1}$, and $k_{i2}$ were determined. The model accurately simulated the uniaxial extension of the skin samples ($R^2 = 99.5\%$) and also predicted the lateral response of some samples with good accuracy ($R^2 = 98\%$).

Groves et al. [47] recently simulated the uniaxial tensile testing of in vitro skin using a combination of a transversely isotropic constitutive law representing the fiber response [48] and an isotropic phenomenological law representing the ground matrix [49]. Weiss et al. [48] developed their model specifically for ligaments, tendons, and cardiac muscle, where the collagen fibers are aligned in one direction with little dispersion. An exponential law modeled the uncrimping of those fibers. Veronda and Westmann [49] developed the isotropic exponential model to simulate the uniaxial response of whole cat skin. While Groves et al. [47] obtained a good fit between the experimental results and the simulation results, three layers of elements were required—each assigned to one of three fiber families to characterize skin's anisotropy. This resulted in a model with 14 material parameters, which is considerable for a model that ignores the viscoelastic characteristics of skin.

### 5.3.3  Eight-Chain Non-Gaussian Network Models

Arruda and Boyce [50] introduced a constitutive model to mechanically characterize elastomers, which was adopted by Bischoff et al. [35] to simulate the stress–stretch behavior of human skin. The model consists of a unit cubic cell, which contains eight collagen fibers linked at the centre and extending to each corner

(Fig. 5.2). Each collagen fiber is modeled as a number of freely-joined links. Using non-Gaussian statistical approaches, an expression for the strain energy of the collagen network is given by

$$W = nk\theta\sqrt{N}\left(\lambda_c\beta_r + \ln\frac{\beta_r}{\sinh\beta_r}\right),$$ (5.5)

where $n$ is the collagen fiber density, $k$ is Boltzmann's constant, $\theta$ is the absolute temperature, $N$ is the free length of the collagen fibers, $\lambda_c$ is the chain stretch, and $\beta$ is the inverse Langevin function. The Langevin function is defined as $L(x) = \coth(x) - (1/x)$.

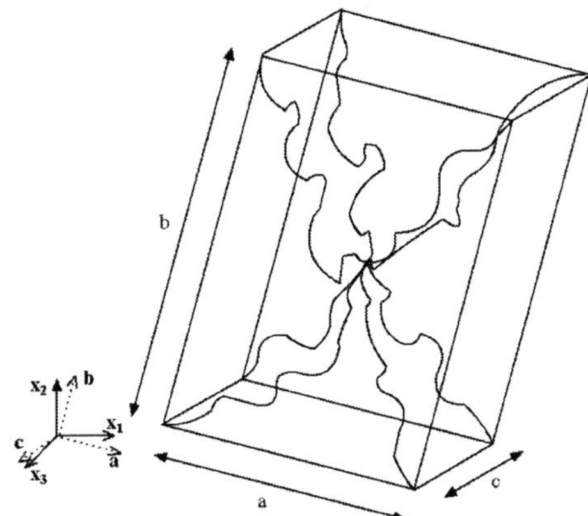


**Figure 5.2**    Eight-chain, three-dimensional unit cell. For the Arruda and Boyce model $a = b = c$; for the Bischoff et al. model, the unit cell dimensions are, in general, unequal.

Model parameter sets were determined that best-fit several experimental tests on skin. In vitro uniaxial tests of normal and scarred human skin [51] were simulated with good accuracy. The predictive capabilities of the model were demonstrated by simulating in vitro uniaxial tensile tests on rat skin in different directions [41]. The isotropic model also provided an estimate of 51 kPa for the maximum in vivo tension in human skin from uniaxial tests [52].

While Bischoff et al. [35] demonstrated that the isotropic Arruda-Boyce model can simulate the anisotropic response of skin by using an anisotropic pre-stress field; it could not simulate the orthotropic characteristics of skin in general such as the biaxial tests of rabbit skin by Lanir and Fung [20]. Bischoff et al. [53] further developed the eight-chain model to characterize the orthotropic behavior of skin. They considered an orthotropic unit cell with unequal dimensions, *a*, *b*, and *c* fixed in space as specified by the orthogonal principal material axes **a**, **b**, and **c** (Fig. 5.2). The collagen fibers are represented in a similar manner to Bischoff et al. [35], while further strain energy terms representing the mutual repulsion of the fibers and the almost incompressible nature of the dermis are added. The strain energy per unit volume is given by

$$W(x) = W_0 + \frac{nk\theta}{4}\left[ N\sum_i^4 \left( \frac{\rho^{(i)}}{N}\beta_\rho^{(i)} + \ln\frac{\beta_\rho^{(i)}}{\sinh\beta_\rho^{(i)}} \right) - \frac{\beta_\rho}{P}\ln\left(\lambda_a^{a^2}\lambda_b^{b^2}\lambda_c^{c^2}\right) \right]$$ (5.6)
$$+ B\{\cosh(J-1)-1\},$$

where $W_0$ is a constant, $\rho^{(i)}$ is the deformed fiber length, $P = \sqrt{a^2 + b^2 + c^2}/2$ is the normalized undeformed fiber length, $\lambda_i = \sqrt{\mathbf{i}^\mathbf{T}\mathbf{Ci}}$, (where $i = a, b, c$), and $B$ is the bulk modulus of skin.

The model simulated the in vitro biaxial extension of rabbit skin with an error of 15.5% (Fig. 5.3).

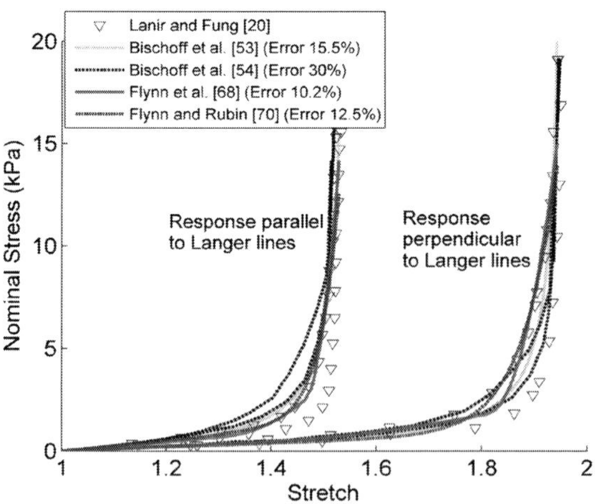


**Figure 5.3**    Simulation of biaxial stretching of rabbit-skin.

Viscoelasticity has been incorporated into the orthotropic eight-chain model using a couple of approaches. Bischoff et al. [54]

considered two parallel fiber networks—one network representing the collagen fibers that are in equilibrium and the other representing a portion of collagen fibers that are realigning themselves with time in the ground substance. Each network consists of an orthotropic unit cell with the strain energy of each described by Eq. 5.2. Viscoelasticity is modeled by using reptation dynamics, a theory that was developed in polymer science, where the fibers are assumed to diffuse along their lengths. This approach was taken in a constitutive model of elastomers [55]. The model simulated the non-linear, anisotropic, and viscoelastic behavior observed in the biaxial stretch tests of Lanir and Fung [20] with an error of 30% (Fig. 5.3). Stress relaxation tests of rabbit skin were also simulated with good accuracy.

Flynn and McCormack [56,57] developed a very similar model that was used to represent the dermis in a multi-layer model of human skin. A limitation of this model is that it contains many material parameters—12 for Flynn and McCormack [58] and 15 for Bischoff et al. [54]. The goal of any constitutive model would be to accurately capture the various properties with as few parameters as possible. Bischoff et al. [54] effectively reduced the number of parameters of the orthotropic-viscoelastic model to eight by, among other things, restricting the dimensions of the unit cells of each network—$(a_A, b_A, c_A)$ and $(a_B, b_B, c_B)$—to be equal to each other. They fitted the model to a biaxial stretch test of rabbit skin [20] with an error of about 30%. This compares to an error of 7.6% when Flynn [59] fitted the model simultaneously to uniaxial and biaxial stretch tests of rabbit skin with no restriction on the material parameters. Therefore, the reduced parameter number comes at the expense of accuracy of fit.

Bischoff [60] proposed a seven-parameter model for soft tissues that is capable of simulating anisotropic and viscoelastic effects. The model contains the orthotropic unit cell of previous models [53,54] but viscoelasticity is incorporated at the fiber level using the theory of quasi-linear viscoelasticity (QLV) [28]. The model simulated various stress relaxation tests of porcine skin to a high accuracy (1.3% error of fit). Representing viscoelasticity in soft tissues such as skin as quasi-linear is only an abstraction in that it does not simulate any particular viscoelastic mechanism. Despite this, the approach does offer good potential for an orthotropic-viscoelastic model with minimal number of parameters.

The orthotropic eight-chain model of Bischoff et al. [53] has been used in tissue remodeling simulations [61]. In this case, the orthotropic unit cell axis gradually realigns in the direction of the maximum principal strain. The model has also been used to simulate skin that has been stretched beyond the physiological limit [62]. The applications of the model are in the area of tissue expansion, which results in extra skin growth to be used in reconstructive surgery.

The worm-like chain model for collagen fibers used in Bischoff [60] has also been used in multi-scale model proposed by Limbert [63]. The 23 parameter model decouples the volumetric, deviatoric stretches in the fiber directions, cross-fiber shear, and fiber-to-fiber or matrix-to-fiber shear stress responses. While the number of parameters is large, the decoupling allows one directly link the parameters to the particular mechanical mode considered using appropriate physical experiments. The model was tested by simulating a biaxial stretch test of rabbit skin performed by Lanir and Fung [20]. Excellent agreement between the model data and experimental data was obtained.

## 5.3.4 Discrete Fiber Icosahedral Structural Models

Many physically-based models simulate the uncrimping and engagement of the collagen fibers using a normal distribution function [37], a Lorentz function [64], or a log-logistic distribution function [65]. In order to calculate the stress–strain relationship, these functions need to be integrated, which can be computationally expensive, especially within a finite element framework [9,66,67]. Similarly, the use of distribution functions to represent the orientation of the collagen fibers within the dermis [8,9,37] can lead to prohibitively expensive integration methods.

To address this, Flynn et al. [68] proposed a discrete six-fiber model with distribution functions to model the collagen fiber undulation, which can be integrated to give analytical strain energy expressions. The six weighted fiber-bundles are each oriented such that it passes through opposing vertices of a regular icosahedron. Each fiber bundle is assumed to consist of a distribution of undulated collagen fibers in parallel with an elastin fiber. The total Cauchy stress response of the composite material is given by

$$\mathbf{T} = -p\mathbf{I} + \sum_{i=1}^{6} w_i \left( \frac{\lambda_i}{J} \rho_0 \left( \frac{dW_e(\lambda_i)}{d\lambda_i} + \frac{dW_c(\lambda_i)}{d\lambda_i} \right) \right) \left( \mathbf{s_i} \otimes \mathbf{s_i} - \frac{1}{3}\mathbf{I} \right), \quad (5.7)$$

where $W_e$ is the elastin fiber strain energy, $W_c$ is the collagen fiber strain energy, $w_{1-6}$ are the weights of the fiber bundles, and $\mathbf{s_i}$ is the deformed orientation of the $i$-th fiber bundle.

The elastin fiber strain energy is modeled using a neo-Hookean function.

Flynn et al. [68] showed that the stress of a collagen fiber bundle at stretch $\lambda$ is given by

$$\lambda \rho_0 \frac{dW_c(\lambda)}{d\lambda} = E_c \int_1^\lambda \int_1^\lambda D(x)\,dx\,d\lambda \qquad (5.8)$$

where $E_c$ is the elastic modulus of a collagen fiber and $D(x)$ is the normalized distribution of undulation.

Flynn et al. [68] considered a step distribution to model the collagen fiber undulation given by

$$D(x) = \begin{cases} 0, & x < x_1 \text{ or } x > x_3 \\ \dfrac{1}{x_3 - x_1}, & \text{otherwise} \end{cases} \qquad (5.9)$$

Substituting Eq. 5.9 into Eq. 5.8 gives

$$\begin{aligned} \lambda \rho_0 \frac{\partial W_c}{\partial \lambda} &= 0, \quad \lambda < x_1 \\ \lambda \rho_0 \frac{\partial W_c}{\partial \lambda} &= E_c \frac{(\lambda - x_1)^2}{2(x_3 - x_1)}, \quad x_1 \le \lambda < x_3 \\ \lambda \rho_0 \frac{\partial W_c}{\partial \lambda} &= E_c \left[ \frac{(x_3 - x_1)}{2} + (\lambda - x_3) \right], \quad \lambda > x_3 \end{aligned} \qquad (5.10)$$

Equation 5.10 is substituted into Eq. 5.7 to give the Cauchy stress response of the soft tissue. The model accurately simulated a suite of soft tissue experiments including biaxial rabbit skin tests [20] (error 8.7%) (see Fig. 5.3) and uniaxial stretching of pig-skin [69] (error 7.6%). The physically-based model parameters include two directly representing the stiffness of the collagen and elastin fibers and a set of weights representing the orientation of the fibers within the tissue.

One limitation of the proposed model is that when the weights $w_{1-6}$ are equal the tissue response is not always isotropic. This means that unequal weights cannot be interpreted as the sole contribution to anisotropy. Flynn and Rubin [70] proposed a discrete-fiber model that is based on a generalized strain invariant, which gives an unambiguous interpretation of the anisotropy when the weights are not equal. Similarly to Flynn et al. [68], six collagen fiber bundles are oriented parallel to the lines connecting opposing vertices of a regular icosahedron. The unit vectors representing these directions are given by

$$\mathbf{N}_1 = \frac{2}{\sqrt{5}}\mathbf{e}_1 + \frac{1}{\sqrt{5}}\mathbf{e}_3;$$

$$\mathbf{N}_2 = \frac{1}{2}\left(1 - \frac{1}{\sqrt{5}}\right)\mathbf{e}_1 + \sqrt{\frac{1}{2}\left(1 + \frac{1}{\sqrt{5}}\right)}\mathbf{e}_2 + \frac{1}{\sqrt{5}}\mathbf{e}_3;$$

$$\mathbf{N}_3 = -\frac{1}{2}\left(1 + \frac{1}{\sqrt{5}}\right)\mathbf{e}_1 + \sqrt{\frac{1}{2}\left(1 - \frac{1}{\sqrt{5}}\right)}\mathbf{e}_2 + \frac{1}{\sqrt{5}}\mathbf{e}_3;$$

$$\mathbf{N}_4 = -\frac{1}{2}\left(1 + \frac{1}{\sqrt{5}}\right)\mathbf{e}_1 - \sqrt{\frac{1}{2}\left(1 - \frac{1}{\sqrt{5}}\right)}\mathbf{e}_2 + \frac{1}{\sqrt{5}}\mathbf{e}_3;$$

$$\mathbf{N}_5 = \frac{1}{2}\left(1 - \frac{1}{\sqrt{5}}\right)\mathbf{e}_1 - \sqrt{\frac{1}{2}\left(1 + \frac{1}{\sqrt{5}}\right)}\mathbf{e}_2 + \frac{1}{\sqrt{5}}\mathbf{e}_3;$$

$$\mathbf{N}_6 = \mathbf{e}_3 \tag{5.11}$$

A generalized symmetric second-order structural tensor $\mathbf{B}$ with non-negative weights $w_i$ is defined by:

$$\mathbf{B}_i = \mathbf{N}_i \otimes \mathbf{N}_i, \quad i = 1,2\ldots6 \text{ (no sum on } i), \tag{5.12}$$

where $\otimes$ denotes the tensor product operator.

From this, a generalized strain invariant is defined by

$$\gamma = (C + C^{-1}) \cdot \sum_{i=1}^{6} w_i B_i - 2 \tag{5.13}$$

The strain energy function is defined as function of this invariant.

$$\rho_0 W = \frac{K}{2}\left[\gamma + \sum_{m=1}^{M}\frac{\gamma_m}{m}\left(\frac{\gamma}{\gamma_m}\right)^m\right],\qquad(5.14)$$

where $\rho_0$ is the reference mass density, $K$ is a positive material constant having the units of stress, $\gamma_m$ are dimensionless non-negative material constants and $M$ is the order of the polynomial expression for the energy. The Cauchy stress can be determined from this strain energy function using the standard operations.

The generalized invariant model simulated the biaxial rabbit-skin (Fig. 5.3) and uniaxial pig-skin tests with errors a little higher than the Flynn et al. [68] model (12% and 17%, respectively) but with the advantage that the weights are a pure measure of the anisotropy of the tissue.

Flynn and Rubin [70] also related the fiber-bundle weights to the continuous fiber distributions that can be measured histologically (references). The calculated pig-skin preferred fiber orientation of 45° to the plane of the skin in the anterior–posterior axis compared favorably with measurements of Jor et al. [71].

## 5.4   Discussion

Significant advancements have been made in the development of physical fiber-matrix models of the dermis. A wide range of models have been presented in this chapter that can simulate the non-linear, anisotropic, and viscoelastic characteristics of the dermis. Further model development will require more experimental data.

The development of structural fiber-matrix models of the dermis requires extensive experimental data sets. The descriptive power of a proposed constitutive model is evaluated by determining the quality of fit between it and experimental deformation data. The predictive power of a proposed model is also an important quality. Useful constitutive models are those that are optimized using an experimental data set and can subsequently predict the mechanical response of the dermis undergoing a rich set of deformations.

Several experimental devices and protocols have been developed to measure particular mechanical properties of skin. Some of these methods, such as suction, torsion, and normal indentation, are unable to quantify the anisotropic response of skin [29,72–75]. Extensometry tests are only able to apply deformations in a limited number of directions [23,76]. In order to characterize the mechanical properties of skin, it is necessary to apply a rich set of deformations to the region of interest such as the micro-robotic probe used by Flynn et al. [32].

Digital image correlation (DIC) has been used to track the deformation of the skin surface [36,39,77,78]. This technique provides a very rich set of experimental data. While, DIC has mostly been used to measure the surface deformation of soft tissues, it has also been used to quantify the deformation of layers of intact porcine skin under simple shear [1]. However, this latter approach is limited to in vitro experiments.

Various non-invasive imaging modalities have been employed to track the subsurface deformations of skin. Ultrasound is frequently used to measure the thickness and motion of the dermis and other layers when the skin surface is deformed [29,73,79]. High frequency ultrasound has been used to measure the strain of deformed skin in vivo [80,81]. While ultrasound can image the skin and subcutaneous tissues down to 1 cm, it has a low resolution on the order of tens of microns and so cannot be used to provide information on the collagen network. Magnetic resonance imaging (MRI) has been used to track the motion of forearm skin layer boundaries [82]. It has similar penetration depths and resolution to ultrasound scanning [83].

Confocal and multi-photon excitation microscopy techniques allow imaging of the papillary dermis and collagen fibers due to their in vivo penetration depths of about 300 micron and resolution of almost histological detail [84–86]. Jor et al. [71] imaged in vitro pig skin using confocal laser scanning microscopy and quantified the orientation and dispersion of the collagen fibers. Optical coherence tomography is a promising technique, which can non-invasively image in vivo skin to 1 mm depths with a resolution of 10 microns [83,87].

Imaging the structure of the dermis using OCT, confocal microscopy, or histological methods [19] has the ability to provide quantitative information on the collagen fiber network. These measurements include its waviness, orientation, dispersion, and volume fraction. Corresponding material parameters in structural dermis-matrix models can then be specified. This reduces the number of parameters that need to be determined though non-linear optimization techniques. The identification of unique material parameter sets is a difficult problem. In some cases, it is possible to similarly fit a model to experimental data using different parameter sets [39,88]. Using an appropriately rich set of deformations improves the identifiability of the parameters and increases the likelihood of determining a unique parameter set [32,88,89].

Structural fiber-matrix constitutive models of the dermis are becoming increasingly important in several research and industrial fields. Future model developments will require a parallel effort in the development of experimental techniques to quantify the three-dimensional mechanical and structural characteristics of the dermis.

## References


1. Gerhardt L, Schmidt J, Sanz-Herrera JA, Baaijens FPT, Ansari T, Peters GWM, and Oomens CWJ (2012). A novel method for visualising and quantifying through-plane skin layer deformations, *J Mech Behav Biomed*, **14**, 199–207.

2. Groves RB, Coulman SA, Birchall JC, and Evans SL (2012). Quantifying the mechanical properties of human skin to optimise future microneedle device design, *Comput Methods Biomech Biomed Eng*, **15**, 73–82.

3. Flynn C (2010). Finite element models of wound closure, *J Tissue Viability*, **19**, 137–149.

4. Lott-Crumpler DA and Chaudhry HR (2001). Optimal patterns for suturing wounds of complex shapes to foster healing, *J Biomech*, **34**, 51–58.

5. Barbenel JC and Evans J (1977). The time-dependent mechanical properties of skin, *J Invest Dermatol*, **69**, 318–320.

6. Tong P and Fung Y (1976). The stress–strain relationship for the skin, *J Biomech*, **9**, 649–657.

7. Ridge MD and Wright V (1966). Mechanical properties of skin: a bioengineering study of skin structure, *J Appl Physiol*, **21**, 1602–1606.

8. Lokshin O and Lanir Y (2009). Micro and macro rheology of planar tissues, *Biomaterials*, **30**, 3118–3127.

9. Gasser TC, Ogden RW, and Holzapfel GA (2006). Hyperelastic modelling of arterial layers with distributed collagen fibre orientations, *J R Soc Interface*, **3**, 15–35.

10. Lanir Y (1987). Skin mechanics, in *Handbook of Bioengineering* (Skalak R, Chien S, eds), McGraw-Hill, New York, pp. 11.1–11.25.

11. Wilkes GL, Brown IA, and Wildnauer RH (1973). The biomechanical properties of skin, *CRC Cr Rev Biotech*, **1**, 453–495.

12. Oxlund H, Manschot J, and Viidik A (1988). The role of elastin in the mechanical properties of skin, *J Biomech*, **21**, 213–218.

13. Odland GF (1991). Structure of the skin, in *Biology of the Skin* (Goldsmith LA, ed), Oxford University Press, Oxford, pp. 3–62.

14. Lee Y and Hwang K (2002). Skin thickness of Korean adults, *Surg Radiol Anat*, **24**, 183–189.

15. Daly CH (1982). Biomechanical properties of dermis, *J Invest Dermatol*, **79**(Suppl 1), 17s–20s.

16. Daly CH and Odland GF (1979). Age-related changes in the mechanical properties of human skin, *J Invest Dermatol*, **73**, 84–87.

17. Dupuytren G (ed) (1835). *Traité théorique et pratique des blessures par armes de guerre*, H. Dumont, Paris.

18. Langer K (1978). On the anatomy and physiology of the skin: II. Skin Tension, *Br J Plast Surg*, **31**, 93–106.

19. Ní Annaidh AN, Bruyere K, Destrade M, Gilchrist MD, Maurini C, Ottenio M, and Saccomandi G (2012). Automated estimation of collagen fibre dispersion in the dermis and its contribution to the anisotropic behaviour of skin, *Ann Biomed Eng*, **40**, 1666–1678.

20. Lanir Y and Fung YC (1974). Two-dimensional mechanical properties of rabbit skin–II. Experimental results, *J Biomech*, **7**, 171–174.

21. Flynn C, Taberner A, and Nielsen P (2011). Measurement of the force–displacement response of in vivo human skin under a rich set of deformations, *Med Eng Phys*, **33**, 610–619.

22. Flynn C, Taberner AJ, Nielsen PMF, and Fels S (2013). Simulating the three-dimensional deformation of in vivo facial skin, *J Mech Behav Biomed*, **28**, 484–494.

23. Wan Abas WAB (1994). Biaxial tension test of human skin in vivo, *Biomed Mater Eng*, **4**, 473–486.

24. Pereira J, Mansour J, and Davis B (1991). Dynamic measurement of the viscoelastic properties of skin, *J Biomech*, **24**, 157–162.

25. Shen ZL, Dodge MR, Kahn H, Ballarini R, and Eppell SJ (2008). Stress–strain experiments on individual collagen fibrils, *Biophys J*, **95**, 3956–3963.

26. Shen ZL, Kahn H, Ballarin R, and Eppell SJ (2011). Viscoelastic properties of isolated collagen fibrils, *Biophys J*, **100**, 3008–3015.

27. Har-Shai Y, Bodner SR, Egozy-Golan D, Lindenbaum ES, Ben-Izhak O, Mitz V, and Hirshowitz B (1996). Mechanical properties and microstructure of the superficial musculoaponeurotic system, *Plast Reconstr Surg*, **98**, 59–73.

28. Fung YC (ed) (1993). *Biomechanics: Mechanical Properties of Living Tissues*, Springer–Verlag, New York.

29. Diridollou S, Patat F, Gens F, Vaillant L, Black D, Lagarde JM, Gall Y, and Berson M (2000). In vivo model of the mechanical properties of the human skin under suction, *Skin Res Technol*, **6**, 214–221.

30. Jacquet E, Josse G, Khatyr F, and Garcin C (2008). A new experimental method for measuring skin's natural tension, *Skin Res Technol*, **14**, 1–7.

31. de Jong LAM (1995). *Pre-Tension and Anisotropy in Skin: Modelling and Experiments*, Master of Science Thesis, Eindhoven University of Technology.

32. Flynn C, Taberner A, and Nielsen P (2011). Modeling the mechanical response of in vivo human skin under a rich set of deformations, *Ann Biomed Eng*, **39**, 1935–1946.

33. Silver FH, Siperko LM, and Seehra GP (2003). Mechanobiology of force transduction in dermal tissue, *Skin Res Technol*, **9**, 3–23.

34. Lanir Y (2009). Mechanisms of residual stress in soft tissues, *J Biomech Eng*, **131**, 044506.

35. Bischoff JE, Arruda EM, and Grosh K (2000). Finite element modeling of human skin using an isotropic, nonlinear elastic constitutive model, *J Biomech*, **33**, 645–652.

36. Evans SL and Holt CA (2009). Measuring the mechanical properties of human skin in vivo using digital image correlation and finite element modelling, *J Strain Anal Eng*, **44**, 337–345.

37. Lanir Y (1979). Rheological behavior of the skin—experimental results and a structural model, *Biorheology*, **16**, 191–202.

38. Lanir Y (1983). Constitutive equations for fibrous connective tissues, *J Biomech*, **16**, 1–12.

39. Jor J, Nash M, Nielsen P, and Hunter P (2011). Estimating material parameters of a structurally based constitutive relation for skin mechanics, *Biomech Model Mechanobiol*, **10**, 767–778.

40. Meijer R, Douven LFA, and Oomens CWJ (1999). Characterisation of anisotropic and non-linear behaviour of human skin in vivo, *Comput Methods Biomech Biomed Eng*, **2**, 13–27.

41. Belkoff SM and Haut RC (1991). A structural model used to evaluate the changing microstructure of maturing rat skin, *J Biomech*, **24**, 711–720.

42. Manschot JFM and Brakkee AJM (1986). The measurement and modelling of the mechanical properties of human skin in vivo-II. The model, *J Biomech*, **19**, 517–521.

43. Shoemaker PA, Schneider D, Lee MC, and Fung YC (1986). A constitutive model for two-dimensional soft tissues and its application to experimental data, *J Biomech*, **19**, 695–702.

44. Holzapfel G and Gasser T (2001). A viscoelastic model for fiber-reinforced composites at finite strains: Continuum basis, computational aspects and applications, *Comput Methods Appl Mech Eng*, **190**, 4379–4403.

45. Vassoler JM, Reips L, and Fancello EA (2012). A variational framework for fiber-reinforced viscoelastic soft tissues, *Int J Numer Methods Eng*, **89**, 1691–1706.

46. Holzapfel GA, Gasser TC, and Ogden RW (2000). A new constitutive framework for arterial wall mechanics and a comparative study of material models, *J Elasticity*, **61**, 1–48.

47. Groves RB, Coulman SA, Birchall JC, and Evans SL (2013). An anisotropic, hyperelastic model for skin: experimental measurements, finite element modelling and identification of parameters for human and murine skin, *J Mech Behav Biomed*, **18**, 167–180.

48. Weiss J, Maker B, and Govindjee S (1996). Finite element implementation of incompressible, transversely isotropic hyperelasticity, *Comput Methods Appl Mech Eng*, **135**, 107–128.

49. Veronda DR and Westmann RA (1970). Mechanical characterization of skin—Finite deformations, *J Biomech*, **3**, 111–124.

50. Arruda EM and Boyce MC (1993). A three-dimensional constitutive model for the large stretch behavior of rubber elastic materials, *J Mech Phys Solids*, **41**, 389–412.

51. Dunn MG, Silver FH, and Swann DA (1985). Mechanical analysis of hypertrophic scar tissue: structural basis for apparent increased rigidity, *J Invest Dermatol*, **84**, 9–13.

52. Gunner CW, Hutton WC, and Burlin TE (1979). The mechanical properties of skin in vivo—a portable hand-held extensometer, *Brit J Dermatol*, **100**, 161–163.

53. Bischoff JE, Arruda EA, and Grosh K (2002). A microstructurally based orthotropic hyperelastic constitutive law, *J Appl Mech-T ASME*, **69**, 570–579.

54. Bischoff J, Arruda E, and Grosh K (2004). A rheological network model for the continuum anisotropic and viscoelastic behavior of soft tissue, *Biomech Model Mechanobiol*, **3**, 56–65.

55. Bergström JS and Boyce MC (1998). Constitutive modeling of the large strain time-dependent behavior of elastomers, *J Mech Phys Solids*, **46**, 931–954.

56. Flynn C and McCormack BAO (2008). Finite element modelling of forearm skin wrinkling, *Skin Res Technol*, **14**, 261–269.

57. Flynn C and McCormack BAO (2009). Simulating the wrinkling and aging of skin with a multi-layer finite element model, *J Biomech*, **43**, 442–448.

58. Flynn C and McCormack BAO (2008). A simplified model of scar contraction, *J Biomech*, **41**, 1582–1589.

59. Flynn, C. (2007). *The Design and Validation of a Multi-layer Model of Human Skin*, PhD Thesis, Institute of Technology, Sligo.

60. Bischoff JE (2006). Reduced parameter formulation for incorporating fiber level viscoelasticity into tissue level biomechanical models, *Ann Biomed Eng*, **34**, 1164–1172.

61. Kuhl E, Garikipati K, Arruda EM, and Grosh K (2005). Remodeling of biological tissue: mechanically induced reorientation of a transversely isotropic chain network, *J Mech Phys Solids*, **53**, 1552–1573.

62. Tepole AB, Gosain AK, and Kuhl E (2012). Stretching skin: the physiological limit and beyond, *Int J Non-Linear Mech*, **47**, 938–949.

63. Limbert G (2011). A mesostructurally-based anisotropic continuum model for biological soft tissues-Decoupled invariant formulation, *J Mech Behav Biomed*, **4**, 1637–1657.

64. Wuyts FL, Vanhuyse VJ, Langewouters GJ, Decraemer WF, Raman ER, and Buyle S (1995). Elastic properties of human aortas in relation to age and atherosclerosis: a structural model, *Phys Med Biol*, **40**, 1577–1597.

65. Zulliger MA, Fridez P, Hayashi K, and Stergiopulos N (2004). A strain energy function for arteries accounting for wall composition and structure, *J Biomech*, **37**, 989–1000.

66. Raghupathy R and Barocas VH (2009). A closed-form structural model of planar fibrous tissue mechanics, *J Biomech*, **42**, 1424–1428.

67. Freed AD, Einstein DR, and Vesely I (2005). Invariant formulation for dispersed transverse isotropy in aortic heart valves: an efficient means for modeling fiber splay, *Biomech Model Mechanobiol*, **4**, 100–117.

68. Flynn C, Rubin MB, and Nielsen P (2011). A model for the anisotropic response of fibrous soft tissues using six discrete fibre bundles, *Int J Numer Meth Biomed Eng*, **27**, 1793–1811.

69. Ankersen J, Birkbeck A, Thomson R, and Vanezis P (1999). Puncture resistance and tensile strength of skin simulants, *Proc Inst Mech Eng H*, **213**, 493–501.

70. Flynn C and Rubin MB (2012). An anisotropic discrete fibre model based on a generalised strain invariant with application to soft biological tissues, *Int J Eng Sci*, **60**, 66–76.

71. Jor JWY, Nielsen PMF, Nash MP, and Hunter PJ (2011). Modelling collagen fibre orientation in porcine skin based upon confocal laser scanning microscopy, *Skin Res Technol*, **17**, pp. 149–159.

72. Delalleau A, Josse G, Lagarde J-M, Zahouani H, and Bergheau JM (2008). A nonlinear elastic behavior to identify the mechanical parameters of human skin in vivo, *Skin Res Technol*, **14**, 152–164.

73. Hendriks FM, Brokken D, Oomens CWJ, Bader DL, and Baaijens FPT (2006). The relative contributions of different skin layers to the mechanical behavior of human skin in vivo using suction experiments, *Med Eng Phys*, **28**, 259–266.

74. Batisse D, Bazin R, Baldeweck T, Querleux B, and Lévêque, J-L (2002). Influence of age on the wrinkling capacities of skin, *Skin Res Technol*, **8**, 148–154.

75. Pailler-Mattei C, Bec S, and Zahouani H (2008). In vivo measurements of the elastic mechanical properties of human skin by indentation tests, *Med Eng Phys*, **30**, 599–606.

76. Delalleau A, Josse G, Lagarde J-M, Zahouani H, and Bergheau JM (2008). Characterization of the mechanical properties of skin by inverse analysis combined with an extensometry test, *Wear*, **264**, 405–410.

77. Parker MD, Azhar M, Gamage TPB, Alvares D, Taberner AJ, and Nielsen PMF (2012). Surface deformation tracking of a silicone gel skin phantom in response to normal indentation, in *2012 Annual International Conference of the IEEE Engineering in Medicine and Biology Society (EMBC)*, pp. 527–530.

78. Malcolm DTK, Nielsen PMF, Hunter PJ, and Charette PG (2002). Strain measurement in biaxially loaded inhomogeneous, anisotropic elastic membranes, *Biomech Model Mechanobiol*, **1**, 197–210.

79. Sutradhar A and Miller MJ (2013). In vivo measurement of breast skin elasticity and breast skin thickness, *Skin Res Technol*, **19**, E191–E199.

80. Vogt M and Ermert H (2005). Development and evaluation of a high-frequency ultrasound-based system for in vivo strain imaging of the skin, *IEEE Trans Ultrason Ferr*, **52**, 375–385.

81. Gahagnon S, Mofid Y, Josse G, and Ossant F (2012). Skin anisotropy in vivo and initial natural stress effect: a quantitative study using high-frequency static elastography, *J Biomech*, **45**, 2860–2865.

82. Tran HV, Charleux F, Rachik M, Ehrlacher A, Ho Ba Tho M-C (2007). In vivo characterization of the mechanical properties of human skin derived from MRI and indentation techniques, *Comput Methods Biomech Biomed Eng*, **10**(6), 401–407.

83. Dalimier E and Salomon D (2012). Full-field optical coherence tomography: a new technology for 3D high-resolution skin imaging, *Dermatology*, **224**, 84–92.

84. Nouveau-Richard S, Monot M, Bastien P, and de Lacharrière O (2004). In vivo epidermal thickness measurement: ultrasound vs. confocal imaging, *Skin Res Technol*, **10**, 136–140.

85. Rajadhyaksha M, Gonzalez S, Zavislan J, Anderson R, and Webb R (1999). In vivo confocal scanning laser microscopy of human skin II: advances in instrumentation and comparison with histology, *J Invest Dermatol*, **113**, 293–303.

86. Masters B and So P (2001). Confocal microscopy and multi-photon excitation microscopy of human skin in vivo, *Opt Express*, **8**, 2–10.

87. Schmitt J, Yadlowsky M, and Bonner R (1995). Subsurface imaging of living skin with optical coherence microscopy, *Dermatology*, **191**, 93–98.

88. Ogden RW, Saccomandi G, and Sgura I (2004). Fitting hyperelastic models to experimental data, *Comput Mech*, **34**, 484–502.

89. Gamage TPB, Rajagopal V, Ehrgott M, Nash MP, and Nielsen PMF (2011). Identification of mechanical properties of heterogeneous soft bodies using gravity loading, *Int J Numer Meth Biomed Eng*, **27**, 391–407.

# Chapter 6

# Cellular-Scale Mechanical Model of the Human *Stratum Corneum*

Roberto Santoprete and Bernard Querleux

*L'OREAL Research & Innovation, Aulnay-sous-bois, France*

RSANTOPRETE@rd.loreal.com

*Stratum corneum* (SC), the typically 15 micron-thick outermost layer of the skin on most parts of the body except palms and soles can be mechanically described as a brick and mortar structure corresponding to a stiff tissue composed of a series of layers of anucleated dead cells, the corneocytes, embedded in an intercellular lipid organization. SC cohesiveness between corneocytes is due to proteic structures named corneodesmosomes.

After reviewing its morphological and mechanical properties at different scales, this chapter details the structurally and physically-based model we have developed. A particular focus is given on the level of complexity of the numerical model regarding the availability and variability of the experimental data.

Results mainly concern (i) a method to extract the unknown mechanical properties of certain SC components by a reverse engineering approach in good agreement with experimental data

*Computational Biophysics of the Skin*
Edited by Bernard Querleux
Copyright © 2014 Pan Stanford Publishing Pte. Ltd.
ISBN  978-981-4463-84-3 (Hardcover),  978-981-4463-85-0 (eBook)
www.panstanford.com

obtained on other epithelial tissues providing a first validation of the model, (ii) a quantitative analysis of the relative impact of the three major SC components upon its mechanical properties at the macroscopic scale, demonstrating that corneodesmosomes should have the largest impact, a few times higher than the impact of lipids, while the corneocytes should have a rather smaller impact; (iii) a better understanding of the role of relative humidity (RH) on SC mechanical properties, by demonstrating that the intercellular spaces, and in particular the corneodesmosomes, are the main responsible for the observed variation of the SC Young's modulus. All these results will give us a better insight on the impact of hydration on SC mechanical properties at different scales.

In brief, our approach aims at providing additional information on new targets to be addressed for better treating some skin diseases as well as designing new skincare products.

## 6.1  Introduction

One major function of the skin is to act as a protective barrier toward environmental factors such as physicochemical penetration of exogenous compounds, microbial invasion, or mechanical insults [1,2]. If this latter aspect is related to the biomechanical properties of the skin, increasing our understanding in this domain also concerns their changes with intrinsic factors such as aging [3,4], ethnic origin [5,6] and/or external environmental factors such as sun exposure [7,8]. It should also be noticed that many dermatological disorders often lead to alterations in the biomechanical properties of the skin [9–11].

Many authors have reported on skin biomechanics using experimental methods [12,13], or numerical modeling [14–16]. Recent results have demonstrated the important role of the outermost layer, the *stratum corneum*, on the mechanical properties of the whole skin [17–20].

This chapter is devoted to the study of the mechanical properties of the SC, and in particular their respective dependence on the morphological and mechanical properties of its main constituents at a cellular scale. It has to be acknowledged that related literature is rather scarce mainly due to the difficulty in assessing the mechanical properties of the constituents and relate them to overall tissue properties.

The approach chosen here aims at combining mechanical and morphological experimental data at different scales to a multi-scale biomechanical model. The method allows us to (i) extract the unknown mechanical properties of certain constituents by inverse analysis, (ii) provide a quantitative link between constituent's properties at a cellular scale and the overall properties of macroscopic tissue, and (iii) better understand the role of relative humidity (RH) on SC mechanical properties and, at the same time, to better highlight the effect of some common moisturizers.

## 6.2 *Stratum Corneum*: Structure and Biomechanics

This section describes the structural and mechanical properties of the SC at both tissue and cellular levels. Data obtained at different scales are necessary for setting up a multiscale model of SC. We use data available in the literature on human skin in vitro, as well as some new experimental data we obtained at both tissue and cellular levels. The data presented here, on both morphological and mechanical properties, were obtained on the same human skin samples for a better coherence between structure and mechanics and, therefore, leading to a more accurate model.

### 6.2.1 Structure

From a mechanical viewpoint, SC can be described as a stiff composite material (Fig. 6.1) composed of 15 to 30 rigid cell layers of about 0.3 to 0.5 μm each in thickness.

Intercellular lipid regions (Fig. 6.2), about 30 to 40 nm thick, are organized as lamellar phases mainly parallel to corneocyte membranes [21].

Corneodesmosomes, which are protein moieties bridging and interconnecting corneocytes include peripheral and non-peripheral corneodesmosomes (Fig. 6.3) [22].

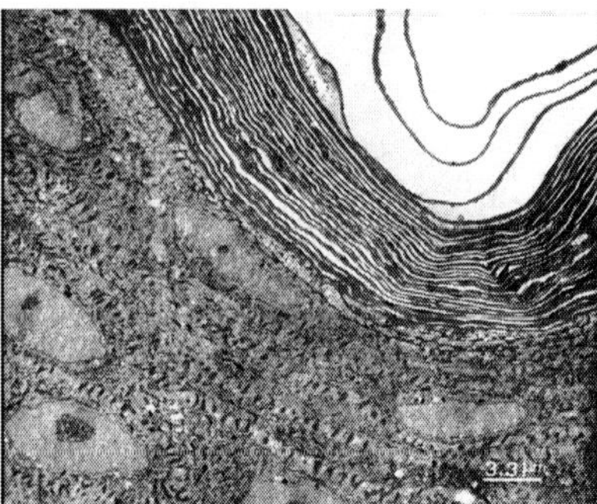

**Figure 6.1** Scanning electron microscopy (SEM) of the outermost part of the skin. SEM image assess the multilayer organization of the *stratum corneum*. The studied SC sample is composed of 22 cell layers

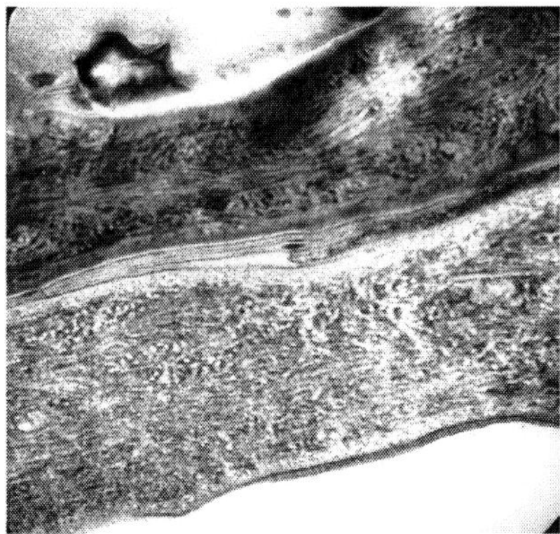

**Figure 6.2** SEM image of the SC intercellular lipids. Lipid bilayers surround the corneocyte membranes.

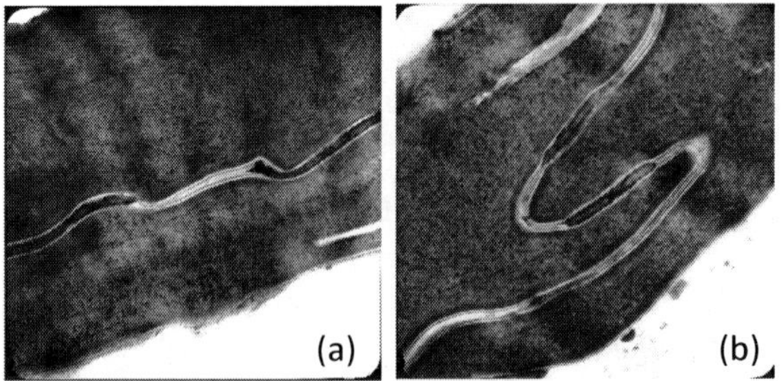



**Figure 6.3** SEM image of corneodesmosomes. (a) Dense areas within the lipid bilayers correspond to non-peripheral corneodesmosomes (CDs). (b) Same dark areas correspond to peripheral CDs.

## 6.2.2   SC Biomechanics at the Macroscopic Scale

Measuring the mechanical properties of the *stratum corneum* in vivo is still an unresolved challenge since all available mechanical methods are sensitive to all skin layers to various extents. Few recent papers aimed at solving the inverse problem by coupling experimental data and a numerical model of the skin, which allowed Young's modulus of the SC in vivo to be predicted in the 1–20 MPa range [20,23]. Such preliminary studies are still in progress and have not yet been fully validated although being in good agreement with in vitro experimental data, which are in the 1–100 MPa range, mainly depending on SC intrinsic and extrinsic conditions as detailed in the next paragraph.

Almost all direct measurements of the SC mechanical properties have been performed in vitro. Longitudinal traction tests, both static [24–31] and dynamic [28,32] are by far the most common methodology, in which Young's modulus of the SC in the direction of the plane of the skin is determined in different environmental conditions (temperature and relative humidity) or following chemical treatment such as delipidation. Most authors reported SC Young's modulus in the 1 to 100 MPa range for static experiments (sometimes higher for very dry SC) and in the range 250–900 MPa for dynamic experiments (frequency >170 Hz). As most biological tissues, SC has a nonlinear viscoelastic anisotropic mechanical behavior.

Since SC can be easily separated from dermis and viable epidermis, a series of publications showed that stress relaxation depended upon the SC physicochemical state and established a major impact of its water content, a more limited impact of the lipid component, and an intermediate role of natural moisturizing factors (NMFs) through their strong influence on the water diffusion process [33–36]. With regard to the impact of corneodesmosomes, delamination experiments have shown a poor correlation with SC cohesiveness which should participate in its mechanical properties [37–39]. These works allowed the values of Young's modulus to be determined in transverse orientation (perpendicular to plane) in the range 1–25 MPa. A weak dependence on the relative humidity was recorded despite the low accuracy of the experiments inherent to the difficulty in deducing the transverse deformations on such a thin tissue.

## 6.2.3 SC Biomechanics at the Microscopic Scale

As key component of SC biomechanics, several studies aimed at characterizing the corneocyte biomechanical properties, mainly through atomic force microscopy (AFM) [18,40–42] or scanning acoustic microscopy [43]. Typical results reported values of Young's modulus in the GPa range (Fig. 6.4), decreasing with the hydration level of the isolated corneocytes.

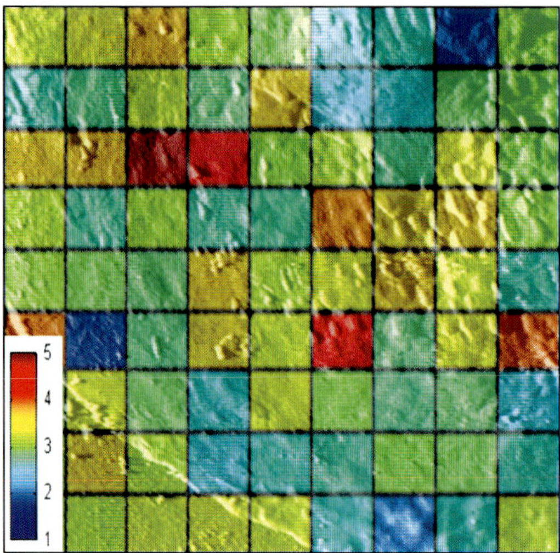

**Figure 6.4** AFM on isolated corneocyte. Fusion of topographic grey image (30 μm × 30 μm) with Young's modulus reconstructed colored map (in GPa). Adapted from [18].

The precise impact of lipids upon SC mechanical properties remains controversial. According to Middleton [44], lipid removal had no consistent effect on SC extensibility, whereas Park and Baddiel stated that it did not influence SC elastic properties [25,26]. In contrast, Lévêque et al. [32] suggested that lipids slightly contributed to the plasticization of the *stratum corneum*. More recently, Potter et al. (unpublished work) using nanoindentation techniques found that lipids contributed to the SC softening at a low RH level and to its stiffening at a higher humidity level, whereby lipids reduce the water accessibility to the hydrophilic sites into the intercellular spaces. To the best of our knowledge, no data is available in the literature on mechanical properties of lipids. At such stage, it can only be assumed that they could be similar to multi-layered films of dioleoylphosphatidylcholine lipids, Young's modulus of which, as measured by AFM nanoindentation falls within the 20–200 kPa range [45].

As regards the third key element, corneodesmosomes, very few studies deal with their mechanical properties and their impact on SC mechanical properties. A pioneering and exploratory work [46] measured the elongation of corneocyte through a micromanipulation experiment between two corneocytes interconnected with a corneodesmosome. A personal discussion with one of the authors suggest that such data should be mostly considered qualitative since at early stages of the micromanipulation technology, the reported values may not be relevant as quantitative data for simulations. Epithelial cadherins, whose spring constants, as measured by AFM pulling-up experiments may help to suggest values ranging between 1 pN/nm [47] and 8 pN/nm [48]. The next paragraph presents the numerical model, the way we used to overcome these limitations.

## 6.3 *Stratum Corneum* Numerical Model

The SC model presented here aims at better understanding the role played by the main microscopic components on the overall SC mechanical properties, as well as determining the unknown mechanical properties of some key components by coupling experimental and simulated data.

Up to our knowledge, all mechanical simulations of the SC consider this layer as a homogeneous isotropic membrane in the framework of a multilayer model of the skin [15–17,49,50]. At a microscopic level, most models of the SC deal with the barrier function, modeling the diffusion phenomena of several compounds through a biphasic membrane, where each phase has a different diffusion coefficient and each interface a different partitioning coefficient [51–53]. From a mechanical viewpoint, we mostly found brick-and-mortar biocomposite models such as nacre, composed of aragonite platelets embedded into an organic proteic matrix [54–56].

Due to the lack of accurate experimental data on the mechanical behavior of major SC components at a cell scale, we favored a mechanical description in the framework of the linear elasticity theory, where most of the tissue-scale tensional experiments referred to are carried out.

## 6.3.1 Structural Description

The model takes into account the multi-layered structure of the SC down to the cellular scale. It is done by coupling two mechanical models: a multi-layer model allowing simulating the overall SC mechanical behavior, and a cellular-scale model that explicitly takes into account the corneocytes, corneodesmosomes and intercellular lipids. This combined multi-scale approach allows a fine representation of the whole SC in terms of cellular-scale components to be achieved without requiring a high computation, which would have been the case when all layers were to be considered at a cellular scale.

Figure 6.5 illustrates the multi-layer mechanical model (on the right), the geometry of which is inspired by electron microscopy images of a transversal section, as previously shown in Fig. 6.1. This model is composed of 22 homogeneous 300 nm-thick cellular layers, representing the cell layers (corneocytes and in-plane intercellular spaces), separated by 21 homogeneous 30 nm-thick intercellular space layers representing the out-of-plane intercellular spaces. Lateral periodic boundary conditions allow an infinitely long SC to be simulated, avoiding the finite size effects due to the boundaries. Each cellular layer is further described in terms of the cellular-scale model.

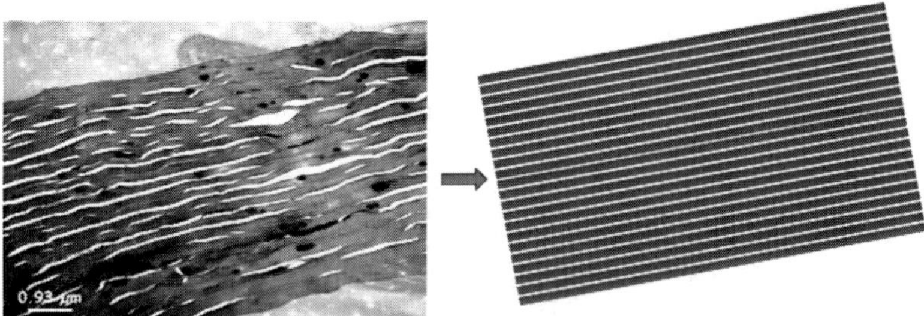

**Figure 6.5**     On left, a transversal section of the SC as seen by electron microscopy. On right, the multi-layered model of the SC.

Its structure is represented in Fig. 6.6. It contains three components: corneocytes, CDs and intercellular lipids. The model's building block, showed in the center, is the representative volume element (RVE) of dimensions 60 μm × 40 μm × 300 nm. Its structure is inspired by SEM images of the SC surface, as shown on the left of the figure, which illustrates the in-plane corneocytes' arrangement. The cell shape has been assumed as hexagonal, of an average lateral size estimated at 60 μm and a 300 nm thickness. By the application of in-plane periodic boundary conditions, one SC cell layer has been modeled. Figure 6.3 shows that the intercellular spaces are composed by lipids and peripheral CDs. Accordingly, as further discussed in the next section, we model these 2 components by a 30 nm-thick homogeneous material (Fig. 6.5, right). In fact, although the CDs are not continuously distributed along the corneocytes, their surface density is large enough to justify, from a mechanical viewpoint, the hypothesis of a continuous material.

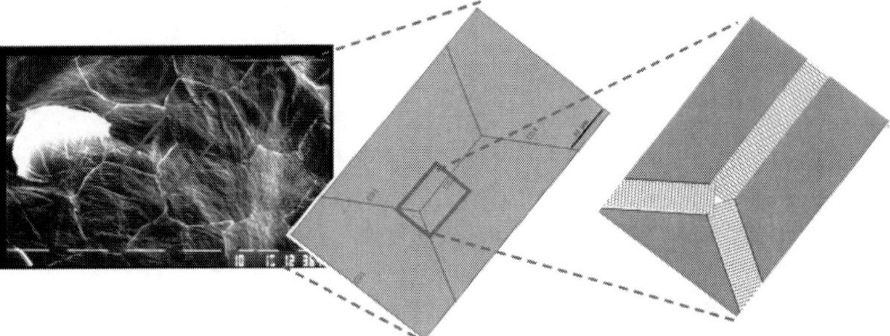

**Figure 6.6**   On left, SEM image of the SC's surface showing the in-plane cell arrangement. At center, model's representative volume element (RVE). On right, a zoom of RVE around the intercellular spaces.

## 6.3.2  Mechanical Model

The mechanical properties of all components in both models were described in the framework of the linear elastic theory. Poisson's ratio has been taken equal to 0.49 for all components, a current hypothesis that accounts for the poor compressibility of the biological materials due to their high water content.

For the cellular-scale model, according to Section 6.2.3, corneocytes were modeled as homogeneous isotropic materials whose Young's modulus was arbitrarily chosen as 1 GPa. As already mentioned in Section 6.3.1, both peripheral and non-peripheral intercellular spaces were modeled as homogeneous domains and were mechanically described as a unidirectional fiber-reinforced material, where the matrix represented the lipid phase, and the fibers the corneodesmosomes. In the framework of the mixture theory, the local stiffness matrix of the peripheral intercellular spaces can be easily deduced. In particular, the resulting longitudinal and transverse Young's modulus $E_l$ and $E_t$, its shear modulus $G_{lt}$ and its Poisson's ratio $\nu_{lt}$ are given by

$$
\begin{aligned}
E_l &= E_{cd}\, V_{cd} + E_{li}\, V_{li} \\[4pt]
\frac{1}{E_t} &= \frac{V_{cd}}{E_{cd}} + \frac{V_{li}}{E_{li}} \\[4pt]
\frac{1}{G_{lt}} &= \frac{V_{cd}}{G_{cd}} + \frac{V_{li}}{G_{li}} \\[4pt]
\nu_{lt} &= \nu_{cd}\, V_{cd} + \nu_{li}\, V_{li},
\end{aligned}
\tag{6.1}
$$

where $G_{cd}$ and $G_{li}$ denote the shear modulus of the corneodesmosomes and the lipids, $\nu_{cd}$ and $\nu_{li}$ their respective Poisson's ratios, and $V_{cd}$ and $V_{li}$ their volume fractions, with $V_{cd} + V_{li} = 1$.

The fibers were considered to be always oriented perpendicularly to the corneocyte's borders. By defining $(x, y, z)$ the reference frame ($z$-direction being perpendicular to the cellular plane) and $(l, t, z)$ the local frame ($l$ being the longitudinal direction parallel to the fibers, $t$ the transverse one) and by considering the cellular-scale model as a ply of a thin laminate, the reference stiffness matrix $Q_{ij}$, defined by

$$
\begin{pmatrix} \sigma_x \\ \sigma_y \\ \tau_{xy} \end{pmatrix}
=
\begin{pmatrix}
Q_{11} & Q_{12} & Q_{16} \\
Q_{12} & Q_{22} & Q_{26} \\
Q_{16} & Q_{26} & Q_{66}
\end{pmatrix}
\begin{pmatrix} \varepsilon_x \\ \varepsilon_y \\ \gamma_{xy} \end{pmatrix},
\tag{6.2}
$$

can be calculated in terms of the local stiffness matrix and the angle $\theta$ of rotation between the two frames ($\theta$ defines the direction of orientation of the fibers) [57]:

$$
\begin{aligned}
Q_{11} &= c^4\,\overline{E}_1 + s^4\,\overline{E}_t + 2c^2 s^2\,(\nu_{tl}\,\overline{E}_1 + 2G_{lt}) \\
Q_{22} &= s^4\,\overline{E}_1 + c^4\,\overline{E}_t + 2c^2 s^2\,(\nu_{tl}\,\overline{E}_1 + 2G_{lt}) \\
Q_{66} &= c^2 s^2\,(\overline{E}_1 + \overline{E}_t - 2\nu_{tl}\,\overline{E}_1) + (c^2 - s^2)^2\,G_{lt} \\
Q_{12} &= c^2 s^2\,(\overline{E}_1 + \overline{E}_t - 4G_{lt}) + (c^4 + s^4)\nu_{tl}\,\overline{E}_1 \\
Q_{16} &= -cs\,[c^2\,\overline{E}_1 - s^2\,\overline{E}_t - (c^2 - s^2)(\nu_{tl}\,\overline{E}_1 + 2G_{lt})] \\
Q_{26} &= -cs\,[s^2\,\overline{E}_1 - c^2\,\overline{E}_t + (c^2 - s^2)(\nu_{tl}\,\overline{E}_1 + 2G_{lt})],
\end{aligned}
\tag{6.3}
$$

where $c = \cos(\theta)$, $s = \sin(\theta)$, $\overline{E}_1 = \dfrac{E_1}{1-\nu_{lt}\,\nu_{tl}}$ and $\overline{E}_t = \dfrac{E_t}{1-\nu_{lt}\,\nu_{tl}}$.

The fiber volume fraction of this composite material was taken equal to the fraction of the corneocyte's surface covered by the corneodesmosomes. According to Skerrow et al. [58] and Chapman and Walsh [59], this fraction is, respectively, 25% and 20% for peripheral and non-peripheral corneodesmosomes in the *stratum compactum*. For the multi-layer mechanical model, the transverse and longitudinal Young's modulus of each cellular layer are given, respectively, by transverse and longitudinal effective Young's modulus of the cellular-scale model, the first one being equal to the corneocyte's modulus (1 GPa) and the second one being numerically determined by simulating a traction experiment on the cellular-scale model. The lipid layers are modeled as a homogeneous fiber-reinforced material, as in the case of intercellular spaces of the cellular-scale model, with fibers oriented perpendicularly to the cell layers. Their Young's modulus is also determined according to the mixture theory.

Corneocytes' interdigitation, as shown on top of Fig. 6.7, increases lateral cohesion between corneocytes. For a typical cell thickness of 0.3 µm, the average contact length, as estimated on several images, is about 3 µm. Therefore, we define an interdigitation coefficient whose value is 10. In order to take into account this increased cohesion without increasing the geometrical complexity of our cellular model, we keep the cell lateral boundaries flat, but we increase their effective Young's modulus by multiplying it by the interdigitation coefficient.

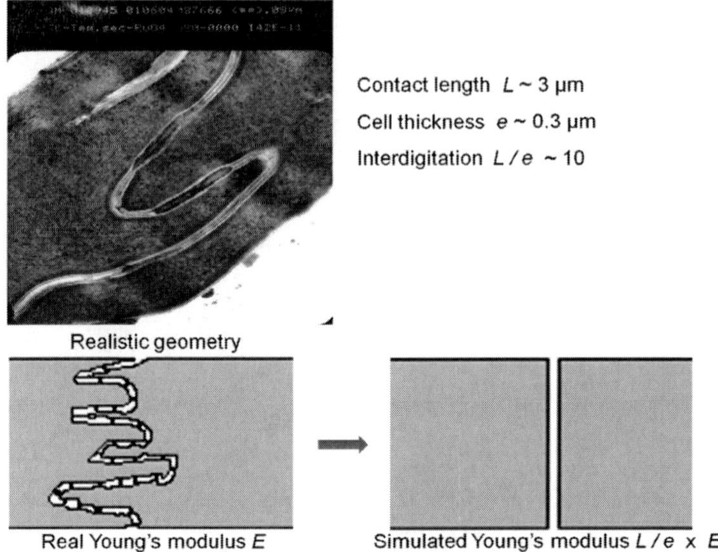


**Figure 6.7**    On top, corneocyte's interdigitation as seen in SEM (internal data). On bottom, this complex geometry is modeled as a planar interface with an increased simulated Young's modulus of the peripheral intercellular spaces of the cellular-scale model.

## 6.3.3    Estimation of Unknown Parameters

As we discussed before, no data are reported on the mechanical properties of corneodesmosomes or intercellular lipids. Instead of using data reported for other tissues, we adjusted the numerical values of Young's modulus for these two constituents, respectively, $E_{cd}$ and $E_{li}$, by fitting experimental data of longitudinal and transverse traction tests, keeping Young's modulus of corneocytes to the fixed value of 1 GPa, obtained by AFM experiments.

The procedure employed was rather simple, we allow $E_{li}$ to vary between 10 Pa and 1 MPa, and $E_{cd}$ between 0.1 kPa and 10 MPa, with the constraint $E_{cd} > E_{li}$. For each couple of values, we calculated the effective SC longitudinal ($E_{||}$) and transverse ($E_{\perp}$) Young's moduli by combining the cellular-scale and the multilayer model. The grid ($E_{cd}$, $E_{li}$) was chosen rather coarse to fit the correct order of magnitude of $E_{||}$ and $E_{\perp}$. A more precise fit would have been useless due to the cellular scale simplifying assumptions, especially with respect to the morphology of corneodesmosomes.

By fitting in with the value $E_{\parallel} \approx 50$ MPa obtained by static extensometry (internal results) and $E_{\perp} \approx 5$ MPa obtained by delamination [39], we estimated $E_{li} \approx 1$–10 kPa and $E_{cd} \approx 10$–100 kPa.

$E_{cd}$ can be expressed in terms of spring constant of a single protein filament and compared to the values of 1 pN/nm [47] and 8 pN/nm [48] obtained on epithelial cadherins by AFM pulling-up experiments. For such a goal, we first assimilated each cadherin to a 30 nm long and a 2 nm thick cylinder. We then considered that each corneodesmosome was formed by a bundle of cadherins whose surface density was about 1000 fibers/$\mu m^2$, a value obtained by image analysis on SEM on cryofractures shown in Fig. 6.8.

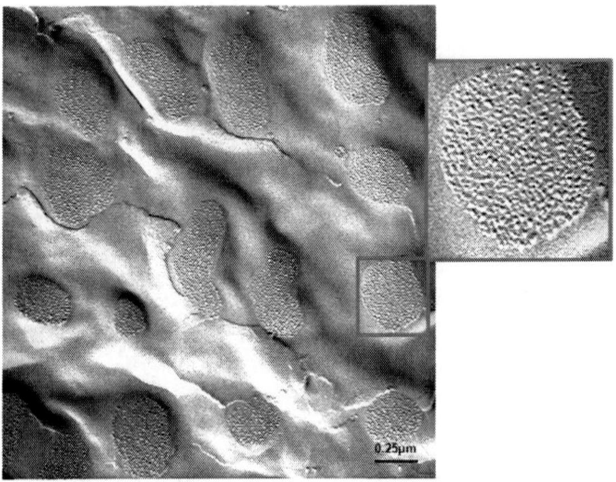


**Figure 6.8**    SEM on cryofractures reveals the intimate structure of corneodesmosomes in terms of a bundle of transmembrane proteins called cadherins.

Under these hypotheses, Young's modulus of each transmembrane protein can be estimated as $E_{pr} \approx 10$–100 MPa. Finally, the protein's spring constant $k$ is derived from the following formula:

$$k \approx E_{pr} \frac{\pi d^2}{4L}, \tag{6.4}$$

where $d$ is the protein's diameter (2 nm) and $L$ its length (30 nm). This gives $k \approx 1$–10 pN/nm, a value fully consistent with the 1 pN/nm [47] and 8 pN/nm [48].

The estimated value of Young's modulus of the intercellular lipids, $E_{li} \approx 1$–10 kPa, appears close to the value 20–200 kPa measured by AFM nanoindentation on lipid films [45], whose multilayered structure reminds the lamellar lipid structure in the SC. This discrepancy could be partially explained by the low impact of $E_{li}$ (compared to $E_{cd}$) on the calculated $E_{||}$ and $E_{\perp}$, as will be shown in the next section, giving rise to a lower accuracy of the retrieved $E_{li}$ with respect to $E_{cd}$.

Therefore, the overall agreement between estimated values of $E_{cd}$, and in a less extent that of $E_{li}$, and the experimental data provides us with a first validation of our model.

## 6.3.4  Relative Impact of the Three SC Major Components

We studied the impact of Young's moduli of the corneocytes $E_c$, the corneodesmosomes $E_{cd}$, and the intercellular lipids $E_{li}$ on both longitudinal ($E_{||}$) and transverse ($E_{\perp}$) SC Young's moduli. With this aim, we started from the values $E_c \approx 1$ GPa, $E_{cd} \approx 100$ kPa, and $E_{li} \approx 1$ kPa, and calculated the corresponding values of $E_{||}$ and $E_{\perp}$. Then we selectively decreased $E_c$, $E_{cd}$, and $E_{li}$ by 10% and recalculated the corresponding values of $E_{||}$ and $E_{\perp}$. Additionally, the impact upon $E_{||}$ and $E_{\perp}$ of the morphology of the intercellular spaces was studied. The latter have been characterized by the ratios $L_{cd}/L_c$, namely the thickness $L_{cd}$ of the peripheral intercellular space divided by the corneocyte's length $L_c$, and the ratio $e_{cd}/e_c$, namely the thickness $e_{cd}$ of the non-peripheral intercellular space divided by the corneocyte's thickness $e_c$. The starting values are $L_{cd} = e_{cd} = 30$ nm, $L_c = 40$ μm and $e_c = 0.3$ μm. All the results of this sensitivity analysis are shown on Table 6.1.

**Table 6.1**  Impact of the mechanical properties of corneocytes, corneodesmosomes and intercellular lipids, and of the morphology of the intercellular spaces, on the longitudinal and transverse SC traction behavior

|  | $E_{||}$ (MPa) | $E_{\perp}$ (MPa) |
|---|---|---|
| $E_c \rightarrow E_c - 10\%$ | 50 → 49.7 (−0.5%) | 5.45 → 5.38 (−1%) |
| $E_{cd} \rightarrow E_{cd} - 10\%$ | 50 → 46.0 (−8%) | 5.45 → 5.07 (−7%) |
| $E_{li} \rightarrow E_{li} - 10\%$ | 50 → 48.5 (−3%) | 5.45 → 5.34 (−2%) |
| $L_{cd}/L_c \rightarrow L_{cd}/L_c - 10\%$ | 50 → 53.5 (+7%) | 5.45 → 5.45 (<$10^{-3}$%) |
| $e_{cd}/e_c \rightarrow e_{cd}/e_c - 10\%$ | 50 → 50.5 (+1%) | 5.45 → 5.94 (+9%) |

These results show that the intercellular spaces play a major role in the SC mechanical properties. In particular,

- corneodesmosomes are the component of highest impact upon both longitudinal and transverse SC mechanical properties. The higher their Young's modulus, the stiffest the SC,
- intercellular lipids have a three to four times lower effect than corneodesmosomes,
- corneocytes have less impact upon the *stratum corneum* overall stiffness, about 10 times lower than corneodesmosomes,
- thickness of the intercellular spaces has an important impact, comparable to that of corneodesmosomes, but opposite, i.e., the lower their thickness, the stiffer the overall SC *stratum corneum*.

The higher impact of the intercellular spaces compared to the cells is a consequence of their much lower stiffness (of the order of $E_{cd} \sim 10$–$100$ KPa versus $\sim$ GPa), which results in much larger stretches and, ultimately, higher sensitivity.

To get a better insight into all these results, we refer to Fig. 6.9, where the cellular layers are assimilated to two elastic parallelepiped-shaped materials connected in series, representing the corneocytes and the intercellular spaces, respectively.

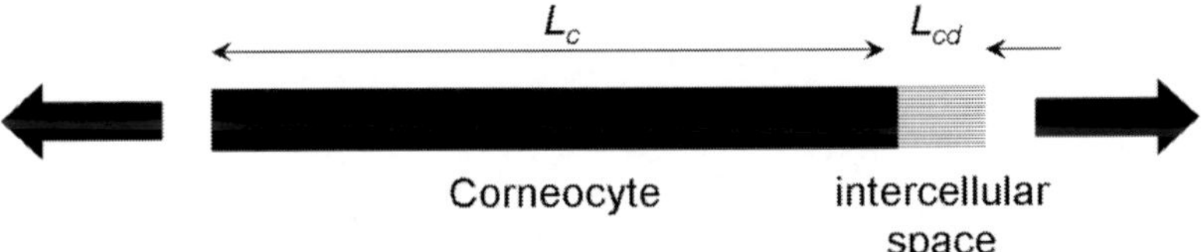


**Figure 6.9**    The SC stretching behavior may be qualitatively derived from the mechanical behavior of two elastic materials connected in series, representing the corneocytes and the intercellular spaces, respectively.

The mechanical behavior under longitudinal stretch of such a bi-component system may be expressed in terms of an equivalent Young's modulus $E_{\parallel}$ as

$$\frac{1}{E_{\parallel}} = \frac{L_{cd}}{L_{cd}+L_c}\frac{1}{E_{cd}} + \frac{L_c}{L_{cd}+L_c}\frac{1}{E_c}, \tag{6.5}$$

where $E_{cd}$ is Young's modulus of the intercellular spaces and $E_c$ that of the corneocytes, all boundary effects having be neglected. From this equation we immediately justify that

- for a SC whose Young's modulus $E_{||}$ under longitudinal stress is in the range 10–100 MPa, Young's modulus $E_{cd}$ of the intercellular spaces lies in the range 10–100 KPa, which is the result of the previous section,

- the intercellular spaces have an impact about 10 times higher than the corneocytes upon the longitudinal mechanical properties as described in Eq. 6.6:

$$\frac{\Delta E_{||}/E_{||}}{\Delta E_{sc}/E_{sc}} \cong \frac{E_{sc}}{E_{||}}\frac{\partial E_{||}}{\partial E_{sc}} = \frac{L_{sc}\,E_c}{L_{sc}\,E_c + L_c\,E_{sc}} \approx 1$$

$$\frac{\Delta E_{||}/E_{||}}{\Delta E_c/E_c} \cong \frac{E_c}{E_{||}}\frac{\partial E_{||}}{\partial E_c} = \frac{L_c\,E_{sc}}{L_c\,E_{sc} + L_{sc}\,E_c} \approx 0.1 \tag{6.6}$$

Results from Eq. 6.6 are consistent with the results of Table 6.1. The same qualitative reasoning allows the strong dependency on $L_{cd}/L_c$ to be justified. At the same time, it justifies the larger dependency of $E_\perp$ on $E_{cd}$ (and $e_{cd}/e_c$) with respect to $E_c$ by replacing $L_{sc}$ and $L_c$ by $e_{sc}$ and $e_c$, respectively.

## 6.3.5 Simulation of Hydrated SC

Hydration has a strong impact upon the SC mechanical properties, as already mentioned. Internal data on uniaxial tensile test on the same samples employed for microstructural analysis showed an increase in Young's modulus $E_{||}$ from 50 ± 20 MPa to 370 ± 60 MPa when relative humidity decreases from 75% to 32%.

Our multi-scale model may help to better understand which components are affected by change in humidity level and, more importantly, which are responsible for the observed variation of the mechanical properties of the tissue.

Nanoindentation measurements on isolated corneocytes [60] indicated that their Young's modulus increased by a factor 2–3 when the relative humidity decreased from 75% to 15%.

The SC mechanical behavior shows that the corneocyte's alterations with relative humidity level cannot explain the large variation observed on the SC mechanical behavior. In fact, assuming that $E_c$ increases from 1 GPa to 2 GPa, $E_{li} \approx 10$ kPa and $E_{cd} \approx 100$ kPa, we find that $E_{||}$ increases by 2% only. Even though $E_c$ increased by one order of magnitude, which is more than what is observed, it would not explain the SC stiffening. Therefore, we conclude that the stiffening of the intercellular spaces is responsible for the observed SC behavior with variations in RH level. In particular, the intercellular spaces stiffen by about one order of magnitude, either due to corneodesmosome or to both corneodesmosome and lipid stiffening of about one order of magnitude. These results are consistent with the experimental data in [25] obtained by nanoindentation measurements, showing that the components involved in the SC softening are mainly corneodesmosomes, glycoproteins and sugars contained in the intercellular spaces, rather than lipids or corneocytes.

We further observe that the model predicts that, for a delipidated SC where the intercellular spaces become thinner, the overall Young's modulus should increase. This is indeed observed in experiments at low humidity level [31].

These results allow the observed behavior of some common moisturizers, such as urea and glycerol to be better explained. In fact, the model predicts that corneodesmosomes are the most effective target for decreasing the SC stiffening. Among the moisturizers mentioned, urea 3% solution is known as the most effective, as it decreases the SC dynamic Young's modulus by about 70%, as measured 2 h after application. Its mode of action is supposed to be the degradation of proteins inside the intercellular spaces, resulting in the weakening of the bonds of corneodesmosomes. On the other hand, glycerol whose softening effect is lower than urea (decrease in SC stiffness by 30–40%), does not have any specific action on corneodesmosomes but rather a hygroscopic effect on the other components.

Although these comparisons with experimental observations of the effects of the RH level are very encouraging, they should not be pushed very far toward more quantitative predictions, since the model is not able to simulate the impact of the lipids on water accessibility to the different components.

## 6.4 Conclusion

We developed the first multiscale model of the SC accounting for its macroscopic overall mechanical behavior, both longitudinal and transverse, in terms of structural and mechanical properties of the main components at a cellular scale, namely corneocytes, corneodesmosomes, and intercellular lipids.

This model allows us to gain better insight into the impact of the different components upon the overall mechanical behavior, by differentiating and quantifying their respective contribution. Corneodesmosomes were found having the largest impact upon the SC mechanical properties, a few times more than the lipids, while the corneocytes have a rather little impact.

Our approach also provides the first estimation of the mechanical properties of corneodesmosomes and intercellular lipids starting from coherent experimental data at both cellular and tissue levels. The good agreement with experimental data obtained on other epithelial tissues provides a first validation of the model.

Finally, we demonstrated that the RH level has an impact upon the mechanical properties of the intercellular spaces, in particular corneodesmosomes, whose modification is the main responsible for the observed variation of the SC Young's modulus.

This coupled experimental-numerical approach can be improved in many ways. First of all, from an experimental viewpoint, further experiments (micropipette, delamination, ...) should be performed to better target the mechanical properties of corneodesmosomes. Alternatively, ex vivo AFM pull-up experiments could provide direct experimental information about these structures. From a numerical viewpoint, a biomechanically more realistic non-linear viscoelastic behavior should be considered for the components, provided that accurate experimental data are available. Furthermore, the impact of additional components, such as corneocyte's membrane or sugars could be taken into account. Finally, a simulation of the mechanisms of action of moisturizers, such as urea or glycerol, could help to better understand the link between a chemical effect and a macroscopic impact.

### Acknowledgments

The authors would like to thank A. M. Minondo, A. Potter, and G. Luengo for fruitful discussions on SC ultrastructure and for providing us electronic and AFM images. F. Servantes-Munhoz is also recognized for her development of the numerical model during her internship in our lab. Finally, we are deeply grateful to P. Tracqui (TIMC-CNRS UMR 5525) for his numerous advices and overall contribution to this work.

## References


1. Marks R (2004). The *stratum corneum* barrier: the final frontier, *J Nutr*, **134**(8 Suppl), 2017S–2021S.

2. Elias PM (2005). *Stratum corneum* defensive functions: an integrated view, *J Invest Dermatol*, **125**(2), 183–200.

3. Escoffier C, de Rigal J, Rochefort A, Vasselet R, Lévêque J-L, and Agache PG (1989). Age-related mechanical properties of human skin: an in vivo study, *J Invest Dermatol*, **93**(3), 353–357.

4. Krueger N, Luebberding S, Oltmer M, Streker M, and Kerscher M (2011). Age-related changes in skin mechanical properties: a quantitative evaluation of 120 female subjects, *Skin Res Technol*, **17**(2), 141–148.

5. Berardesca E, de Rigal J, Lévêque J-L, and Maibach HI (1991). In vivo biophysical characterization of skin physiological differences in races, *Dermatologica*, **182**(2), 89–93.

6. Wesley NO and Maibach HI (2003). Racial (ethnic) differences in skin properties: the objective data, *Am J Clin Dermatol*, **4**(12), 843–860.

7. Richard S, de Rigal J, de Lacharrière O, Berardesca E, and Lévêque J-L (1994). Noninvasive measurement of the effect of lifetime exposure to the sun on the aged skin, *Photodermatol Photoimmunol Photomed*, **10**(4), 164–169.

8. Oba A and Edwards C (2006). Relationships between changes in mechanical properties of the skin, wrinkling, and destruction of dermal collagen fiber bundles caused by photoaging, *Skin Res Technol*, **12**(4), 283–288.

9. Dobrev HP (1999). In vivo study of skin mechanical properties in patients with systemic sclerosis, *J Am Acad Dermatol*, **40**(3), 436–442.

10. Dobrev H (2007). In vivo study of skin mechanical properties in Raynaud's phenomenon, *Skin Res Technol*, **13**(1), 91–94.

11. Seirafi H, Farsinejad K, Firooz A, Davoudi SM, Robati RM, Hoseini MS, Ehsani AH and Sadr B (2009). Biophysical characteristics of skin in diabetes: a controlled study, *J Eur Acad Dermatol Venereol*, **23**(2), 146–149.

12. Agache P and Humbert P (eds) (2004). *Measuring the Skin*, 2nd ed, Springer-Verlag, Berlin Heidelberg.

13. Serup J, Jemec GBE, and Grove GL (eds) (2006). *Handbook of Non-Invasive Methods and the Skin*, 2nd ed, CRC Press, Boca Raton.

14. Jor JW, Parker MD, Taberner AJ, Nash MP, and Nielsen PM (2013). Computational and experimental characterization of skin mechanics: identifying current challenges and future directions, *Wiley Interdiscip Rev Syst Biol Med*, **5**(5), 539–556.

15. Limbert G (2014). State-of-the-art constitutive models of skin biomechanics, in *Computational Biophysics of the Skin* (Querleux B, ed), Chapter 4, Pan Stanford Publishing, Singapore.

16. Flynn C (2014). Fiber-matrix models of the dermis, in *Computational Biophysics of the Skin* (Querleux B, ed), Chapter 5, Pan Stanford Publishing, Singapore.

17. Magnenat-Thalmann N, Kalra P, Lévêque J-L, Bazin R, Batisse D, and Querleux B (2002). A computational skin model: fold and wrinkle formation, *IEEE Trans Inf Technol Biomed*, **6**(4), 317–323.

18. Potter A, Luengo G, Santoprete R, and Querleux, B (2009). *Stratum corneum* biomechanics, in *Skin Moisturization*, 2nd ed (Rawlings AV and Leyden JJ, eds), Informa Healthcare, New York, pp. 259–278.

19. Lévêque J-L and Audoly B (2013). Influence of *Stratum corneum* on the entire skin mechanical properties, as predicted by a computational skin model, *Skin Res Technol*, **19**(1), 42–46.

20. Hara Y, Masuda Y, Hirao T, and Yoshikawa N (2013). The relationship between the Young's modulus of the *stratum corneum* and age: a pilot study, *Skin Res Technol*, **19**(3), 339–345.

21. Bouwstra JA and Gooris GS (2010). The lipid organisation in human *stratum corneum* and model systems, *Open Dermatol J*, **4**(1), 10–13.

22. Simon M, Bernard D, Minondo AM, Camus C, Fiat F, Corcuff P, Schmidt R, and Serre G (2001). Persistence of both peripheral and non-peripheral corneodesmosomes in the upper *stratum corneum* of winter xerosis skin versus only peripheral in normal skin, *J Invest Dermatol*, **116**(1), 23–30.

23. Querleux B (28–30 November 2012). *Combining Experiments and Simulations for a Better Understanding of Skin Properties*, paper presented at the World Congress of the International Society for Biophysics and Imaging of the Skin, Copenhagen, Denmark, Book of Abstracts, p. 27.

24. Wildnauer RH, Bothwell JW, and Douglass AB (1970). *Stratum corneum* biomechanical properties. I. Influence of relative humidity on normal and extracted human *stratum corneum*, *J Invest Dermatol*, **56**(1), 72–78.

25. Park AC and Baddiel CB (1972). Rheology of *stratum corneum*—I: a molecular interpretation of the stress-strain curve, *J Soc Cosmet Chem*, **23**, 3–12.

26. Park AC and Baddiel CB (1972). Rheology of *stratum corneum*—II: a physico-chemical investigation of factors influencing the water content of the *stratum corneum*, *J Soc Cosmet Chem*, **23**, 13–21.

27. Papir YS, Hsu H-K, and Wildnauer RH (1975). The mechanical properties of the *stratum corneum*. I. The effect of water and ambient temperature on the tensile properties of newborn rat *stratum corneum*, *Biochim Biophys Acta*, **399**, 170–180.

28. Rasseneur L, de Rigal J, and Lévêque J-L (1982). Influence des différents constituants de la couche cornée sur la mesure de son élasticité, *Int J Cosmet Sci*, **4**, 247–260.

29. Druot P, Rochefort A, Oytana C, and Agache P (1985). In vitro stress relaxation tests of human *stratum corneum*, *Bioeng Skin*, **1**, 141–156.

30. Rochefort A, Druot P, Leduc M, Vasselet R, and Agache P (1986). A new technique for the evaluation of cosmetics effect on mechanical properties of *stratum corneum* and epidermis in vitro, *Int J Cosmet*, **8**, 27–36.

31. Koutroupi KS and Barbenel JC (1990). Mechanical and failure behaviour of the *stratum corneum*, *J Biomech*, **23**, 281–287.

32. Lévêque J-L, Escoubez M, and Rasseneur L (1987). Water-keratin interaction in human *stratum corneum*, *Bioeng Skin*, **3**, 227–242.

33. Wolfram MA, Wolejsza NF, and Laden K (1972). Biomechanical properties of delipidized *stratum corneum*, *J Invest Dermatol*, **59**(6), 421–426.

34. Wilkes GL, Wildnauer RH (1973). Structure-property relationships of the *stratum corneum* of human and neonatal rat. II. Dynamic mechanical studies, *Biochim Biophys Acta*, **304**, 276–289.

35. Takahashi M, Machida Y, and Tsuda Y (1985). The influence of hydroxyl acids on the rheological properties of *stratum corneum*, *J Soc Cosmet Chem*, **36**, 177–187.

36. Rawlings AV, Watkinson A, Harding CR, Ackerman C, Banks J, Hope J, and Scott IR (1995). Changes in *stratum corneum* lipid and desmosome structure together with water barrier function during mechanical stress, *J Soc Cosmet Chem*, **46**, 141–151.

37. Levi K, Baxter J, Meldrum H, Misra M, Pashkovski E, and Dauskardt RH (2008). Effect of corneodesmosome degradation on the inter-

cellular delamination of human *stratum corneum*, *J Invest Dermatol*, **128**(9), 2345–2347.

38. Wu KS, Van Osdol WW, and Dauskardt RH (2006). Mechanical properties of *stratum corneum*: effects of temperature, hydration and chemical treatment, *Biomaterials*, **27**(5), 785–795.

39. Wu KS, Stefik MM, Ananthapadmanabhan KP, and Dauskardt RH (2006). Graded delamination behavior of human *stratum corneum*, *Biomaterials*, **27**(34), 5861–5870.

40. Yuan Y and Verma R (2006). Measuring microelastic properties of *stratum corneum*, *Colloids Surf B*, **48**(1), 6–12.

41. Gaikwad RM, Vasilyev SI, Datta S, and Sokolov I (2010).Atomic force microscopy characterization of corneocytes: effect of moisturizer on their topology, rigidity, and friction, *Skin Res Technol*, **16**(3), 275–282.

42. Beard JD, Guy RH, and Gordeev SN (2013). Mechanical tomography of human corneocytes with a nanoneedle, *J Invest Dermatol*, **133**(6), 1565–1571.

43. Gardner TN and Briggs GA (2001). Biomechanical measurements in microscopically thin stratum comeum using acoustics, *Skin Res Technol*, **7**(4), 254–261.

44. Middelton JD (1968). The mechanism of water binding in the *stratum corneum*, *Br J Dermatol*, **80**(7), 437–450.

45. Ngwa W, Chen K, Sahgal A, Stepanov EV, and Luo W (2008). Nanoscale mechanics of solid-supported multilayered lipid films by force measurement, *Thin Solid Films*, **516**, 5039–5045.

46. Lévêque J-L, Poelman MC, de Rigal J, and Kligman AM (1988). Are corneocytes elastic? *Dermatologica*, **176**(2), 65–69.

47. Du Roure O, Buguin A, Feracci H, and Silberzan P (2006). Homophilic interactions between cadherin fragments at the single molecule level: an AFM study, *Langmuir*, **22**(10), 4680–4684.

48. Waschke J, Menendez-Castro C, Bruggeman P, Koob R, Amagai M, Gruber HJ, Drenckhahn D, and Baumgartner W (2007). Imaging and force spectroscopy on desmoglein 1 using atomic force microscopy reveal multivalent $Ca^{2+}$-dependent, low-affinity trans-interaction, *J Membrane Biol*, **216**, 83–92.

49. Hendriks F, Brokken D, Oomens C, Bader D, and Baaijens F (2006). The relative contribution of different skin layers to the mechanical behavior of human skin in vivo using suction experiments, *Med Eng Phys*, **28**, 259–266.

50. Kuwazuru O, Saothong J, and Yoshikawa N (2008). Mechanical approach to aging and wrinkling of human facial skin based on multistage buckling theory, *Med Eng Phys*, **30**(4), 516–522.

51. Barbero AM and Frasch HF (2005). Modeling of diffusion with partitioning in *stratum corneum* using a finite element model, *Ann Biomed Eng*, **33**, 1281–1292.

52. Feuchter D, Heisig M, and Wittum G (2006). A geometry model for the simulation of drug diffusion through the *stratum corneum*, *Comput Visual Sci*, **9**, 117–130.

53. Wang T-F, Kasting GB, and Nitsche JM (2006). A multiphase microscopic diffusion model for *stratum corneum* permeability. I. Formulation, solution, and illustrative results for representative compounds, *J Pharm Sci*, **95**, 620–648.

54. Katti K, Katti DR, Tang J, Pradhan S, and Sarikaya M (2005). Modeling mechanical responses in a laminated biocomposite. Part II. Nonlinear responses and nuances of nanostructure, *J Mater Sci*, **40**, 1749–1755.

55. Qi HJ, Bruet BJF, Palmer JS, Ortiz C, and Boyce MC (2005). Micromechanics and macromechanics of the tensile deformation of nacre, in *Mechanics of Biological Tissues* (Holzapfel GA and Ogden RW, eds), Springer-Verlag, Graz, 190–203.

56. Barthelat F, Tang H, Zavattieri PD, Li C-M, and Espinosa HD (2007). On the mechanics of mother-of-pearl: a key feature in the material hierarchical structure, *J Mech Phys Solids*, **55**, 306–337.

57. Kollar LP and Springer GS (eds) (2003). *Mechanics of Composite Structures*, Cambridge University Press, Cambridge.

58. Skerrow CJ, Clelland DG, and Skerrow D (1989). Changes to desmosomal antigens and lectin-binding sites during differentiation in normal human epidermis: a quantitative ultrastructural study, *J Cell Sci*, **92**, 667–677.

59. Chapman SJ and Walsh A (1990). Desmosomes, corneosomes and desquamation. An ultrastructural study of adult pig epidermis, *Arch Dermatol Res*, **282**(5), 304–310.

60. Potter A, Luengo G, Baltenneck C, Pavan S, and Loubet J-L (11–13 July 2007). *Measuring Mechanical Properties of Stratum Corneum and Isolated Corneocytes at a Sub-Micron Length Scale*, paper presented at the *Stratum corneum* V conference, Cardiff, Book of Abstracts, p. 15.

# PART 3

# SKIN BARRIER

# Chapter 7

# Mathematical Models of Skin Permeability: Microscopic Transport Models and Their Predictions

**Gerald B. Kasting[a] and Johannes M. Nitsche[b]**

[a]*Winkle College of Pharmacy, University of Cincinnati Academic Health Center, Cincinnati, USA*
[b]*Department of Chemical and Biological Engineering, University at Buffalo, The State University of New York, Buffalo, USA*

Gerald.Kasting@uc.edu

## 7.1  Introduction

Quantitative attempts to interpret skin permeability in terms of mathematical models date back to Scheuplein as nicely summarized in his reviews of the subject [1,2]. The first microscopic transport models for *stratum corneum* were published by Yotsuyanagi and Higuchi in 1972 [3] and the Alza group in 1975 [4]. The former established the intrinsically multiphase nature of the tissue barrier, alternating between cellular (aqueous) and intercellular (lipid) lamallae, and the latter developed a more complete two-dimensional theory for diffusion through the microstructure, spurring a great deal of additional interest. Since that time, quantitative models at several levels of detail—quantitative structure–permeability

*Computational Biophysics of the Skin*
Edited by Bernard Querleux
Copyright © 2014 Pan Stanford Publishing Pte. Ltd.
ISBN 978-981-4463-84-3 (Hardcover), 978-981-4463-85-0 (eBook)
www.panstanford.com

relationships, compartment kinetic models, diffusion models based on homogeneous membrane theory, and microscopic transport models—have been explored. A thorough review as of 2011 may be found in Mitragotri et al. [5].

It is not the authors' intention to review this field in a manner similar to Ref. [5]. Rather, we focus here on microscopic transport models and the homogenization thereof to build effective medium models [6]. We draw largely from our own work in this area but offer selected comparisons in order to highlight the importance of the microstructural details and the transport and partition properties assigned to each component thereof.

## 7.2 Review of Layer-Specific Properties and Models

From a biological point of view, skin has two layers: epidermis and dermis. However, from a morphological or transport perspective, three layers must be distinguished: *stratum corneum*, viable epidermis, and dermis. Each of these layers is discussed briefly in the following text. One must also recognize that human skin is pierced with three types of appendages: hair follicles and their associated sebaceous glands (pilosebaceous units), eccrine sweat glands, and apocrine sweat glands. The nature and density of these appendages vary sharply with body site. This review will not specifically address skin appendages other than to note that they are important for the transport of hydrophilic solutes [5] and, possibly, for all solutes at short times [1,2,7,8]. They are often described in terms of a "porous" or "polar" pathway through the *stratum corneum* [9–12]. An as-yet-unpublished microscopic transport model of the hair follicle is also available for study [13].

### 7.2.1  *Stratum Corneum*

It has been recognized for some time that the composite nature of the *stratum corneum*, with dried, cornified cells (corneocytes) interspersed in a matrix of structured lipids [4,14–16], is responsible for its remarkable barrier function (Fig. 7.1). However, the precise contribution of each component to the barrier and the associated possibilities for transport pathways has been the subject of a longstanding debate. The term "bricks-and-mortar" [4] combined with early observations that lipophilic permeants and even some putative hydrophilic ones [17] were generally found in intercellular spaces prompted many workers to conclude that the corneocytes were effectively impermeable to most solutes. However, others have noted that water swells corneocytes [18–21] and amino acids and other natural moisturizing factor components are depleted from the outer *stratum corneum* layers by washing [22]. Recent two-photon fluorescence microscopy studies also support the presence of diffusible solutes within corneocytes [23].

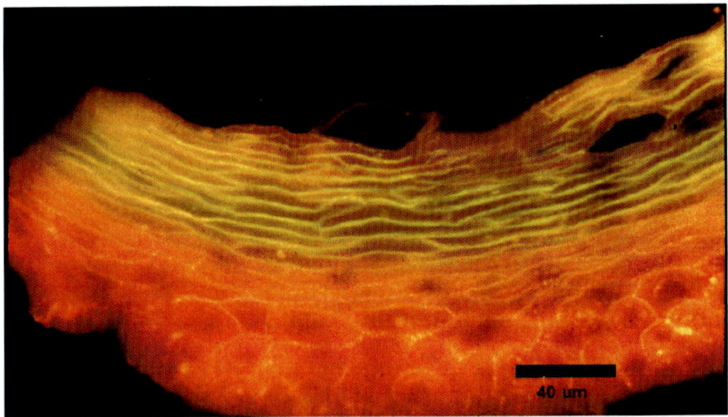


**Figure 7.1** Fluorescence micrograph of alkali-swollen human epidermis stained with Nile Red. The non-polar *stratum corneum* lipids fluoresce in the yellow range, whereas the more polar epidermal lipids are more orange-red. Reprinted from [24] with permission from AAPS.

The microscopic representation of *stratum corneum* discussed herein is shown in Fig. 7.2 and has been fully described elsewhere [25,26]. The key features that distinguish this model from other entries in this field are (1) incorporation of anisotropic lipid bilayers between the corneocytes with two limiting lipid arrangements, (2) provision for swelling of the system in the transverse direction to describe both partially hydrated and fully hydrated *stratum corneum*, and (3) a corneocyte phase with diffusion and partition properties developed from a combination of experimental data [27] and fiber matrix diffusion theory [26]. The combination of these features with a sophisticated, variable-grid finite difference numerical solution and parameterization thereof into a readily-computed form [26] gives this model unique properties not yet achieved in alternative representations.

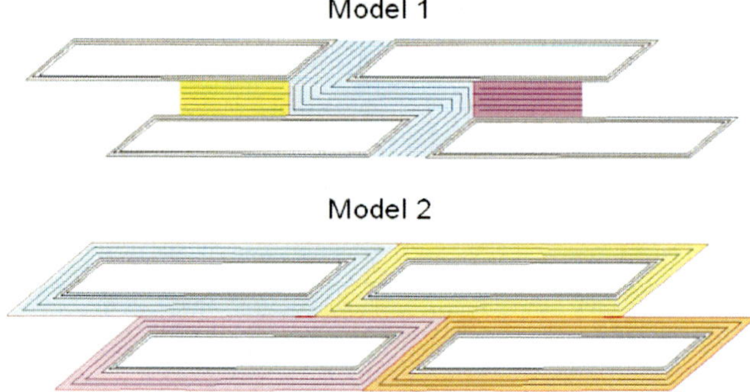



**Figure 7.2** Two-dimensional microstructure of *stratum corneum* microscopic model developed in [25,26] and discussed herein. Six anisotropic lipid bilayers (magnified in the diagram) fill the intercellular spaces. The assumed lipid configurations either allow transverse transport via continuous lateral diffusion within the bilayers (Model 1) or require at least one transverse hopping step at each cell layer (Model 2).

Discussion so far refers to the mobile (freely diffusible) penetrating solute. Pioneering work by Raykar, Anderson, and coworkers [28–30] quantified significant solute binding to corneocyte-phase keratin, which increases solute holdup beyond the diffusible holdup in the water that hydrates the corneocytes. More recently, Hansen et al. [31] developed a more detailed breakdown into fractions bound to interior (keratin) protein and corneocyte envelope proteins, as well as distinguishing accessible and inaccessible aqueous compartments. This was followed by publication of an experimental database on keratin binding that includes a predictive component [32]. A particularly significant paper by Anissimov and Roberts [33] showed that explicit inclusion of binding (in terms of a bound solute concentration in addition to the freely diffusible concentration) is essential to properly calculating transient dermal absorption. Seif and Hansen [34] established an in vitro model employing purified keratin powder that further quantifies binding kinetics. Frasch et al. [35] discussed the importance of keratin binding in properly interpreting theophylline diffusion through skin, and Nitsche and Frasch [36] discussed the implications of slow reversible binding for homogenization schemes. It is becoming clear that slow solute binding to keratin in the *stratum corneum* is the missing element needed to accurately describe transient dermal absorption, and to resolve unexplained transients in models that do not include it [37].

## 7.2.2 Viable Epidermis

Viable epidermis is a cellular tissue that changes continuously from the basal layer to the granular layer as the terminal differentiation of the constituent keratinocytes progresses. It does not have a blood supply, drawing its energy by diffusive exchange with the atmosphere (primarily $O_2$) and the dermis. A typical depiction is shown in Fig. 7.3.

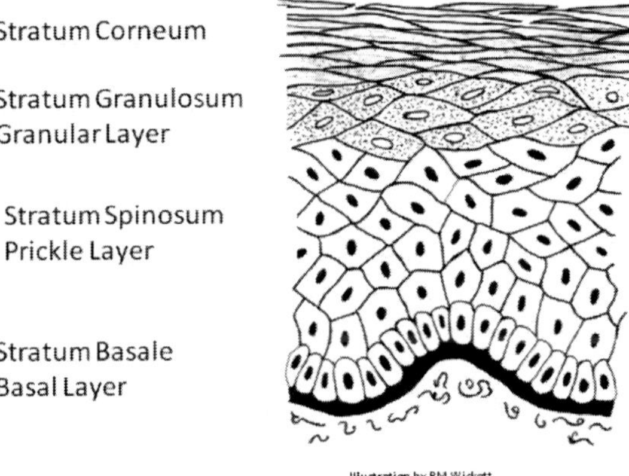


**Figure 7.3** Artist's representation of epidermis showing the four recognized layers and the associated morphological changes in the continually differentiating tissue. Illustration courtesy of Robin M. Wickett.

Because it is difficult to isolate, few direct measurements of solute transport in viable epidermis have been made. Since the rate-limiting barrier for most small solutes is the *stratum corneum*, the most common treatment of viable epidermis in skin transport models has been to combine it with dermis as an aqueous barrier in series with the *stratum corneum* [38–41]. A slightly more sophisticated approach acknowledges the difference in perfusion between viable epidermis and dermis but still does not differentiate between the primarily cellular and acellular nature, respectively, of the two tissues [42,43]. This approximation still may be suitable for many applications involving small molecules, but it is unsatisfactory for mechanistic analysis of their pharmacological or toxicological activity within the tissue [44]. Furthermore, experimental evidence that viable epidermis provides a significant diffusion barrier for macromolecules has recently been presented [45,46].

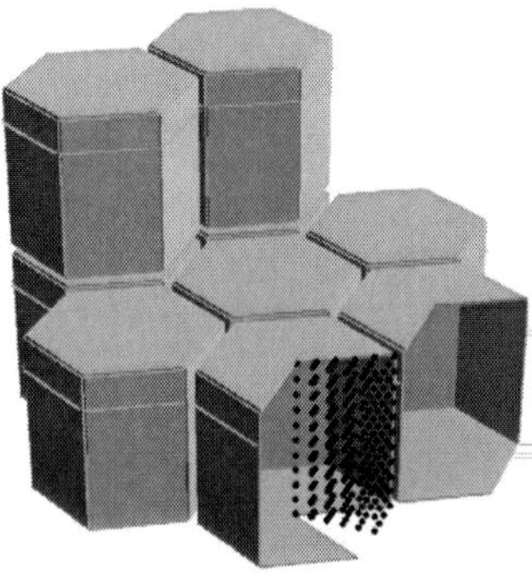

**Figure 7.4**    Hexagonal cellular model components for the viable epidermis microtransport model described in [47]. The "cells" are given two aspect ratios, a taller one corresponding to basal and spinous layers and a flatter one corresponding to the granular layer. Provision for solute transport via both extracellular fluid and transcellular pathways (including both gap junctions and tight junctions) is included in the model.

To address these needs, we have recently developed a microscopic transport model for viable epidermis with a cellular architecture involving keratinocytes in the shape of hexagonal prisms (Fig. 7.4) [47]. Cell membranes are represented as anisotropic lipid bilayers with passive diffusion properties drawn from the phospholipid membrane literature on permeability [48,49], lateral diffusion [50], and anisotropic diffusion [51]. Transport through and around these membrane barriers is analyzed using a finite difference approach. Provision for direct cell-to-cell transport via gap junctions [52–54] and impedance of extracellular fluid transport via tight junctions [55] are included within the model framework.

Example calculations are presented for water, L-glucose (a small, passively transported hydrophilic solute), and hydrocortisone (a larger lipophilic solute with low-to-moderate protein binding characteristics). Extension of this work to encompass a larger range of solutes including highly protein-bound species is envisioned. This type of microscopic model may eventually provide a detailed picture of solute distribution within the tissue and, in particular, freely diffusing solute concentrations at the site of action of haptens or other pharmacophores.

### 7.2.3   Dermis

Dermis is a largely acellular tissue comprising an aqueous "ground substance" dispersed in a matrix of collagen and elastin fibers, a small cellular population including fibroblasts and mast cells, and a complex network of blood and lymphatic vessels [56]. The primary structural protein is collagen, which occupies some 30% of the dermal volume. The "ground substance" is an aqueous mileau of glycosaminoglycans (GAGs) and proteoglycans, which provide the water-holding capacity for the tissue along with a variety of important biological functions. Dermis has an upper, papillary layer, which is highly perfused with blood capillaries and a lower, reticular layer, which contains most of the structural protein (Fig. 7.5). There are two significant fiber networks to consider: one comprising primarily collagen and having a relatively coarse mesh and the other associated with the proteoglycans having a much finer mesh.

Solute transport in the dermis has been described at several levels of complexity. The compartment models referenced in [5] have been used to interpret the phenomenon loosely termed local enhanced transdermal delivery [57–59]. The data from one of these studies [57] were later reanalyzed by Kretsos et al. using a diffusion model with a uniformly distributed capillary clearance [60]. This model was subsequently developed into a predictive tool using dermis diffusion, partition and clearance data from a combination of in vitro and in vivo studies [61]. The model and associated data [62,63] emphasized the importance of binding to soluble proteins in describing solute transport through the tissue (Fig. 7.6). Ibrahim et al. expanded on this concept by including a more physiologically accurate solute exchange between blood capillaries and dermis,

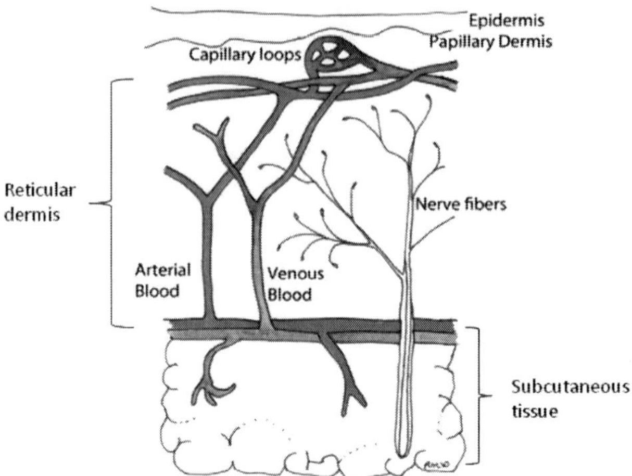



**Figure 7.5**    Artist's representation of skin highlighting the papillary and reticular layers of the dermis and the associated blood supply and nerves. Despite these structures and others, including fibroblasts, mast cells, sweat glands, and pilosebaceous units, the tissue is largely acellular. Illustration courtesy of Robin M. Wickett.

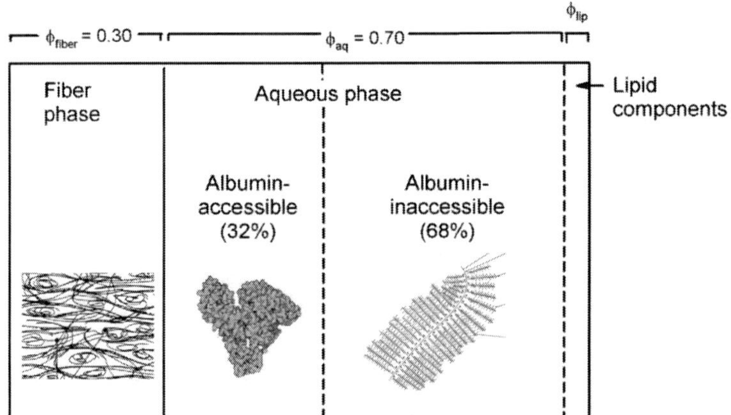



**Figure 7.6**    Conceptual partition model for dermis employed by Kretsos et al. [61]. The tissue was divided into a solute-inaccessible fibrous region, a region accessible to small solutes only and a region accessible to both large and small solutes based on data from Bert et al. [71,72]. The volume of the lipid component, which is much smaller than that reported by Bert et al., was adjusted to best match in vitro dermis/water partition data.

as well as lymphatic clearance [64]. The latter is important for estimating the clearance of macromolecules and migrating dendritic cells from the dermis as well as that of small, highly protein-bound solutes. Although rigorous hydrodynamic theory exists addressing hindered diffusion in idealized arrays of fibers [65–69] and hydraulic permeability within bimodal arrays generically representative of collagen/proteoglycan matrices [70], it has yet to be applied to solute diffusion in structures specifically mimicking dermis.

Anissimov and Roberts [73] and also Dancik et al. [74] have taken a somewhat different tack in describing transport in dermis. These investigators have used a diffusion model with uniform clearance to analyze both ex vivo skin biopsy [73] and in vivo microdialysis [74] data. These investigators report that satisfactory interpretation of solute concentrations in skin can only be achieved if a substantial element of convective transport is included in the analysis. They achieve this result by increasing the diffusion coefficients of the solutes in the dermis by approximately a factor of 10 and re-interpreting them as dispersion coefficients. There is sound theoretical basis for such a replacement [6,75,76]. Physically, one can interpret this as solute uptake in the papillary dermis and redistribution in the reticular dermis by the blood and lymph. Such a mechanism does offer an explanation for local enhanced transdermal delivery, which had previously been described using compartment models [57–59]. However, transdermal fluxes assumed by Anissimov and Roberts [73] to achieve the fits to the skin biopsy data are unusually high for intact human skin (GBK, JMN, unpublished). So the matter is not fully resolved.

A true, albeit simplified, microtransport model for dermis was developed by Kretsos [77], working as a student in JMN's laboratory at the State University of New York at Buffalo (UB). It was later published by Kretsos and Kasting [78] during Kretsos's postdoctoral tenure at the University of Cincinnati (UC). A depiction of the absorbing capillary microarray is shown in Fig. 7.7.

The analysis showed that the absorption pattern from this array can be well approximated by a uniform dispersed first-order clearance. Thus, the latter approximation seems a sound one for solute uptake in the papillary dermis. However, the capillary loop structure is unique to this layer, and a different pattern may come into play in the less highly perfused reticular dermis. The seeds for such a distinction have been sewn by Cevc and Vierl [79], who developed a model for the spatial distribution of the microvasculature in the dermis.

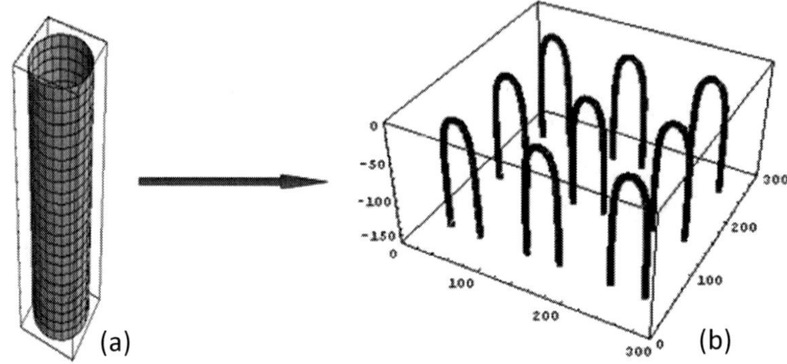



**Figure 7.7**  Framework of the capillary loop microtransport model for dermis presented in Ref. [78]. The Starling flux equations applying to a single Krogh's cylinder (a) were adapted for a regular array of U-shaped capillaries embedded in an otherwise homogeneous medium (b). The analysis shows that the absorption pattern from this array can be well approximated by a uniform dispersed first-order clearance.

## 7.3　Analysis of Three *Stratum Corneum* Microscopic Transport Models

The validity of predictions from microscopic transport models hinges on two distinct aspects of their construction: (1) accurate depiction of the microstructure and (2) accurate estimation of microphase transport and partition coefficients. In order for predictions from the simpler, homogenized versions of these models (e.g., [42]) to also be valid, a third condition—conformity with the requirements of effective medium theory [6]—must also be met. Most simply stated, the central such requirement is that the time scale of the microscopic transport processes is much less than that for transport across the macroscopic system [25]. Equivalently, the macroscopic tissue layer must comprise a large number $N$ of the microscopic unit cells. For a brick-and-mortar model using tetrakaidekahedral corneocytes, Muha et al. [80] found that the error associated with a homogenized representation of the *stratum corneum* is only 14% for $N = 5$, i.e., the number of cell layers does not have to be large. Naegel et al. [81] earlier came to a similar conclusion for cuboidal corneocytes. For biological systems it is our experience that the second requirement—accurate estimation of the microphase properties—is often the most difficult to ensure. To illustrate this point, we consider three *stratum corneum* microscopic transport models sharing similar microstructures but employing very different choices for the microphase properties. The models considered here are those of Johnson et al. [82], Chen et al. [83,84], and our own [25–27]. All models have associated data and analysis [20,21,24,50,85–87] to which the reader are referred for details. For convenience, we will refer to these models as the MIT, CAU, and UB/UC models, respectively, reflecting the institutional affiliations of the developers.

### 7.3.1 *Stratum Corneum* Microstructure

Figure 7.8 shows the major microstructural features of the three skin diffusion models. All models comprise an ordered, two-dimensional array of corneocytes embedded in a lipid matrix with a nearly equivalent number of corneocyte layers ($N = 15$–16). Two-dimensional arrays have been termed "ribbon" geometries [80,81]; vis-à-vis more complex three-dimensional models, they are generally less permeable, and can be regarded as establishing an upper limit on barrier properties. The relevant dimensions are listed in Table 7.1. The MIT and CAU models share identical geometries but differ in the properties assigned to the lipid and corneocyte phases. The UB/UC model has slightly shorter corneocytes and wider lipid regions with a higher corneocyte offset ratio $\omega = d_l/d_s$. The value $\omega \cong 4$ in the UB/UC model was based on an analysis of tortuosity in alkali-swollen human *stratum corneum*, whereas the value $\omega = 8$ derives from rodent (mouse ear) *stratum corneum* [24]. The UB/UC model is also the only one for which the dimensions change as the skin hydrates. The corneocytes swell slightly in the lateral dimension and substantially in the transverse direction [24], whereas the lipid regions do not [88]. The acute angle $\varphi$ associated with the intercellular lipid "necks" between corneocytes (Fig. 7.8b) provides a plausible mechanism for this anisotropic swelling behavior without requiring an associated variation in lipid density. The swelling feature avoids the logical inconsistency present in the MIT and CAU models of using dimensions associated with partially hydrated skin while calibrating the model with steady-state permeability data from aqueous solutions, a test system that always results in fully hydrated skin.

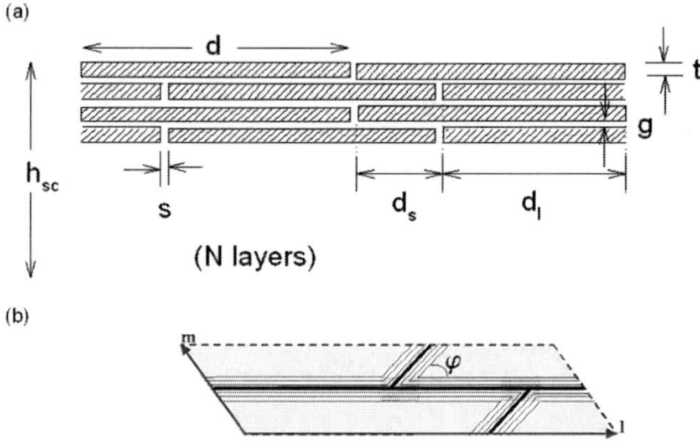

**Figure 7.8**    Two-dimensional microstructure of *stratum corneum* microscopic models discussed in the text. All models employed periodic boundary conditions in the lateral direction and 15–16 corneocyte/lipid composite layers ($N$ = 15 or 16) in the transverse directions. Six anisotropic lipid bilayers (magnified in the diagram) fill the intercellular space in the MIT and UB/UC models; the CAU lipid phase is isotropic. The transverse thickness $t$ (and consequently $h_{sc}$) varies with skin hydration state in the UB/UC model but is fixed at the partially hydrated *stratum corneum* value of 0.8 µm in the others.

**Table 7.1**    Properties of the three *stratum corneum* microtransport models discussed in the text

| Property | MIT | CAU | UB/UC partial hydration | UB/UC full hydration |
|---|---|---|---|---|
| $N$ | 15 | 16 | 15 | 15 |
| $d$, um | 40 | 40 | 30 | 31.2 |
| $t$, um | 0.8 | 0.8 | 0.8 | 2.8 |
| $s$, nm | 75 | 75 | 91 | 91 |
| $g$ | 75 | 75 | 91 | 91 |
| $\omega\ (d_l/d_s)$ | 8 | 8 | ~4.0 | ~4.3 |

| Property | MIT | CAU | UB/UC partial hydration | UB/UC full hydration |
|---|---|---|---|---|
| $\varphi$, degrees | 90 | 90 | 20 | 50 |
| $h_{sc}$, µm | 13.1 | 13.9 | 13.4 | 43.4 |
| Permeable corneocytes? | No | Yes | Yes | Yes |
| Anisotropic lipids? | Yes | No | Yes | Yes |
| Accomodates hydrophilic solutes? | No | Yes | No | No |

## 7.3.2 Transport Properties and Predictions

These properties will be discussed in terms of four representative skin permeants ranging from highly lipophilic (testosterone) to highly hydrophilic (sucrose). The permeants and their physical properties relevant for model calculations are shown in Table 7.2. The properties of each model associated with these compounds are assembled in the Appendix in Tables 7.A1–7.A3 and discussed below.

**Table 7.2**     Permeants considered in the analysis

| Compound | MW | log $K_{oct}$ |
|---|---|---|
| Testosterone | 288.4 | 3.32 |
| Caffeine | 194.2 | −0.07 |
| Water | 18.01 | −1.38 |
| Sucrose | 342.3 | −3.70 |

## 7.3.2.1 MIT model

Johnson et al. [82] created the first *stratum corneum* model allowing for anisotropic diffusion in the lipid phase, but assumed an impermeable corneocyte phase. The consequences of these assumptions have been discussed at some length [25] and will be recapitulated here. Their construction implicitly assumes a lipid configuration that is equivalent to Model 1 (Fig. 7.2). If the lipids wrap around the cells as in Model 2 (Fig. 7.2), then the transverse mass transfer coefficient for hopping between bilayers must, in their construction, be inconsequential [82]. Under these restrictions, these investigators concluded that lateral diffusion in the *stratum corneum* lipids is rate-limiting for transport of solutes across the tissue. Johnson et al. explicitly excluded large hydrophilic solutes like sucrose from their analysis because they correctly realized that a purely lipid pathway model would not accommodate such solutes. Small hydrophilic solutes like water or moderately hydrophilic compounds like caffeine fell within the scope of the model.

There are several concerns with the MIT model. Partitioning of hydrophilic compounds, notably water, into the tissue is highly underpredicted. The lateral diffusivity of water in the lipid phase required to match the permeability and partition data is about 60% of its self-diffusivity (i.e. diffusivity of water in water), an unlikely outcome for an array of ordered lipids. The predicted time lags for achievement of steady-state diffusion (Table 7.A3) are remarkably short—about 100 min for testosterone, 10 min for caffeine, and 4 s for water. Experimental studies of diffusion through excised split-thickness human skin in one of the authors' laboratories have yielded time lags of 550 ± 40 min for testosterone ($n$ = 24) [37] and 31 ± 14 min ($n$ = 38) for water [26]. The MIT investigators acknowledged the time lag issue in their original report [82]. They, in fact, reported time lags that were about 16-fold shorter than those reported here; however, the method by which they were calculated was incorrect. This discrepancy was pointed out earlier by Frasch and Barbero [89].

Despite these limitations, the MIT work introduced the concept of anisotropic transport in the lipid phase and provided a plausible correspondence between *stratum corneum* permeability and their own lateral diffusivity measurements for fluorescent probes in isolated *stratum corneum* lipids [50].

### 7.3.2.2   UB/UC model

This model, created in the authors' laboratories, retains the concept of anisotropic diffusion in the lipid phase but also includes permeable corneocytes. It addresses many of the concerns in the MIT model, yet shares some of its limitations. In particular, transport of ionized or highly hydrophilic neutral solutes through the *stratum corneum* is not addressed by either model. This raises concerns if the model is to be employed in the context of risk assessment for, say, metal allergens or cationic hair dyes, potentially hazardous substances that contact the skin in various occupational settings.

As the developers, we could say a lot of good things about this model but will refrain from doing so here. We emphasize, however, the key tenet of anisotropic transport in the lipid phase. This is a known phenomenon in phospholipid membranes [49,51,90,91], and there is every reason to believe it should also apply to *stratum corneum* lipid bilayers. It is computationally difficult to treat, which we believe to be the primary reason most investigators have not considered this feature. Our analysis suggests (Table 7.A2 and Refs. [25,26]) that the extent of anisotropy is several hundred-fold to several thousand-fold, depending on molecular size, with transverse diffusion being much slower than lateral diffusion. Thus, the rate-limiting step for diffusion of most permeants across the *stratum corneum* is intramembrane transbilayer hopping, in stark disagreement with the conclusions drawn from the MIT and CAU models.

It will be noted that the predictions of the UC/UB model for the macroscopic transport and partition properties of the selected test permeants (Table 7.A3) have some limitations. A comparison of the hydrated skin model predictions (Column 6) with the experimental data in Column 2 shows that the model overpredicts the *stratum corneum*/water partition coefficient $(K_{sc})$ and permeability coefficient $(k_p)$ for testosterone and underpredicts the time lag $(t_L)$. For caffeine $K_{sc}$ is about right, $k_p$ is underpredicted and $t_L$ is overpredicted. Water is handled fairly well in these calculations with steady (unchanging) tissue structure and properties; however, it should be noted that simulation of the swelling dynamics associated with transient exposures to water or aqueous formulations is not presently possible. Transport of sucrose across the *stratum corneum* is grossly underpredicted, reinforcing the fact that a model that requires solute transit across intact, highly anisotropic lipid bilayers will not admit large polar solutes. A separate, aqueous-continuous pathway is required. In our estimation, this is probably the reason the model underestimates caffeine transport as well. Using earlier estimates of polar pathway permeability (e.g., [38] and the Robinson model in [92]) this smaller, moderately hydrophilic solute $(\log K_{oct} = -0.07)$ is expected to have comparable transport through polar and lipid pathways in the *stratum corneum*.

The above argument highlights the difficulty in correctly interpreting macroscopic transport behavior in complex structures such as *stratum corneum*. Skin permeabilities and, especially, time lags to achievement of steady-state transport, are highly sensitive to the heterogeneous nature of the tissue. When the additional phenomenon of slowly reversible binding is also added to the picture [33,34] the interpretation of time lags becomes problematical [35]. Only by carefully identifying and characterizing the contributing factors does an accurate predictive picture emerge.

### 7.3.2.3 CAU model

This is the most recent entry in the class of predictive skin microscopic transport models. The original formulation appeared in 2008 [83] and the most recent summary in 2013 [85]. The CAU model borrows some features from the MIT and UB/UC entries, employs a lipid diffusion model from Mitragotri [93], but introduces a new approximation for corneocyte phase diffusivities. As a consequence, this model is able to match the steady-state flux and associated skin permeability of large, highly hydrophilic solutes such as sucrose, raffinose, and mannitol, in addition to accommodating lipophilic solutes. The investigators have emphasized this point in their research reports [84,85].

It is of interest to examine how this is accomplished. The CAU model assumes isotropic diffusion in the lipid phase, with diffusivities comparable to the lateral diffusivities in the MIT and UB/UC models (Table 7.A2). Corneocytes are permeable, and the bulk of the transport for most compounds is transcellular [84]. Since transverse diffusion in the lipids is much more facile than in the UB/UC model (see $k_{trans}\delta$ entries in Table 7.A2), the corneocytes must impart most of the diffusive resistance. This is accomplished by modifying a fiber matrix diffusion model originally developed for interpreting protein diffusion in agarose gels [69]. By adjusting the parameters $\alpha$ and $\beta$ in this model to match bulk skin permeability data for 8 selected solutes [84], the investigators achieved hindrance factors of $\sim 10^{-6}$ for diffusion in corneocytes versus aqueous diffusion for all solutes (Table 7.A1). The plausibility of this approximation is defended in [84] and includes citations of work from Heisig et al. [94] and Naegel et al. [95].

However, is this approximation correct? The original fiber matrix model proposed by Johnson et al. [69] yielded hindrance factors on the order of $10^{-1}$ for macromolecules diffusing in dilute aqueous gels. The revised model [84] yields hindrance factors of $10^{-6}$ for small molecules in a keratin matrix with a fiber volume fraction (fully hydrated) of ~0.19 [25–27]. It is hard to support such estimates for hindered aqueous diffusion based on established theory (to say nothing of intuition regarding molecular mobility with a very moderate degree of blockage by cylindrical obstacles). Indeed, estimation of corneocyte phase diffusivity in [26] using another fiber matrix approach, supported by literature studies [65,96,97] with a carefully constructed extrapolation to denser matrices [98], led to the much higher diffusivity values ($D_{cor}$) shown in Table 7.A2. The CAU model leads to plausible time lags for lipophilic and moderately hydrophilic compounds, but yields a value of 15.4 h for sucrose (Table 7.A3). Tang et al. reported a time lag of 3.9 h for sucrose in excised pig skin [10], which has a thicker *stratum corneum* than human skin. Furthermore, Peck et al. [99] determined steady-state permeabilities for these compounds through human epidermal membrane by sampling four times within the first 12 h, suggesting their time lags were much shorter than 14 h. The CAU model also fails to explain the different temperature dependence of skin permeability exhibited by hydrophilic and lipophilic permeants [100,101], which suggests that the primary barrier for lipophilic solutes resides in a lipid rather than aqueous microenvironment. The well-known large increase in *stratum corneum* permeability following delipidization [1,2] is also hard to reconcile with a model in which the corneocytes provide the primary barrier to transport.

### 7.3.3  Targets for Future Research

In our experience, there is an ongoing interest in better computational models for many biological systems, and skin is certainly included in this list. Other chapters in this book deal with computational approaches to describe mechanical and cosmetic aspects of skin. For skin permeability and absorption, we find dermal toxicology and risk assessment to be the biggest drivers for research. Both industrial and government sponsors are looking for practical tools to evaluate risk for a variety of dermal exposure scenarios, and for compounds dissolved in complex industrial, dermatological or cosmetic matrices. Formulation thermodynamics as well as effects of the components on skin permeability are difficult to predict with current technology. These deficiencies can be addressed. We believe the area is ripe for further research to broaden the range of ingredients, formulations and exposure scenarios for which predictive permeation modeling may be applied.

From a technical perspective, several points stand out. Although the geometrical and mathematical sophistication of brick-and-mortar models has reached a high level [80,81], the physicochemical inputs have sometimes lagged behind; in particular these models still assume isotropic lipid-phase diffusion [80,81,102]. The basis for a significant impact of slow binding processes in the *stratum corneum* corneocyte phase has been laid [32–36], yet none of the developed microscopic models incorporate this feature. The entries of Mitragotri [103] and the CAU group [83–85,87] notwithstanding, appropriate meshing of the polar and lipid pathways through the *stratum corneum* remains an unresolved problem. Finally the impact of formulation components on *stratum corneum* permeability, while extensively characterized from a phenomenological perspective, remains a difficult challenge for *a priori* prediction.

## Appendix:  Selected Transport and Partition Coefficients for Three Stratum Corneum Microscopic Models

**Table 7.A1**  Corneocyte-phase properties of the microscopic *stratum corneum* models for four representative solutes

| Property | MIT | CAU | UB/UC partial hydration | UB/UC full hydration |
|---|---|---|---|---|
| *Testosterone* | | | | |
| $D_{\mathrm{cor}} \times 10^6$, $\mathrm{cm^2s^{-1}}$ | —[a] | 7.68E-06 | 0.884 | 3.71 |
| $K_{\mathrm{cor}}$ | 0 | 17.6 | 0.216 | 0.750 |
| *Caffeine* | | | | |
| $D_{\mathrm{cor}} \times 10^6$, $\mathrm{cm^2s^{-1}}$ | —[a] | 1.28E-05 | 1.85 | 5.87 |
| $K_{\mathrm{cor}}$ | 0[b] | 0.979 | 0.274 | 0.768 |
| *Water* | | | | |
| $D_{\mathrm{cor}} \times 10^6$, $\mathrm{cm^2s^{-1}}$ | —[a] | 2.08E-04 | 3.32 | 19.2 |
| $K_{\mathrm{cor}}$ | 0 | 0.828 | ~0.40[c] | 0.81[c] |

| Property | MIT | CAU | UB/UC partial hydration | UB/UC full hydration |
|---|---|---|---|---|
| *Sucrose* | | | | |
| $D_{cor} \times 10^6$, cm$^2$s$^{-1}$ | —[a] | 6.13E-06 | 1.08 | 4.17 |
| $K_{cor}$ | 0 | 0.808 | 0.232 | 0.755 |

*Note:* These properties represent those of the freely diffusing or unbound solute except where noted.

[a]Not applicable to this model.

[b]Investigators acknowledged the presence of water in the corneocytes; however, its contribution to transport across the *stratum corneum* was considered to be negligible.

[c]Water is a special case in the UB/UC model. These properties represent effective values reflecting both free and bound water. $D_{cor}$ was calculated from Eq. 13 in Ref. [20] using a value of $D_{11} = 27.4 \times 10^{-6}$ cm$^2$s$^{-1}$ for the self-diffusivity of water at 32°C and a binding constant $\kappa = 0.30$. The $D_{11}$ value was estimated from the pulsed field NMR data in [104] and the water viscosity data in [105].

**Table 7.A2** Lipid-phase properties of the microscopic *stratum corneum* models for four representative solutes

| Property | MIT | CAU | UB/UC partial hydration | UB/UC full hydration |
|---|---|---|---|---|
| *Testosterone* | | | | |
| $D_{lat} \times 10^9$, cm$^2$s$^{-1}$ | 11.3[a] | 14.2 | 3.93 | 11.8 |
| $k_{trans}\delta \times 10^9$, cm$^2$s$^{-1}$ | — | [14.2][b] | 0.477E-03 | 1.43E-03 |
| $K_{lip}$ | 334 | 211 | 210 | 210 |
| *Caffeine* | | | | |
| $D_{lat} \times 10^9$, cm$^2$s$^{-1}$ | 113 | 76.3 | 9.02 | 27.1 |
| $k_{trans}\delta \times 10^9$, cm$^2$s$^{-1}$ | — | [76.3][b] | 2.12E-03 | 6.34E-03 |
| $K_{lip}$ | 0.885 | 0.893 | 0.377 | 0.377 |
| *Water* | | | | |
| $D_{lat} \times 10^9$, cm$^2$s$^{-1}$ | 16,400 | 6390 | 2660 | 7990 |
| $k_{trans}\delta \times 10^9$, cm$^2$s$^{-1}$ | — | [6390][b] | 0.685 | 2.05 |
| $K_{lip}$ | 0.0894 | 0.108 | 0.0328 | 0.0328 |

| Property | MIT | CAU | UB/UC partial hydration | UB/UC full hydration |
|---|---|---|---|---|
| *Sucrose* | | | | |
| $D_{lat} \times 10^9$, $\mathrm{cm^2 s^{-1}}$ | — | 5.91 | 2.86 | 8.57 |
| $k_{trans}\delta \times 10^9$, $\mathrm{cm^2 s^{-1}}$ | — | $[5.91]^b$ | 0.235E-03 | 0.706E-03 |
| $K_{lip}$ | 15.4E-04 | 25.7E-04 | 4.33E-04 | 4.33E-04 |

*Note*: The product $k_{trans}\delta$ is an estimate of the transverse diffusivity $D_{trans}$ required to produce an equivalent diffusive resistance for traversing a lipid bilayer of width $\delta$. The value of $\delta$ in *stratum corneum* lipids is 13 nm [25].

[a]Values estimated as in [82] from experimental permeabilities and their Eq. 11, but using the log $K_{oct}$ values in Table 7.2.

[b]Lipid-phase diffusion in the CAU model is isotropic.

**Table 7.A3**   Macroscopic transport properties associated with the microscopic *stratum corneum* models for four representative solutes

| Property | Experimental values[a] | MIT | CAU | UB/UC Partial hydration | UB/UC Full hydration |
|---|---|---|---|---|---|
| *Testosterone* | | | | | |
| $D_{sc} \times 10^{12}$, $\mathrm{cm^2 s^{-1}}$ | | 47.2 | 68.2 | 19.9 | 559 |
| $K_{sc}$ | $7.32^b$ | 29.2 | 18.2 | 51.87 | 18.51 |
| $k_p \times 10^5$, $\mathrm{cm\,h^{-1}}$ | $220^c, 536^c$ | $[378]^d$ | 321 | 278 | 859 |
| $t_L$, h | $9.2^e$ | 1.68 | 1.31 | 4.16 | 1.56 |
| *Caffeine* | | | | | |
| $D_{sc} \times 10^{12}$, $\mathrm{cm^2 s^{-1}}$ | | 471 | 35.1 | 1.76 | 37.4 |
| $K_{sc}$ | $2.59^b$ | 0.0773 | 1.82 | 4.28 | 2.12 |
| $k_p \times 10^5$, $\mathrm{cm\,h^{-1}}$ | $10.0^c, 32^f$ | $[10.0]^g$ | 16.5 | 2.03 | 6.56 |
| $t_L$, h | $4.0^g, 0.83^f$ | 0.169 | 2.56 | 47.1 | 23.3 |
| *Water* | | | | | |
| $D_{sc} \times 10^{12}$, $\mathrm{cm^2 s^{-1}}$ | | 68,500 | 1000 | 591 | 2800 |
| $K_{sc}$ | $0.78^h, 0.795^i$ | 0.00781 | 0.595 | 0.358 | 0.782 |
| $k_p \times 10^5$, $\mathrm{cm\,h^{-1}}$ | $147^d$ | $[147]^d$ | 154 | 57.0 | 182 |
| $t_L$, h | $0.30^j, 0.52^k$ | 0.00116 | 0.090 | 0.140 | 0.311 |

| Property | Experimental values[a] | MIT | CAU | UB/UC Partial hydration | UB/UC Full hydration |
|---|---|---|---|---|---|
| *Sucrose* | | | | | |
| $D_{sc} \times 10^{12}$, $cm^2 s^{-1}$ | | 55900[l] | 5.83 | 0.00130[l] | 0.0105[l] |
| $K_{sc}$ | | 1.35E-04[l] | 0.87 | 0.766 | 0.920 |
| $k_p \times 10^5$, cm h$^{-1}$ | 2.07[c] | [2.07][d] | 1.31 | 2.69E-04[l] | 8.06E-04[l] |
| $t_L$, h | 3.9[g] | 0.00142[l] | 15.4 | 63500[l] | 82500[l] |

[a]All values apply to fully hydrated skin. The list is representative rather than comprehensive.

[b][27] and references therein.

[c][82] and references therein.

[d]Median of reported values in [82]. The MIT group [82] did not estimate $k_p$, but rather estimated $D_{lat}$ from the experimental value of $k_p$.

[e][37] Split-thickness human skin ($n$ = 24); value is discussed in text.

[f][106]. Nitsche and Frasch (unpublished) reanalyzed the data in Fig. 7.1 of this report and estimated $t_L$ = 2.5 h.

[g][107] and references therein. The sucrose value was obtained on full-thickness pig skin.

[h][20].

[i]Based on data in Table 7.2 of [86] and conversions given in [21].

[j][108].

[k][26].

[l]Values marked with this superscript indicate that these predictions are not within the scope of the model. They are included in the table to show why the lipid-continuous MIT and UB/UC models must be supplemented with a polar pathway contribution in order to describe the permeation of large, hydrophilic solutes.

## Acknowledgments

Support for this work from the US National Institute for Occupational Safety and Health (NIOSH) and Cosmetics Europe (formerly COLIPA) is gratefully acknowledged. The conclusions drawn here reflect the opinions of the authors and have not been endorsed by either NIOSH or Cosmetics Europe.

## References

1. Scheuplein RJ and Blank IH (1971). Permeability of the skin, *Physiol Rev*, **51**, 702–747.

2. Scheuplein RJ (1978). Skin permeation, in *The Physiology and Pathophysiology of the Skin* (Jarrett A, ed), Academic Press, New York, pp. 1669–1752.

3. Yotsuyanagi T and Higuchi WI (1972). A two phase series model for the transport of steroids across the fully hydrated *stratum corneum*, *J Pharm Pharmacol*, **24**, 934–941.

4. Michaels AS, Chandrasekaran SK, and Shaw JE (1975). Drug permeation through human skin: theory and in vitro experimental measurement, *AIChE J*, **21**, 985–996.

5. Mitragotri S, Anissimov YG, Bunge AL, Frasch HF, Guy RH, Hadgraft J, Kasting GB, Lane ME, and Roberts MS (2011). Mathematical models of skin permeability: an overview, *Int J Pharm*, **418**, 115–129.

6. Brenner H and Edwards DA (1993). *Macrotransport Processes*, Butterworth-Heinemann, Boston.

7. Scheuplein RJ (1967). Mechanism of percutaneous absorption II. Transient diffusion and the relative importance of various routes of skin penetration, *J Invest Dermatol*, **48**, 79–88.

8. Ho CK (2004). Probabilistic modeling of percutaneous absorption for risk-based exposure assessments and transdermal drug delivery, *Stat Methodol*, **1**, 47–69.

9. Tang H, Mitragotri S, Blankschtein D, and Langer R (2001). Theoretical description of transdermal transport of hydrophilic permeants: application to low-frequency sonophoresis, *J Pharm Sci*, **90**, 545–568.

10. Tang H, Blankschtein D, and Langer R (2002). Prediction of steady-state skin permeabilities of polar and nonpolar permeants across excised pig skin based on measurements of transient diffusion: characterization of hydration effects on the skin porous pathway, *J Pharm Sci*, **91**, 1891–1907.

11. Kushner J IV, Blankschtein D, and Langer R (2008). Evaluation of hydrophilic permeant transport parameters in the localized and non-localized transport regions of skin treated simultaneously with low-frequency ultrasound and sodium lauryl sulfate, *J Pharm Sci*, **97**, 906–918.

12. Kushner J IV, Blankschtein D, and Langer R (2007). Evaluation of the porosity, the tortuosity, and the hindrance factor for the transdermal delivery of hydrophilic permeants in the context of the aqueous pore pathway hypothesis using dual-radiolabeled permeability experiments, *J Pharm Sci*, **96**, 3263–3282.

13. Dancik Y (2006). *Mathematical Models of Diffusion through and Near Skin Appendages: Hair Follicle and Eccrine Sweat Gland Pathways*, Ph.D. thesis, Department of Chemical and Biological Engineering, State University of New York, Buffalo.

14. Elias PM (1983). Epidermal lipids, barrier function, and desquamation, *J Invest Dermatol*, **80**, 44s–49s.

15. Grayson S and Elias PM (1982). Isolation and lipid biochemical characterization of *stratum corneum* membrane complexes: implications for the cutaneous permeability barrier, *J Invest Dermatol*, **78**, 128–135.

16. Elias PM, Goerke J, and Friend DS (1977). Mammalian epidermal barrier layer lipids: composition and influence on structure, *J Invest Dermatol*, **69**, 535–546.

17. Bodde HE, van den Brink I, Koerten HK, and de Haan FHN (1991). Visualization of in vitro percutaneous penetration of mercuric chloride transport through intercellular space versus cellular uptake through desmosomes, *J Control Rel*, **15**, 227–236.

18. Warner RR, Stone KJ, and Boissy YL (2003). Hydration disrupts human *stratum corneum* ultrastructure, *J Invest Dermatol*, **120**, 275–284.

19. Bouwstra JA, de Graaff A, Gooris GS, Nijsse J, Wiechers JW, and van Aelst AC (2003). Water distribution and related morphology in human *stratum corneum* at different hydration levels, *J Invest Dermatol*, **120**, 750–758.

20. Kasting GB, Barai ND, Wang T-F, and Nitsche JM (2003). Mobility of water in human *stratum corneum*, *J Pharm Sci*, **92**, 2326–2340.

21. Kasting GB and Barai ND (2003). Equilibrium water sorption in human *stratum corneum*, *J Pharm Sci*, **92**, 1624–1631.

22. Robinson M, Visscher M, Laruffa A, and Wickett R (2010). Natural moisturizing factors (NMF) in the *stratum corneum* (SC). II. Regeneration of NMF over time after soaking, *J Cosmet Sci*, **61**, 23–29.

23. Kushner J IV, Kim D, So PTC, Blankschtein D, and Langer RS (2007). Dual-channel two-photon microscopy study of transdermal transport in skin treated with low-frequency ultrasound and a chemical enhancer, *J Invest Dermatol*, **127**, 2832–2846.

24. Talreja PS, Kasting GB, Kleene NK, Pickens W, and Wang T-F (2001). Visualization of lipid barrier and measurement of lipid path length in human *stratum corneum*, *AAPS Pharm Sci*, **3**, Article 13.

25. Wang T-F, Kasting GB, and Nitsche JM (2006). A multiphase microscopic diffusion model for *stratum corneum* permeability. I. Formulation, solution and illustrative results for representative compounds, *J Pharm Sci*, **95**, 620–648.

26. Wang T-F, Kasting GB, and Nitsche JM (2007). A multiphase microscopic diffusion model for *stratum corneum* permeability. II. Estimation of physicochemical parameters, and application to a large permeability database, *J Pharm Sci*, **96**, 3024–3051.

27. Nitsche JM, Wang T-F, and Kasting GB (2006). A two-phase analysis of solute partitioning into the *stratum corneum*, *J Pharm Sci*, **95**, 649–666.

28. Anderson BD, Higuchi WI, and Raykar PV (1988). Heterogeneity effects on permeability-partition coefficient relationships in human *stratum corneum*, *Pharm Res*, **5**, 566–573.

29. Anderson BD and Raykar PV (1989). Solute structure–permeability relationships in human *stratum corneum*, *J Invest Dermatol*, **93**, 280–286.

30. Raykar PV, Fung M-C, and Anderson BD (1988). The role of protein and lipid domains in the uptake of solutes by human *stratum corneum*, *Pharm Res*, **5**, 140–150.

31. Hansen S, Naegel A, Heisig M, Wittum G, Neumann D, Kostka K-H, Meiers P, Lehr C-M, and Schaefer UF (2009). The role of corneocytes in skin transport revised—a combined computational and experimental approach, *Pharm Res*, **26**, 1379–1397.

32. Hansen S, Selzer D, Schaefer UF, and Kasting GB (2011). An extended database of keratin binding, *J Pharm Sci*, **100**, 1712–1726.

33. Anissimov YG and Roberts MS (2009). Diffusion modelling of percutaneous absorption kinetics: 4. Effects of a slow equilibration process within *stratum corneum* on absorption and desorption kinetics, *J Pharm Sci*, **98**, 772–781.

34. Seif S and Hansen S (2012). Measuring the *stratum corneum* reservoir: desorption kinetics from keratin, *J Pharm Sci*, **101**, 3718–3728.

35. Frasch HF, Barbero AM, Hettick, JM, and Nitsche JM (2011). Tissue binding affects the kinetics of theophylline diffusion through the *stratum corneum* barrier layer of skin, *J Pharm Sci*, **100**, 2989–2995.

36. Nitsche JM and Frasch HF (2011). Dynamics of diffusion with reversible binding in microscopically heterogeneous membranes: general theory and applications to dermal penetration, *Chem Eng Sci*, **66**, 2019–2041.

37. Kasting GB, Miller MM, and Talreja PS (2005). Evaluation of *stratum corneum* heterogeneity, in *Percutaneous Absorption* (Bronaugh RL and Maibach HI, eds), Taylor & Francis, New York, pp. 193–212.

38. Kasting GB, Smith RL, and Anderson BD (1992). Prodrugs for dermal delivery: solubility, molecular size, and functional group effects, in *Prodrugs: Topical and Ocular Drug Delivery* (Sloan KB, ed), Marcel Dekker, New York, pp. 117–161.

39. Bunge AL and Cleek RL (1995). A new method for estimating dermal absorption from chemical-exposure. 2. Effect of molecular weight and octanol-water partitioning, *Pharm Res*, **12**, 88–95.

40. Cleek RL and Bunge AL (1993). A new method for estimating dermal absorption from chemical exposure. 1. General approach, *Pharm Res*, **10**, 497–506.

41. Kruse J, Golden D, Wilkinson S, Williams F, Kezic S, and Corish J (2007). Analysis, interpretation, and extrapolation of dermal permeation data using diffusion-based mathematical models, *J Pharm Sci*, **96**, 682–703.

42. Dancik Y, Miller MA, Jaworska J, and Kasting GB (2012). Design and performance of a spreadsheet-based model for estimating bioavailability of chemicals from dermal exposure, *Adv Drug Deliv Revs*, **65**, 221–236.

43. Kasting GB, Miller MA, and Bhatt V (2008). A spreadsheet-based method for estimating the skin disposition of volatile compounds: application to *N,N*-diethyl-*m*-toluamide (DEET), *J Occup Environ Hyg*, **10**, 633–644.

44. Basketter DA, Pease C, Kasting GB, Kimber I, Casati S, Cronin MTD, Diembeck W, Gerberick GF, Hadgraft J, Hartung T, Marty J-P, Nikolaidis E, Patlewicz GY, Roberts D, Roggen E, Rovida C, and van de Sandt H (2007). Skin sensitisation and epidermal disposition. The relevance of epidermal bioavailability for sensitisation hazard identification/ risk assessment, *ATLA*, **35**, 137–154.

45. Raphael AP, Meliga SC, Chen X, Fernando GJP, Flaim C, and Kendall MAF (2013). Depth-resolved characterization of diffusion properties within and across minimally-perturbed skin layers, *J Control Rel*, **166**, 87–94.

46. Andrews SN, Jeong E, and Prausnitz MR (2012). Transdermal delivery of molecules is limited by full epidermis, not just *stratum corneum*, *Pharm Res*, **30**, 1099–1109.

47. Nitsche JM and Kasting GB (2013). A microscopic multiphase diffusion model of viable epidermis permeability, *Biophys J*, **104**, 2307–2320.

48. Nitsche JM and Kasting GB (2013). A correlation for 1,9-decadiene/water partition coefficients, *J Pharm Sci*, **102**, 136–144.

49. Nitsche JM and Kasting GB (2013). Permeability of fluid-phase phospholipid bilayers: assessment and useful correlations for permeability screening and other applications, *J Pharm Sci*, **102**, 2005–2032.

50. Johnson ME, Berk DA, Blankschtein D, Golan DE, Jain RK, and Langer RS (1996). Lateral diffusion of small compounds in human *stratum corneum* and model lipid bilayer systems, *Biophys J*, **71**, 2656–2668.

51. Wasterby P, Oradd G, and Lindblom G (2002). Anisotropic water diffusion in macroscopically oriented lipid bilayers studied by pulsed magnetic field gradient NMR, *J Magnet Resonance*, **157**, 156–159.

52. Safranyos RGA, Caveney S, Miller JG, and Peterson NO (1987). Relative roles of gap junction channels and cytoplasm in cell-to-cell diffusion of fluorescent tracers, *Proc Nat Acad Sci USA*, **84**, 2272–2276.

53. Weber PA, Chang H-C, Spaeth KE, Nitsche JM, and Nicholson BJ (2004). The permeability of gap junction channels to probes of different size is dependent on connexin composition and permeant-pore affinities, *Biophys J*, **87**, 958–973.

54. Nitsche JM, Chang H-C, Weber PA, and Nicholson BJ (2004). A transient diffusion model yields unitary gap junctional permeabilities from images of cell-to-cell fluorescent dye transfer between Xenopus oocytes, *Biophys J*, **86**, 2058–2077.

55. Brandner JM, Kief S, Wladykowski E, Houdek P, and Moll I (2006). Tight junction proteins in the skin, *Skin Pharmacol Physiol*, **19**, 71–77.

56. Kretsos K and Kasting GB (2005). Dermal capillary clearance: physiology and modeling, *Skin Pharmacol Physiol*, **18**, 55–74.

57. Singh P and Roberts, MS (1993). Iontophoretic transdermal delivery of salicylic acid and lidocaine to local subcutaneous structures, *J. Pharm. Sci.*, **82**, 127–131.

58. Singh P and Roberts MS (1993). Dermal and underlying tissue pharmacokinetics of salicylic acid after topical administration, *J Pharm Biopharm*, **21**, 337–373.

59. Singh P and Roberts MS (1996). Local deep tissue penetration of compounds after dermal application: structure-tissue penetration relationships, *J Pharmacol Exp Therapeut*, **279**, 908–917.

60. Kretsos K, Kasting GB, and Nitsche JM (2004). Distributed diffusion-clearance model for transient drug distribution within the skin, *J Pharm Sci*, **93**, 2820–2835.

61. Kretsos K, Miller MA, Zamora-Estrada G, and Kasting GB (2008). Partitioning, diffusivity and clearance of skin permeants in mammalian dermis, *Int J Pharm*, **346**, 64–79.

62. Ibrahim R and Kasting GB (2010). Improved method for determining partition and diffusion coefficients in human dermis, *J Pharm Sci*, **99**, 4928–4939.

63. Ibrahim R and Kasting GB (2012). Partitioning and diffusion of parathion in human dermis, *Int J Pharm*, **435**, 33–37.

64. Ibrahim R, Nitsche JM, and Kasting GB (2012). Dermal clearance model for epidermal bioavailability calculations, *J Pharm Sci*, **101**, 2094–2108.

65. Clague DS and Phillips RJ (1996). Hindered diffusion of spherical macromolecules through dilute fibrous media, *Phys Fluids*, **8**, 1720–1731.

66. Phillips RJ (2000). A hydrodynamic model for hindered diffusion of proteins and micelles in hydrogels, *Biophys J*, **79**, 3350–3353.

67. Phillips RJ, Dean WM, and Brady JF (1989). Hindered transport of spherical macromolecules in fibrous membranes and gels, *AIChE J*, **35**, 1761–1769.

68. Phillips RJ, Dean WM, and Brady JF (1990). Hindered transport in fibrous membranes and gels: effect of solute size and fiber configuration, *J Colloid Interface Sci*, **139**, 363–373.

69. Johnson EM, Berk DA, Jain RK, and Deen WM (1996). Hindered diffusion in agarose gels: test of effective medium model, *Biophys J*, **70**, 1017–1026.

70. Clague DS and Phillips RJ (1997). A numerical calculation of the hydraulic permeability of three-dimensional disordered fibrous media, *Phys Fluids*, **9**, 1562–1572.

71. Bert JL, Mathieson JM, and Pearce RH (1982). The exclusion of human serum albumin by human dermal collagenous fibres and within human dermis, *Biochem J*, **201**, 395–403.

72. Bert JL, Pearce RH, and Mathieson JM (1986). Concentration of plasma albumin in its accessible space in postmortem human dermis, *Microvasc Res*, **32**, 211–223.

73. Anissimov YG and Roberts MS (2011). Modelling dermal drug distribution after topical application in human, *Pharm Res*, **28**, 2119–2129.

74. Dancik Y, Anissimov YG, Jepps OG, and Roberts MS (2012). Convective transport of highly plasma protein bound drugs facilitates direct

penetration into deep tissues after topical application, *Brit J Clin Pharmacol*, **73**, 564–578.

75. Taylor GI (1953). Dispersion of soluble matter in solvent flowing slowly through a tube, *Proc Royal Soc London A*, **219**, 186–203.

76. Aris R (1956). On the dispersion of a solute in a fluid flowing through a tube, *Proc Royal Soc London A*, **235**, 67–77.

77. Kretsos K (2003). *Transport Phenomena in the Human Skin*, Ph.D. thesis, Department of Chemical Engineering. State University of New York, Buffalo.

78. Kretsos K and Kasting GB (2007). A geometrical model of dermal capillary clearance, *Math Biosci*, **208**, 430–453.

79. Cevc G and Vierl U (2007). Spatial distribution of cutaneous microvasculature and local drug clearance after drug application on the skin, *J Control Rel*, **118**, 18–26.

80. Muha I, Naegel A, Stichel S, Grillo A, Heisig M, and Wittum G (2011). Effective diffusivity in membranes with tetrakaidekahedral cells and implications for the permeability of human *stratum corneum*, *J Membr Sci*, **368**, 18–25.

81. Naegel A, Heisig M, and Wittum G (2009). A comparison of two- and three-dimensional models for the simulation of the permeability of human *stratum corneum*, *Eur J Pharm Biopharm*, **72**, 332–338.

82. Johnson ME, Blankschtein D, and Langer R (1997). Evaluation of solute permeation through the *stratum corneum*: lateral bilayer diffusion as the primary transport mechanism, *J Pharm Sci*, **86**, 1162–1172.

83. Chen LJ, Lian GP, and Han LJ (2008). Use of "bricks and mortar" model to predict transdermal permeation: model development and initial validation, *Ind Eng Chem Res*, **47**, 6465–6472.

84. Chen L, Lian G, and Han L (2010). Modeling transdermal permeation. Part I. Predicting skin permeability of both hydrophobic and hydrophilic solutes, *AIChE J*, **56**, 1136–1146.

85. Chen L, Han L, and Lian G (2013). Recent advances in predicting skin permeability of hydrophilic solutes, *Adv Drug Deliv Rev*, **65**, 295–305.

86. Wang L, Chen L, Lian G, and Han L (2010). Determination of partition and binding properties of solutes to *stratum corneum*, *Int J Pharm*, **398**, 114–122.

87. Lian G, Chen L, Pudney PDA, Melot M, and Han L (2010). Modeling transdermal permeation. Part 2. Predicting the dermatopharmacokinetics of percutaneous solute, *AIChE J*, **56**, 2551–2560.

88. Bouwstra JA, Gooris GS, van der Spek JA, and Bras W (1991). Structural investigations of human *stratum corneum* by small angle X-ray scattering, *J Invest Dermatol*, **97**, 1005–1012.

89. Frasch HF and Barbaro AM (2003). Steady-state flux and lag time in the *stratum corneum* lipid pathway: results from finite element models, *J Pharm Sci*, **92**, 2196–2207.

90. Lieb WR and Stein WD (1971). The molecular basis of simple diffusion within biological membranes, *Curr Top Membr Trans*, **11**, 1–39.

91. Lieb WR and Stein WD (1986). Simple diffusion across the membrane bilayer, in *Transport and Diffusion Across Cell Membranes* (Stein WD, ed), Academic Press, Inc., Orlando, pp. 69–112.

92. Wilschut A, ten Berge WF, Robinson PJ, and McKone TE (1995). Estimating skin permeation. The validation of five mathematical skin penetration models, *Chemosphere*, **30**, 1275–1296.

93. Mitragotri S (2002). A theoretical analysis of permeation of small hydrophobic solutes across the *stratum corneum* based on scaled particle theory, *J Pharm Sci*, **91**, 744–752.

94. Heisig M, Lieckfeldt R, Wittum G, Mazurkevich G, and Lee G (1996). Non steady-state descriptions of drug permeation through *stratum corneum*. I. The biphasic brick and mortar model, *Pharm Res*, **13**, 421–426.

95. Naegel A, Hansen S, Neumann D, Lehr C-M, Schaefer UF, Wittum G, and Heisig M (2007). In-silico model of skin penetration based on experimentally determined input parameters. Part II. Mathematical modelling of in-vitro diffusion experiments. Identification of critical input parameters, *Eur J Pharm Biopharm*, **68**, 368–379.

96. Tomadakis MM and Sotirchos SV (1993). Transport properties of random arrays of freely overlapping cylinders with various orientation distributions, *J Chem Phys*, **98**, 616–626.

97. Mottram JT and Taylor R (1987). Thermal conductivity of fibre-phenolic resin composites. Part II: numerical evaluation, *Compos Sci Tech*, **29**, 211–232.

98. Wang T-F (2003). *Microscopic Models for the Structure and Permeability of the Stratum Corneum Barrier Layer of Skin*, Ph.D. thesis, Department of Chemical Engineering, State University of New York, Buffalo.

99. Peck KD, Ghanem A-H and Higuchi WI (1994). Hindered diffusion of polar molecules through and effective pore radii estimates of intact and ethanol treated human epidermal membranes, *Pharm Res*, **11**, 1306–1314.

100. Peck KD, Ghanem A-H, and Higuchi WI (1995). The effect of temperature upon the permeation of polar and ionic solutes through human epidermal membrane, *J Pharm Sci*, **84**, 975–982.

101. Mitragotri S (2007). Temperature dependence of skin permeability to hydrophilic and hydrophobic solutes, *J Pharm Sci*, **96**, 1832–1839.

102. Rim JE, Pinsky PM, and van Osdol WW (2009). Multiscale modeling framework of transdermal drug delivery, *Ann Biomed Eng*, **37**, 1217–1229.

103. Mitragotri S (2003). Modeling skin permeability to hydrophilic and hydrophobic solutes based on four permeation pathways, *J Control Rel*, **86**, 69–92.

104. Holz M, Heil SR, and Saccob A (2000). Temperature-dependent self-dffusion coefficients of water and six selected molecular liquids for calibration in accurate 1H NMR PFG measurements, *Phys Chem Chem Phys*, **2**, 4740–4742.

105. Kestin J, Mordechal S, and Wakeham WA (1978). Viscosity of liquid water in the range -8 to 150 deg C, *J Phys Chem Ref Data*, **7**, 941–948.

106. Akomeah F, Martin G, and Brown M (2007). Variability in human skin permeability in vitro: comparing penetrants with different physicochemical properties, *J Pharm Sci*, **96**, 824–834.

107. Barbero AM and Frasch HF (2006). Transcellular route of diffusion through *stratum corneum*: results from finite element models, *J Pharm Sci*, **95**, 2186–2194.

108. Scheuplein RJ (1965). Mechanism of percutaneous absorption I. Routes of penetration and the influence of solubility, *J Invest Dermatol*, **45**, 334–346.

# Chapter 8

# Cellular Scale Modelling of the Skin Barrier

**Arne Nägel, Michael Heisig, Dirk Feuchter, Martin Scherer, and Gabriel Wittum**

*Frankfurt University, Goethe Center for Scientific Computing, Kettenhofweg 139, 60325 Frankfurt am Main, Germany*

wittum@gcsc.uni-frankfurt.de

Computational modelling and simulation of penetration processes in the skin barrier on multiple biological scales in space and time is increasingly being recognized as a powerful tool to develop and to refine hypotheses, focus experiments, and enable more accurate predictions. One area of the ongoing research effort is physiology-based transport models. On the one hand, these are based on first principles and describe processes in the skin mathematically in terms of conservation equations. On the other hand, these models employ detailed morphology information and are thus capable of exploiting relationships between form and function. Particularly, such models provide an understanding how microscopic physiological structure and heterogeneity govern penetration. In this chapter, we describe microscopic geometry models of the skin cells (e.g. corneocytes) and the lipid bilayers of the *stratum corneum* (SC).

*Computational Biophysics of the Skin*

Edited by Bernard Querleux

Copyright © 2014 Pan Stanford Publishing Pte. Ltd.

ISBN 978-981-4463-84-3 (Hardcover), 978-981-4463-85-0 (eBook)

www.panstanford.com

The particular focus is on geometries based on tetrakaidekahedra (TKD). These polyhedra with 14 faces have certain desirable features for the generic construction of cellular membranes. We provide a detailed geometric description of these membranes, which is complemented by examples of computations in the simulation system UG.

## 8.1  Introduction

The *stratum corneum* (SC) (see Fig. 8.1a) is the outermost skin layer of the epidermis of mammals. It consists of corneocytes and a lipid matrix. The corneocytes are dead, keratinized, fully differentiated skin cells that arise from the underlying keratinocytes. The corneocytes are embedded in a matrix of lipid bilayers (Fig. 8.1b). The SC incorporates the main barrier function of the skin. It protects the human body against the ingress of pathogens and preserves it also from death by dehydration. The protection against the ingress of xenobiotics is achieved by slowing the diffusion of the substances through the SC. This is the result of the special arrangement and geometry of the corneocytes and the chemical properties of the lipid matrix. Micrographs of the SC show that the corneocytes are arranged in staggered columns with different overlapping (see Figs. 8.1 and 8.2).

The overlap of the cells depends on the body region and the differing mechanical stresses. The corneocytes are closely packed, flexible and provide an excellent protective function. The lipid matrix consists of free lipid bilayers and lipids, which are covalently bound to the corneocytes. The anchoring of covalently bound lipids occurs via transmembrane proteins [9]. During the keratinocyte differentiation in the *stratum granulosum* lipids are extruded into the intercellular space, and transform into lipid bilayers with lamellar structure [2,10]. The SC is composed of 10–15 layers of flattened corneocytes according to the body region and has a thickness of about 0.02 mm [4] (see Figs. 8.1a,b).

For the numerical simulation of drug diffusion in the SC many different mathematical models exist. They differ in both the physical description, and also in the geometry model of the corneocytes and of the extracellular lipid matrix. One popular two-dimensional geometry model is the "brick and mortar" geometry in which corneocytes are represented as bricks and the lipid matrix as mortar (see Fig. 8.2, bottom left) [4]. This model thus takes into account the overlap of the corneocytes. Wang et al. [11] gives a survey of existing brick-and-mortar models (cf. Table 1 of [11]). Obviously, three-dimensional geometry models are also desirable because they can represent the SC more realistic than a two-dimensional model.

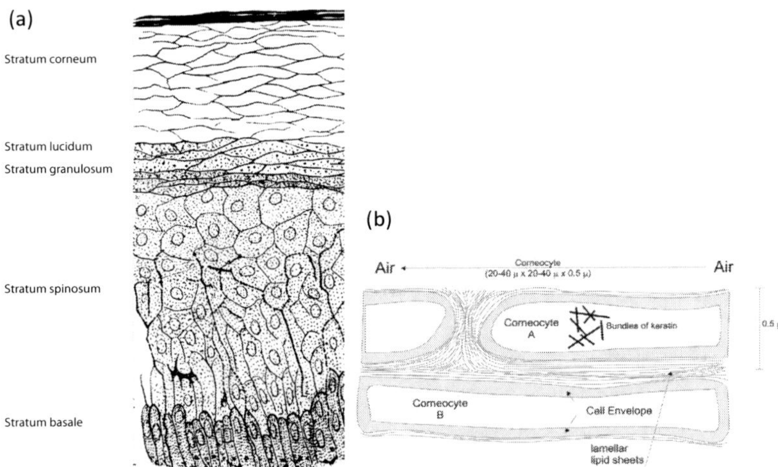


**Figure 8.1**    (a) Layers of the epithelial skin layer: the epidermis. Modified from [1]. (b) Magnified sketch of two corneocytes A and B with lipid matrix. The lamellar structure of the lipid matrix is indicated, as well as the network of keratins within the corneocytes. Reprinted from [2] with permission from BioMed Central.

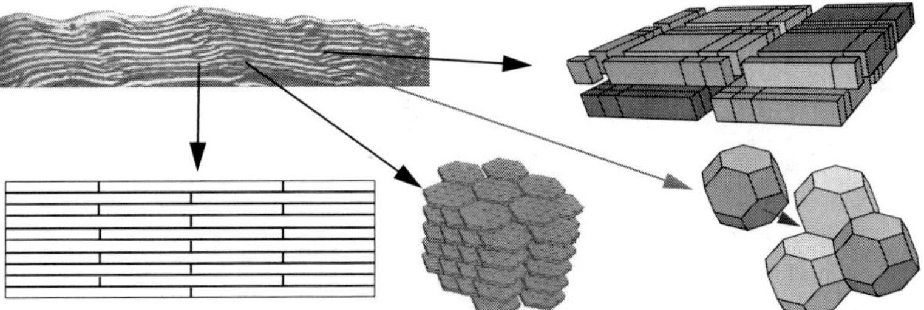

**Figure 8.2**    Light micrograph and four different geometric models of the SC: Top left: Light micrograph. Reprinted from [3] with permission from Elsevier. Bottom left: 2D-Brick-and-mortar model [4,5]. Top right: 3D-Cuboid model [6]. Bottom center: 3D-Model with hexagonal prisms [7]. Bottom right: 3D-Tetrakaidekahedron [8].

The issue "Modeling the human skin barrier—towards a better understanding of dermal absorption", which was published recently in the journal *Advanced Drug Delivery Reviews*, provides an overview of different mathematical models as well as the state of the art of computational research tools that are employed for modelling dermal absorption. We refer for further details, e.g. existing two- and three-dimensional geometry models for the SC, to several articles in this issue (e.g. [12–16]).

In this work, we will focus on geometries based on tetrakaidekahedra (TKD) to model the corneocytes in the SC, because the experimentally observed geometry of the corneocytes is very similar to the space-filling polyhedron tetrakaidekahedron (see Fig. 8.3b), which has an almost optimal surface to volume ratio and is a solution of the Kelvin problem (cf. Section 8.3). The geometry model was suggested in [8,17,53], and later on applied successfully in [18,19].

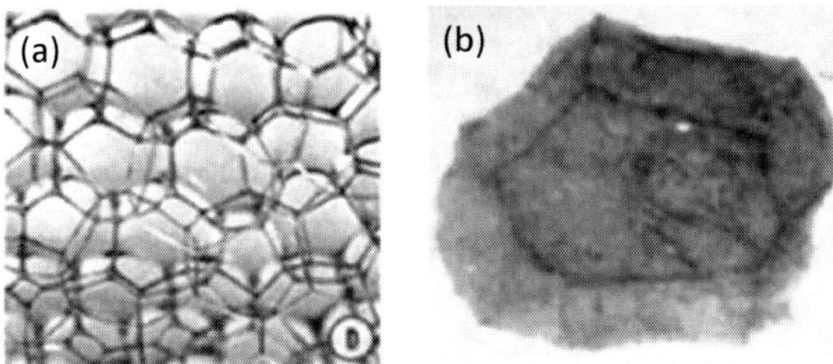


**Figure 8.3**  (a) Micrograph of soap foam with a tetrakaidekahedron like structure. Reprinted from [20] with permission from Nature Publishing Group. (b) Single corneocyte. Reprinted from [21] with permission from Nature Publishing Group.

This work is organized as follows: Section 8.2 provides an extended motivation for the tetrakaidekahedral geometry model of the SC. Section 8.3 then describes the geometry of the tetrakaidekahedron mathematically. In particular, we introduce the necessary parameters for characterizing tetrakaidekahedra. Finally, we provide a mathematical model in Section 8.4 and conclude with computational results in Section 8.5.

## 8.2  Motivation for a *Stratum Corneum* Geometry Model with Tetrakaidekahedra

Using microscopic examination of frozen sections of the SC in the 60s the shape of the corneocytes was assumed being hexagonal

[3,22]. Recent studies confirm this structure [23–27]. In 1975 Menton [20,28] first presented such three-dimensional models of the corneocytes with tetrakaidekahedra (see Fig. 8.5). He based this geometrical arrangement on the similarity of micrographs of the SC (see Fig. 8.2, top left) with the spatial arrangement of soap foam (see Fig. 8.3a). The soap foam is arranged, as the SC, in overlapping columns. This geometry is similar to stacked tetrakaidekahedra (see Fig. 8.2, lower right) [29].

Physically one can explain the formation of the tetrakaide-kahedron form of the corneocyte cells as follows: During the differentiation the keratinocytes in the epidermis are packed denser because they are displaced upwards. Due to its surface tension and mutual pressure, the cells obtain a geometric configuration in which they can be packed with an almost optimal surface to volume ratio to minimize the otherwise occurring forces and without gaps. During the differentiation the cuboidal and irregular arranged keratinocytes with different size change to similarly sized and flat corneocytes, which have a columnar arrangement [30,20] (cf. Figs. 8.2 and 8.4a). Also gaps outside the corneocytes are unlikely due to the pressure. The cells have a staggered arrangement and are interdigitated. Such an interdigitating arrangement saves surface. It is tight, elastic and offers an ideal protection.

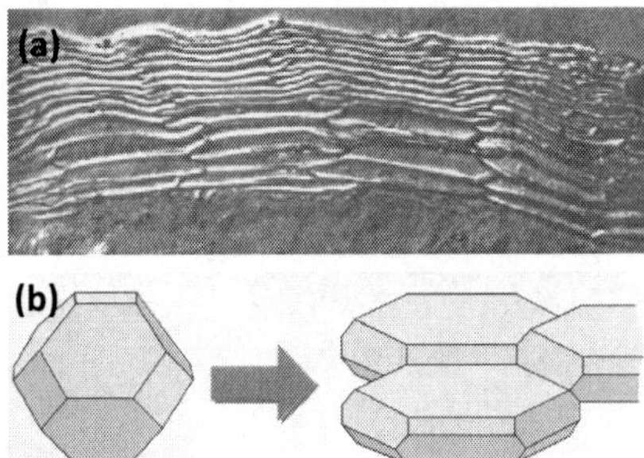


**Figure 8.4**    (a) LM-micrograph of the *stratum corneum*. Reprinted from [3] with permission from Elsevier. (b) Corneocyte model with tetrakaidekahedra, adapted from [33].

Menton as well as Pleswig and Marples presented various micrographs of corneocytes, e.g. [20] cf. Fig. 18, [21] cf. Fig. 3D. Menton also referred to micrographs of elder pith [31] and cork cells [32]. Menton also made experiments with soap foam, showing that foam bubbles are also be arranged in columns and that they overlap. In case of soap foam bubbles the arrangement is similar to highly composite tetrakaidekahedra (see Fig. 8.3a). Based on his reflections on the origin, size and arrangement of corneocytes and his experiments with soap foam [28], Menton proposed a model for the SC geometry with interdigitating cells based on tetrakaidekahedra.

Lord Kelvin introduced the term "tetrakaidekahedron" for a body with 14 faces. The name can be derived from the Greek in which "tetra" means four and "deka" means 10. As part of his research in 1887 Kelvin experimented with soap foam on the search for an ideal geometric arrangement. Kelvin looked for an answer how to divide the space into equal-sized cells with the smallest possible partition ("Kelvin problem") [34–36]. The common solution before Kelvin was a decomposition with rhombic dodekahedra (see Fig. 8.5c). Kelvin came to the conclusion that his problem could be solved with a partition into tetrakaidekahedra with six quadrilateral and eight hexagonal faces ("Kelvin cells") (see Figs. 8.4b and 8.5a,b).

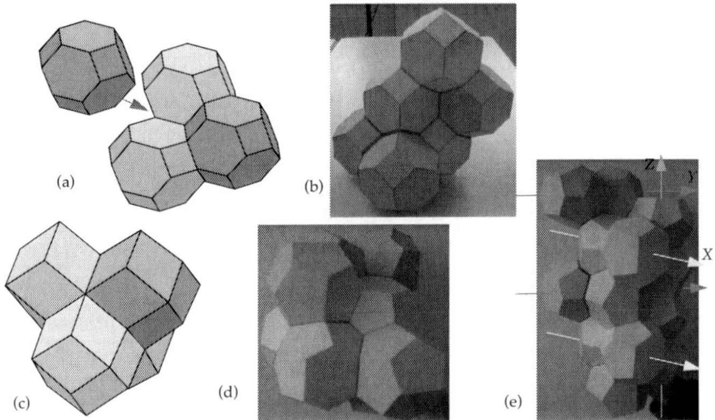

**Figure 8.5**  Three space decompositions without gaps with polyhedra of equal volume: (a) Kelvin tetrakaidekahedra, (b) paper model of the Kelvin-decomposition, (c) rhombic dodekahedra, (d) paper model of the Weaire–Phelan decomposition [40,36, 41] –> Base unit of 3 × 2 Goldberg tetrakaidekahedra and 2 pentagonal dodekahedra, (e) paper model of 2 base units of the Weaire–Phelan decomposition [40,36,41].

Kelvin built on the work of Joseph Plateau [37]. The "Plateau rules" state, that in a border of the foam always three surfaces of the bubble meet at junctions at an angle of 120°, which is the angle in a regular hexagon ("Plateau border"). On the other hand, at a node four plateau borders meet at an angle of 109.47°. This angle is the tetrahedral angle, which is of fundamental importance for the arrangement of all organic compounds in the nature. Thus, the four binding partners of carbon are tetrahedrally arranged to keep the binding energy minimal. Arrangements with greater than four borders per node, or more than three faces at a border are considered to be unstable and tend to transform themselves according to the rules. Thus, the decomposition with the rhombic dodekahedron in Fig. 8.5c is considered as unstable, since eight borders intersect at a node [38,39]. The decomposition of the space with tetrakaidekahedra, however, is stable according to the Plateau rules since only four edges intersect at a node. As already stated, tetrakaidekahedra can be packed without gaps, i.e. 100% tight (see Figs. 8.4b and 8.5a,b).

In search of a solution how to partition the space into cells of a specified volume, such that the total area of the interfaces between the cells is minimal, Kelvin found a package with tetrakaidekahedra. The arrangement proposed by Kelvin has a 0.7% less total area than the complete rhombic decomposition of dodekahedra and was assumed to be ideal for a century, until in 1994, when D. Weaire and R. Phelan presented a solution that has a further 0.3% reduction in total area (see Figs. 8.5d,e and [40,36,41,39]).

Here, however, a hybrid decomposition of equal sized but not identical cells is used. This decomposition consists of dodekahedra with pentagonal faces and so-called Goldberg tetrakaidekahedra. These tetrakaidekahedra have 14 faces: 2 hexagonal and 12 pentagonal (five-sided) faces. In Fig. 8.5e the Goldberg tetrakaidekahedra have a columnar arrangement in the $X$ direction, in the $Y$ direction, and in the $Z$ direction. In the void spaces remaining between these columns pentagonal dodekahedra fit. A basic unit of the Weaire–Phelan decomposition consists of 3 × 2 ($X,Y,Z$) Goldberg tetrakaidekahedra and two dodekahedra.

Recently, Inayat et al. [29] showed that the tetrakaidekahedron geometry represents the foam structure better than the cubic, Weaire–Phelan or pentagonal dodekahedron geometry. The TKD model is the most suitable model to describe the geometrical configuration of the foam structures.

In addition to the arrangement of and decomposition by polyhedra, it is important to investigate the ratio of surface to volume in single polyhedra and, furthermore, which convex polyhedra have a preferably large volume with a minimum surface. Goldberg [42] provides a lower bound estimate for the relation between volume and surface areas in convex polyhedra:

$$\frac{A^3}{V^2} \geq u(n) = \frac{36\pi n(n-1)}{(n-2)^2},$$ (8.1)

where $A^3/V^2$ is a dimensionless ratio between surface area $A$ and volume $V$, and $n$ is the number of faces of the polyhedron. The larger $n$, the smaller the limit $u(n)$. Asymptotically $(n \to \infty)u(n)$ approaches the surface to volume ratio of a sphere, i.e. $36\pi = A_S^3/V_S^2$.

A small value for the ratio $A^3/V^2$ is advantageous, for example, to have a low evaporation surface or to save expensive surface material. Table 8.1 presents values for $A^3/V^2$ and for the Goldberg estimate $u(n)$ for the tetrakaidekahedron, the sphere, as well as the five *Platonic bodies*: icosahedron, dodekahedron, octahedron, hexahedron (cube), and tetrahedron (Fig. 8.6). The ratio $A^3/V^2$ for the tetrakaidekahedron is smaller than for the octahedron, tetrahedron and hexahedron. It is very close to the surface to volume ratio of the regular dodekahedron.

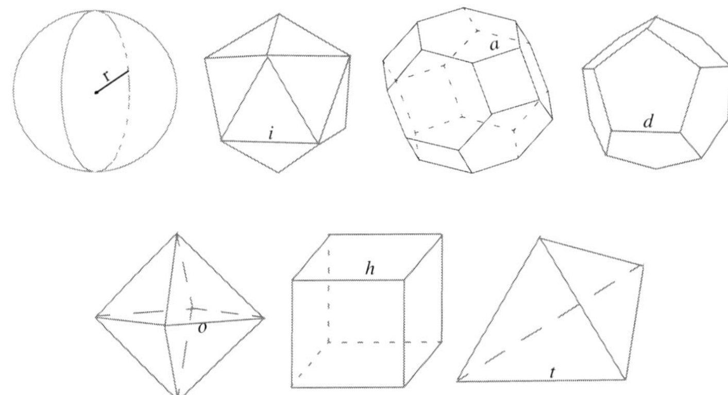


**Figure 8.6**  Sphere, icosahedron, tetrakaidekahedron, dodekahedron, octahedron, cube, and tetrahedron.

The last column in Table 8.1 compares the surfaces of the bodies with identical volume. The surface $A_S$ of a sphere S with volume $V_S$ is compared to the surface $A_{TKD}$ of a tetrakaidekahedron which has the same volume as the sphere S, i.e. $V_{TKD} = V_S$. For the Platonic bodies appropriate comparisons of the surfaces with $V_S = V_I = V_O = V_D = V_C = V_T$ are made.

**Table 8.1** Surface and volume analysis for the five platonic bodies, sphere and tetrakaidekahedron

| Body | Area $A$ | Volume $V$ | $A^3/V^2$ | $n$ | $u(n)$ | $A$ if ($V_S = V_I = V_D = V_{TKD} = V_O = V_C = V_T$) |
|---|---|---|---|---|---|---|
| Sphere | $A_S = 4\pi r^2$ | $V_S = \dfrac{4}{3}\pi r^3$ | $36\pi$ | $\infty$ | $36\pi$ | $A_S = A_S \cdot 1.000$ |
| Icosahedron | $A_I = 5\sqrt{3}i^2$ | $V_I = \dfrac{5}{12}(3+\sqrt{5})i^3$ | 136.460 | 20 | 132.645 | $A_I = A_S \cdot 1.064$ |
| Tetrakaidekahedron | $A_{TKD} = (6+12\sqrt{3})a^2$ | $V_{TKD} = 8\sqrt{2}a^3$ | 150.123 | 14 | 142.942 | $A_{TKD} = A_S \cdot 1.099$ |
| Dodekahedron | $A_D = 3\sqrt{(5(5+2\sqrt{5}))}d^2$ | $V_D = \dfrac{1}{4}(15+7\sqrt{5})d^3$ | 149.858 | 12 | 149.288 | $A_D = A_S \cdot 1.098$ |
| Octahedron | $A_O = 2\sqrt{3}o^2$ | $V_O = \dfrac{1}{3}\sqrt{2}o^3$ | 187.061 | 8 | 175.929 | $A_O = A_S \cdot 1.182$ |
| Cube | $A_C = 6\,h^2$ | $V_C = h^3$ | 216.000 | 6 | 212.058 | $A_C = A_S \cdot 1.241$ |
| Tetrahedron | $A_T = \sqrt{3}t^2$ | $V_T = \dfrac{1}{12}\sqrt{2}t^3$ | 374.123 | 4 | 339.292 | $A_T = A_S \cdot 1.490$ |

In this comparison, the tetrakaidekahedron performs very well and does not even need more than 10% surface area than the sphere. Although spheres have the best surface to volume ratio, spheres cannot be packed 100% tight. The space filling in the densest packing of spheres by Kepler is $\pi/\sqrt{18} \approx 74\%$ [43,44]. With regular icosahedra, regular dodekahedra, regular octahedra and regular tetrahedra [45] a 3D tesselation is also not possible. Unlike to these polyhedra, an arrangement with tetrakaidekahedra is without gaps and has the aforementioned surface-minimization property. Motivated by this desirable feature, we will introduce a geometry concept based on a uniform decomposition with tetrakaidekahedra in the next Section.

## 8.3 Tetrakaidekahedron Model

This section describes the geometric properties of tetrakaideka-hedra. Subsection 8.3.1 presents a parameterization as introduced earlier in [17]. In Subsection 8.3.2, we introduce nested tetrakaid-ekahedra, which allow constructing the lipid matrix between the corneocytes.

### 8.3.1 Parameters of a Tetrakaidekahedron

A single tetrakaidekahedron is depicted in Fig. 8.7. It is specified uniquely by information about the length $a$, the height $h$ and the distance $w$ of two parallel edges $p_j$ and $q_j$. The angles, the volume and the surface can be deduced from these values. The value $s$ is a measure for the overlap of two adjacent tetrakaidekahedra.

$$s = \frac{\sqrt{3}}{3}(w - 2a) \tag{8.2}$$

The overlap $s$ is maximal for $a \to 0$:

$$s_{\max} = \frac{w}{\sqrt{3}} \tag{8.3}$$

For a convex tetrakaidekahedron the following inequality is necessary:

$$w \geq 2a \tag{8.4}$$

For $w = 2a$ the overlap $s$ vanishes and we obtain an octahedron with opposite two hexahedral faces. If Eq. 8.4 is violated, the TKD degenerates, i.e. is no longer convex.

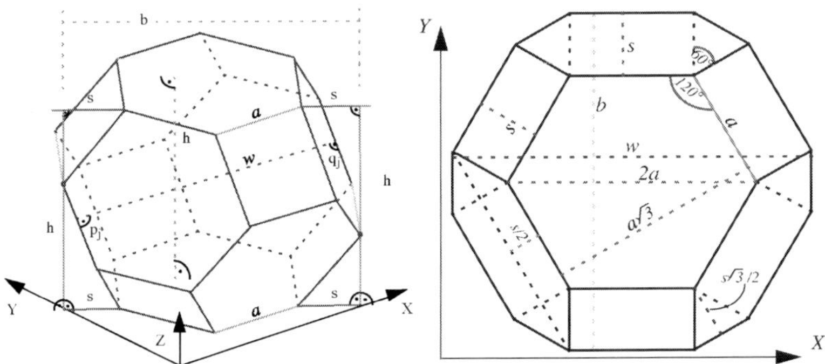

**Figure 8.7**   Angles and lengths in a unit tetrakaidekahedron [8]. 3D view (left), top view (right). $a$: edge length of the base hexagon, $h$: height of tetrakaidekahedron, $w$: distance between two parallel edges $p_j$ and $q_j$, $d$: largest distance between two edges, $s$: overlap of two adjacent tetrakaidekahedra.

The width $b$ is the horizontal distance between two edges of $p_j$ and $q_j$.

$$b = \frac{\sqrt{3}}{3}(2w - a) = 2s + a\sqrt{3} \tag{8.5}$$

The variable $\omega$ indicates the relative horizontal overlap [46].

$$\omega = \frac{s}{b} = \frac{1}{2 + \sqrt{3}\,\dfrac{a}{s}} < \frac{1}{2} \tag{8.6}$$

The variable $d$ defines the largest distance between two points of the tetrakaidekahedron.

$$d = \frac{1}{3}\sqrt{h^2 + 12(a^2 - aw + w^2)^2} = \sqrt{a^2 + b^2 + \frac{1}{9}h^2}$$

$$= \sqrt{a^2 + \frac{1}{3}(2w - a)^2 + \frac{1}{9}h^2} \tag{8.7}$$

The angle $\alpha$ includes a side hexagon and a vertically adjacent hexagon.

$$\alpha = 2\pi - \gamma - \beta \tag{8.8}$$

The angle $\beta$ includes a basis hexagon and a side rectangle.

$$\beta = \frac{\pi}{2} + \arccos\frac{h}{\sqrt{h^2 + 3(w - 2a)^2}} \tag{8.9}$$

The angle $\gamma$ includes a basis hexagon and a side rectangle

$$\gamma = \frac{\pi}{2} + \arccos\frac{2h}{\sqrt{4h^2 + 3(w - 2a)^2}} \tag{8.10}$$

### 8.3.2  Parameter for the Lipid Matrix Tetrakaidekahedron

Feuchter [8] modelled the extracellular lipid matrix of corneo-cytes by a second tetrakaidekahedron, which is nested to the tetrakaidekahedron of the corneocyte (see Fig. 8.8). Let $C_i$ denote tetrakaidekahedron of the corneocyte. Moreover, assume that a lipid layer thickness $\theta_l$, i.e. distance between two corneocytes $C_i$ is given. In order to parameterize the outer tetrakaidekahedron $T_i$, its values for $a_l$, $h_l$, and $w_l$ must be related to the values for $a$, $h$, and $w$ of $C_i$.

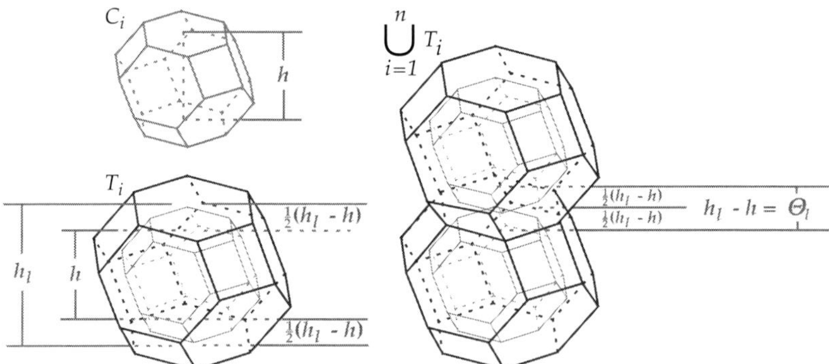


**Figure 8.8**  Interior corneocyte $C_i$ and surrounding tetrakaidekahedron of the lipid matrix $T_i$. The definition of lipid thickness $\theta_l$ is shown (from [8]).

#### 8.3.2.1  Thickness of the lipid layer

The distance between the tetrakaidekahedron of the corneocyte $C_i$ with the height $h$, and the tetrakaidekahedron of the lipid layer $T_i$

with the height $h_l$ is at the top and the bottom (seen from the basis hexagon) ½$(h_l - h)$ respectively. Thus, we have (Fig. 8.8):

$$h_l = h + \theta_l \tag{8.11}$$

### 8.3.2.2 Base edge length

The tetrakaidekahedra of corneocyte and lipid matrix are constructed such that they have equal angles (see Fig. 8.9). Correspondingly, the edge length $a_l$ can be defined using the angles $\beta_l = \beta$ and $\gamma_l = \gamma$ as well as the lipid thickness $\theta_l$. We obtain

$$a_l = \frac{\sqrt{3}}{3}\left(\sqrt{3}a + \frac{\theta_L}{2\tan\dfrac{\beta}{2}} + \frac{\theta_L}{2\tan\dfrac{\gamma}{2}}\right) \tag{8.12}$$

The second term in this sum results from the following observation: The increment from $a$ to $a_l$ on the right side in Fig. 8.9 is related to the angle $\beta_l$ between base hexagon and side rectangle of the lipid tetrakaidekahedron. More precisely, it is obtained by dropping a perpendicular from the angle bisector to the edge. The same is true for the angle $\gamma_l$ yielding the third term.

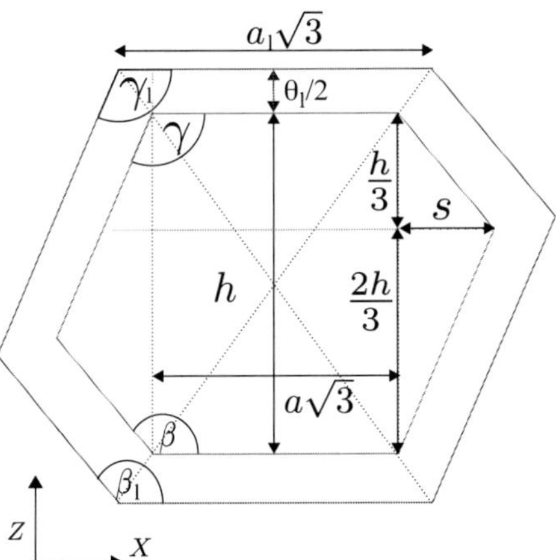


**Figure 8.9**   Cross section of inner and outer tetrakaidekahedron (or corneocyte and lipid matrix) with angle bisectors for $\beta_l = \beta$ and $\gamma_l = \gamma$. The distance between the tetrakaidekahedron for corneocyte and lipid matrix is $\theta_l/2$ (modified from [53]).

### 8.3.2.3 Diameter

For the calculation of $w_l$ we proceed as follows. First, note that Eq. 8.9 yields

$$\beta = \frac{\pi}{2} + \arccos\frac{h}{\sqrt{h^2 + 3(w - 2a)^2}}$$

$$\beta_l = \frac{\pi}{2} + \arccos\frac{h_l}{\sqrt{h_l^2 + 3(w_l - 2a_l)^2}}. \tag{8.13}$$

Using the identity $\beta = \beta_l$, we also obtain the identity of (the square of) the arguments of arccos and thus,

$$w_l = h_l \cdot \frac{\sqrt{3s}}{h} + 2a_l \tag{8.14}$$

## 8.4 Mathematical Model

### 8.4.1 Model Equations

The previous Section 8.3 introduced a geometry concept to construct an artificial SC membrane. This can be used for physiology-based computations [16,18–19]. We will now state this more formally. The geometry parts being identified with lipids and corneocytes, i.e. the cells $C_i$ and the lipids $L_i = T_i \backslash C_i$ from the previous Subsection, are abstractly represented by subdomains $\Omega_{\mathrm{LIP}}$ and $\Omega_{\mathrm{COR}}$. In each of the subdomains, it is assumed that transport is due to diffusion:

$$\partial_t c_i(x,t) + \nabla \cdot \left[ -D_i(x)\nabla c_i(x,t) \right] = 0 \tag{8.15}$$

Between the subdomains, on the interface $\Gamma := \overline{\Omega_{\mathrm{LIP}}} \cap \overline{\Omega_{\mathrm{COR}}}$, the fluxes are continuous, whereas concentrations may be discontinuous due to partitioning according to Nernst's law:

$$\left[ -D_{\mathrm{COR}}\nabla c_{\mathrm{COR}} \right] \cdot \vec{n_i} + \left[ -D_{\mathrm{LIP}}\nabla c_{\mathrm{LIP}} \right] \cdot \vec{n_j} = 0, \tag{8.16}$$

$$c_{\mathrm{COR}} = K_{\mathrm{COR/LIP}} c_{\mathrm{LIP}}. \tag{8.17}$$

This formulation describes transport by a partial differential equation. The equations and transmission conditions must, of course, be complemented by initial and boundary conditions.

## 8.4.2 Periodic Identification for a Finite Number of Layers

The artificial membrane used for skin modelling stretches infinitely into the $x$- and $y$-directions but only features a finite number of layers in the $z$-direction. Technically, this is accomplished by appropriate periodic boundary conditions.

We start with the cell B depicted in Fig. 8.10. This cell has top and bottom surfaces $\Gamma_{\mathrm{TOP}}$ and $\Gamma_{\mathrm{BOT}}$ indicated in grey. Moreover, it features three pairs of side surfaces shown below. Each of these pairs allows for a mutual identification of points through a shift in the $x$–$y$ plane. Staggering several of these base cells vertically yields a membrane with a finite number of layers.

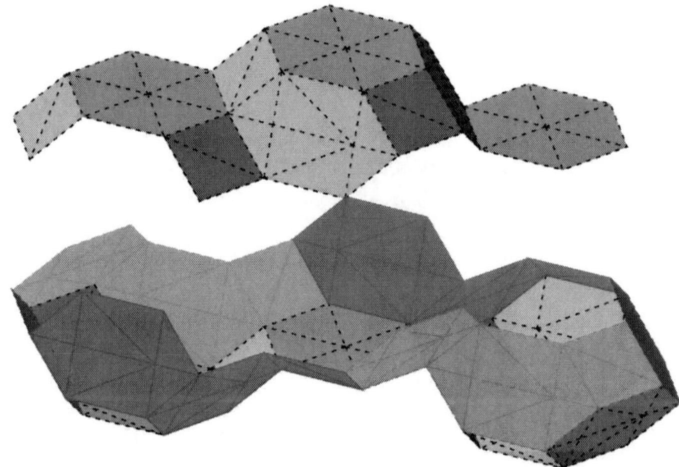

**Figure 8.10** Periodic identification for membranes with a finite number of layers: Faces on the sides (light, medium, and dark grey) are identified pairwise periodically. Cells are staggered on top/bottom faces.

## 8.4.3 Periodic Identification for an Infinite Number of Layers

One motivation for choosing TKD-shaped cells is the property that they provide a space filling in three dimensions. Through an identification of boundary faces, one can use a TKD membrane to construct a computational domain $Y$ that is *similar* to the torus $[0,1]^3$

$\subset \mathbb{R}^3$. Two geometric objects $G_1$ and $G_2$ are called similar, if there is an affine-linear mapping $f : \mathbb{R}^3 \to \mathbb{R}^3, x \mapsto Ax + b$, such that $f(G_1) = G_2$. This transformation is accomplished as follows:

(1) Given an infinite number of cells in all spatial directions, one first identifies a set of three adjacent cells as depicted in Fig. 8.11. This set corresponds to the three cells presented in Fig. 8.10, which are aligned along the $x$-axis. Among all cells, we have three different classes (0,1,2) depending on the $z$-coordinate of their top plate. One readily verifies that the selected set contains one cell for each class.

(2) Starting from these cells, we construct a rectangular box whose interior includes the centres of the three cells as depicted in Fig. 8.11a. It is selected such that two opposite edges can be identified. For the sake of illustration, the coloured lines indicate the shift directions of the three periodicities from Fig. 8.10.

(3) The same process is carried over to the third dimension. Again, the selected cells are embedded in a rectangle. Note that the cells at the heights 0 and 1 are not contained completely. The part outside of the rectangle is included by identification with the part below the opposite face however.

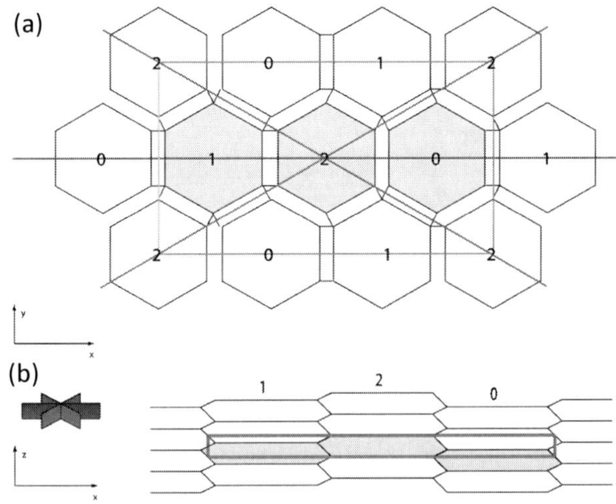

**Figure 8.11** Construction of a periodicity cell Y: (a) Illustration in the $x$-$y$-plane, (b) Illustration in the $x$-$z$-plane. Reprinted from [19] with permission from Elsevier.

### 8.4.4  Homogenization for an Infinite Number of Layers

Let us assume that $K_{COR}$, $K_{LIP}$ are constant and that $K_{COR/LIP} = K_{COR}/K_{LIP}$ holds. One verifies easily that the original system in Eqs. 8.15–8.17 may be restated as

$$\partial_t K(y)u(x,t) + \nabla \cdot \left[ -D(y)K(y)\nabla u(x,t) \right] = 0 \qquad (8.18)$$

Here the concentrations are replaced by $c_i(t,x) = K_i(x)u_i(t,x)$ and the function $u$ is defined piecewise by the functions $u_i$.

In this setting, standard results from homogenization theory, e.g. [47], may be applied. We now consider domains $\Omega$ that consist of many cells of type $Y$. Figure 8.11 provides an example, but we are primarily interested in cases where $\Omega$ and $Y$ have different length scales. In this case, we define a small-scale variable $y = x/\varepsilon \in Y$ for the periodic structures. The method of asymptotic expansion is to write the solution as a function:

$$u_\varepsilon(t,x,y) = u^{(0)}(t,x,y) + \varepsilon\, u^{(1)}(t,x,y) + \cdots$$

Averaging the equation over $Y$, one obtains that $u^{(0)}$ is the solution of

$$\partial_t K^* u(x,t) + \nabla \cdot \left[ -\mathbb{D}^* \nabla u(x,t) \right] = 0.$$

This equation includes an averaged[1] porosity

$$K^* = \langle K \rangle \qquad (8.19)$$

and an averaged diffusion tensor $\mathbb{D} = (D_{ij}^*)_{i,j=1}^3$. The latter is defined by

$$D_{ij}^* = \left\langle DK \left( \nabla_y w_i + e_i \right) \left( \nabla_y w_j + e_j \right) \right\rangle \qquad (8.20)$$

The functions $w_j : Y \to \mathbb{R}$, $j \in \{1,2,3\}$, are $Y$-periodic functions which are given as the solution of

$$\nabla_y \cdot \left[ -D(y)K(y)\nabla_y (e_j + \nabla_y w_j) \right] = 0. \qquad (8.21)$$

These functions are unique up to a constant and characterize the small scale fluctuations in the sense that

---

[1] For any function $f : Y \to \mathbb{R}$, let $\langle f \rangle = \int_Y f(y)dy / \int_Y 1\,dy$ denote the average of $f$ on $Y$.

$$u^{(1)} = \sum_{j=1}^{3} \frac{\partial u}{\partial x_j}(t, x) w_j(y).$$

## 8.5 Computational Results

The PDEs presented were implemented in the software toolbox UG [48]. Space has been discretized by a vertex-centred finite volume scheme; the time integrator for transient problems has been an implicit Euler method. All results were checked for grid convergence. We refer to [46,16] for further details.

### 8.5.1 Example of a Transient Simulation

For the sake of illustration, let us consider the transient problem stated in Eqs. 8.15–8.17. Corneocytes are characterized by $a = 5$ μm, $w = 30$ μm, $h = 1$ μm and $d = 0.1$ μm. The artificial membrane has 10 layers of cells identified as described in Subsection 8.4.2. Figure 8.12 shows the evolution of drug concentration for $a = 5$ μm with the representative values $D_{LIP} = 10^{-8}$ cm$^2$/h, $D_{COR}/D_{LIP} = 10^{-5}$, and $K_{COR/LIP} = 1$.

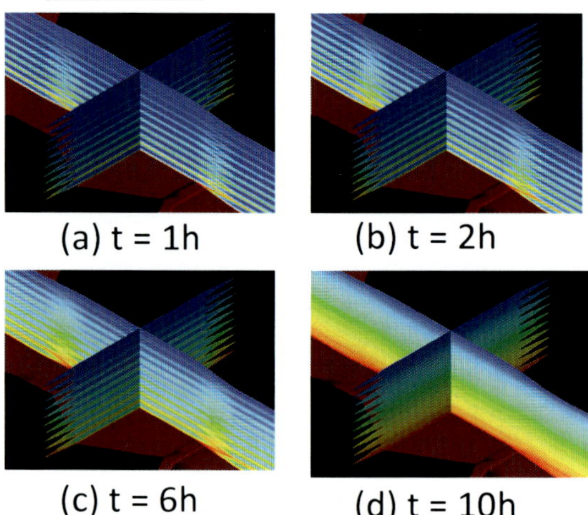


**Figure 8.12** Evolution of drug concentration through SC.

For (moderately) hydrophilic substances, we expect an effective drug transport along an intra-corneocyte pathway: After diffusing along the lipid bilayers first Fig. 8.12(a), the substance enters the corneocytes and permeates vertically (b). The corneocytes fill up in a sponge-like way (c), until finally the steady state is reached (d).

## 8.5.2 Theoretical Results for Homogenized Membranes

Solving Eq. 8.21 on a periodic geometry identified according to Subsection 8.4.3 yields a diffusion tensor from Eq. 8.20. Due to symmetry the off-diagonal entries vanish, i.e. $D_{ij} = 0$, $i \neq j$. The diagonal entries now represent the anisotropy of the cells. They can be represented as functions:

$$D_{11}(\phi) = D_{22}(\phi) = D_{\mathrm{LIP}}\alpha_{\mathrm{LAT}}(\phi), \quad D_{33}(\phi) = D_{\mathrm{LIP}}\alpha_{\mathrm{TRANS}}(\phi) \tag{8.22}$$

depending on $\phi = K_{\mathrm{COR/LIP}}D_{\mathrm{COR}}/D_{\mathrm{LIP}}$. The relation is plotted in Figs. 8.13a,b, respectively. The corneocytes are parameterized as in Subsection 8.5.1 with the edge length $a$ and thus the horizontal cell overlap now being variable.

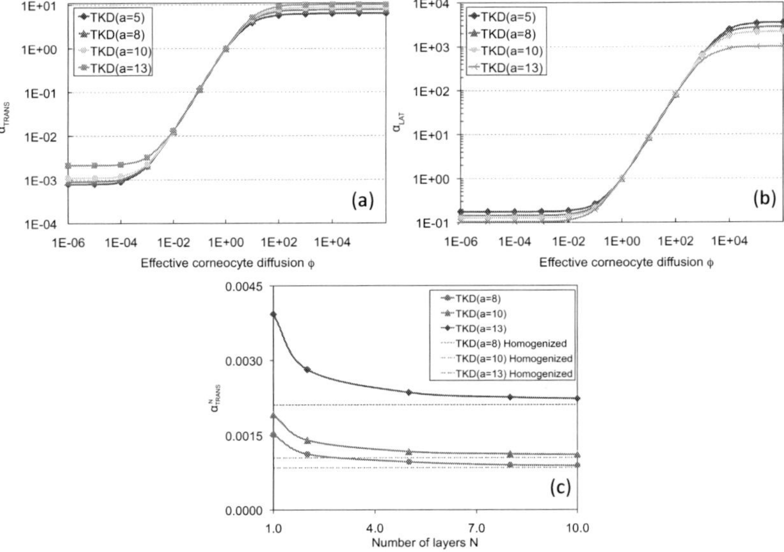


**Figure 8.13** (a) and (b): Relationship between effective corneocyte diffusion $\phi$ and anisotropy factors $\alpha_{\mathrm{LAT}}$ and $\alpha_{\mathrm{TRANS}}$. (c): For an increasing number of layers $\alpha_{\mathrm{TRANS}}^{N}(\phi)$ approaches $\alpha_{\mathrm{TRANS}}(\phi)$ (Illustration for $\phi = 0.0001$). Modified reprint from [19] with permission from Elsevier.

For a membrane with $N$ horizontal layers, we define $\alpha_{\text{TRANS}}^{N}$ as the ratio of the flux through a membrane with diffusivity $\phi$ and of the flux through a homogeneous membrane ($\phi = 1$). The solution of Eq. 8.20 can be regarded as the asymptotic limit of the solutions of Eq. 8.21 for $\varepsilon \to 0$, i.e. for membranes with a large number of cells in all spatial directions. Theoretically, we may thus conclude that $\alpha_{\text{TRANS}}^{N}(\phi)$ approaches the homogenized value $\alpha_{\text{TRANS}}(\phi)$ for the number of layers $N \to \infty$. This is visualized in Fig. 8.13c for $\phi = 0.0001$.

### 8.5.3  Application

Various studies proved the applicability of microscopic models for both finite and infinite dose in vitro experiments [49,50]. These works are based on microscopic diffusion models. The model compounds used were flufenamic acid and caffeine. For the description of lateral diffusion, these models, which feature a cellular resolution, are less suitable, due to the horizontal length scale of the diffusion cell.

Extending the previously mentioned work [51] thus also employed a homogenized (macroscopic) diffusion model. This was built from a two-dimensional model for a Franz cell with cylindrical coordinates and compartments for donor chamber, *stratum corneum* and deeper skin layers (DSL, viable epidermis and dermis). The goal is to match experimentally determined mass profiles which show the (relative amount of) mass in each compartment as a function of time.

The study is based on experimental input parameters determined in [52]. However, since the diffusion coefficient in the SC was only determined in transversal direction, this was not directly applicable for estimating the amount of lateral diffusion. As an alternative, the diffusion coefficients $D_{\text{SC,LAT}}$ and $D_{\text{SC,TRANS}}$ were determined by one parameter least squares fit on Eq. 8.22 w.r.t. $\phi$. In a refinement, regression was also performed for a three parameter model, which also adjusted $D_{\text{DSL}}$, $K_{\text{SC/DON}}$, and, indirectly $K_{\text{SC/DSL}}$.

Table 8.2 provides the input parameters; the values for $D_{\text{SC,TRANS}}$ are close to the values between $3.95 \times 10^{-8}$ cm$^2$/h and $7.98 \times$

$10^{-8}$ cm$^2$/h observed in [52]. Figure 8.14 shows the resulting mass profiles.

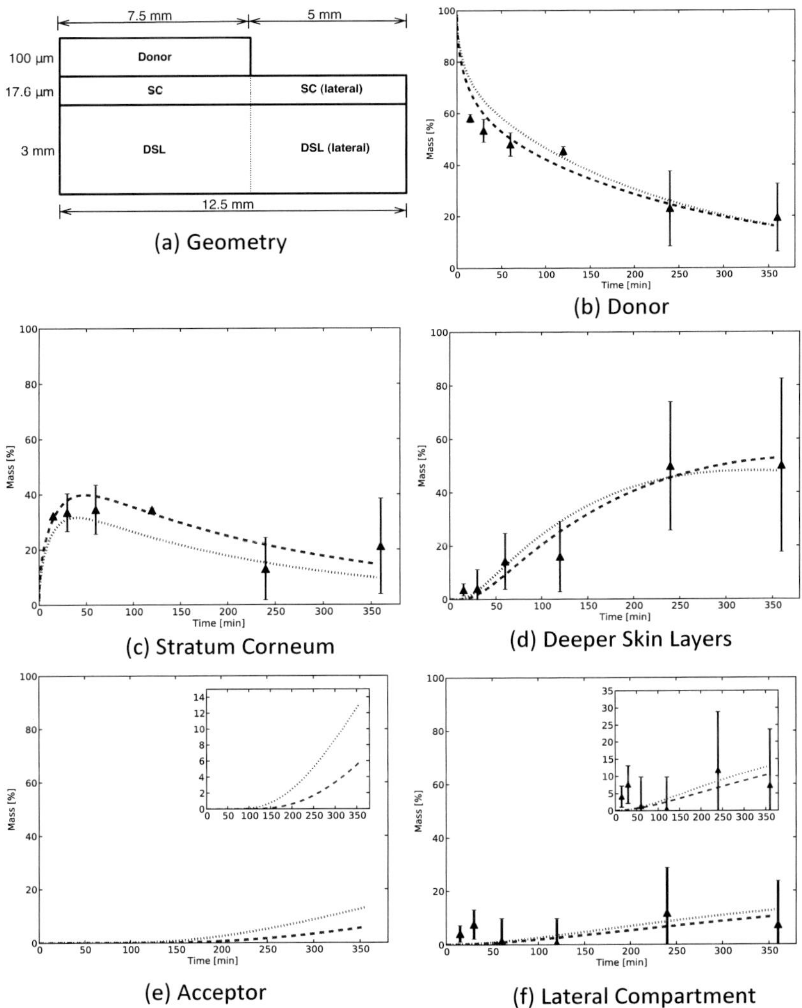



**Figure 8.14** Franz cell diffusion model with lateral diffusion. (a) Sketch of geometry. FFA mass profiles over time for (b) Donor compartment, (c) SC compartment, (d) DSL compartment, (e) Acceptor compartment, (f) Lateral compartment. Experimental data (triangle), and homogenized diffusion models (thin dashes: 1 parameter fit, thick dashes: 3 parameter fit) (modified from [51]).

**Table 8.2**     Parameters for MACRO Franz cell model *w*/lateral diffusion

| Parameter | MACRO (1) | | | MACRO (3) | | |
|---|---|---|---|---|---|---|
| $D_{DON}$ [cm$^2$/h] | 2.47 | $\times$ 10$^{-2}$ | # | 2.47 | $\times$ 10$^{-2}$ | # |
| $D_{SC,LAT}$ [cm$^2$/h] | 2.00 | $\times$ 10$^{-5}$ | a | 1.98 | $\times$ 10$^{-5}$ | b |
| $D_{SC,TRANS}$ [cm$^2$/h] | 10.43 | $\times$ 10$^{-7}$ | a | 7.72 | $\times$ 10$^{-7}$ | b |
| $D_{DSL}$ [cm$^2$/h] | 4.90 | $\times$ 10$^{-3}$ | § | 3.26 | $\times$ 10$^{-3}$ | b |
| $K_{SC/DON}$ | 5.88 | | § | 8.54 | | b |
| $K_{SC/DSL}$ | 3.00 | | § | 4.36 | | b |

#: from Ref. 51; §: from Ref. 52; a: determined by one parameter fit; b: determined by three parameter fit.

# References


1. Gray H (ed) (1913). *Gray's Anatomy: Descriptive and Applied*, Lea & Febiger, Philadelphia.

2. Marquez-Lago TT, Allen DM, and Thewalt J (2010). A novel approach to modelling water transport and drug diffusion through the *stratum corneum*, *Theor Biol Med Model*, **7**(1), 33–58.

3. Menton DN and Eisen AZ (1971). Structure and organization of mammalian *stratum corneum*, *J Ultra Mol Struct R*, **35**, 247–264.

4. Elias PM (1983). Epidermal lipids, barrier function, and desquamation, *J Invest Dermatol*, **80**, 44–49.

5. Heisig M, Lieckfeldt R, Wittum G, Mazurkevich G, and Lee G (1996). Non-steady-state descriptions of drug permeation through *stratum corneum*. I. The biphasic brick-and-mortar model, *Pharm Res*, **13**, 421–426.

6. Wagner C (2007). *Dreidimensionale digitale Rekonstruktion des humanen Stratum corneum der Haut in Kombination mit substantieller Diffusion durch das Stratum corneum*, Dissertation (in German), Tierärztliche Hochschule Hannover.

7. Goodyer CE, Wood J, and Berzins M (2008). Mathematical modelling of chemical diffusion through skin using grid-based PSEs, in *Modeling, Simulation and Optimization of Complex Processes* (Bock HG, Kostina E, Phu HX, and Rannacher R, eds), Springer Berlin, Heidelberg, Berlin, Heidelberg, pp. 249–258.

8. Feuchter D (2008). *Geometrie- und Gittererzeugung für anisotrope Schichtengebiete*, Dissertation (in German), Ruprecht-Karls-Universität Heidelberg.

9. Swartzendruber DC, Wertz PW, Madison KC, and Downing DT (1987). Evidence that the corneocyte has a chemically bound lipid envelope, *J Invest Dermatol*, **88**(6), 709–713.

10. Kuempel D, Swartzendruber DC, Squier CA, and Wertz PW (1998). In vitro reconstitution of *stratum corneum* lipid lamellae, *Biochim Biophys Acta*, **1372**(1), 135–140.

11. Wang T-F, Kasting GB, and Nitsche JM (2006). A multiphase microscopic diffusion model for *stratum corneum* permeability. I. formulation, solution, and illustrative results for representative compounds, *J Pharm Sci*, **95**, 620–648.

12. Anissimov YG, Jepps OG, Dancik Y, and Roberts MS (2013). Mathematical and pharmacokinetic modelling of epidermal and dermal transport processes, *Adv Drug Del Rev*, **65**, 169–190.

13. Dancik Y, Miller MA, Jaworska J, and Kasting GB (2013). Design and performance of a spreadsheet-based model for estimating bioavailability of chemicals from dermal exposure, *Adv Drug Del Rev*, **65**, 221–236.

14. Frasch HF and Barbero AM (2013). Application of numerical methods for diffusion-based modeling of skin permeation, *Adv Drug Del Rev*, **65**, 208–220.

15. Jepps O, Dancik Y, Anissimov YG, and Roberts MS (2013). Modeling the human skin barrier—Towards a better understanding of dermal absorption, *Adv Drug Del Rev*, **65**, 152–168.

16. Naegel A, Heisig M, and Wittum G (2013) Detailed modelling of skin penetration—an overview, *Adv Drug Deliv Rev*, **65**, 191–207.

17. Feuchter D, Heisig M, and Wittum G (2006). A geometry model for the simulation of drug diffusion through the *stratum corneum*, *Comput Visual Sci*, **9**, 1–14.

18. Naegel A, Heisig M, and Wittum G (2009). A comparison of two- and three-dimensional models for the simulation of the permeability of human *stratum corneum*, *Eur J Pharm Biopharm*, **72**, 332–338.

19. Muha I, Naegel A, Stichel S, Grillo A, Heisig M, and Wittum G (2011). Effective diffusivity in membranes with tetrakaidekahedral cells and implications for the permeability of human *stratum corneum*, *J Membr Sci*, **368**, 18–25.

20. Menton DN (1975). A minimum-surface mechanism to account for the organization of cells into columns in the mammalian epidermis, *Am J Anat*, **145**, 1–22.

21. Plewig G and Marples R (1970). Regional differences of cell sizes in the human *stratum corneum*. Part I, *J Invest Dermatol*, **54**(1), 13–18.

22. Christophers E and Kligman AM (1964). Visualization of the cell layers of the *stratum corneum*, *J Invest Dermatol*, **42**, 407–409.

23. König K (2000). Multiphoton microscopy in life sciences, *J Microsc*, **200**, 83–104.

24. König K and Riemann I (2003). High-resolution multiphoton tomography of human skin with subcellular spatial resolution and picosecond time resolution, *J Biomed Opt*, **8**, 432–439.

25. Richter T, Müller JH, Schwarz UD, Wepf R, and Wiesendanger R (2001). Investigation of the swelling of human skin cells in liquid media by tapping mode scanning force microscopy, *Appl Phys A*, **72**(Suppl), S125–S128.

26. Richter T, Peuckert C, Sattler M, König K, Riemann I, Hintze U, Wittern K-P, Wiesendanger R, and Wepf R (2004). Dead but highly dynamic: the *stratum corneum* is divided into three hydration zones, *Skin Pharmacol Physiol*, **17**, 246–257.

27. Schätzlein A and Cevc G (1998). Non-uniform cellular packing of the *stratum corneum* and permeability barrier function of intact skin: a high-resolution confocal laser scanning microscopy study using highly deformable vesicles (Transfersomes), *Br J Dermatol*, **138**, 583–592.

28. Menton DN (1976). A liquid film model of tetrakaidekahedral packing to account for the establishment of epidermal cell columns, *J Invest Dermatol*, **66**(5), 283–291.

29. Inayat A, Freund H, Zeiser T, and Schwieger W (2011) Determining the specific surface area of ceramic foams: the tetrakaidekahedra model revisited, *Chem Eng Sci*, **66**, 1179–1188.

30. Christophers E (1971). Die epidermale Columnärstruktur—Voraussetzungen und möglicher Entstehungsmechanismus, *Z Zellforsch*, **114**, 441–450.

31. Lewis FT (1923). The typical shape of polyhedral cells in vegetable parenchyma and in the restoration of the shape following cell-division, *Proc Am Acad Arts Sci*, **58**, 537–552.

32. Lewis FT (1928). The shape of cork cells: a simple demonstration that they are tetrakaidekahedral, *Science*, **68**, 625–626.

33. Fritsch P (ed) (2004). *Dermatologie Venerologie—Grundlagen Klinik Atlas* (in German), Springer, Heidelberg.

34. Kelvin WT (1887). On the division of space with minimal partitional area, *Philos Mag*, **24**, 503–514.

35. Kelvin WT (1894). On the homogeneous division of space, *Proc R Soc*, **55**, 1–16.

36. Weaire D (ed) (1997). *The Kelvin Problem: Foam Structures of Minimal Surface Area*, Taylor & Francis, London.

37. Plateau J (ed) (1873). *Statique expérimentale et théorique des liquides soumis aux seules forces moléculaires*, Gauthier-Villars, Paris.

38. Thompson DW (ed) (1917). *On Growth and Form*, Dover reprint of 1942 2nd ed. (1st ed., 1917).

39. Ziherl P and Kamien D (2001). Maximizing entropy by minimizing area: towards a new principle of self-organization, *J Phys Chem B*, **105**, 10147–10158.

40. Weaire D and Phelan R (1994). A counterexample to Kelvin's conjecture on minimal surfaces, *Phil Mag Lett*, **69**, 107–110.

41. Weaire D and Hutzler S (eds) (1999). *The Physics of Foams*, Clarendon Press, Oxford.

42. Goldberg M (1935). The isoperimetric problem for polyhedra, *Tohoku Math J*, **40**, 226–236.

43. Kepler J (1611). Strena seu de nive sexangula (in Latin), Festschrift on New Year's day.

44. Leppmaier M (1997). *Kugelpackungen von Kepler bis heute* (in German), Vieweg, Braunschweig.

45. Fuchs A (1999). *Optimierte Delaunay-Triangulierungen zur Vernetzung getrimmter NURBS-Körper* (in German), Shaker Verlag Aachen, pp. 55–58.

46. Naegel A, Heisig M, and Wittum G (2011) Computational modeling of the skin barrier, *Methods Mol Biol*, **763**, 1–32.

47. Bensoussan A, Lions J, and Papanicolau G (eds) (1978). *Asymptotic Analysis for Periodic Structures*, North-Holland, Amsterdam.

48. Vogel A, Reiter S, Rupp M, Nägel A, and Wittum G (2013), UG 4—A novel flexible software system for simulating PDE based models on high performance computers, *Comput Visual Sci*, accepted for publication.

49. Naegel A, Hansen S, Neumann D, Lehr CM, Schaefer UF, Wittum G, and Heisig M (2008). In-silico model of skin penetration based on

experimentally determined input parameters. Part II: mathematical modelling of in-vitro diffusion experiments. Identification of critical input parameters, *Eur J Pharm Biopharm*, **68**, 368–379.

50. Naegel A, Hahn T, Schaefer UF, Lehr C-M, Heisig M, and Wittum G (2011). Finite dose skin penetration: a comparison of concentration-depth profiles from experiment and simulation, *Comput Visual Sci*, **14**(7), 327–339.

51. Selzer D, Hahn T, Naegel A, Heisig M, Kostka KH, Lehr CM, Neumann D, Schaefer UF, and Wittum G (2013). Finite dose skin mass balance including the lateral part: comparison between experiment, pharmacokinetic modeling and diffusion models, *J Control Release*, **165**, 119–128.

52. Hansen S, Henning A, Naegel A, Heisig M, Wittum G, Neumann D, Kostka K-H, Zbytovska J, Lehr CM, and Schaefer UF (2008). In-silico model of skin penetration based on experimentally determined input parameters. Part I: Experimental determination of partition and diffusion coefficients, *Eur J Pharm Biopharm*, **68**, 352–367.

53. Scherer M (2012). Modellierung des Schwellens von Korneozyten im Stratum Corneum. Diplomarbeit, Goethe-Universität Frankfurt (in German).

# Chapter 9

# Molecular Scale Modeling of Human Skin Permeation

Sophie Martel and Pierre-Alain Carrupt

*School of Pharmaceutical Sciences, University of Geneva, University of Lausanne, Quai Ernest Ansermet, 30, 1211 Geneva 4, Switzerland*

Pierre-Alain.Carrupt@unige.ch

The skin represents a potential pathway through which chemicals can access the systemic circulation. Thus, many efforts are currently devoted to evaluate the permeation across the skin as non-invasive route for drug administration in the pharmaceutical industry or as the principal partner for chemicals in cosmetic industry.

Experimental procedures evaluating the human skin permeation are expensive and time-consuming and involve ethical considerations. In vitro alternative solutions were then proposed to provide accurate information on skin permeation as early as possible in products development. However, depending on the stage of the discovery process, tools able to screen a very large number of molecules prior to their synthesis are highly required. In silico tools such as the decision tree of Flynn and the quantitative structure–permeation relationships (QSPeR) offer fast and low-cost predictions of transdermal permeation and allow the selection of the most interesting compounds.

*Computational Biophysics of the Skin*

Edited by Bernard Querleux

Copyright © 2014 Pan Stanford Publishing Pte. Ltd.

ISBN 978-981-4463-84-3 (Hardcover), 978-981-4463-85-0 (eBook)

www.panstanford.com

In this review, in vitro and in silico models used to predict skin penetration of new chemical entities at a molecular level will be introduced and discussed. First, a brief description of relevant components of the skin barrier associated with a good prediction of permeation and a reminder on the main mechanisms relevant for skin penetration will be done. Then in vitro models (retention (chromatographic)-based models, artificial membranes (e.g., Franz cells, PAMPA techniques), cell-based techniques (keratinocyte cells), and in vitro approaches using human skin (e.g., Franz cells)) will be exposed. Finally, the most pertinent in silico models will be reviewed. The discussion will focused on the relevance of parameters regarding the skin composition and mechanisms of transport, and the predictability/usefulness of such models.

## 9.1 Introduction

The assessment of skin permeation is crucial for the estimation of the potential of transdermal drug delivery, for the evaluation of the risk associated with dermal contacts with toxic substances and in the cosmetics industry. In toxicology risk assessment, if no experimental dermal absorption data are available for a substance, European regulatory authorities assume 10% dermal absorption for compounds having a molecular weight (MW) higher than 500 Da and an 1-octanol/water partition coefficient (log $P_{oct}$) lower than −1 or higher than 4. In other cases, dermal absorption is assume to be maximal (100%) [1]. Yet many molecules that fall in the 100% dermal absorption according to this rule are not 100% absorbed. Since 2006, a new legislation for registration of chemicals has been accepted and entered in force in June 2007: REACH (Registration, Evaluation, Authorization and restriction of CHemicals) [2]. Until 2017, all substances will need to be evaluated in term of environmental and health safety. This means that a large number of chemicals will have to be tested regarding their skin absorption in accordance with the manner that they will be used.

Skin penetration aspects are also very important in cosmetic and drug discovery fields. On the one hand, chemicals are not expected to pass through the skin barrier and reach the systemic circulation. On the other hand, the skin represents a potential door for drugs to reach the blood. Advantages of transdermal drug delivery over oral administration are the avoidance of hepatic metabolism, a predictable and extended duration of pharmacological activity, and a better patient compliance. Therefore, there is a great need of methods that provide accurate and high throughput information for registration and/or screening purpose.

Percutaneous penetration studies include a number of in silico, in vitro, and in vivo models characterized by increasing complexity. Of course, in vivo models, even if considered as the gold standard in absorption studies, are difficult to apply for evident ethical, cost, and time reasons. Therefore, many alternative methods were developed to predict the skin permeation of chemicals. One of the best alternatives to in vivo studies is the ex vivo approach based on human or animal skin. However, since 2009 animal testing for cosmetics for instance is prohibited and therefore numerous studies were conducted to develop in vitro skin absorption testing [3]. Of course, faster and low-cost are in silico methods. Thus, many mathematical models have been reported that can be categorized into two classes: empirical and mechanistic models. The former are based on experimental data and correlate linearly (often multilinear models, called quantitative structure permeability relationships (QSPeR), or non-linearly (based on an artificial neural network (ANN), for instance) with relevant descriptors related to skin permeation. Mechanistic models are based on well-established physical laws [4]. In fact, most mathematical models for the prediction of skin permeability are empirical and only few are mechanistic.

In this review, in vitro and in silico models used to predict skin penetration of new chemical entities at a molecular level will be reviewed. First, a brief description of relevant components of the skin barrier associated with a good prediction of permeation and a reminder on the main mechanisms relevant for skin penetration will be done. Then ex vivo approaches using human skin and in vitro models (retention (chromatographic)-based models, artificial membranes, cell-based techniques) will be described. Finally, the most relevant or most recent empirical models used for human skin permeability prediction will be discussed.

## 9.2 Skin Barrier

The skin protects the body against uncontrolled water loss and minimizes the entrance of external agents and UV radiation [5]. The skin is composed of several anatomically distinct layers, which have been defined as epidermis, dermis, and hypodermis. The *stratum corneum* (SC) is the superficial region of epidermis and its 10–20 μm thickness provides the rate-controlling barrier for diffusion for almost all compounds [6]. Underlying the SC is the viable epidermis, a dynamic, constantly self-renewing tissue in which the loss of the cells from the surface of the SC is balanced by cell growth in the lower epidermis. It is composed of basal, spinous (prickle) and granular cell layers, which represent different states of differentiation of keratinocytes [7]. The anucleated corneocytes are the last sequence of the keratinocyte differentiation which led the desquamation.

The dermis (1–2 mm thick) is an acellular collagen-based connective tissue that supports the many blood vessels, lymphatic channels, and nerves and provides mechanical support. The dermis thus represents the gateway to the systemic circulation for absorbed molecules. Finally, the hypodermis, directly adjacent to the dermis, is below the vascular system and as such is not relevant to percutaneous penetration toward the systemic circulation, and functions as a fat storage layer [7–9].

### 9.2.1 *Stratum Corneum*: Composition and Organization

The protective function of the skin is largely provided by the *stratum corneum*, the outermost layer of the skin. The SC water permeability is 1000 times lower than the majority of other biomembranes and the basis of this exceptional property relies on the SC lipid composition and organization [10]. SC consists of dead, flat keratin-filled cells (corneocytes) surrounded by a mixture of intercellular lipids assembled in a "brick and mortar" structure (Fig. 9.1). Connecting the corneocytes are protein structures called corneodesmosomes, which contribute to SC cohesion. Ceramides, free fatty acids, cholesterol, and cholesterol sulfate are the main constituents of SC. Nine different ceramides have been identified in the human SC [11]. Ceramides are a combination of fatty acid and a sphingoid base, joined by an amide bond between the carboxyl group of the fatty acid and the amino group of the base. The fatty acid moiety can be

$\alpha$-hydroxylated or non-hydroxylated, while the sphingoid moiety is a sphingosine or a phytosphingosine [12,13].

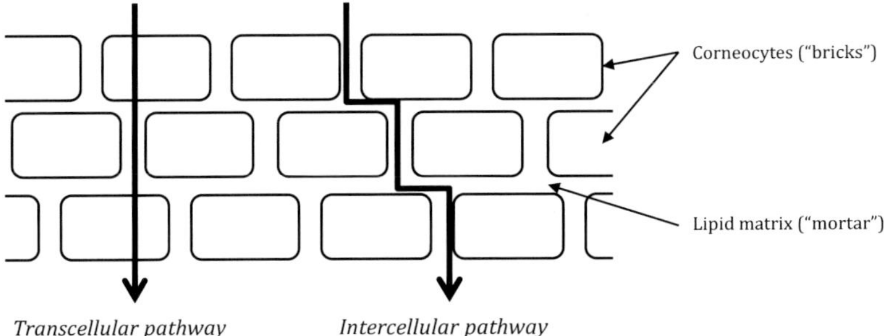


**Figure 9.1**  Schematic structure of *stratum corneum* and the two main permeation routes of solutes.

The free fatty acids present in the SC are mainly saturated acids with a chain length of C22 and C24. Cholesterol and cholesterol sulfate play an important role in the desquamation of corneocytes [14]. In aged epidermis the decreased synthesis of cholesterol accelerates the desquamation of the SC, which is responsible for the observed thicker SC and increased scaling [15,16].

## 9.2.2  Skin Permeability Pathways

Two pathways through the SC intact barrier may be identified: the intercellular lipid route *via* the lipid matrix between the corneocytes, and the transcellular route across the corneocytes and the intercellular lipid matrix (Fig. 9.1). It was shown that the passive diffusion through the lipid matrix between the corneocytes is the major determinant of percutaneous transport rate for hydrophobic molecules [17,18].

Recently, two different intercellular transport pathways have been proposed for hydrophobic solutes according to their size [19]: free-volume diffusion through lipid layers and lateral diffusion along lipid bilayers. The first model is based on the scaled particle theory [20] and describes the diffusion of small hydrophobic solutes (MW < 400) in terms of jumps between free-volume pockets that are opened by density fluctuations in the lipid bilayers. According to this theory the probability of formation of these cavities is supposed to decrease rapidly as the solute size exceeds the lipid size (the dynamic of solutes is slower in this case than that of the lipids) and, as a consequence, the mechanism of diffusion of larger solutes (Mw > 400) is assumed to be controlled by the dynamic of lipids themselves (lateral diffusion of SC lipid bilayers).

For small polar molecules, no relation has been observed between skin permeability and 1-octanol/water partition coefficients (log $P_{oct}$). This observation has suggested that these molecules permeate the skin through an "aqueous" or a "polar" pathway [17]. Moreover other experimental evidence such as the observed relationship between urea permeability and electrical resistance through human epidermal membrane also support the presence of porous permeation pathway [21]. The first attempt to associate the porous pathway with the skin structure was made by Mitragotri [19], who hypothesized that the pores through which highly hydrophilic solutes (log $P_{oct}$ < –2) permeate the skin were imperfections present in the lipid bilayers. The author also proposed that transdermal transport of large hydrophilic solutes such as sucrose, could be explained by diffusion through hair follicles and sweat ducts ("shunt" pathways). However, the limited experimental permeation data for polar compounds do not allow a systematic study focusing upon the porous/polar pathway.

## 9.3 Experimental Methods for Human Skin Permeability Prediction

### 9.3.1 Ex vivo Human or Animal Skin Permeability

The most common methods for the evaluation skin permeation use diffusion cells [22]. The classic diffusion cell (i.e., Franz cell) consists of donor and acceptor compartments separated by a skin sample [23,24]. Although these experiments cannot fully reproduce in vivo conditions particularly with respect to metabolism, distribution and blood supply, their major advantage is that experimental conditions can be controlled precisely, such that the only variables are membranes and the tested compounds [25,26]. Although human excised skin is the membrane of choice and considered the "gold standard" in skin permeability studies, it is not always easily available and creates ethical interrogations. Furthermore, the high variability of sources has been reported depending on many factors such as gender, age, race, and also anatomical site of sampling [27,28].

In this context, many animal skins were tested as alternative to human skin. The main reported models used monkey, pig, guinea pig, rat, and mice skin as well were reviewed by El Maghraby et al. [29]. Regarding all studies together, it is clear that there is a difference between permeability through human skin and animal skin whatever the type of animal considered. Furthermore, this difference is clearly specific for a given permeant. However, to summarize, the best results were probably obtained with skin of primates. This model, however, remains costly and restricted. It has been shown that porcine ear skin is a good alternative to human skin in permeability studies even if it remains also costly. Porcine ear possesses characteristic close to human skin with respect to thickness of SC and epidermis, follicular structure and hair density [30]. More generally, pig skin is widely used for skin permeability studies [27,31–35] due to the structural similarity and permeability characteristic compared to human skin. In addition, relatively low inter-specie variabilities were observed with miniaturized pig models [31,36]. The cheaper models remain rodent model and in particular rat for which hairless animals are available to eliminate the problem of fur. Furthermore, lower inter-individual variations were observed compared to human skin [37]. Even if this model presents relatively higher permeability characteristic than human skin [37], it represents a good alternative for skin diffusion studies in early development stage and formulation investigations.

Even if standardized protocols were established to reduce variations in predictive testing of chemicals as illustrated by the OECD guideline 428 [38], since 2009 animal testing for cosmetics for instance is prohibited and therefore numerous studies were conducted to developed in vitro skin absorption testing.

## 9.3.2 In vitro Models to Predict Skin Penetration

### 9.3.2.1 Reconstructed skin from keratinocytes

Different reconstructed skin models exist and part of them widely used in pharmaceutical and cosmetic industries are commercially available. Two main categories of models can be differentiated: epidermal models and full-thickness (FT) skin models. Basically, epidermal models are based on the growth of human keratinocytes on appropriate membrane such as polycarbonate or collagen matrix in a culture medium at the air–liquid interface. After proliferation of cells, the exposition at the interface air–liquid showed to ensure a stratification and a vertical differentiation of cells that lead to a functional skin layer [39]. SkinEthic™ HRE (human reconstructed epidermis) (SkinEthic Laboratories, Nice, France) [40], EpiSkin™ (L'Oréal, Paris, France, EpiSkin™ is produced and marketed by SkinEthic laboratories, Nice, France), and EpiDerm™ (MatTek corporation, Ashland, Ma, USA) are the most used epidermal models. These three models were compared in a study with respect to their morphology, lipids composition, permeability properties and bio-chemical markers [41]. To summarize, it was concluded that their general structure and composition bear a close resemblance to human skin even if ceramides/phospholipids ratio was generally slightly different between cell culture and native human skin. The compilation of available permeability results on these models also shows a considerably more permeable behavior than human skin meaning that the models provide a relatively weak barrier function that can be explained by the variations in ceramide proportions. However, the culture models appear to be useful for transport studies since the ranking of permeation through the models reflects the permeation through human skin and the variability is lower than the variability of native human skin models. Others models also exist such as EST-1000 (CellSystems™, St Katharine, Germany) or RHE [42] but less used and/or supported by few information. A different model based on rat epidermal keratenocytes (REK) [43–45] has also been developed. Compared to human-based keratinocyte models reported above, REK can be easily maintained and it was shown that the permeability of corticosterone, a lipophilic solute, was close to the permeability measured in intact human skin.

Epidermal models by definition only mimic upper part of full skin and it is well admitted that dermis also plays a role in permeability of solutes especially for lipophilic substances. Besides, it was outlined that full skin models much more converged toward the in vivo situation [41,46]. Full-thickness skin equivalents are mainly constructed from the growth of keratinocytes either on de-epidermized dermis (DED) removed from intact human skin or on dermal equivalents constituted of fibroblasts embedded in a collagen gel [47]. As for epidermal models, after proliferation of keratinocytes on the top of the DED or dermal equivalent, cells can differentiate by the exposure to the air. Both techniques lead to the a functional barrier containing an epidermis and a dermis, which resemble the full-thickness skin [48]. More models exist in this category compared to epidermal models. Few of them are keratinocytes seeded on DED. Most of the published or marketed models are keratinocytes seeded on fibroblasts embedded in collagen. In commercially available models useful for permeation studies, we can cite EpiDerm™ FT (MatTek corporation, Ashland, Ma, USA) and Phenion™ Full-Thickness (Henkel, Düsseldorf, Germany) [47]. With Phenion™ FT, testosterone and caffeine as well as benzoic acid and nicotine were tested and compared to the permeability measured on pig skin using diffusion cells and epidermal models. If permeability on cultured cells was again higher than on pig skin, the lipophilic testosterone was efficiently slowdown compared to data obtained on epidermal models that has been explained by the presence of dermis equivalent forming a reservoir [47]. However, compared to EpiDerm™, SkinEthic™, and EpiSkin™, Phenion™ has a little bit weaker barrier function for more hydrophilic compounds.

Of course, unlike human excised skin, these models do not contain blood vessels, hair follicles, or sweat glands that can significantly change permeability properties. Indeed, Brain et al. [49] have pointed out numerous problems inherent to in vitro models even full-thickness models. In vivo, the dermis is perfused by vasculature implying a potential rapid remove of the permeants. Furthermore, it has been argued that the in vitro aqueous environment of the dermis tends to slowdown lipophilic compounds, whereas in vivo the situation is different. The authors also concluded that SC membrane or epidermal models should be more relevant in permeability studies in particular for lipophilic compounds.

However, in a practical point of view, of course, these models suffer from limitations and remain experiment-sensitive. Indeed, when dealing with cell cultures, many factors can affect results. In the case of keratinocytes, the final model properties are widely dependent on culture conditions such as medium composition or environmental humidity. Besides, many studies varying these parameters were conducted for many years mainly to optimize skin equivalents [48,50]. However, majority of these models are commercially available and ready to use, manufactured in multiwell plates (12, 24, and/or 96 wells). Therefore, these models can be advantageously used even in a screening compounds or formulation testing mode.

### 9.3.2.2 Artificial membranes

To avoid variability inherent to biological materials, several synthetic membranes have been used with diffusion cells techniques: solid membranes such as cellulose acetate [51,52] and polydimethylsiloxane (PDMS) [53–55], organic liquid-supported membranes containing hydrocarbons, long-chain alcohols or isopropyl myristate [24,56,57], and skin lipids [58,59]. The transport across the different membranes is usually determined by monitoring the delivery rate of chemical permeated into the receptor solution or its rate loss from the donor [21,25,60]. Due to the throughput of the technique, often small series of compounds were tested in such diffusion studies. The membrane-coated fiber (MCF) approach was also proposed to predict skin absorption from chemicals or biological mixture based on the measurement of the strength of the molecular interactions of the molecules with the membranes [61]. Hypothesizing that a single MCF will characterize one pattern of molecular interactions, a multiple MCF having different pattern of molecular interactions should simulate skin absorption. For a series of compounds with a wide range of physicochemical properties, the partition into the membrane from the liquid vehicle was measured for three artificial membranes (PDMS for lipophilic interactions, CarboWax for hydrogen bonding interactions and polyacrylate (PA) for $\pi$-electron interactions). It was shown that the correlation between the partitioning in a unique membrane (PDMS, or CarboWax or PA) with $\log k_{\mathrm{p}}$ was pretty poor ($r^2$ from 0.39 for CarboWax to 0.61 for PA) meaning that one membrane is a limited model to predict skin absorption. However, when merging information given by all three membranes, correlation was highly improved (Eq. 9.1):

$$\log k_{\mathrm{p}} = -0.124 \log P_{\mathrm{PDMS}} + 1.91 \log P_{\mathrm{PA}} - 1.17 \log P_{\mathrm{wax}} - 2.34$$

$$n = 25; \quad r^2 = 0.93; \quad F = 93 \tag{9.1}$$

More recently, high throughput techniques using artificial membranes emerged for skin permeability measurements. Parallel artificial membrane permeability assay (PAMPA) is a recent procedure developed for a rapid determination of passive transport permeability which is gaining acceptance in pharmaceutical research [62]. Originally it was developed for gastro-intestinal track permeability prediction [62]. In PAMPA, a 96-well filter plate coated with a liquid artificial membrane is used to separate two compartments, one containing a buffer solution of compounds to be tested (defined as donor compartment) and the other an initial fresh buffer solution (defined as acceptor compartment) assembled in a "sandwich-like" configuration. After a fixed incubation time, sample concentrations are measured in the donor and acceptor compartments.

For skin permeability prediction two different artificial membranes have been developed. The first one, "PAMPA-skin", was made of silicone oil and isopropyl myristate [63,64]. Results have shown a good correlation between log $k_p$ and effective permeability coefficient (log $P_e$) for a series of 69 structurally diverse compounds. Furthermore, when plotting the quantity of compound that reached the acceptor compartment and the quantity of compound trapped in the artificial membrane, it was possible to discriminate: (i) compounds with negligible membrane retention and low permeation (no or very few quantity of compound found in the acceptor compartment). These compounds also have a low $k_p$; (ii) compounds with low or negligible retention on the artificial membrane and high permeation (high quantity of compound found in acceptor compartment); and (iii) compounds with high membrane retention and low permeation. Compounds of these two latter classes are all compounds with high $k_p$ values. Moreover, the retention was shown to well correlate with SC/water partition coefficients (log $P_{SC}$) for a limited number of compounds for which log $P_{SC}$ were available. This means that this membrane retention should reflected the affinity of compounds for SC.

By analogy, a second artificial membrane has been developed for skin permeability prediction based on PAMPA technique [65]. The membrane (Skin-PAMPA$^{TM}$) was constituted of certramide, cholesterol, stearic acid and silicon oil. If the composition of the membrane sounds more "*stratum corneum*-like" with synthetic derivatives of natural and expensive ceramides (certramides) and fatty acids, the correlation between human skin permeability log $k_p$

and permeability coefficients log $P_e$ was comparable to the original PAMPA-skin.

### 9.3.2.3 Chromatographic-based approaches

Chromatographic approaches are extensively used for partition coefficients determination notably 1-octanol-water partition coefficients [66–70]. Even if in comparison with oral drug absorption, few chromatographic studies deal with percutaneous penetration; particular stationary phases or specific experimental conditions have been used to assess skin barrier permeability.

Studies based on immobilized artificial membrane columns (IAMs) have been published. IAM phases are silica-based columns with, initially, phospholipids bounded covalently. The retention factor ($k_{IAM}$) derived from retention time obtained on columns based on phosphatidylcholine (PC) linked to a silica propylamine surface has been compared to human skin permeability coefficients ($k_p$). Various results and conclusions were obtained: For a series of steroids and for five compounds that permeate the skin under their ionized form, a correlation was obtained between both parameters [71]. On the other hand, weak correlation was obtained for a series of phenolic acids [71] and for a series of structurally diverse compounds [72]. In fact, for most authors, the retention on IAM columns is not sufficient to predict drug penetration whatever the biological membrane (e.g., intestinal, blood-brain or cutaneous barrier) since this parameter is largely correlated to log $P_{oct}$ only [73]. Thus, the addition of other descriptors (e.g., molecular weight or hydrogen bonding) is generally needed to enhance the correlations [74–76]. To specifically reach skin permeability information, keratin has been immobilized on silica support [77,78]. Indeed, once again no direct correlation has been obtained between retention factor $k_{keratin}$ and $k_p$. Furthermore, the relationship between $k_{keratin}$ and $k_p$ was even worse than with $k_{IAM}$. However, retentive properties of immobilized keratin were specific and different from the one of other stationary phases and therefore provided information regarding the basic skin protein keratin.

Biopartitioning micellar chromatography (BMC) was also proposed to predict skin permeability [79,80]. BMC consists of polyoxyethylene (23) lauryl ether (Brij35) micellar mobile phase, and a C18 stationary phase. If no correlation was obtained between human skin permeability coefficient log $k_p$ and retention factor log $k_{BMC}$ of 42 diverse compounds, the latter parameter has proved to be useful in QSAR analysis. Indeed, different physicochemical parameters (steric parameters such as molecular weight, refractivity and volume, electronic parameters such as polarizability, molar total charge and H bond capacity and physical parameters such as water solubility and melting point) were tested as additional descriptors to predict skin permeability [80]. Finally, after eliminating non-significant and intercorrelated parameters, the 42 $k_p$ values ($k_p$ ranging from –5 to 0 cm/h) were correlated to log $k_{BMC}$ and melting point (MP) as shown by Eq. 9.2:

$$\log k_p = 1.3 \log k_{BCM} - 0.008 \, MP - 3.3$$

$$n = 42; \quad r^2 = 0.83; \quad s = 0.51; \quad F = 93 \tag{9.2}$$

Since the chromatographic retention depends on the ionization degree of the solute, this model was also used to predict pH effect on skin permeability for 12 ionized non-steroidal anti-inflammatory drugs and the local anesthesic lidocaine using the same Eq. 9.2 [81]. Not surprisingly, predicted log $k_p$ increases (resp. decreases) for basic (resp. acidic) compounds when pH increases. Of course, no experimental $k_p$ pH-profiles exist for ionizable solutes, so it is hard to evaluate the predictiveness of such model.

Finally, a last separative technique has been tested to emulate biological barrier namely liposome electrokinetic chromatography (LEKC). LEKC is based on experimental setup of capillary electrophoresis. Liposomes are suspended in buffer solution and act as pseudo stationary phase. Liposomes become the site of partitioning for solutes. As for BMC technique, no or slight direct correlation was observed but the retention parameter log $k$ there obtained was a useful parameter for QSAR studies of skin permeability [82,83]. For instance, Wang et al. [82] added, to log $k_{LEKC}$, the molecular weight (MW), the number of OH and NH, O, and N ($n_{OHNH+ON}$ as a representative parameter for H bond capacity) in the multiple linear regression to predict skin permeability. They also compared results with liposomes with (Eq. 9.3) and without (Eq. 9.4) cholesterol and obtained the following models:

$$\log k_{\mathrm{p}} = 0.43 \log k_{\mathrm{LECK,chol}} - 0.84\frac{\mathrm{MW}}{100} - 0.12 n_{\mathrm{OHNH+ON}} + 0.03$$

$$n = 23; \quad r^2 = 0.90; \quad s = 0.46 \tag{9.3}$$

$$\log k_{\mathrm{p}} = 0.49 \log k_{\mathrm{LECK,not\ chol}} - 0.83\frac{\mathrm{MW}}{100} - 0.12 n_{\mathrm{OHNH+ON}} + 0.11$$

$$n = 23; \quad r^2 = 0.89; \quad s = 0.48 \tag{9.4}$$

As claimed by the authors, the statistical fit obtained was better (in particular in presence of cholesterol) than with the Potts and Guy basic equation (see Section 9.4.2.1) involving log $P$ and MW. Because for some models based on Potts and Guy equation, the input log $P$ value is a calculated log $P$, the slight improvement that provides the LEKC models are relatively low compared to the required time and solute quantity involved.

## 9.4 In silico Models to Predict Skin Penetration

The development of mathematical models to describe and predict skin permeability has been a fertile area of research. Although much progress has been made in the last decades, the understanding of permeation processes and the development of (Q)SAR models or more specifically QSPeR to interpret skin permeation are hindered by the complex nature of the skin barrier [84] mainly associated with the highly ordered intercellular lipid matrix of the SC, which is the essential layer providing excellent barrier properties [11]. The transport of compounds through a membrane can be easily described using Fick's first law [25]:

$$J = \frac{D_{\mathrm{M}} \cdot P_{\mathrm{M}}}{h} \cdot \Delta C_{\mathrm{M}} = k_{\mathrm{p}} \cdot \Delta C_{\mathrm{M}}, \tag{9.5}$$

where $J$ is the flux, $D_{\mathrm{M}}$ the diffusion coefficient into the membrane, $P_{\mathrm{M}}$ the partition coefficient of the solute between the membrane and the aqueous phase, $h$ the diffusional path length, i.e., the thickness of the membrane, $\Delta C_{\mathrm{M}}$ the difference in concentrations between both sides of the membrane, and $k_{\mathrm{p}}$ the permeability coefficient.

Typically, the steady-state flux and the $k_p$ are assessed from an in vitro experiment in which the donor concentration of the penetrant is maintained (more or less) constant while the receiver phase provides "sink" conditions. Over time, therefore, the flux increases to reach a steady-state value ($J$). $k_p$ is simply calculated from the slope of the linear portion of the graph of the cumulative amount penetrated as a function of time.

Hence, in addition to the thickness of the membrane, permeability through human skin depends on the solute diffusivity through and affinity with the membrane, mainly the SC. It is well known that diffusivity is in general size-dependent (small molecules diffuse more rapidly than large molecules). Molecular size and polar interactions have also an impact on the skin/water partition coefficient that can describe the affinity of the solute for the membrane. That is why these parameters were selected in QSPeRs studies on skin penetration.

## 9.4.1 Reliable Data for Skin Prediction Models

The first important point to consider before performing QSAR models is the initial dataset. Hence, the quality of the model will, of course, mainly depend on the quality of the data taken. However, large consistent datasets are very hard to obtain because skin permeability measurements are so labor intensive.

Different databases exist for skin penetration prediction purpose. Some databases gather permeability coefficients from several studies, and some others focus on SC/water partition coefficients. Ideally, permeability coefficients should be taken from in vivo experiments performed according to well-standardized protocols or even better from a single laboratory. Of course, this "perfect" database constituted of a large number of compounds presenting a wide range of properties does not exist because such experiments are often performed for others purposes than QSPeR studies.

Originally, the most widely used database was the Flynn database [85], which considered the permeability coefficients from 94 compounds for which permeability coefficients, mostly derived from human skin in vitro experiments, were listed (only three permeability values were obtained from in vivo experiments). In this database, values were taken from a large number of publications and therefore inter-laboratory variability inevitably appeared [86, 87]. A detailed look on the values highlighted some critical points [88]. Indeed, permeability coefficients were obtained from studies performed at different temperatures (from 24 to 37°C) and different ionization states (i.e., compounds were not all fully under their neutral form). Yet it is a source of error since permeability highly depends on these two parameters. Indeed, the effect of temperature on log $k_p$ modified the quality of the modeling of skin permeability. For lipophilic compounds, skin permeability has a positive correlation with temperature. For low molecular weight hydrophilic compounds, penetration actually decreases as temperature increases [89]. However, this Flynn database exhibits a broad range of properties (18 < MW < 7 65; –2.3 < log $P_{oct}$ < 5.5) and therefore a relatively broad range of skin permeability values (–9.7 < log $k_p$ < –3.5) [90]. However, few compounds exhibit a log $P$ higher than 4 and lower than 0 (Fig. 9.2). Therefore, as demonstrated in different publications where predictive models have been recalculated from Flynn dataset or part of the dataset [86–88,90], variation in experimental conditions can explain outliers [91] and some permeability values should be evaluated before being included in models.

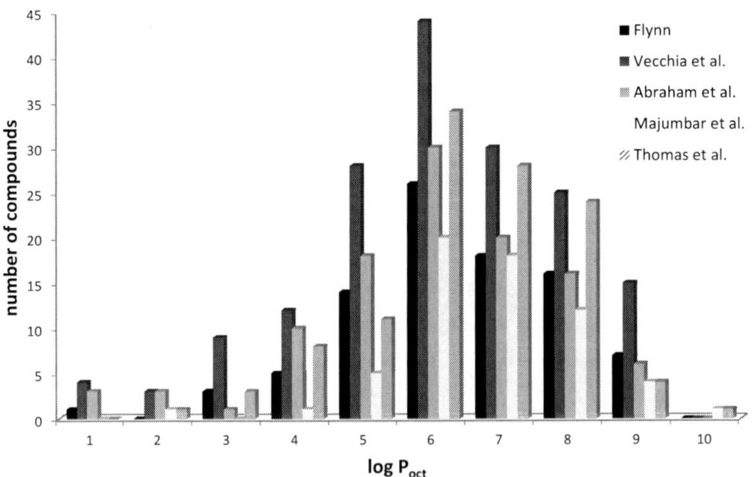



**Figure 9.2**  Repartition of compounds lipophilicity (log $P_{oct}$) of 5 widely used databases in QSPeR studies (Flynn [85], Vecchia et al. [88], Abraham et al. [94], Majumbar et al. [95], and Thomas et al. [96]).

Since then, many authors have worked on the update and/or extension of the Flynn database, which has also been reviewed by Cronin et al. [92]. For instance, in 2003, Vecchia and Bunge proposed a fully validated database for both permeability coefficients ($k_p$) and water/SC partition coefficients (log $P_{SC}$) after a detailed re-analysis of the Flynn database. They highly extended the database as shown in Figs. 9.2 and 9.3. However, the repartition of compounds along log $P_{oct}$ and MW values remain identical to the repartition provided by Flynn database. They also listed important criteria for data validation that should be taken into account [88,93]. Permeability coefficients were validated according to five criteria: (i) temperature must be known and comprised between 20 and 40°C, (ii) more than 10% of unionized form of the tested compound must be present, (iii) a validated log $P_{oct}$ must exist, (iv) the measurement must have been made at a steady-state, and (v) the donor and acceptor fluids do not compromise the skin barrier [88].

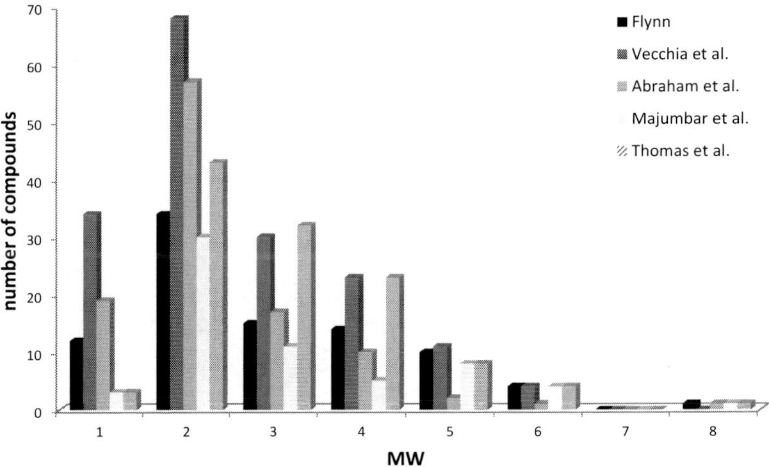


**Figure 9.3**    Repartition of compounds molecular weight (MW) of five widely used databases in QSPeR studies (Flynn [85], Vecchia et al. [88], Abraham et al. [94], Majumbar et al. [95], and Thomas et al. [96]).

Abrahams and Martins [94] also listed 119 compounds with $k_p$ corrected for ionization (neutral species) and temperature (37°C). In this database, new compounds were added compared to the original Flynn database in particular hydrophilic compounds that were missing in the Flynn database (e.g., urea, mannitol, and raffinose). Also values for steroids were substituted by the more recent values from Jonhson et al. [86] that were considered more preferable values [86,91]. Indeed, it was observed in many studies that the remove of these compounds from dataset or more recent experimental values for steroids improved considerably QSPeR models and these latter values are now considered as the correct ones.

Majumdar et al. [95] and Thomas et al. [96] edited and extended the Flynn database. The edited Flynn database is a selection of 62 compounds from the Flynn database for which solubilities in water and maximum fluxes from water through human skin in vitro are known or can be calculated for QSAR purpose [95]. This selection was extended with 52 compounds from nine contributors (the total number of contributors to this extended database was therefore 15) [96]. In this database, compounds were not excluded regarding their ionization state or because of the skin thickness. Therefore, a mix of data obtained on heat-separated epidermis and full skin were included [95,96]. This edited and extended Flynn database is one of the database that exhibit more compounds with "extreme" log $P_{oct}$ and MW (Figs. 9.2 and 9.3) that were missing in the previous databases. This extended edited database (as well as the edited database) was used to study the effect of water solubility of solutes on their flux through human skin in vitro (and not $k_p$) performing QSPeR analysis based on Roberts and Sloan equation using aqueous and lipidic solubilities of solutes as independent variables [97]. And in this study it was shown that the thickness of the skin (SC, epidermis, or full skin) as well as the ionization level of solutes did not appear to pejorate the fits of the data.

Others extended databases have been also published by different authors. However, it is important to mention that some of them include non-experimental data. For instance, Kirchner et al. [98] published permeability coefficients for 114 compounds incorporating much of the Flynn database and additional compounds from Occupational Safety and Health Association. It was later observed that 63 of permeability coefficients were calculated log $k_p$ with a modified Potts and Guy equation [99]. Furthermore, new data for steroids were not included, whereas steroids were represented in the dataset. As clearly mentioned by Frasch et al. this database must not be used for QSPeR model developments as it would a model of model [99].

Therefore, before performing models based on experimental skin permeability coefficients, readers should keep attention to different criteria. And it is important to remind that originally the Flynn database was not designed for QSAR purpose and therefore do not intent to provide data as accurate as expected for such purposes. More recent databases such as the one of Vecchia and Bunge are of better quality in term of suitability for modeling.

More recently, Lee and co-workers [100] published a new database containing 44 non-proprietary compounds for which they measured in house the log $P_e$ using Franz cell diffusion and human skin. Therefore, it constitutes a quite large database of standardized measurements. Contrary to other databases, the vehicle used for this study was 45% polyethylene glycol (PEG 400)/65% phosphate buffer saline (PBS) (w/v) instead of the normal water. Indeed, it is considered that water does not simulate what is typical in topical discovery project applications. Further PEG may resolve some solubility issues. Lastly, permeability studies were performed with cassettes of solutes that, of course, improve the throughput. Each cassette also contained an internal standard (3-isobutyl-1-methylxanthine (IBMX)) that eliminates the need to normalize data for each cassette over many different skin sources and therefore reducing variability.

Recently, Buist et al. [101] measured 15 permeability coefficients according to the standard protocols in agreement with the OECD test guideline 428 [38]. Assays were performed using diffusion cells and skin from female donor aged from 29 to 53 years. Even if the number of compounds seems relatively low, the originality is that permeability measurements were measured in two experimental conditions: with a large and a small donor solution volume to represent infinite and finite dose experiments, respectively. Indeed, usually $k_p$ is determined under infinite dose conditions by dividing the measured flux by the initial concentration in the donor compartment (under steady state conditions). Infinite conditions means that the concentration of the solute applied to the skin does not change significantly over time. However, in practice, skin exposure occurs under finite conditions. Furthermore, different concentrations in the donor compartment were tested for seven substances.

At this state, it is important to note that almost all databases provide only few (if any) representative compounds of very low or very high lipophilicity (Figs. 9.2 and 9.3). Therefore, models developed on the basis of these databases should therefore be limited to a moderate range of lipophilicity. That is why recently, Moss and co-workers [102] merged 142 $k_p$ values from different sources. Unfortunately, no table is provided with the complete database but it can be estimated from figures that compounds log $P$ provide a Gaussian repartition centered on log $P$ around 2. It should be noted that some $k_p$ values (13) were extracted from [103] for which the measurements were made using Franz cells but with porcine skin.

## 9.4.2 Models Based on Molecular Properties

The assessment of a global predictive model requires, besides consistent and reliable data, that the process to be modeled occurs with the same mechanism for all tested compounds [104]. As shown before, it is reasonable to believe that the passive diffusion pathway through the SC controls the permeation of most compounds whose permeation through human skin has been experimentally determined. Many quantitative-structure–permeation relationships (QSPeRs) models have been developed by researchers to model passive percutaneous penetration of exogenous chemicals.

### 9.4.2.1 Models based on lipophilicity and molecular size

The most popular predictive model is the equation proposed by Potts and Guy [17]. Based on 93 compounds of the 94 included in the Flynn database, they simply described the human skin permeability coefficient as a linear combination of 1-octanol/water partition coefficient (log $P_{oct}$) and permeant size (molecular weight (MW) or molecular volume (MV)). They therefore reported the following Eq. 9.6:

$$\log k_p = 0.75 \log P_{oct} - 0.0061 MW - 6.3$$

$$n = 93; \quad r^2 = 0.67, \tag{9.6}$$

where (as in the following equations) $n$ is the number of permeability coefficients (observations), and $r^2$ is the square of the correlation coefficient.

This model has been built based on the original Flynn database, for which, as mentioned above, steroids values were criticized. After the evidence of error on experimental values and the publication of new ones, Cronin et al. re-analyzed the dataset with also more accurate log $P$. New data for steroids only concern part of steroids published in Flynn database. As there was significant evidence that the quality of permeability coefficients of steroids was poor, Cronin also removed from the dataset the 19 steroids for which no new data were available. He therefore obtained the following Eq. 9.7 [105]:

$$\log k_p = 0.61 \log P_{oct} - 0.0058 \mathrm{MW} - 2.54$$

$$n = 75; \quad r^2 = 0.75; \quad s = 0.63; \quad F = 112, \tag{9.7}$$

where (as in the following equations) $s$ is the standard error and $F$ the Fisher statistic.

This approach has also been applied to larger databases. For instance Buchwald and Bodor [106] analyzed 98 compounds from experimental permeability values published by Wilschut et al. [107] and Johnson et al. [86] with refined steroids permeability values (new values were updated and some steroids without new data were removed). Furthermore, in this dataset, permeability values were corrected for ionized compounds. Applying the Potts and Guy equation, they obtained the following relationship (Eq. 9.8):

$$\log k_p = 0.60 \log P_{oct} - 0.0052 \mathrm{MW} - 6.02$$

$$n = 98; \quad r^2 = 0.75; \quad s = 0.59; \quad F = 144 \tag{9.8}$$

They also demonstrated by subdividing the whole dataset in subgroups of compounds with increased molecular size (the Van der Waals volume was there considered) the good correlation between log $k_p$ and log $P_{oct}$ within each size subgroups. Nevertheless, the statistical fit obtained with this extended dataset provides no improvement compared to the model proposed by Cronin et al. built on 75 compounds.

Interestingly, Lee et al. [100] published, based on their 61 compounds with permeability values measured in house using Franz cells, the following model (Eq. 9.9):

$$\log k_{\mathrm{p}} = 0.39C\log P - 0.0055\mathrm{MW} - 0.23$$

$$n = 61; \quad r^2 = 0.53 \tag{9.9}$$

The statistical fit is worse compared to previous models. Furthermore, the in vitro permeability values were obtained in a different vehicle than the standardized water. Indeed, log $k_{\mathrm{p}}$ were obtained with PEG 400 as vehicle. This considerably impacts the model since the partition of the solute between the SC and the vehicle is, of course, different.

Cronin et al. [108] and Kichner et al. [98] have analyzed 114 permeability coefficients published originally by Kichner et al. After removing seven outliers (two steroids (estriol and hydrocortisone), propylene chloride (the only positive permeability value), atropine and etorphine (with complex fused rings), digitoxin and sucrose (able to form much more hydrogen bonds than all other compounds)), the correlation based on log $P_{\mathrm{oct}}$ and MW was statistically much better than the one published by Potts and Guy. However, as mentioned in the previous paragraph, it has also been seen that a large number of permeability data were calculated leading to a biased statistical model [99].

Just for comparison, the mechanistic (non-empirical) model of Mitragotri et al. [20] used a slightly different parameter as molecular size descriptor namely the solute radius, $r$, that can be calculated using the empirical correlation between $r$ and MW: $4/3\pi r^3 = 0.91$ MW. Based on the database published by Johnson et al. [86] and on the scaled particle theory (that allows the calculation of the work required to create a cavity for solute diffusion in lipid bilayers) they obtained the following Eq. 9.10:

$$\log k_{\mathrm{p}} = 5.6 \cdot 10^{-6} P_{\mathrm{oct}}^{0.7} \exp(-0.46r^2) \tag{9.10}$$

This model was tested on 124 compounds [109] from four sources already mentioned in this chapter, namely Flynn (1990) [85], Johnson et al. (1997) [86], Patel and co-workers (2002) [110], and Wilschut et al. (1995) [107]. After transformation of the Mitragotri equation, Lian et al. [109] obtained the following model (Eq. 9.11):

$$\log k_{\mathrm{p}} = 0.7 \log P_{\mathrm{oct}} - 0.0072 \mathrm{MW}^{2/3} - 5.25$$

$$n = 203; \quad r^2 = 0.70 \tag{9.11}$$

This mechanistic model leads to an equation similar to the statistically derived empirical QSPR equations mentioned above. The main difference is that for the Mitragotri model the power index of the molecular weight is 2/3, slightly lower than 1. This model was shown to correctly predict permeability coefficient for small solutes (MW < 400 Da). When MW increases, it approaches the molecular size of lipids constituting SC barrier. Indeed, mathematical model was constructed based on the assumption that solute moves in a stationary frame of lipid molecules, assumption that may not be valid when solute size becomes comparable to the size of lipids themselves and therefore the model cannot be used for bigger molecules. Furthermore, Mitragotri model is found to under-predict the skin permeability of the hydrophilic compounds by few orders of magnitudes. Generally, this is also the case for other models [109].

More recently, Berge et al. [111] proposed a non-linear model for the prediction of permeability coefficient through the skin. Based on the assumption that two pathways can occurred through the SC (the main barrier) the transcellular route through corneocytes and the intercellular route through the extracellular lipids, the permeability through human skin can be decomposed in two terms: $k_{\mathrm{p,SC\text{-}intercellular}}$ and $k_{\mathrm{p,SC\text{-}transcellular}}$. From the experimental $k_{\mathrm{p}}$ values taken from Vecchia et al. [112], using $\log P_{\mathrm{oct}}$ and MW as independent variables and applying an iterative non-linear fit, they obtained the following model:

$$k_{\mathrm{p}} = k_{\mathrm{p,SC\text{-}intercellular}} + k_{\mathrm{p,SC\text{-}transcellular}} \tag{9.12}$$

with

$$k_{\mathrm{p,SC\text{-}intercellular}} = 10^{\left[-2.59 + 0.732 \log P_{\mathrm{oct}} - 0.0068 \mathrm{MW}\right]} \tag{9.13}$$

and

$$k_{\mathrm{p,SC\text{-}transcellular}} = \frac{0.043}{\mathrm{MW}^{1.361}}$$

$$n = 182; \quad r^2 = 0.682 \tag{9.14}$$

This model was derived from observations on the skin permeation of non-ionized substances from aqueous solutions. And as noted by the authors the validity is therefore limited to this kind of compounds. In fact, this model seems a priori more complex than others. However, its application remains simple since the input parameters are identical. However, it was often criticized the colinearity between log $P$ and MW (e.g. [106]) for compounds considered in skin permeability studies. If it is the case, therefore when MW increases, log $P$ increases, and looking at both Eqs. 9.13 and 9.14, it appears that $k_{p,SC\text{-transcellular}}$ could therefore be negligible or even low for a large number of molecules (exception should appear for big molecules with low lipophilicity). Then considering the predominant $k_{p,SC\text{-intercellular}}$, coefficients obtained are, in fact, similar to most of models developed and described above (Eqs. 9.6–9.8, for instance).

All these studies highlight the great importance of lipophilicity and molecular size of compounds in permeability through human skin. Vecchia et al. [88] listed different published models based on log $P_{oct}$ and molecular size. And it was clear that almost all of them were able to predict human skin permeability at least for compounds with low molecular weight. On the contrary, when MW increases, less of the published models were able to predict accurately the skin penetration. This can be explained by the usually low number of compounds with high MW and more generally limited range in compounds properties in the databases explored. Therefore, reader should first clearly identified the limitation of the model to be used and in particular avoid the prediction of permeability coefficients for compounds outside of the range of dataset used to build the model in term of compound's properties. Nevertheless, these equations remain simple to apply for an early fast evaluation of the potential ability of compounds to cross the human skin.

### 9.4.2.2 Models considering H bond capacities

Because a colinearity between log $P_{oct}$ and MW can be observed when studying the different dataset dealing with skin penetration (e.g. [106]), many authors proposed to considered H bond capacity of the solutes in QSPeR studies.

Potts and Guy [113] proposed a new empirical model based on H bond donor ($\Sigma\alpha_2^H$) and acceptor ($\Sigma\beta_2^H$) capacities and molecular volume (MV, Van der Waals volume). Based on 37 compounds taken from the Flynn database (only permeability coefficients measured at temperatures close to 25°C) with log $P$ ranging from −1.4 to 4.2 and MW ranging from 18 to 158, the following Eq. 9.15 was obtained:

$$\log k_{p} = 0.0257\text{MW} - 1.74\,\Sigma\alpha_2^{H} - 3.85\;\Sigma\beta_2^{H} - 4.89$$

$$n = 37; \;\; r^2 = 0.94; \;\; s = 0.24; \;\; F = 169 \tag{9.15}$$

It is clear regarding Eq. 9.15 that H bond capacity of the solute plays an important role in the permeability though human skin by restricting the penetration.

As noted by the authors, this model can only be adequate for compounds for which the permeability is limited by the SC barrier. This model cannot be used for very lipophilic compounds for whose penetration is determined by the underlying viable skin tissue.

Buchwald and Bodor [106] introduced a H bond–related parameter, namely $N$, to predict skin permeability. $N$ was first described in the prediction of log $P$ and is a positive integer increased in an additive manner by each functional group of the molecule [114]. Mostly all polar, oxygen- and nitrogen-containing simple functions increase $N$ by 2 units, while those in an aromatic environment increase its value by 1. Model for human skin penetration prediction was therefore built based on 98 compounds with permeability values from Wilschut et al. [107] database with steroids values from Johnson et al. [86] and corrected for ionization when necessary. Therefore, they obtained the fully predictive model described by the following Eq. 9.16 based on Van der Waals volume ($V_e$) and H bond–related parameter ($N$):

$$\log k_{p} = 0.013V_{e} - 0.49N - 5.94$$

$$n = 98; \;\; r^2 = 0.72; \;\; s = 0.62; \;\; F = 124 \tag{9.16}$$

Compared to Potts and Guy model on the 98 compounds (Eq. 9.8), the fit is not improved by using $N$ and $V_e$. For predictive estimation of skin permeability, the advantage of such model is the simplicity of parameters involved. Both are easily calculable. According to the authors, in opposite to Potts and Guy approach, the Eq. 9.16 does not use apparently interrelated parameters. However, it was noted by Geinoz and co-workers [90] that, in fact, for the 98 compounds tested here, there was a correlation between $N$ and $V_e$ with an $r^2$ of 0.85. Indeed, both parameters have no interrelatedness in a physicochemical point of view, but it can be imagined that in the global set of compounds, compounds that have a high number of heteroatoms (leading to a high $N$ parameter) may be the biggest compounds of the set.

Solvatochromic analysis (LSER) have been widely used in correlations with biological, chemical and physical properties involving solute-solvent interactions for a large number of chemicals [115]. They are based on the solvatochromic parameters developed by Taft, Kamlet, Abraham, and co-workers [116–119]. The general form of LSER equation includes a cavity/bulk term (such as a calculated Van der Waals volume, $V_w$) and the so-called solvatochromic parameters such as dipolarity/polarizability $\pi^*$, hydrogen-bond donor acidity $\alpha$, and H bond acceptor basicity $\beta$. Abraham et al. proposed a first model [120] on 22 solutes extracted from the Flynn database, including steroids for which, as already mentioned in this chapter, permeability values were criticized. Later a fairly good permeation model for 119 solutes [94] based on the general linear free-energy relationship (LFER) below was published:

$$\log k_p = c + eE + sS + aA + bB + vV, \tag{9.17}$$

where $k_p$ is the human skin permeability coefficient, $E$ is the solute excess molar refractivity, $S$ is the dipolarity/polarizability, $A$ and $B$ the hydrogen bond acceptor and donor activity, respectively, and $V$ is the molecular volume.

The 119 permeability values used as dependent variables were corrected for ionization and temperature (37°C). Furthermore, new data from Jonhson et al. [86] for steroids were included in the dataset. Solvatochromic parameters were obtained from previously published results based on partition coefficients in different water/solvent system. The molecular volume corresponds here to the Mc Gowan volume that can be calculated [121]. The model leads to the following equation:

$$\log k_p = -5.426 - 0.106E - 0.473S - 0.473A - 3.000B + 2.296V$$

$$n = 119; \quad r^2 = 0.83; \quad s = 0.46; \quad F = 112 \tag{9.18}$$

The main factors influencing $\log k_p$ are hydrogen bond basicity that decreases $\log k_p$ and solute volume that increases $\log k_p$. In this study, compounds $\log P$ were ranging from $-1.5$ to $5.5$ and MW from 18 to 765 that is larger than the ranges observed in the Potts and Guy study [113]. In addition, LSER equation was also applied to $\log P_{SC}$ prediction for a reduced set of 45 compounds (only compounds with experimental $\log P_{SC}$ available) leading to the following equation:

$$\log P_{SC} = 0.341 + 0.341E - 0.206S - 0.024A - 2.178B + 1.850V$$

$$n = 45; \quad r^2 = 0.93; \quad s = 0.22; \quad F = 97 \tag{9.19}$$

Based on their home-made measurements using Franz cells and human skin on 61 drugs (among which 44 are non-proprietary), Lee et al. [100] proposed a model also including parameters related to H bond donor and acceptor capacities. The model is described by Eq. 9.20:

$$\log k_p = -0.0022\text{PISA} - 0.35\text{donorHB} - 0.26\text{accptHB} - 5.84\text{glob},$$

$$+0.27\text{EA(eV)} + 6.62$$

$$n = 61; \quad r^2 = 0.77 \tag{9.20}$$

where PISA is the $\pi$ (carbon and attached hydrogen) component of the solvent-accessible surface area, donorHB is the estimated number of hydrogen bonds that would be donated by the solute in solution, accptHB is the estimated number of hydrogen bonds that would be accepted by the solute in solution, glob is the globularity descriptor and is equal to $4 * \pi * r^2/\text{SASA}$ where $r$ is the radius of a sphere with a volume equal to the molecular volume and SASA is the solvent-accessible surface area (glob is equal to 1.0 for a spherical molecule), and EA(eV) is the quantum mechanically calculated electron affinity. All the descriptors used in this model were calculated with QikProp (Schrödinger, New York, USA).

After normalization of the multilinear regression coefficients, Eq. 9.17 becomes

$$\log k_p = -0.43\text{PISA} - 0.70\text{donorHB} - 1.01\text{accptHB} - 0.49\text{glob}$$

$$+0.30\text{EA(eV)} + 0.77$$

$$n = 61; \quad r^2 = 0.77 \tag{9.21}$$

All descriptors have an impact on the skin permeability in particular solute HB bond acceptor capacity that slow down the permeability as already shown in other models. However, the influence of this parameter is less significant. According to the authors, this could be due to the presence of PEG 400 in the vehicle. Indeed, all others presented models consider water a vehicle and it is easy to imagine that such difference can significantly change the partitioning of the solute toward vehicle and skin barrier because the relative H bond donor capacity of the vehicle in presence of PEG 400 is reduced compared to water vehicle.

### 9.4.2.3　Considering solubility parameters

Solubility parameters were used to predict the maximal flux ($J_{max}$). Considering that $J_{max}$ was a relevant clinical parameter for human skin absorption, research groups modeled this dependent variable using different physicochemical parameters including solubility values. In 2007, Majumdar et al. [95] proposed the following model to predict the maximal flux through human skin (Eq. 9.22) based on a previous study of Roberts and Sloan [97]:

$$\log J_{max} = 0.73 \log S_{oct} + 0.27 \log S_{aq} - 0.005\, MW - 3.01$$

$$n = 62; \quad r^2 = 0.93; \quad s = 0.37; \quad F = 274 \tag{9.22}$$

The experimental values of $J_{max}$ were taken from the Flynn database except for steroids and constituted the "edited Flynn database" (see Section 9.5.1 for details). This model was also extended later by the same group to the "extended edited database" (Eq. 9.23) [96]:

$$\log J_{max} = 0.58 \log S_{oct} + 0.41 \log S_{aq} - 0.0044\, MW - 2.57$$

$$n = 114; \quad r^2 = 0.89; \quad s = 0.40; \quad F = 139 \tag{9.23}$$

Models were also performed on the same data using different independent variables ($S_{oct}$ only, MW only, both MW, and $S_{oct}$) that were not including aqueous solubility as independent variable and results obtained were worse in all cases. In the extended model [96] it was also highlighted that the $S_{aq}$ parameter was much more important in the prediction of $J_{max}$ than previously found. In fact, it is not really surprising that solubility values can play an important role in the flux predictions. Finally, $S_{oct}$ and $S_{aq}$ replace lipophilicity parameters that were widely recognized to impact on the skin absorption. This is also confirmed by the fact that $S_{oct}$ alone (as well as $S_{aq}$ alone) were not sufficient to predict the maximal flux [95,96] that is perfectly coherent with the dependence of skin permeability to 1-octanol/water partition coefficients.

### 9.4.2.4  3D-QSARs

Although predictive models have been developed, the use of 2D descriptors in QSPeRs analysis do not take into account the tri-dimensional aspects of molecular structures, thus limiting the development of more realistic models especially for flexible molecules.

The calculation of molecular properties from 3D molecular interaction fields (MIFs) has generated a novel approach to correlate 3D molecular structures with pharmacokinetic and physicochemical properties [122]. These fields describe the variation of interaction energy between a target molecule and a chemical probe moved in a 3D grid constructed around the target. The total interaction energy is calculated at each point of the 3D grid. Since the information contained in 3D molecular fields is related to the interacting partners, the amount of information in MIFs is clearly greater than that in one- or two-dimensional computed molecular descriptors. The GRID force field [123–125] is one of the most widely used computational tool to map the molecular surfaces of molecules and macro-molecules.

A probe is a small molecule or chemical fragment, e.g., a water molecule, a methyl group, a carboxylate group or a carbonyl oxygen atom. The water probe is used to simulate the enthalpy part of the solvation–desolvation processes. The hydrogen-bonding carbonyl and amide probes and the hydrophobic probe (called DRY in the GRID force field) are used to simulate interactions with the polar headgroups and the hydrophobic core of biological membranes, respectively, or with polar or hydrophobic regions in proteins. As GRID probes are selective, their use allows to collect data on molecular property fields, which can be used in QSAR, 3D-QSAR, and selectivity studies [126–129].

The Molecular Lipophilicity Potential (MLP) is a transformation of log $P_{oct}$ values (conceptually one-dimensional representations) into three-dimensional representations [130,131]. The MLP describes the combined lipophilic influence of all fragments in a molecule on its environment and can be calculated at any given point in space around a molecule. From this potential the hydrophilic ($MLP_{hi}$) and hydrophobic ($MLP_{ho}$) fields can be extracted. To explore three-dimensional H bonding properties, a computational tool—the molecular hydrogen-bonding potentials (MHBPs)—has recently been created [132], comprising a H bonding donor potential ($MHBP_{do}$) and a H bonding acceptor potential ($MHBP_{ac}$). The information contained in 3D molecular fields is very large. Moreover, when various compounds are studied at the same time, a simple graphic analysis and visualization of the fields generated by each single compound is no longer sufficient to highlight the useful information. In this case, appropriate chemometric methods are needed to condense and extract the desired information. Chemometrics comprises the application of multivariate statistics, mathematics, and computational methods to chemical results. Principal component analysis (PCA) allows to summarize the information provided by the numerous variables (PCA) and principal component regression (PCR) or partial least squares (PLS) are very useful techniques to correlate them with a biological activity (PCR and PLS) or property (for instance $k_p$) [133].

3D-QSPeR models were established based on the MIFs extracted from GRID force fields in addition to four shape descriptors namely $V$ (molecular volume), $S$ (molecular surface), $R$ (rugosity) and $G$ (globularity) [134,135]. 75 compounds for which $k_p$ values were obtained from the Vecchia et al. [112] database (fully validated database) were used. Different models were built using the (a) $V$, $S$, $R$, $G$, and fields extracted from the four probes water, DRY, amide and carbonyl, (b) $V$, $S$, $R$, $G$, and $MLP_{hi}$, $MLP_{ho}$, $MHPB_{do}$, $MHBP_{ac}$, (c) merging fields from models (a) and (b). Based on the observations made from these three models, only more relevant molecular fields were kept to build the final model that comprises $V$, $S$, $R$, $G$, $GRID_{DRY}$ (molecular field extracted from DRY probe), $MLP_{ho}$, $MHBP_{do}$, and $MHBP_{ac}$. Correlating log $k_p$ predicted with this model and experimental log $k_p$ values, the statistical fit was pretty good with an $r^2 = 0.81$, $s = 0.48$, $F = 308$ [135,136]. This model highlighted that good skin permeation is related with localized polar interactions and low hydrogen-bond capacity. In addition, solute lipophilicity should be high and preferentially delocalized to improve permeability of compounds through human skin. If this computational method is easy to apply, the interpretation should be made with caution.

This 3D approach was also used to predict mice skin permeation [137] and also to interpret the permeability mechanisms through artificial membranes and relate them to in vivo situation [55,64].

It is important to note that, of course, in this kind of model, the molecule conformation may influence the $k_p$ prediction. Therefore, at the opposite of the 2D-model, attention should be paid to the initial step dealing with conformational analysis. Although various algorithms exist to obtain 3D structures from 2D geometries, they are based on specific rules to derive gas phase conformations, which may be sometimes irrelevant for the analysis of pharmacokinetic data.

### 9.4.2.5 Others models (non-linear)

Linear or more generally multilinear models by definition assume that descriptors taken into account are linearly correlated to the skin permeability. Recently, several authors estimated that methods based on linear regression analysis may not be the best way to develop QSPeR. The rationale for non-linear models is that if lipophilicity is too low or too high, then absorption will in general be poor, and significantly lower than that of molecules with intermediate lipophilicities which is not modeled by QSPeR. Indeed, in models exposed above, log $P_{oct}$ has a positive impact on skin permeability coefficients. As such these models fail to fully represent the apparently non-linear relationship between a molecule's physicochemical parameters and its permeability across the skin. It has been shown that the greatest difference between experimental and predicted values was found at the highest log $P$ values [103].

Other statistical methods were therefore proposed avoiding the linear dependence of descriptors assumption. For instance, ANN or Gaussian process (GP) is suitable for extracting non-linear effects of descriptors. Here are some examples of nonlinear models proposed for human skin permeability prediction purposes.

Degim et al. [138] considered the partial charge of solute in addition to the log $P_{oct}$ and MW on a set of 40 compounds and used the ANN methodology to correlate the descriptors with log $k_p$ for a series of 40 compounds (small molecules and drugs) from [107] which were obtained using Franz diffusion cells. Based on the same data, a multilinear model was first built by the same authors [139] and they obtained an $r^2$ of 0.67. After optimization of ANN model, they obtained a relationship between experimental and predicted log $k_p$ with an $r^2$ of 0.997. This is, of course, the highest $r^2$ for a predictive skin permeability model. However, the applicability of this model, build only to fit or maybe overfit experimental data, seems very low and its interpretation is very hard. However, it also reveals that there is no need to increase the number of descriptors to be able to predict skin penetration.

Later, Chen et al. [4] used the Abraham descriptors as input in another ANN model. They collected 215 $k_p$ values (small chemicals and drugs with log $k_p$ ranging from –5.22 to –0.85, log $P_{oct}$ ranging from –2.11 to 7.6 and MW ranging from 18 to 518 Da) from literature [85,110,140] and compared to the corresponding multilinear relationship model. Once again when the multilinear analysis gave an $r^2$ of 0.70, the ANN model was highly improved to an $r^2$ of 0.83. By running the ANN keeping four descriptors constant mean value and varying the last descriptors, they also tried to explain the influence of each descriptor. In fact, the same conclusions as the ones already shown with the multilinear analysis were observed. The H bond capacity (donor and acceptor) as well as the polarity of compounds are not favorable for the solutes skin permeability. At the opposite, the Mc Gowan volume and the excess molar refraction are favorable for a good permeation of a solute. The better fit obtained with ANN model tends to show the non-linearity between Abraham descriptors and skin permeability.

In 2009, Moss and colleagues [102] tested two models: a single layer neural (SLN) network and the other one base on GP method. Their models were first based on two significant descriptors (log $P_{oct}$ and MW) and second based on four additional descriptors namely the melting point, SP (a solubility parameter representative of the solubility in SC), HA and HB (the count of the number of H bond acceptor and donor on the molecule). It was demonstrated that even with two descriptors, GP and SLN models were more performant (on a statistically basis) than the linear Potts and Guy approach. Second, the GP method provided the better fit for the dataset considered. It is important to note that in this case the dataset was extended mainly by completing the data with compounds with much higher lipophilicities that were lacking in the "traditional" databases used in QSPeR analysis [103]. Using this extended dataset the original Potts and Guy approach gave an $r^2$ of 0.36 instead of the $r^2$ higher than 0.7 provided in others studies. This kind of model should therefore be more efficient for lipophilic compounds than linear ones described earlier in the chapter.

An alternative artificial intelligence method was also proposed for skin permeability prediction: genetic programming in which a long list of QSAR parameters (17) were taken as input, among which log $P_{oct}$, H bond information, charges parameters, MW, solubility parameter, and molecular shape indexes. Permeability data for 22 compounds were taken from [141] themselves taken in different "traditional" literature references. They obtained a model with an $r^2$ of 0.91 which is pretty good with a final equation including only 3 parameters (from the 17 initially employed) namely the number of H bonding heteroatoms, the sum of atomic charges on the H bonding heteroatoms and the second-order molecular shape index [142]. However, many issues could be highlighted: (a) The number of compounds used was very low; (b) the 22 compounds were only steroids (64%) and alcohols (36%); (c), steroids $k_p$ values were taken from the criticized published data [143,144]. However, new data have been published that are unanimously considered more relevant (see Section 9.4.1). Therefore, many cautions should be taken when considering this useless model.

In general, these models lack of transparency since they act as a "black box" with input data and output data. They are often more difficult to interpret than linear models. Furthermore, they are much more difficult to apply that the simple Potts and Guy approach for instance. However, the better fits usually observed with these non-linear models tend to show, when they do not reflect overfitting problems, that the classically used descriptors are not so linearly related to skin penetration.

## 9.5 Conclusion

The main difficulty in predicting human skin permeability is to build an accurate model. Indeed, if in vivo experimental techniques exist for human skin permeability measurements, legislation as well as cost and time are drastic obstacles for accurate data acquisition. Of course, many experimental alternatives have been proposed to bypass, first, in vivo testing and, second, the use of tissues from animal or human origins. Efficient experimental models based on non-biological materials have proven to well predict human skin permeability. On the other side, the development of mathematical models to describe and predict skin permeability has been a fertile area of research. In the literature, many models were developed but the choice of the dataset used for mathematical modeling is crucial in skin permeability predictions. Several authors tented to rationalize experimental data and offer databases that have been constructed correcting permeability values according to parameters such as temperature, ionization, or skin thickness. These "validated" databases should be chosen preferentially even if, nowadays again, high-quality data are required. Using a predictive model, therefore, requires a well identification of its limitations. For instance, it is important to keep in mind that in most (if not all) models developed, "extreme" lipophilicity is inexistent or very rare. And it was shown that an accurate model can becomes very poor when dealing with compounds providing the lowest or highest log $P$. However, most of the models developed are based on the dependency of skin permeability to lipophilicity and molecular weight a relevant choice since passive diffusion through the SC is considered the main limiting route for solutes. Some models also proposed other parameters such as solubility and H bond capacities, which are highly related to lipophilicity of compounds. More complex are the 3D-QSPeR models. However, they take into account the three-dimensional structures that can be influent in particular for flexible molecules. Of course, these models involved much more descriptors than only log $P_{oct}$ and MW, but these descriptors are easy to obtain and the final models are easy to interpret. Much more difficult to interpret are the non-linear models based on ANN or GP principles, as they act as "black-boxes" and due to the non-linear dependence of descriptors regarding the skin permeability. However, the statistical results obtained with the large majority of these models, highlighted that probably, the dependence of usually used descriptors (e.g., log $P_{oct}$, MW) is not absolutely linear. Linear models such as the well-known Potts and Guy equation can be considered a simplified approach. However, for screening purpose in drug or cosmetic discovery as well as for risk assessment, these simple approaches, if well applied regarding their limitations, are really competitive.

# References


1. Guidance Document on Dermal Absorption (2004). European Commission Health and Consumer Protection Directorate-General.

2. Regulation (EC) (2007). No 1907/2006 of the European Parliament and of the Council of 18 December 2006.

3. Regulation (EC) (2009). No 1223/2009 of the European Parliament and of the Council.

4. Chen L, Lian G, and Han L (2007). Prediction of human skin permeability using artificial neural network (ANN) modeling, *Acta Pharmacol Sin*, **28**, 591–600.

5. Hadgraft J (2001). Skin, the final frontier, *Int J Pharm*, **224**, 1–18.

6. Hadgraft J and Guy RH (2003). Feasibility assessment in topical and transdermal delivery: mathematical models and in vitro studies, in *Transdermal Drug Delivery* (Guy RH and Hadgraft J, eds), Marcel Dekker, Inc., New York, pp. 1–23.

7. Bouwstra JA, Honeywell-Nguyen PL, Gooris GS, and Ponec M (2003). Structure of the skin barrier and its modulation by vesicular formulations, *Prog Lip Res*, **42**, 1–36.

8. Ritschel WA and Hussain AS (1988). The principles of permeation of substances across the skin, *Meth Fin Exp Clin Pharmacol*, **10**, 39–56.

9. Maibach HI, Feldmann RJ, Milby TH, and Serat WF (1971). Regional variation in percutaneous penetration in Man. Pesticides, *Arch Environ Health*, **23**, 208–211.

10. Potts RO and Francoeur ML (1991). The influence of *stratum corneum* morphology on water permeability, *J Invest Dermatol*, **96**, 495–499.

11. de Jager MW, Gooris GS, Dolbnya IP, Bras W, Ponec M, and Bouwstra JA (2004). Novel lipid mixtures based on synthetic ceramides reproduce the unique *stratum corneum* lipid organization, *J Lipid Res*, **45**, 923–932.

12. Wertz PW, Miethke MC, Long SA, Strauss JS, and Downing DT (1985). The composition of the ceramides from human *stratum corneum* and from comedones, *J Invest Dermatol*, **84**, 419–412.

13. Stewart ME and Downing DT (1999). A new 6-hydroxy-4-sphingenine-containing ceramide in human skin, *J Lipid Res*, **40**, 1434–1439.

14. Haratake A, Komiya A, Horikoshi T, Uchiwa H, and Watanabe S (2006). Acceleration of de novo cholesterol synthesis in the epidermis

influences desquamation of the *stratum corneum* in aged mice, *Skin Pharmacol Physiol*, **19**, 275–282.

15. Haratake A, Ikenaga K, Katoh N, Uchiwa H, Hirano S, and Yasuno H (2000). Topical mevalonic acid stimulates De Novo cholesterol synthesis and epidermal permeability barrier homeostasis in aged mice, *J Invest Dermatol*, **114**, 247–252.

16. Ghadially R, Brown BE, Hanley K, Reed JT, Feingold KR, and Elias PM (1996). Decreased epidermal lipid synthesis accounts for altered barrier function in aged mice, *J Invest Dermatol*, **106**, 1064–1069.

17. Potts RO and Guy RH (1992). Predicting skin permeability, *Pharm Res*, **9**, 663–669.

18. Hadgraft J (2004). Skin deep, *Eur J Pharm Biopharm*, **58**, 291–299.

19. Mitragotri, S. (2003). Modeling skin permeability to hydrophilic and hydrophobic solutes based on four permeation pathways, *J.Control Release*, **86**, 69–92.

20. Mitragotri S (2002). A theoretical analysis of permeation of small hydrophobic solutes across the *stratum corneum* based on scaled particle theory, *J Pharm Sci*, **91**, 744–752.

21. Peck KD, Ghanem AH, and Higuchi WI (1985). The effect of temperature upon the permeation of polar and ionic solutes through human epidermal membrane, *J Pharm Sci*, **84**, 975–962.

22. Friend DR (1992). In vitro skin permeation techniques, *J Control Release*, **18**, 235–248.

23. Moser K, Kriwer K, Naik A, Kalia YN, and Guy RH (2001). Passive skin penetration enhancement and its quantification in vitro, *Eur J Pharm Sci*, **52**, 103–112.

24. Hadgraft J and Ridout G (1987). Development of model membranes for percutaneous absorption measurements. I. Isopropyl myristate, *Int J Pharm*, **39**, 149–156.

25. Barry BW (ed) (1983). *Dermatological Formulations*, Marcel Dekker, Inc., New York.

26. Brain KR, Walters KA, and Watkinson AC (2002). Methods for studying percutaneous absorption, in *Dermatological and Transdermal Formulations* (Walters KA, ed), Marcel Dekker, Inc., New York, pp. 197–269.

27. Barbero AM and Frasch HF (2009). Pig and guinea pig skin as surrogates for human in vitro penetration studies: a quantitative review, *Toxicol in Vitro*, **23**, 1–13.

28. Finnin B, Walters KA, and Franz TJ (2011). In vitro skin permeation methodology, in *Transdermal and Topical Drug Delivery: Principles and Practice*, John Wiley & Sons, Inc., Hoboken, pp. 85–108.

29. El Maghraby GM, Barry BW, and Williams AC (2008). Liposomes and skin: from drug delivery to model membranes, *Eur J Pharm Sci*, **34**, 203–222.

30. Jacobi U, Kaiser M, Toll R, Mangelsdorf S, Audring H, Otberg N, Sterry W, and Lademann J (2007). Porcine ear skin: an in vitro model for human skin, *Skin Res Technol*, **13**, 19–24.

31. Takeuchi H, Tersaka S, Sakurai T, Furuya A, Urano H, and Sugibayashi K (2011). Variation assessment for in vitro permeabilities through Yucatan micropig skin, *Biol Pharm Bull*, **34**, 555–561.

32. Fujii M, Yamanouchi S, Hori N, Iwanaga N, Kawaguchi N, and Matsumoto M (1997). Evaluation of Yucatan micropig skin for use as an in vitro model for skin permeation study, *Biol Pharm Bull*, **20**, 249–254.

33. Sekkat N, Kalia YN, and Guy RH (2004). Porcine ear skin as a model for the assessment of transdermal drug delivery to premature neonates, *Pharm Res*, **21**, 1390–1397.

34. Vallet V, Cruz C, Josse D, Bazire A, Lallement G, and Boudry I (2007). In vitro percutaneous penetration of organophosphorus compounds using full-thickness and split-thickness pig and human skin, *Toxicol in Vitro*, **21**, 1182–1190.

35. Koizumi A, Fujii M, Kondoh M, and Watanabe Y (2004). Effect of *N*-methyl-2-pyrrolidone on skin permeation of estradiol, *Eur J Pharm Biopharm*, **57**, 473–478.

36. Qvist MH, Hoeck U, Kreilgaard B, Madsen F, and Frokjaer S (2000). Evaluation of Göttingen minipig skin for transdermal in vitro permeation studies, *Eur J Pharm Sci*, **11**, 59–68.

37. Takeuchi H, Mano Y, Terasaka S, Sakurai T, Furuya A, Urano H, and Sugibayashi K (2011). Usefulness of rat skin as a substitute for human skin in the in vitro skin permeation study, *Exper Anim*, **60**, 373–384.

38. OECD Guideline for the Testing of Chemicals (2004). Skin absorption: in vitro method.

39. Mak VHW, Cumpstone MB, Kennedy AH, Harmon CS, Guy RH, and Potts RO (1991). Barrier function of human keratinocyte cultures grown at the air–liquid interface, *J Invest Dermatol*, **96**, 323–327.

40. Rosdy M and Clauss LC (1990). Terminal epidermal differentiation of human keratinocytes grown in chemically defined medium on inert filter substrates at the air–liquid interface, *J Invest Dermatol*, **95**, 409–414.

41. Netzlaff F, Lehr C M, Wertz PW, and Schaefer UF (2005). The human epidermis models EpiSkin-, SkinEthic- and EpiDerm-: an evaluation of morphology and their suitability for testing phototoxicity, irritancy, corrosivity, and substance transport, *Eur J Pharm Biopharm*, **60**, 167–178.

42. Poumay Y, Dupont F, Marcoux S, Leclercq-Smekens M, Hérin M, and Coquette A (2004). A simple reconstructed human epidermis: preparation of the culture model and utilization in in vitro studies, *Arch Dermatol Res*, **296**, 203–211.

43. Marjukka Suhonen T, Pasonen-Seppänen S, Kirjavainen M, Tammi M, Tammi R, and Urtti A (2003). Epidermal cell culture model derived from rat keratinocytes with permeability characteristics comparable to human cadaver skin, *Eur J Pharm Sci*, **20**, 107–113.

44. Pasonen-Seppänen S, Suhonen MT, Kirjavainen M, Suihko E, Urtti A, Miettinen M, Hyttinen M, Tammi M, and Tammi R (2001). Vitamin-C enhances differentiation of a continuous keratinocyte cell line (REK) into epidermis with normal *stratum corneum* ultrastructure and functional permeability barrier, *Histochem Cell Biol*, **116**, 287–297.

45. Pasonen-Seppänen S, Suhonen MT, Kirjavainen M, Miettinen M, Urtti A, Tammi M, and Tammi R (2001). Formation of permeability barrier in epidermal organotypic culture for studies on drug transport, *J Invest Dermatol*, **117**, 1322–1324.

46. Nakamura M, Rikimaru T, Yano T, Moore KG, Pula PJ, Schofield BH, and Dannenberg Jr AM (1990). Full-thickness human skin explants for testing the toxicitiy of topically applied chemicals, *J Invest Dermatol*, **95**, 325–332.

47. Ackermann K, Lombardi Borgia S, Korting HC, Mewes KR, and Schäfer-Korting M (2010). The phenion- full-thickness skin model for percutaneous absorption testing, *Skin Pharmacol Physiol*, **23**, 105–112.

48. Van Gele M, Geusens B, Brochez L, Speeckaert R, and Lambert J (2011). Three-dimensional skin models as tools for transdermal drug delivery: challenges and limitations, *Exp Opin Drug Del*, **8**, 705–720.

49. Brain KR, Walters KA, and Watkinson AC (1998). Investigation of skin permeation in vitro, in *Dermal Absorption and Toxicity Assessment* (Roberts MS and Walters KA, eds), Marcel Dekker, Inc., New York, pp. 161–187.

50. Asbill C, Nim N, El-Kattan A, Creek K, Wertz P, and Michniak B (2000). Evaluation of a human bio-engineered skin equivalent for drug permeation studies, *Pharm Res*, **17**, 1092–1097.

51. Barry BW and Brace AR (1977). Permeation of oestrone, oestradiol, oestriol and dexamethasone across cellulose acetate membrane, *J Pharm Pharmacol*, **29**, 397–400.

52. Barry BW and El Eini DI (1976). Influence of non-ionic surfactants on permeation of hydrocortisone, dexamethasone, testosterone and progesterone across cellulose, *J Pharm Pharmacol*, **28**, 219–227.

53. Jetzer WE, Huq AS, Ho NFM, Flynn GL, Duraiswamy N, and Condie Jr L (1986). Permeation of mouse skin and silicone rubber membranes by phenols: relationship to in vitro partitioning, *J Pharm Sci*, **75**, 1098–1103.

54. Garrett ER and Chemburkar PB (1968). Evaluation, control, and prediction of drug diffusion through polymeric membranes, *J Pharm Sci*, **57**, 944–948.

55. Geinoz S, Rey S, Boss G, Bunge AL, Guy RH, Carrupt PA, Reist M, and Testa B (2002). Quantitative structure–permeation relationships for solute transport across silicone membranes, *Pharm Res*, **19**, 1622–1629.

56. Hadgraft J and Ridout G (1988). Development of model membranes for percutaneous absorption measurements. II. Dipalmitoyl phosphatidylcholine, linoleic acid and tetradecane, *Int J Pharm*, **42**, 97–104.

57. Santi P, Catellani PL, Colombo P, Ringard-Lefebvre C, Barthélémy C, and Guyot-Hermann AM (1991). Partition and transport of verapamil and nicotine through artificial membranes, *Int J Pharm*, **68**, 43–49.

58. Kai T, Isami T, Kurosaki Y, Nakayama T, and Kimura T (1993). Keratinized epithelial transport of b-blocking agents. II. Evaluation of barrier property of *stratum corneum* by using model lipid systems, *Biol Pharm Bull*, **16**, 284–287.

59. Matsuzaki K, Imaoka T, Asano M, and Miyajima K (1993). Development of a model membrane system using startum corneum lipids for estimations of drug skin permeability, *Chem Pharm Bull*, **41**, 575–579.

60. Lovering EG and Black DB (1974). Diffuion layer effect on permeation of phenylbutazone through polydimethylsiloxane, *J Pharm Sci*, **63**, 1399–1402.

61. Xia XR, Baynes RE, Monteiro-Riviere NA, and Riviere JE (2007). An experimentally based approach for predicting skin permeability of chemicals and drugs using a membrane-coated fiber array, *Toxicol Appl Pharmacol*, **221**, 320–328.

62. Kansy M, Senner F, and Gubernator K (1998). Physicochemical high throughput screening: parallel artificial membrane permeation assay in the description of passive absorption processes, *J Med Chem*, **41**, 1007–1010.

63. Ottaviani G, Martel S, and Carrupt PA (2006). Parallel artificial membrane permeability assay: a new membrane for the fast prediction of passive human skin permeability, *J Med Chem*, **49**, 3948–3954.

64. Ottaviani G, Martel S, and Carrupt PA (2007) In silico and in vitro filters for the fast estimation of skin permeation and distribution of new chemical entities, *J Med Chem*, **50**, 742–748.

65. Sinko B, Garrigues TM, Balogh GT, Nagy ZK, Tsinman O, Avdeef A, and Takacs-Novak K (2012). Skin-PAMPA: a new method for fast prediction of skin penetration, *Eur J Pharm Sci*, **45**, 698–707.

66. Martel S, Guillarme D, Henchoz Y, Galland A, Veuthey JL, Rudaz S, and Carrupt PA (2008). Chromatographic approaches for measuring log P, in *Drug Properties: Measurement and Computation* (Mannhold R, ed), Wiley-VCH, Weinheim, pp. 331–356.

67. Martel S, Gasparik V, and Carrupt PA (2009). In silico tools and in vitro HTS approaches to determine lipophilicity during the drug discovery process, in *Hit and Lead Profiling* (Faller B, and Urban L, eds), Wiley-VCH, Weinheim, pp. 91–107.

68. Nicoli R, Martel S, Rudaz S, Wolfender JL, Veuthey JL, Carrupt PA, and Guillarme D (2010). Advances in LC platforms for drug discovery, *Exp Opin Drug Del*, **5**, 475–489.

69. Kaliszan R, Nasal A, and Bucinski A (1994). Chromatographic hydrophobicity parameter determined on an immobilized artificial membrane column: relationships to standard measures of hydrophobicity and bioactivity, *Eur J Med Chem*, **29**, 163–170.

70. Nasal A and Kaliszan R (2006). Progess in the use of HPLC for evaluation of lipophilicity, *Curr Comput Aided Drug Des*, **2**, 327–340.

71. Nasal A, Sznitowska M, Bucinski A, and Kaliszan R (1995). Hydrophobicity parameter from high-performance liquid chromatography on an immobilized artificial membrane column and its relationship to bioactivity, *J Chromatogr A*, **692**, 83–89.

72. Barbato F, Cappello B, Miro A, La Rotonda MI, and Quaglia F (1998). Chromatographic indexes on immobilized artificial membranes for the prediction of transdermal transport of drugs, *Farmaco*, **53**, 655–661.

73. Taillardat-Bertschinger A, Barbato F, Quercia MT, Carrupt PA, Reist M, La Rotonda MI, and Testa B (2002). Structural properties governing

retention mechanisms on immobilized artificial membrane (IAM) HPLC-columns, *Helv Chim Acta*, **85**, 519–532.

74. Kotecha J, Shah S, Rathod I, and Subbaiah G (2008). Prediction of oral absorption in humans by experimental immobilized artificial membrane chromatography indices and physicochemical descriptors, *Int J Pharm*, **360**, 96–106.

75. Yoon CH, Kim SJ, Shin BS, Lee KC, and Yoo SD (2006). Rapid screening of blood-brain barrier penetration of drugs using the immobilized artificial membrane phosphatidylcholine column chromatography, *J Biomol Screen*, **11**, 13–20.

76. de Jager M, Groenink W, Bielsa I, Guivernau R, Andersson E, Angelova N, Ponec M, and Bouwstra J (2006). A novel in vitro percutaneous penetration model: evaluation of barrier properties with P-aminobenzoic acid and two of its derivatives, *Pharm Res*, **23**, 951–960.

77. Turowskil M and Kaliszan R (1997). Keratin immobilized on silica as a new stationary phase for chromatographic modelling of skin permeation, *J Pharm Biomed Anal*, **15**, 1325–1333.

78. Turowski M and Kaliszan R (1997). Keratin immobilized on silica as a new stationary phase for chromatographic modelling of skin permeation, *J Pharm Biomed Anal*, **15**, 1325–1333.

79. Escuder-Gilabert L, Martinez-Pla JJ, Sagrado S, Villanueva-Camanas RM, and Medina-Hernandez MJ (2003). Biopartitioning micellar separation methods: modelling drug absorption, *J Chromatogr B*, **797**, 21–35.

80. Martinez-Pla JJ, Martin-Biosca Y, Sagrado S, Villanueva-Camanas RM, and Medina-Hernandez MJ (2003). Biopartitioning micellar chromatography to predict skin permeability, *Biomed Chromatogr*, **17**, 530–537.

81. Martinez-Pla JJ, Martin-Biosca Y, Sagrado S, Villanueva-Camanas RM, and Medina-Hernandez MJ (2004). Evaluation of the pH effect of formulations on the skin permeability of drugs by biopartitioning micellar chromatography, *J Chromatogr A*, **1047**, 255–262.

82. Wang Y, Sun J, Liu H, Liu J, Zhang L, Liu K, and He Z (2009). Predicting skin permeability using liposome electrokinetic chromatography, *Analyst*, **134**, 267–272.

83. Xian DL, Huang KL, Liu SQ, and Xiao JY (2008). Quantitative retention-activity relationship studies by liposome electrokinetic chromatography to predict skin permeability, *Chin J Chem*, **26**, 671–676.

84. Hadgraft J and Lane ME (2005). Skin permeation: the years of enlightenment, *Int J Pharm*, **305**, 2–12.

85. Flynn GL (1990). Physicochemical determinants of skin absorption, in *Principles of Route-to-Route Extrapolation for Risk Assessment* (Gerrity TR and Henry CJ, eds), Elsevier, Amsterdam, pp. 93–127.

86. Johnson ME, Blankschtein D, and Langer R (1995). Permeation of steroids through human skin, *J Pharm Sci*, **84**, 1144–1146.

87. Degim IT, Pugh WJ, and Hadgraft J (1998). Skin permeability data: anomalous results, *Int J Pharm*, **170**, 129–133.

88. Vecchia BE and Bunge A (2003). Evaluating the transdermal permeability of chemicals, in *Transdermal Drug Delivery* (Guy RH and Hadgraft J, eds), Marcel Dekker, Inc., New York, pp. 25–55.

89. Keshwani DR, Jones DD, and Brand RM (2005). Review: Takagi-Sugeno fuzzy modeling of skin permeability, *Cutan Ocul Toxicol*, **24**, 149–163.

90. Geinoz S, Guy RH, Carrupt PA, and Testa B (2004). Quantitative structure–permeation relationships (QSPeRs) to predict skin permeation: a critical review, *Pharm Res*, **21**, 83–92.

91. Moss GP and Cronin MTD (2002). Quantitative structure–permeability relationships for percutaneous absorption: re-analysis of steroid data, *Int J Pharm*, **238**, 105–109.

92. Cronin MTD and Hewitt M (2007). In silico models to predict passage through the skin and other barriers, in *Comprehensive Medicinal Chemistry II. Volume 5: ADME-Tox Approaches* (Taylor JB and Triggle DJ, eds), John Moores University, Liverpool, pp. 725–744.

93. Vecchia BE and Bunge AL (2003). Partitioning of chemicals into skin: results and predictions, in *Transdermal Drug Delivery* (Guy RH and Hadgraft J, eds), Marcel Dekker, Inc., New York, pp. 143–198.

94. Abraham MH and Martins F (2004). Human skin permeation and partition : general linear free-energy relationship analyses, *J Pharm Sci*, **93**, 1508–1523.

95. Majumdar S, Thomas J, Wasdo S, and Sloan KB (2007). The effect of water solubility of solutes on their flux through human skin in vitro, *Int J Pharm*, **329**, 25–36.

96. Thomas J, Majumdar S, Wasdo S, Majumdar A, and Sloan KB (2007). The effect of water solubility of solutes on their flux through human skin in vitro: an extended Flynn database fitted to the Roberts-Sloan equation, *Int J Pharm*, **339**, 157–167.

97. Roberts WJ and Sloan KB (1999). Correlation of aqueous and lipid solubilities with flux fro prodrugs of 5-fluorouracil, theophylline, and 6-mercaptopurine: a Potts-Guy approach, *J Pharm Sci*, **88**, 515–522.

98. Kirchner LA, Moody RP, Doyle E, Bose R, Jeffery J, and Chu I (1997). The prediction of skin permeability by using physicochemical data, *ATLA*, **25**, 359–370.

99. Frasch HF and Landsittel DP (2002). Regarding the sources of data analyzed with quantitative structure-skin permeability relationship methods (commentary on "Investigation of the mechanism of flux across human skin in vitro by quantitative structure–permeability relationships"), *J Pharm Sci*, **15**, 399–403.

100. Lee PH, Conradi R, and Shanmugasundaram V (2010). Development of an in silico model for human skin permeation based on a Franz cell skin permeability assay, *Bioorg Med Chem Lett*, **20**, 69–73.

101. Buist HE, van Burgsteden JA, Freidig AP, Maas WJM and van de Sandt JJM (2010). New in vitro dermal absorption database and the prediction of dermal absorption under finite conditions for risk assessment purposes, *Regul Toxicol Pharmacol*, **57**, 200–209.

102. Moss GP, Sun Y, Prapopoulou M, Davey N, Adams R, Pugh WJ, and Brown MB (2009). The application of Gaussian processes in the prediction of percutaneous absorption, *J Pharm Pharmacol*, **61**, 1147–1153.

103. Moss GP, Gullick DR, Cox PA, Alexander C, Ingram MJ, Smart JD, and Pugh WJ (2006). Design, synthesis and characterization of captopril prodrugs for enhanced percutaneous absorption, *J Pharm Sci*, **58**, 167–177.

104. Moss GP, Dearden JC, Patel H, and Cronin MTD (2002). Quantitative structure–permeability relationships (QSPRs) for percutaneous absorption, *Toxicol in Vitro*, **16**, 299–317.

105. Cronin MTD (2005). The prediction of skin permeability using quantitative structure–activity relationship methods, in *Dermal Absorption Models in Toxicology and Pharmacology* (Riviere JE, ed), pp. 113–134.

106. Buchwald P and Bodor N (2001). A simple, predictive, structure-based skin permeability model, *J Pharm Pharmacol*, **53**, 1087–1098.

107. Wilshut A, ten Berge WF, Robinson PJ, and McKone TE (1995). Estimating skin permeation. The validation of five mathematical skin permeation models, *Chemosphere*, **30**, 1275–1296.

108. Cronin MTD, Dearden JC, Moss GP, and Murray-Dickson G (1999). Investigation of the mechanism of flux across human skin in vitro by quantitative structure–permeability relationships, *Eur J Pharm Sci*, **7**, 325–330.

109. Lian G, Chen L, and Han L (2008). An evaluation of methematical models for predicting skin permeability, *J Pharm Sci*, **97**, 584–598.

110. Patel H, ten Berge W, and Cronin MTD (2002). Quantitative structure–activity relationships (QSARs) for the prdiction of skin permeation of exogenous chemicals, *Chemosphere*, **48**, 603–613.

111. ten Berge W (2009). A simple dermal absorption model: derivation and application, *Chemosphere*, **75**, 1440–1445.

112. Vecchia BE, and Bunge A (2003). Skin absorption databases and predictive equations, in *Transdermal Drug Delivery* (Guy RH, and Hadgraft J, eds), Marcel Dekker, Inc., New York, pp. 57–141.

113. Potts RO and Guy RH (1995). A predictive algorithm for skin permeability: the effects of molecular size and hydrogen bond activity, *Pharm Res*, **12**, 1628–1633.

114. Bodor N and Buchwald P (1997) Molecular size based approach to estimate partition properties for organic solutes, *J Phys Chem B*, **101**, 3404–3412.

115. Kamlet MJ, Doherty RM, Famini GR, and Taft RW (1987). Linear solvation energy relationships. Local empirical rules or fundamental laws of chemistry? The dialogue continues. A challenge for the chemometricians, *Acta Chem Scand Ser B*, **B41**, 589–598.

116. Kamlet MJ and Taft RW (1976). The solvatochromic comparison method. I. The b-scale of solvent hydrogen-bond acceptor (HBA) basicities, *J Am Chem Soc*, **98**, 377–383.

117. Taft RW and Kamlet MJ (1976). The solvatochromic comparison method. 2. The a-scale of solvent hydrogen-bond donor (HBD) acidities, *J Am Chem Soc*, **98**, 2886–2894.

118. Abraham MH and Chadha HS (1996). Application of a solvation equation to drug transport properties, in *Lipophilicity in Drug Action and Toxicology* (Pliska V, Testa B, and van de Waterbeemd H, eds), VCH Publishers, Weinheim, 311–337.

119. Abraham MH (1993). Scales of solute hydrogen-bonding: their construction and application to physicochemical and biochemical processes, *Chem Soc Rev*, 73–83.

120. Abraham MH, Chadha HS, and Mitchell RC (1995). The factors that influence skin penetration of solutes, *J Pharm Pharmacol*, **47**, 8–16.

121. Abraham MH and McGowan JC (1987). The use of characteristic volumes to measure cavity terms in reversed phase liquid chromatography, *Chromatographia*, **23**, 243–246.

122. Cruciani G, Crivori P, Carrupt PA, and Testa B (2000). Molecular fields in quantitative structure permeation relationships: the VolSurf approach, *J Mol Struct (Theochem)*, **503**, 17–30.

123. Wade RC, Clark KJ, and Goodford PJ (1993). Further development of hydrogen bond functions for use in determining energetically favorable binding sites on molecules of known structure. 1. Ligand probe groups with the ability to form two hydrogen bonds, *J Med Chem*, **36**, 140–147.

124. Wade RC and Goodford PJ (1993). Further development of hydrogen bond functions for use in determining energetically favorable binding sites on molecules of known structure. 2. Ligand probe groups with the ability to form more than two hydrogen bonds, *J Med Chem*, **36**, 148–156.

125. Boobbyer DNA, Goodford PJ, McWhinnie PM, and Wade RC (1989). New hydrogen-bond potentials for use in determining energetically favorable binding sites on molecules of known structure, *J Med Chem*, **32**, 1083–1094.

126. Cruciani G and Watson KA (1994). Comparative molecular field analysis using GRID force-field and GOLPE variable selection methods in a study of inhibitors of glycogen, *J Med Chem*, **37**, 2589–2601.

127. Pastor M and Cruciani G (1995). A novel strategy for improving ligand selectivity in receptor-based drug design, *J Med Chem*, **38**, 4637–4647.

128. Clementi S, Cruciani G, Fifi P, Riganelli D, Valigi R, and Musumarra G (1996). A new set of principal properties for heteroaromatics obtained by GRID, *Quant Struct-Act Relat*, **15**, 108–120.

129. Goodford PJ (1985). A computational procedure for determining energetically favorable binding sites on biologically important macromolecules, *J Med Chem*, **28**, 849–857.

130. Gaillard P, Carrupt PA, Testa B, and Boudon A (1994). Molecular lipophilicity potential, a tool in 3D-QSAR. Method and applications, *J Comput Aided Mol Des*, **8**, 83–96.

131. Carrupt PA, Gaillard P, Billois F, Weber P, Testa B, Meyer C, and Pérez S (1996). The molecular lipophilicity potential (MLP): a new tool for log P calculations and docking, and in comparative molecular field analysis (CoMFA), in *Lipophilicity in Drug Action and Toxicology* (Pliska V, Testa B, and van de Waterbeemd H, eds), VCH Publishers, Weinheim, pp. 195–217.

132. Rey S, Caron G, Ermondi G, Gaillard P, Pagliara A, Carrupt PA, and Testa B (2001). Development of molecular hydrogen bonding potentials

(MHBPs) and their application to structure permeation relations, *J Mol Graph Model*, **19**, 521–535.

133. Jurs PC (1990). Chemometrics and multivariate analysis in analytical chemistry, in *Reviews in Computational Chemistry* (Lipkowitz KB and Boyd DB, eds), VCH Publishers, New York, pp. 169–212.

134. Geinoz S (2002). Assessment of Drug Permeation :Theory, Methods and Applications to Skin and Bacteria Thesis, University of Lausanne.

135. Bajot, F. (2006) 3D Solvatochromic Models to Derive Pharmacokinetic in silico Profiles of New Chemical Entities, PhD Thesis, University of Geneva.

136. Bajot F, Geinoz S, Rey S, Cruciani G, Guy RH, and Carrupt PA (2008). The Volsurf approach in structure–permeation relationships: molecular interaction fields focused on specific intermolecular interactions, *In preparation*.

137. Weber H, Steimer U, Mannhold R, and Cruciani G (2001). Synthesis, in vitro skin permeation studies, and PLS-analysis of new naproxen derivatives, *Pharm Res*, **18**, 600–607.

138. Degim T, Hadgraft J, Ibasmis S, and Özkan Y (2003). Prediction of skin penetration using artificial neural network (ANN) modeling, *J Pharm Sci*, **92**, 656–664.

139. Pugh WJ, Degim IT, and Hadgraft J (2000). Epidermal permeability-penetrant structure relationships. 4. QSAR of permeant diffucion across human *stratum corneum* in terms of molecular weight, H-bonding and electronic charge, *Int J Pharm*, **197**, 203–211.

140. Johnson ME, Blankstein D, and Langer R (1997). Evaluation of solute permeation through the *stratum corneum*: lateral bilayer diffusion as the primary transport mechanism, *J Pharm Sci*, **86**, 1162–1172.

141. Ghafourian T and Fooladi S (2001). The effect of structural QSAR parameters on skin penetration, *Int J Pharm*, **217**, 1–11.

142. Chung KK and Do DK (2010). Modelling the effect of structural QSAR parameters on skin penetration using genetic programming, *Adv Nat Sci Nanosci Nanotechnol*, **1**, 035003.

143. Scheuplein RJ, Blank IH, Baruner GJ, and MacFarlane DJ (1969). Percutaneous absorption of steroids, *J Invest Dermatol*, **52**, 63–70.

144. Scheuplein RJ (1965). Mechanism of percutaneous adsorption. I. Routes of penetration and the influence of solubility, *J Invest Dermatol*, **45**, 334–346.

# Chapter 10

# Accessing the Molecular Organization of the *Stratum Corneum* Using High-Resolution Electron Microscopy and Computer Simulation

**Lars Norlén,[a] Jamshed Anwar,[b] and Ozan Öktem[c]**

[a]*Department of Cell and Molecular Biology, Karolinska Institutet, and Dermatology Clinic, Karolinska University Hospital, 171 77 Stockholm, Sweden*
[b]*Chemical Theory and Computation, Department of Chemistry, University, Lancaster Lancaster LA1 4YB, United Kingdom*
[c]*Department of Mathematics, KTH Royal Institute of Technology, 100 44 Stockholm, Sweden*

lars.norlen@ki.se

The superficial-most layer of skin—the *stratum corneum* or as sometimes referred to as the horny layer—represents the main barrier toward delivery of drugs through skin. The secret behind the horny layer's barrier properties lies in its structural organization. It is composed of keratin-filled cells embedded in an extracellular fat matrix that is largely impermeable to both lipophilic and hydrophilic compounds.

The molecular organization of the *stratum corneum* components is still an outstanding problem despite being both fundamentally and clinically significant. There is a need to develop methodology

*Computational Biophysics of the Skin*
Edited by Bernard Querleux
Copyright © 2014 Pan Stanford Publishing Pte. Ltd.
ISBN 978-981-4463-84-3 (Hardcover), 978-981-4463-85-0 (eBook)
www.panstanford.com

that yields molecular level resolution of the *stratum corneum* components in their native state, without introducing artifacts due to staining or dehydration processes. We review here the recent success of the combined approach of using high-resolution cryo-electron microscopy coupled with computer simulation of the electron microscope images to elucidate the molecular organization of the *stratum corneum*'s lipid matrix in its native state. This combined approach has significant potential to access the structure of the other key components of the skin's *stratum corneum*. Having a model of the *stratum corneum* with appropriate molecular detail could serve to get insights into the normal physiology of skin as well as into the pathology of skin diseases like eczema, psoriasis and "dry skin," and it could facilitate the development and optimization of transdermal drug delivery. Given the potential of the combined imaging and simulation approach, we present technical details of the methodology including electron microscopy (EM) simulation and electron tomography (ET) regularization. These methods are set to have a significant impact in the quest to develop a better understanding of the molecular level organization characterizing biological tissues in situ.

## 10.1   Introduction

Terrestrial life was only made possible through the adaptive evolution of a waterproof barrier in the integument of organisms. In man, like in other land-living vertebrates, this barrier is essentially constituted by a uniquely organized fat matrix between the cells of the horny layer of skin.

The fat matrix is remarkably robust, as the barrier properties remain unaltered upon changes in environmental conditions, such as water activity, temperature, and mechanical stress. It represents the major permeability barrier toward both hydrophilic and lipophilic compounds.

Ever since the realization that the extracellular space is filled with lipid material [1–3], skin lipids have been the subjects of much research interest. The core questions have been the chemical composition and the nature of the molecular organization of these lipids. While the chemical composition of the skin lipids has been defined for some time [4], but refined continuously [5], how the different types of lipids are organized has been a hot, contentious topic for an extended period. Indeed, no less than six distinct models of lipid organization have been proposed involving either a repeat bilayer with bands with the same width or a repeat triple-sandwich type layer. The essential difficulty has been that the lipid molecular organization in its *native state* has not been accessible to experimental methods. Thus, researchers have had to modify their skin samples in different ways (e.g., by chemical fixation, staining and dehydration) during preparation for experimentation, or have chosen to study the skin lipid organization in vitro in reconstituted model systems. This has led to differing results depending on the methods and model systems employed.

Not having a native reference for the molecular organization of the skin lipids has limited our fundamental understanding of the skin both in healthy and disease states, and hampered technological progress in areas such as development of treatments for skin disease, transdermal drug delivery, dealing with toxicity from topical exposure to chemicals, and the development of non-invasive diagnostic sensors.

A recent breakthrough has come from the use of very-high-magnification cryo-electron microscopy of vitreous skin section (CEMOVIS) [6–7]. This technique can yield high-resolution images of the skin lipids in situ and in their *near native state*. The attainable resolution is exceptional, being about ~1 nm. However, despite the advance, this resolution is still marginally insufficient to reveal the organization of the individual lipid molecules. In view of this limitation, we recently brought to bear the powerful inter-disciplinary combination of CEMOVIS, electron microscopy simulation, and molecular modeling, onto the challenge of resolving the molecular organization of the skin lipids. This combination proved to be a remarkably effective in identifying the molecular organization of the skin lipids [7–8].

We review here the basis for the combined approach involving cryo-electron microscopy coupled with simulation. Section 10.2 outlines the application of the methodology to the elucidation of the molecular organization of the skin lipids and briefly presents the elucidated lipid organization and its significance. We then present technical aspects of the methodology including high-resolution cryo-electron microscopy, a brief introduction to modeling of data, cryo-electron tomography, tomographic regularization and electron microscopy simulation.

The elucidation of the molecular organization of the skin lipids, important as it may be, was but a first step toward building a complete molecular model for the *stratum corneum* that also includes the corneocytes. Outstanding questions in this respect are the nature of the molecular level structure of the corneocyte keratin filament network and the interfacial corneocyte cell envelope. In Section 10.8, we explore the potential application and further development of the combined approach of cryo-electron microscopy coupled with simulation to elucidate the molecular organization of the remaining key *stratum corneum* components.

## 10.2 Skin Lipids

The skin lipids consist of a heterogeneous mixture of saturated, long-chain ceramides (CERs), free fatty acids (FFAs), and cholesterol (CHOL) in a roughly 1:1:1 molar ratio [4]. More than 300 different species have been identified in the ceramide fraction alone [5].

The key characteristic features of the *stratum corneum* lipid composition [4] are (i) extensive compositional heterogeneity with broad, but invariable, chain length distributions (20–32C; peaking at 24C) in the ceramide fatty acid and free fatty acid fractions, (ii) almost complete dominance of saturated very long hydrocarbon chains (C20:0–C32:0), and (iii) substantial relative amount of cholesterol (about 30 mol%).

Six different models for the molecular organization of the *stratum corneum* lipid matrix had been proposed earlier. The first model was presented by Swartzendruber et al. in 1989 [9]. It was based on the broad:narrow:broad electron lucent band pattern observed in RuO4 stained *stratum corneum*, and consisted of triple-band units with ceramides in fully extended conformation (i.e., with the ceramide sphingoid- and the fatty acid parts pointing in opposite directions). Each triple-band unit was composed of one narrow central band and two broad peripheral bands. The central band expressed hydrocarbon chain interdigitation and contained no cholesterol. The peripheral bands expressed no chain interdigitation but contained cholesterol. Later, Forslind [10] presented a model based on lateral lipid domain segregation. It consisted of stacked lipid bilayers composed of ceramides in folded conformation (i.e., with the ceramide sphingoid- and the fatty acid parts pointing in the same direction). Each bilayer expressed thickness changes due to laterally segregated crystalline and liquid crystalline domains. Combining data derived from conventional electron microscopy and SAXD, Bouwstra et al. [11] presented a model consisting of triple-band units with a 13 nm repeat period. Each triple-band unit was composed of one narrow central band and two broad peripheral bands. The central band expressed interdigitating omega-esterified polyunsaturated fatty acids of ceramide EOS, short chain ceramides in folded conformation and cholesterol. The two peripheral bands expressed long chain ceramides in folded conformation and cholesterol. Reinterpreting the band patterns of RuO4 stained *stratum corneum*, Hill and Wertz [12] proposed a model similar to that of Bouwstra et al. [11], but with uniform thicknesses of the three bands constituting the triple-band units. Based on SAXD experiments on skin lipid model systems in vitro, McIntosh [13] presented a model consisting of twin-band (double bilayer) units with a 13 nm repeat period, with an asymmetric cholesterol distribution, and with equal thicknesses of the constituent bands. Recently, Schröter et al. [14] presented a model based on neutron scattering experiments on skin lipid model systems in vitro. It consisted of lamellar units of equal thickness, composed of mixed ceramides in folded and extended conformation, and with a homogenous cholesterol distribution. All bands were spanned by the fatty acid chains of ceramide EOS.

## 10.3 Molecular Structure Determination in situ

### 10.3.1 The Procedure

The new procedure for molecular structure determination in situ involves four distinct steps: cryo-electron microscopy of vitreous skin section (CEMOVIS) to yield high-resolution images of the skin lipid organization (Fig. 10.1); development of potential molecular models for the organization of the skin lipids (Fig. 10.2); simulation of electron micrographs resulting from the proposed molecular models (Fig. 10.2); and confrontation of the simulated micrographs with those observed experimentally to identify a molecular organization which is consistent with the observed data (Fig. 10.3).

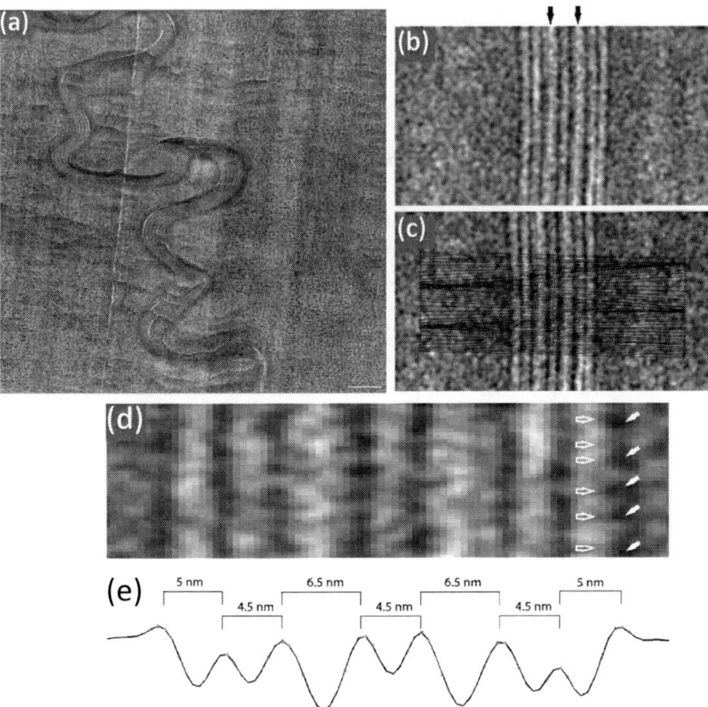

**Figure 10.1** The CEMOVIS intensity pattern of the *stratum corneum* extracellular lipid matrix consists of folded stacked layers. (a) Medium magnification CEMOVIS micrograph of the interface between two cells in the midpart of *stratum corneum*. Note that in CEMOVIS the tissue is unstained, and that the pixel intensity is directly related to the local electron density of the sample. The stacked lamellar pattern represents the extracellular lipid matrix. Dark ~10 nm dots represent keratin intermediate filaments filling out the intracellular space. (b) High-magnification CEMOVIS micrograph of the extracellular space in the midpart of *stratum corneum*. The averaged intensity profile of the lipid matrix was obtained by fuzzy distance based image analysis. The red stars in (b) represent the manually chosen start and end points for fuzzy distance based path growing. (c) The red line represents the traced out path. Stacked lines mark extracted intensity profiles. (d) Enlarged area of the central part of (b). (e) Reversed averaged pixel intensity profile obtained from the extracted area in (c). Peaks in (e) correspond to dark bands and valleys to lucent bands in (d). Black arrows in (b) denote electron lucent narrow bands at the centre of the 6.5 nm bands. Section thickness ~50 nm (a–d). Scale bar (a): 100 nm. Pixel size in (a–d): 6.02 Å.

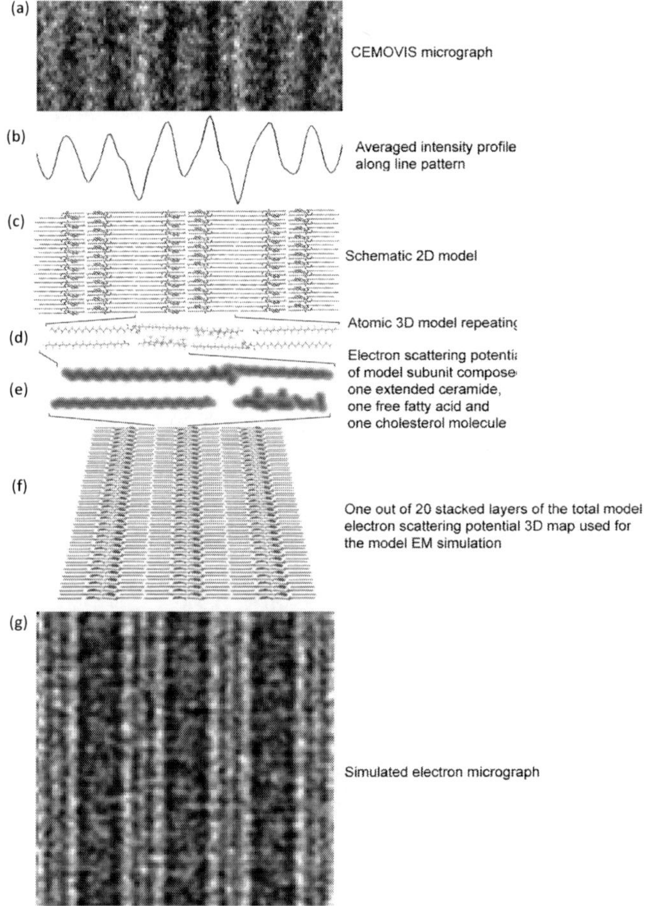


**Figure 10.2** Electron microscopy simulation of the *stratum corneum* extracellular lipid matrix. (a) High-magnification CEMOVIS micrograph of the extracellular space in the midpart of *stratum corneum*. (b) Corresponding averaged intensity profile obtained by fuzzy distance based path growing (cf. Figs. 10.1b,c). (c) Schematic 2D illustration of ceramides (tetracosanyl-phytosphingosine (C24:0)) in fully extended conformation with cholesterol associated with the ceramide sphingoid part and free fatty acids (lignoceric acid (C24:0)) associated with the ceramide fatty acid part. (d) Atomic 3D model of the repeating unit composed of two mirrored subunits, each composed of one fully extended ceramide-, one cholesterol- and one free fatty acid molecule. (e) Calculated electron scattering potential of one model subunit. (f) Calculated electron scattering potential 3D maps of the topmost layer out of 20 superimposed layers used to generate the simulated electron micrograph (g). Defocus (a, g): –2.5 μm. Pixel size in (a, g): 3.31 Å.

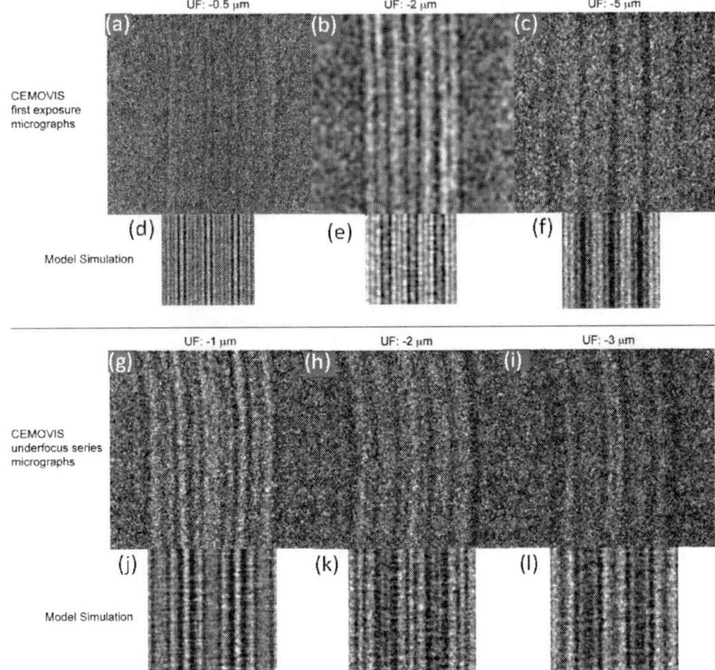



**Figure 10.3** Electron microscopy simulation of alternating fully extended ceramides with selective localization of cholesterol to the ceramide sphingoid part. (a–c) High-magnification CEMOVIS micrographs (first exposition images) of the extracellular space in the midpart of *stratum corneum* obtained at –0.5 µm (a), –2 µm (b) and –5 µm (c) defocus. (d–f) represents corresponding atomic 3D model (cf. Fig. 10.5) electron microscopy simulation images recorded at –0.5 µm (d), –2 µm (e) and –5 µm (f) defocus. (g–i) Sequential CEMOVIS micrograph defocus-series obtained at very high magnification (1.88 Å pixel size). Note the fine changes in interference patterns caused by gradually increasing the microscope's defocus during repeated image acquisition at a fixed position. (j–l) represents corresponding atomic 3D model (cf. Fig. 10.2) electron microscopy simulation images recorded at –1 µm (j), –2 µm (k) and –3 µm (l) defocus. Pixel size in (c, f): 3.31 Å, in (b, e): 6.02 Å, and in (a, d, and g–l): 1.88 Å.

## 10.3.2 Cryo-Electron Microscopy of Vitreous Sections

In CEMOVIS, a biological specimen with a thickness of up to about 200 µm [15] is fixed by means of ultrarapid (~20 ms) cooling (below

–140°) under high pressure (~2000 bar) [16]. The high-pressure frozen, vitrified sample is then cut into ultrathin (20–30 nm nominal thickness) sections in a cryo-microtome, and finally observed in the cryo-electron microscope. In this way, the nanostructure of biological tissues can be studied in their native fully hydrated state, without chemical fixation or staining. The native tissue is preserved down to the molecular level, and the micrograph pixel intensity is directly related to the local electron density of the specimen.

Biomolecules generally possess little difference in electron density, as they are essentially composed of atoms with similar atomic weight (carbon, nitrogen, and oxygen). However, for orderly arranged molecular assemblies, such as lipid tails and headgroups in membranes, even small differences in shape and atomic composition may be amplified because of interference effects that appear in the image phase contrast. During image acquisition, phase contrast is made visible using defocus. At high-magnification, complex interference patterns can be resolved in the CEMOVIS micrographs [7]. Exploiting this, CEMOVIS micrographs can be recorded repeatedly at very high magnification at the same position of the skin sample while increasing stepwise the microscope's defocus, thus ensuring that differences in the recorded micrographs are due exclusively to the different defocuses used.

### 10.3.3 Modeling and Simulation of the Skin Lipid Organization

As a starting point for building different testing models we selected the predominant lipid component of each of the of the *stratum corneum*'s three major lipid classes, namely C24 ceramide NP (the predominant ceramide), cholesterol, and a C24 free fatty acid (the predominant free fatty acid). We constructed 16 distinct candidate molecular organizations, representing all the essential variations that are consistent with the twin-peak repeats separated by a deeper (low intensity) trough in the observed cross–sectional electron density. The molecular organizations were generated by packing individual molecules in their low energy conformations in a small unit cell and which was then repeatedly replicated in the *x*, *y* and *z* axes to yield a periodic structure. These periodic structures served as model organizations for each of the 16 candidate models (Figs. 10.4a–c).

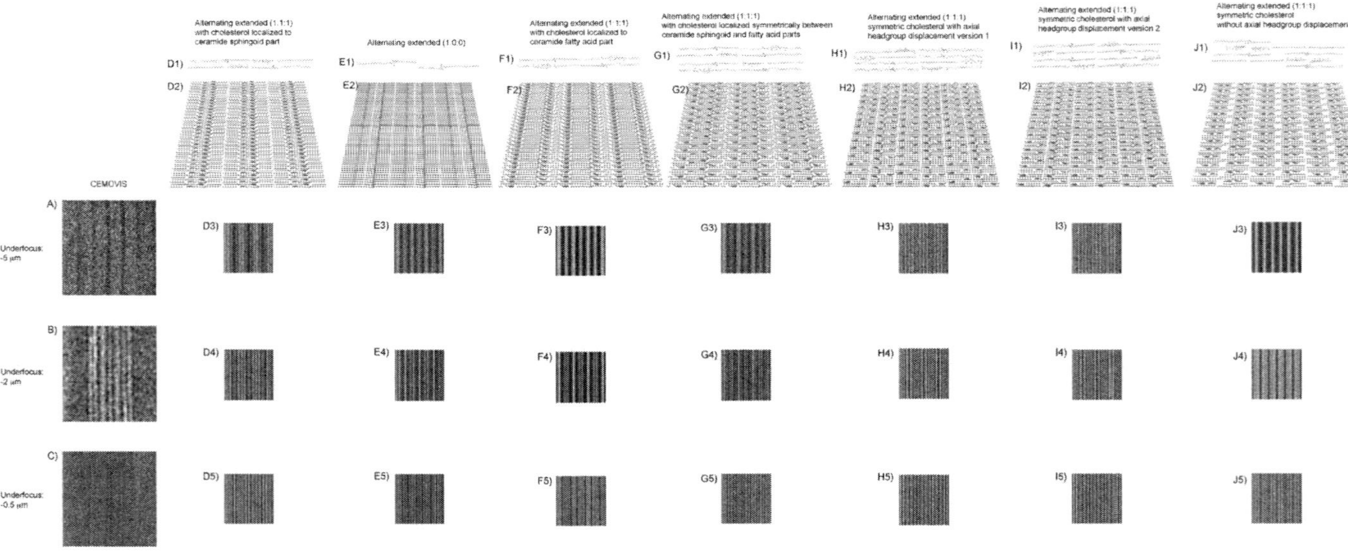



**Figure 10.4a** Electron microscopy simulation results from 7 fully extended ceramide bilayer models with varying cholesterol distribution. (A–C) CEMOVIS micrographs of the *stratum corneum* extracellular lipid matrix acquired at –5 µm (A), –2 µm (B), and –0.5 µm (C) defocus. (D3–J5) Corresponding simulated electron micrographs obtained from 7 fully extended ceramide models. (D1–J1) Repeating units for each simulated model. (D2–J2) Calculated electron scattering potential 3D maps of the topmost layer out of 20 superimposed layers used to generate each individual simulated micrograph (D3–J5).

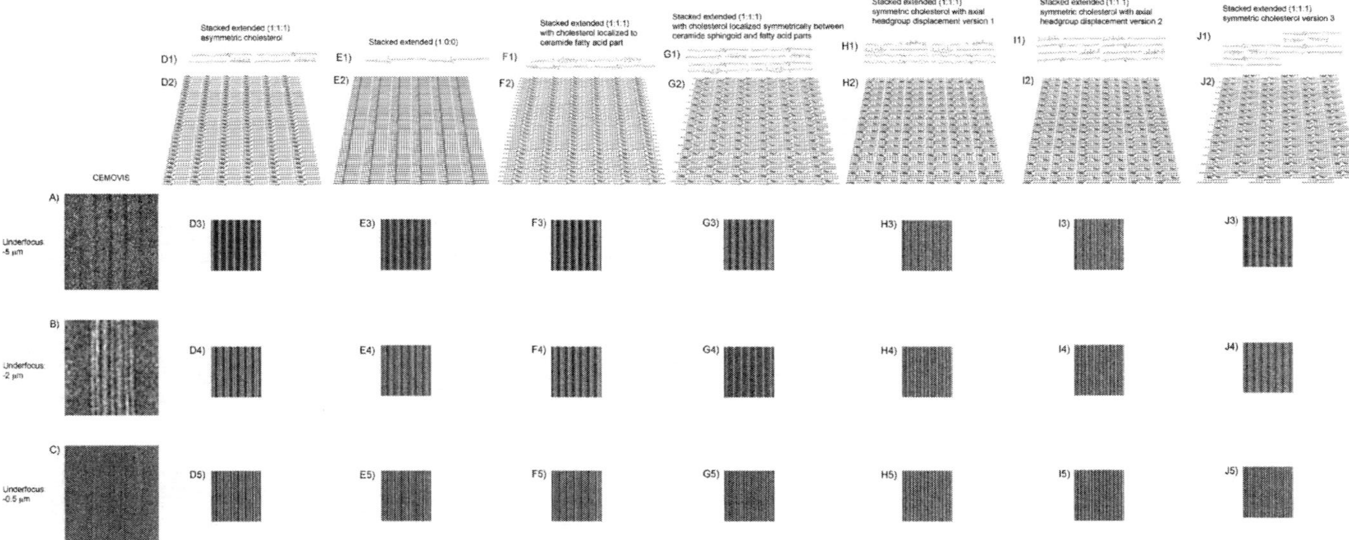

**Figure 10.4b** Electron microscopy simulation results from 7 fully extended ceramide stacked monolayer models with varying cholesterol distribution. (A–C) CEMOVIS micrographs of the *stratum corneum* extracellular lipid matrix acquired at −5 μm (A), −2 μm (B), and −0.5 μm (C) defocus. (D3–J5) Corresponding simulated electron micrographs obtained from 7 stacked fully extended ceramide models. (D1-J1) Two repeating units for each simulated model. (D2–J2) Calculated electron scattering potential 3D maps of the topmost layer out of 20 superimposed layers used to generate each individual simulated micrograph (D3–J5).

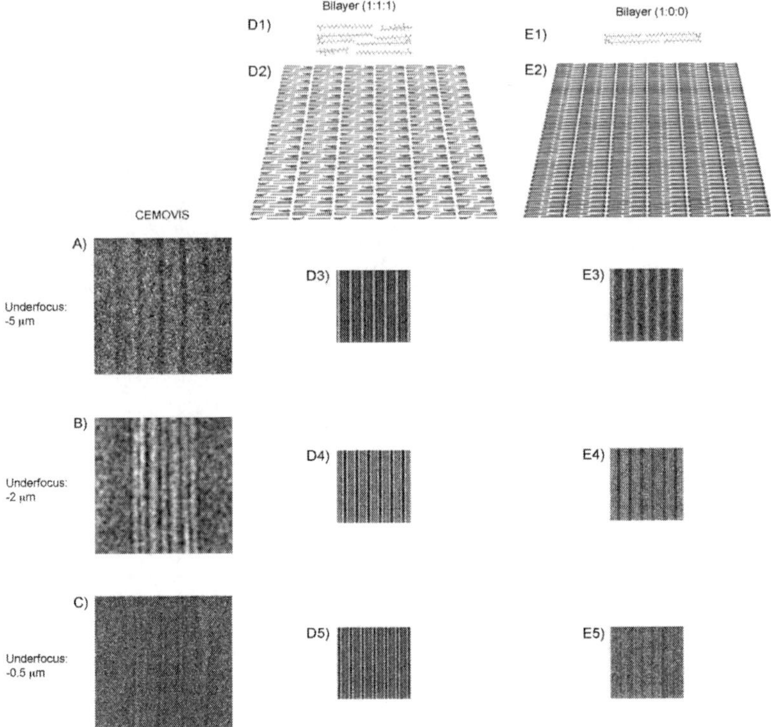


**Figure 10.4c** Electron microscopy simulation results from 2 folded ceramide bilayer models with and without the presence of cholesterol. (A–C) CEMOVIS micrographs of the *stratum corneum* extracellular lipid matrix acquired at –5 µm (A), –2 µm (B), and –0.5 µm (C) defocus. (D3–E5) Corresponding simulated electron micrographs obtained from 2 folded ceramide models. (D1–E1) Repeating units for each simulated model. (D2–E2) Calculated electron scattering potential 3D maps of the topmost layer out of 20 superimposed layers used to generate each individual simulated micrograph (D3–E5).

For each of the 16-candidate model molecular organization, we simulated electron micrograph images using a newly developed transmission electron microscopy (TEM) simulator program [17] (Figs. 10.4a–c). The first part of the program is a phantom generator that can read one or more atomic models in the RCSB Protein Data Bank (PDB) format and construct a model scenario with molecules at defined positions. An electron scattering potential map is then generated with a background structure and potential corresponding to that of vitrified water. The second part of the program simulates the interaction between the potential map and the electron beam, the optical transformation effect of the lens system of the microscope, and the image formation on the detector. Parameters defining optical properties of the microscope, e.g., acceleration voltage, aberration constants and defocus, and the point spread function of the detector were set to mimic the conditions in the real experiments. Finally, the simulated micrographs were compared with the real data. This approach showed to be highly discriminating between different lipid organization models.

### 10.3.4 Toward a Complete Molecular Model of the *Stratum Corneum*

The elucidation of the molecular organization of the skin lipids is but a first step toward building a complete model for the *stratum corneum* that also includes the corneocytes. One should bear in mind that the *stratum corneum* lipid matrix, being a highly organized 2D molecular assembly, is a comparatively simple and well-disposed system for molecular structure determination in situ. For more complex 3D molecular assemblies, such as the corneocyte keratin filament network and the corneocyte cell envelope, the number of candidate atomic models to be considered for high-resolution (0.5–1 nm) CEMOVIS defocus series/EM simulation based structure determination could be very large. Consequently, there will be a need for restricting the number of different molecular model candidates for electron microscopy simulation. One way of doing this is to only consider molecular models that are consistent with medium resolution (2–5 nm) 3D reconstructions of the corneocyte keratin filaments and the corneocyte cell envelope, obtained by cryo-electron tomography of vitreous sections in situ (TOVIS).

### 10.3.5 Tomography of Vitreous Sections

Another cryo-electron microscopy based technique that has considerable potential for accessing the native molecular structure of skin components is tomography of vitreous sections (TOVIS) [6]. This is particularly so as most bio-structures have a distinct 3D molecular arrangement, unlike the largely two-dimensionally arranged *stratum corneum* lipid matrix [7].

In electron tomography (ET), the 3D structure of an object is reconstructed from a series of 2D electron micrographs recorded at different angles. In the simplest setting, such 2D micrographs can be thought of as representing projections of the scattering potential, which in turn describes the 3D structure we seek. Then, reconstruction is performed using a mathematical technique called filtered back-projection [18]. When ET is performed on thin vitreous sections of biological tissues like skin, it is termed TOVIS.

The major factors limiting the resolution in TOVIS 3D reconstruction are a low signal to noise ratio, missing data at high tilt angles, inaccurate image alignment due to inhomogeneous section shrinkage, mass loss under electron exposure, and density spillover from strongly scattering structures located close to the reconstructed area. The signal-to-noise ratio in tomographic low-dose cryo-electron micrographs is well below one because of the low electron doses tolerated by vitreous tissue sections. Further, limitations in the range of tilt angle (typically ±70°) prevent stable inversion during filtered back-projection. This leads to instability in the 3D reconstruction procedure with a resulting resolution worse than expected from the data sampling [19]. The problem of missing data needed for the 3D reconstruction is further augmented in tissue TOVIS because of the diminishing signal-to-noise ratio caused by the increasing relative amount of inelastic scattering at higher tilt angles. This also renders high-tilt images more difficult to align accurately. Finally, density spillover from strongly scattering structures present in the surroundings of the reconstructed region is particularly prominent in tissue TOVIS. Consequently, for proper interpretation of TOVIS data, there is a need for mathematical data regularization procedures [6].

## 10.4 Molecular Organization of the Skin Lipids and Its Significance

According to our CEMOVIS defocus series/EM simulation based structure determination [7], the skin lipids' basic molecular organization is that of stacked bilayers of fully extended ceramides with the sphingoid moieties interfacing. Both cholesterol and the free fatty acids are selectively distributed: cholesterol at the ceramide

sphingoid end and the free fatty acids at the ceramide fatty acid end
(Fig. 10.5).

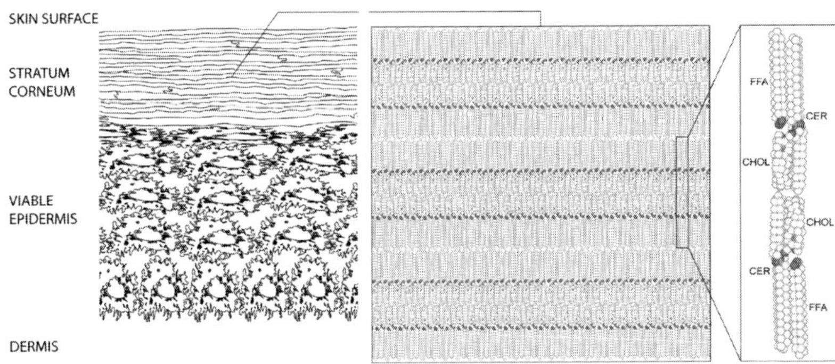


**Figure 10.5**  Schematic drawing of skin. Left: schematic cellular-scale drawing of epidermis. Mid part: molecular-scale drawing of the lamellar lipid matrix occupying the space between the cells of the *stratum corneum*. Right: atomic model of the lipid matrix repeating unit, composed of two mirrored subunits, each composed of one fully extended ceramide-(CER), one cholesterol-(CHOL) and one free fatty acid (FFA) molecule.

The major physiological consequence of this molecular organization is that the fat matrix will be largely impermeable to both hydrophilic and lipophilic substances, because of the condensed state and the presence of alternating lipophilic (alkyl chain) and hydrophilic (headgroup) regions. It will be resistant toward both hydration and dehydration because of the absence of exchangeable water between lipid leaflets. Macroscopically, the structure allows for horny layer cell cohesion and simultaneously for lateral displacement of horny layer cells to accommodate skin bending. At the molecular level, the individual extended bilayers are free to slide with respect to each other, making the fat matrix pliable. The fat matrix thus meets the barrier needs of skin by being simultaneously impermeable and robust.

It is possible that the horny layer's unique fat organization possesses unique physicochemical properties that could be exploited for transdermal drug delivery. By studying more in detail different physicochemical properties of the fully extended ceramide bilayer system one may hopefully propose new venues for drug delivery through the fat matrix. One approach is to use computational molecular modeling combined with in vitro model experiments.

## 10.5 Introduction to Modeling of Data and Simulation

Let us first address an important philosophical issue. How can it be that one can extract molecular level information using computer modeling while the resolution of the original data is insufficient to discriminate the individual molecules? How is modeling able to extend the limited resolution to the molecular level? From where exactly does this additional value come from? The enhanced capability arises as a result of bringing additional information to the problem. We know, for example, the molecular structure of the lipid molecules that comprise the lipid matrix and we know their relative proportions. For each of the molecules we know the atom types and the ideal bond lengths and angles; thus, the 3D molecular structure is very much defined. Flexible molecules can adopt different conformations but one can identify the low energy conformations and consider each of these as potential structures. The problem is thus akin to being asked to assemble a metal contraption from a limited number of component bits, given only a low-resolution picture of the assembled object. Contrast this with the challenge of creating the object on being given the choice of use of any parts from a vast metal scrap-yard.

While modeling is the general term, the term *simulation* is often used for models that have certain sophistication and represent the physical process or phenomena of interest in its entirety. The modeling of data, in its most general form, involves the development of a mathematical model to describe the data. The model may be based on first principles with no parameters or, as is more general, it may involve a number of adjustable parameters that are varied to enable the model to best describe the observed data. Formally, the model may be defined by the function $f(x; b_1, b_2, ..., b_n) = f(x; \mathbf{b})$ where the function $f$ depends on a single variable $x$, and $b_1, b_2, ..., b_n$ is the set of adjustable parameters that can also be represented by the vector $\mathbf{b}$. The model here is 1D, being only dependent on $x$. An example could be the electron density across the cross section (the reaction coordinate $x$) of lipid lamellae. The model function may also be subject to a set of constraints, which for instance may limit the values that the parameters can take. For a multidimensional model the function would take the form $f(x_1, x_2 ..., x_m; b_1, b_2 ..., b_n)$ $= f(\mathbf{x}; \mathbf{b})$ where the model depends on $m$ variables $x_1, x_2, ..., x_m$ ($\mathbf{x}$) and $n$ adjustable parameters $b_1, b_2 ..., b_n$ ($\mathbf{b}$). An electron micrograph image for example would be represented by a 2D model in which the pixel intensity at any given point is given by $f(x, y; b_1, b_2, ..., b_n)$ where $(x, y)$ are the Cartesian coordinates and $b_1, b_2, ..., b_n$ are the adjustable parameters in the model. The latter could be, for instance, the atomic/molecular coordinates of the atoms/molecules in the model that may be varied.

The match between the model and the observed data is usually guided by least squares minimization, which coincides with the maximum likelihood method when noise in data is independent and Gaussian. The least squares method attempts to estimate those parameter values that minimize the sum of the deviations between the observed data $f^{\mathrm{obs}}$ and the calculated data $f^{\mathrm{calc}}$. Thus, the theoretical data is calculated using the model and compared with the experimentally observed data, the parameters are then adjusted until the calculated data best fits the observed data. The least squares function $M(\mathbf{b})$ takes the following form:

$$M(\mathbf{b}) = \sum_{i=0}^{n\text{-points}} \left[ f^{\mathrm{obs}}(\mathbf{x}_i) - f^{\mathrm{calc}}(\mathbf{x}_i; \mathbf{b}) \right]^2, \tag{10.1}$$

where $f^{\mathrm{obs}}(\mathbf{x}_i) - f^{\mathrm{calc}}(\mathbf{x}_i; \mathrm{b})$ is the deviation between the $i$-th observed and calculated data point, and the summation is over all data points. As only the extent of the deviation is important (rather than its sign) the function is squared to remove the sign. The function $M(\mathbf{b})$ is minimized w.r.t. $\mathbf{b}$—hence the term "least squares"—to yield the value of the parameters $\mathbf{b}$.

The data modeling approach outlined above is highly successful when the number of data points is larger than the number of parameters. It is applied widely and underpins, among other application domains, the whole of crystallography—where the interest is similar to that at hand, i.e., the determination of the molecular structure and packing. The X-ray or neutron diffraction or scattering data does not directly reveal atomic positions; rather the diffraction/scattering arising from a proposed molecular structure/packing is modeled, and the model structure manipulated until it best describes the data. The assumption then is that the modeled structure characterizes the structure of the sample. Therefore, to extract the molecular organization of the lipids from the CEMOVIS data, one would need to be able to simulate the electronic microscopy process in its entirety, including the interference effects of de-focusing—hence the development and use of the electron microscope simulator in our study to elucidate the skin lipid organization.

Models can also be based on first principles. These tend to have a strong physical basis and ideally have no adjustable parameters. The goal is not to fit observed data, but rather to gain insights or to independently predict the phenomenon or process of interest. Thus, such models are not employed to extract information from data, but rather can serve as independent checks on the extracted information, assuming that the model is a good representation. Molecular dynamics (MD) simulation, which is a powerful computational method for modeling the emergent behavior of molecular assemblies, falls in the category of a first principle model. We expect molecular simulation to play an increasing role in enhancing our molecular-level understanding of the skin and to form the basis for the development of in silico skin models.

Simulation is now firmly established as one of the major pillars of modern science and engineering, complementing traditional experimental and theoretical approaches. It is routinely used in many parts of science and industry to support, and sometimes replace, experimentation. It can have a dramatic effect on the discovery process, reducing the need for costly experiments and increasing the speed with which new discoveries can be made. We believe simulation is set to play an increasingly important role in skin research, from understanding physiological processes, linking structure to function, modulating transport, to developing new treatments for skin disease.

## 10.6  Introduction to Electron Tomography 3D Reconstruction

In order to access the native molecular 3D organization of skin components like the *stratum corneum* keratin network and corneocyte cell envelope, the cryo-electron microscopy–based technique tomography of vitreous sections (TOVIS) may be particularly useful [6]. Below follows an introduction to electron tomography (ET) and computational tomographic 3D reconstruction.

The basic principle in tomography is to recover the 3D structure of an object from a series of 2D data. The data is acquired by probing the object with a particle/wave travelling along a known direction and then measuring the intensity generated from the reflected and/or transmitted portion of this wave.

The idea in tomography is that the particle/wave interacts with the object and thereby carries information about its structure. By repeatedly probing the same region of the object, one "views" this structure several times from different directions. A key step in the reconstruction process is to relate the data in some known and unambiguous way to the structure one seeks. This is commonly referred to as the forward problem, which among others requires one to model the aforementioned interaction with sufficient accuracy. If necessary, one needs to add models that describe how the instrumentation further distorts the measurements.

For transmission electron microscopy (TEM) imaging of weakly scattering amorphous specimens, it is common to model the specimen classically and the electrons quantum mechanically. Thus, we are dealing with an electron wave that scatters against a specimen. The corresponding forward model is frequently referred to as the image formation model. It is often based on the assumption that the wave function for the scattered electron is expressible in terms of a projection of the electrostatic potential (projection assumption). The influence of TEM optics and detector is modeled by convolutions, both linear operators, and the intensity is linearized. Further details and discussions about the validity of these assumptions are given in the section below about simulation of the image formation.

## 10.6.1 The 3D Reconstruction Problem in the Linear Setting

Assuming a linear image formation model, the 3D tomographic reconstruction problem can be phrased as solving a system of linear equations. To see this more clearly, let $x$ denote the variable representing the 3D structure of the specimen that we seek to recover and $y$ is the series of 2D TEM images that one collects in the microscope.[a] Since we have a linear image formation model, the data $y$ is related to $x$ by a linear transformation, which we call $T$. For TEM imaging $T$ will, in the simplest case, represent a projection, but it may also include blurring due to optics, detector response, etc. The linear transformation $T$ is known and does not depend on the specimen, but it does depend on the geometrical arrangement guiding the data collection.

The task of simulating a series of TEM images $y$ in absence of noise and measurement errors is now expressible as calculating

$$Y = T(x). \tag{10.2}$$

Analogously, reconstructing the 3D structure $x$ of the specimen requires us to solve the above equation for $x$ given a data set $y$ and a forward model $T$.

## 10.6.2 Concept of Ill-Posedness and Regularization

In most applications of tomography, including ET, the number of unknowns and the number of equations are not the same in the above system of linear equations. Therefore, most likely there are no solutions to this equation. In this situation, the common procedure is to relax the notion of a solution, e.g., by seeking least-squares solutions. This frequently occurs in science, the most well-known situation being when one seeks to fit a straight line through a set of points in the plane. It is highly unlikely to find a straight line passing through all points, i.e., there are no solutions, and one needs to settle for the "best line." The latter is frequently chosen as the line that minimizes the residual errors (least-squares solution, see discussion Section 10.5). The issue of lack of solutions in ET can be addressed in the same way.

An issue, however, with seeking least-squares solutions is that, in the under-determined case (i.e., there are more unknowns than equations) one ends up with infinitely many such solutions. Furthermore, these may be overly sensitive to errors in the data, i.e., small variations in data are amplified during the reconstruction process. In such situations, the reconstruction problem is said

---

[a]Note that $y$ is not a single 2D micrograph, it is a set of 3D micrographs typically forming a tilt-series.

to be *ill-posed*. An alternative way of understanding the issue of ill-posedness is to investigate the behavior of the eigenvalues of the matrix representing *T*. If they drop-off rapidly toward zero, the matrix is highly ill-conditioned and straightforward matrix inversion becomes unfeasible due to instability.

To solve an ill-posed reconstruction problem requires using a method for selecting a unique solution that is robust against noise and errors in data. A *regularization method* is a mathematical framework for doing this. The idea is to construct a family of well-posed problems whose solutions "converge" to a least-squares (or maximum likelihood) solution of the ill-posed problem as the data error tend to zero. The formal definition involves quite a lot of mathematical machinery; see, for example, [20]. The important take-home message here is that regularization methods are systematic methods for avoiding over-fitting and they may be constructed quite differently. The suitability of a regularization method for a specific problem at hand depends on (i) its ability to account for *a priori knowledge* about the true (but unknown) solution, (ii) the accuracy of the underlying forward model,[b] (iii) its ability to account for the statistical nature of the noise in data, and (iv) the possibility to properly weigh the influence of the a priori information against the need to fit measured data.

On a final note, it must be mentioned that essentially all tomographic reconstruction problems are ill-posed. There are, however, degrees of ill-posedness depending on the sensitivity of the inversion to noise and measurements errors. This can be measured by considering how fast the aforementioned eigenvalues drop off. *Moderate ill-posedness* refers to the case when they drop-off relatively slowly, whereas a fast drop-off corresponds to *severe ill-posedness*, indicating a high degree of sensitivity to noise and measurements errors. It turns out that the degree of ill-posedness is an important criterion in choosing the "right" regularization method. As an example, many tomographic reconstruction problems arising in medical imaging are moderately ill-posed, so it is enough to use a regularization method that is based on the assumption that noise is high-frequency whereas true object features of interest are low frequency.

---

[b]This deals with how well *T* models the relation between the structure we seek and measured data in absence of noise and measurement errors.

### 10.6.3  Ill-Posedness in ET

The most significant difficulty that arises when ET is applied to TEM data recorded from biological specimens is the *dose problem*. It limits the total number of images that can be taken and arises due to specimen damage during electron exposure.

Next, all data collection schemes in ET give rise to *missing data* since they cannot provide images acquired from uniformly distributed directions. This is well known to lead to severe ill-posedness. Furthermore, for a given positioning of the specimen, only a sub-region of it is subject to electron exposure, so we are dealing with region of interest data, also called *local tomography*, which implies that the 3D specimen structure (encoded by the scattering potential) is not uniquely determined, regardless of the quality of the data at our disposal unless prior information of the sample can be used.

Taken together, the above factors strongly indicate that the reconstruction problem in ET is severely ill-posed. Thus, a reliable and useful reconstruction method must include regularization, either by reconstructing only some information about the specimen that can be stably retrieved, or, alternatively, introduce prior information about the specimen into the reconstruction scheme.

There are, however, further difficulties associated with ET that needs to be dealt with. Due to the complex stochastics of the data, it is challenging to provide a priori estimates of the data error[c] to a sufficient degree of accuracy. Many regularization methods require reliable a priori estimates of the data error to properly weigh the influence of the a priori information against the need to fit measured data. Finally, in ET there are parameters whose values needs to be set if one seeks optimal performance in recovering the 3D specimen structure (scattering potential). One example is parameters that determine the values of the scattering potential outside the 3D region of interest. Since we have local tomography, data will be influenced from those parts. The simplest is to set the scattering potential to zero (or constant) in those regions. This assumption is perhaps not that big of a problem for in vitro specimens, but more problematic for in situ specimens where there is a lot of structures outside the 3D region of interest that contribute to the data. Another

---

[c]The data error is here simply defined as the discrepancy between measured data and data one would have measured in absence of noise and measurement errors, the latter being unknown of course.

such nuisance parameter is the amplitude contrast ratio that accounts for the "absorption effect" on the flux of elastically scattered electrons due to inelastic scattering (see Section 10.7.3).

## 10.6.4 Reconstruction Methods

All reconstruction methods used in ET that the authors are aware of are implicitly (or explicitly) based on the projection assumption (see Section 10.7.4). Therefore, 3D reconstruction from a series of 2D projection data (inversion of the ray transform) is a central theme.

## 10.6.5 Early Development

As already mentioned, 1968 marked the beginning of ET with the publication of several independent papers all based on the above mentioned projection assumption. 3D structures of specimens with helical symmetry were reconstructed in the seminal paper [21]. Similar work, that made use of symmetry in the specimen under study, was done in [22]. In [23], one also made the observation that reconstruction of an arbitrary specimen (not necessarily symmetric) is possible given TEM micrographs from a sufficient number of directions.

The reconstruction schemes in these early papers are all based on the Fourier slice theorem, a rather natural choice bearing in mind that the latter result was known among crystallographers. The Fourier slice theorem relates the 2D Fourier transform of projection data to the 3D Fourier transform of the specimen structure. More precisely, let us take the 2D Fourier transform of the 3D specimen structure along a given direction. Next, take its 2D Fourier transform. Then this equals the restriction of the 3D Fourier transform of the same specimen structure restricted to a central section orthogonal to that direction. In a tilt-series we acquire 2D images, or projections, along many different directions. Hence, we sample many different sections of Fourier space and 3D reconstruction can be in principle achieved by Fourier inversion. In practice however, this approach is associated with some difficulties. ET data collection geometries correspond to sampling the 3D Fourier transform of the specimen on a polar grid in 2D sections. The numerical scheme for inverting the 3D Fourier transform that is necessary to recover the specimen structure therefore involves an interpolation from such a polar grid to a rectilinear grid. It turns out that interpolation in Fourier space is non-trivial, especially so for ET where there is a limited number of projections. Fourier methods were therefore soon replaced by the *filtered backprojection* (*FBP*) *method*.

In the 1970s, much attention was paid to the development of other algorithms for 3D reconstruction from a series of 2D projection data. Among others, this included iterative methods such as *algebraic reconstruction technique* (*ART*) and *simultaneous iterative reconstruction technique* (*SIRT*).

Despite this promising start, ET as an imaging technology did not experience the rapid development and deployment like its counterpart in medical imaging. One reason was the difficulties connected with collecting good data. In fact, only rather recently is it possible to routinely collect high quality tilt-series that can be used for ET. Another reason is the difficulties associated with the 3D reconstruction problem in ET (see description in the previous section).

## 10.6.6 Established Methods

In contrast to the rapid development in sample preparation and instrumentation, development in 3D reconstruction methods for ET has been relatively slow. The current established methods are essentially refinements of FBP, ART, and SIRT that were introduced in the early 1970s, and those that have gained widespread use can be categorized into *analytic* and *iterative methods*.

### 10.6.6.1 Analytic methods

The underlying principle in analytic methods is to express the inverse of $T$ analytically and then regularize that expression by some clever scheme. This is only feasible if the inverse is expressible in closed form, which is, for example, possible when $T$ represents a projection of the specimen 3D structure. In this part, we therefore consider this case.

An obvious attempt at reconstructing the 3D object structure at a fixed point in 3D space is to average all projection data that this point is projected upon. Repeating this for all 3D points of interest gives us a 3D structure. This scheme, henceforth called *backprojection*, thus allows us to generate a 3D structure from a series of 2D projection images and is sometimes referred to as *direct backprojection* [24]. The backprojection is a natural candidate for an inverse of the projection *T*. It turns out that this is almost the case. To get an inverse, one must appropriately weight (filter) the projection data before averaging in 3D. This leads to the FBP method, which is also known as *weighted backprojection* (*WBP*) [18].

FBP/WBP has become the standard method for 3D reconstruction in ET, both in life sciences and material sciences. A popular approach is to combine FBP/WBP with post-processing in order to remove speckle and enhance features with fairly impressive results [25–28].

### 10.6.6.2 Iterative methods

The underlying principle in iterative methods is to generate a sequence (iterates) of intermediate 3D reconstructions that in the limit converges to a least squares solution. For ill-posed problems, such as the one we have in ET, this is not desirable since it corresponds to over-fitting. Hence, regularization is by early stopping. One can also regularize further by introducing a relaxation factors. This controls the stability and convergence rate of the iterative process (under-relaxation increases the stability while over-relaxation increases the rate of convergence).

ART and SIRT are the most popular iterative methods in ET. Neither is, however, invented by the EM community. ART is simply the well-known Kaczmarz method for solving (over-or underdetermined) linear systems [29]. Similarly, SIRT is simply the Landweber iteration for solving linear ill-posed problems [30]. Convergence criteria for both methods are by now well understood for many imaging modalities.

ART was introduced to the EM community in [31] and SIRT in [18]. They both became practically applicable to ET only after regularization through early stopping and strong over-relaxation. A further development for ART came when it was combined with a clever way to represent "blobs" in the 3D reconstruction [32]. Likewise, SIRT with early stopping has been successfully applied to ET [33–34] and is now considered the golden standard method. SIRT is widely available in both free-ware software packages for 3D reconstruction for ET, such as IMOD, as well as commercial offerings, such as Inspect 3D from FEI.

### 10.6.6.3 Comparing analytic and iterative methods

Both ART and SIRT are expected to give similar quality of reconstruction, but they may have different requirements on computational resources. In fact, in general it is not to be expected that any of these methods are superior to the other in terms of image quality.

Analytic methods are computationally more efficient. On the other hand, since analytic methods are based on analytically inverting the forward model $T$, they are specifically tailored to a particular measurement geometry and forward model. This limits their applicability to situations where the influence of TEM optics and detectors has to be ignored, or accounted for in a pre-processing step prior to 3D reconstruction. ART and SIRT on the other hand work for arbitrary data acquisition geometries and any linear forward model $T$, so one can include more accurate physics models, such as optics and detector models, as well as more measurement geometries. The latter is perhaps of most interest for single particle methods, another modality for 3D EM imaging.

On a final note, to quantify what is meant by a "better reconstruction" is far from trivial. It is naive to claim that the Fourier Shell Correlation (FSC) is the only way to quantify image quality. One approach is to mimic how such issues are settled within the medical imaging community [35]. The idea is to test methods systematically using an array of quantifiers (called figure-of-merits). By first calibrating the parameter settings in the reconstruction methods to be tested against a training set, one can then make objective and statistically sound comparisons using an array of figure-of-merits (which may of course include FSC numbers). This approach was, for example, applied to test FBP/WBP against ART and SIRT in ET [32]. An issue with this approach is that almost all figure-of-merits are calculated by comparing 3D reconstructions against some ground truth. Hence, one must test with simulated data where the ground truth (phantom) is known, so access to a good simulator is important.

### 10.6.7 Recent Developments

An alternative approach, called constrained maximum entropy tomography (COMET), is to use relative entropy regularization [36–37]. Here, the regularization parameter itself is "updated" in an iterative scheme together with the prior, which encodes the prior knowledge about the solution.

Discrete tomography has been applied to ET with reasonable success [38] and its usage within statistical regularization theory for defining Gibbs priors is provided in [39]. It must be emphasized that discrete tomography in its current form is mostly used in ET applied to material sciences. Finally, recently there have been attempts at using a variant of total variation (TV) regularization with an additional attempt at accounting for the missing data region [40].

Next, there has also been some progress in analytic approaches, i.e., non-iterative reconstruction schemes of FBP type. It turns out that when the detector size is large (large-field TEM imaging), the projection assumption must be replaced in order to account for the fact that the imaging electrons follow curvilinear trajectories. The ray transform (projection) in the forward model is then replaced with a generalized ray transform that projects along curves. The corresponding FBP method is discussed in [41]. A very different approach to analytic inversion is taken in [42–43]. The non-uniqueness and ill-posedness mentioned before point to using a reconstruction method that regularizes by reconstructing only some information about the specimen 3D structure that can be stably retrieved. It turns out that one can retrieve most boundaries of sub-structures in the specimen. This leads to a new FBP type of analytic reconstruction method applicable to ET. One can, furthermore, describe those edges that are stably visible from the limited data obtained using specific data collection geometries.

## 10.7 Introduction to Electron Microscopy (EM) Simulation

### 10.7.1 Usages of Simulation in EM Imaging in Life Sciences

Our new experimental approach allowing for molecular structure determination directly in situ in native tissues, and used in its first application to determine the basic molecular organization of the *stratum corneum* lipid matrix [7], is based on combining cryo-EM with EM-simulation. EM-simulation is here used to interpret the EM data. Below follows a short introduction to EM-simulation in the life sciences. In contrast to material science applications, EM simulators have so far not been widely used in the life sciences.

The usefulness of an EM simulator depends on its ability to faithfully replicate relevant aspects of the EM imaging process. A vital part is the *phantom generator* that provides a model (phantom) of the specimen whose image is to be simulated. Another is the simulation of the *image formation*, which includes the interaction between the electron and specimen, as well as models of the source, electron optical elements, energy filters, detectors and other parts of the EM that influences the image. Both are discussed in more detail in the sections that follow.

An accurate simulator can have many usages for a scientist involved in EM imaging. One is in assisting the identification and characterization of biostructures by comparing experimental micrographs against simulated ones generated from a molecular phantom. In a more advanced analysis, the phantom generator part of a simulator can be used in the docking process where atomic models are fitted into structural maps obtained by means of 3D EM. Yet another usage of a simulator is in the development of novel EM techniques and procedures. For example, it will be possible to easily and cost-effectively investigate the impact of new data collection techniques and improved instrumentation. In addition, simulation will be helpful in the development and evaluation of computational techniques, both for 3D reconstruction as well as for 2D and 3D image processing. In addition, a simulator could also help in assessing whether an EM imaging study is feasible in answering a specific biological question. This underlying biological question translates into a structural question, which then is to be answered by means of EM imaging. One can now perform an in silico study where the first step is to pick molecules of the same size and scattering power and arranging them in a way that mimics the structural question. Next, simulate EM data. And if you cannot answer your question based on such simulated data, you will probably not be able to answer it from experimental data either.

From a *stratum corneum* and skin barrier perspective, our main interest in a simulator is related to *model-based 3D recon-struction*. Here, the idea is to systematically compare simulated and experimental images in order to characterize the *stratum corneum*'s molecular 3D organization. More precisely, consider a case where the major portion of the specimen is built up by a regular arrangement of specific molecules, almost like a crystal. Furthermore, assume the 3D structure of these molecular building blocks, e.g., lipid molecules or keratin molecules in the *stratum corneum*, is known, e.g., by means of X-ray crystallography. The open question is then to determine the *3D arrangement* of the lipid- and keratin molecules. If it turns out that a small change in the 3D arrangement results in detectable changes in simulated micrographs, then one can seek to recover the 3D arrangement by systematically comparing simulated images against experimental ones.

## 10.7.2  Present State of EM Simulators in Life Sciences

Ideally, all components of a simulator should be accurately modeled, followed by testing and validation against experimental data. This is, however, a non-trivial and quite resource intensive task, so the most efficient option would be that the scientific community agrees upon a common software platform for simulation, which then is well supported, validated, and maintained. This is, e.g., the case with GATE; a highly accurate open source software framework dedicated to simulation of a wide range of medical imaging and radiotherapy modalities. The software is developed and maintained within OpenGATE, an international consortium involving academia, industry, and end users.

To our knowledge, the EM community lacks an established framework for EM simulation similar to the above-mentioned GATE framework. Instead, at regular intervals, various research groups develop and release simulators for specific EM modalities, seemingly unaware of what is available, and with varying degree of quality and completeness. These software suits do often have several shortcomings. First, the phantom generator is either lacking or too simplistic. One example is that phantom generators do not properly account for the physics governing how atomistic (such as those given in PDB files) and continuum (such as for aqueous parts) models are to be merged and translated into models for scattering relevant for EM simulation. Next, the model for the noise many times has no clear connection to the physical sources of randomness; it is often taken as Gaussian additive noise. There is also no calibration protocol for setting values of simulation parameters. Finally, the software is insufficiently tested and/or validated against experimental data. Some simulators do, however, properly address these issues. One such is TEM simulator [17], a simulator for TEM imaging of weakly scattering amorphous specimens, such as thin unstained vitreous sections of native skin. The paper [17] also contains a short review of TEM simulators in both material and life sciences with respect to their usefulness in life sciences bearing in mind the above-mentioned issues.

### 10.7.3  Phantom Generator

The phantom generator is the part of an EM simulator that starts out form user-provided specification (which should not require a user to list every single atom), and generates a model of the specimen (phantom) useable by an EM simulator for generating micrographs. Thus, the assumptions and approximations that are used in this process needs to be consistent with those used later on for modeling the interaction between the incident high-energy electrons and the atoms making up the specimen.

EM imaging is inherently quantum mechanical and makes use of the wave properties of the incident high-energy electrons. We will begin by assuming that the incident electron and the specimen form a closed system neglecting any interaction with the environment. Now, a central part is the *interaction potential* of the system consisting of the incident electron and all particles making up the specimen. In this context, a phantom generator models the interaction potential given a specification of the specimen and the energy of the incident electrons. Now, unlike other diffraction phenomena, such as X-ray and neutron diffraction, electrons are charged particles and interact with matter through the Coulomb forces. In the context of electron diffraction, we can safely assume that the particles of the specimen are electrons and nuclei (i.e., we do not account in detail for the other sub-atomic particles). With this assumption in place, it is possible to write the interaction potential as one part accounting for the nuclei and another accounting for the electrons in the specimen. Next, the contribution from the nuclei is commonly modeled by the isolated atom superposition approximation [44]. This approach already accounts for part of the overlap between atoms in the specimen, so the amount of charge distribution associated with the chemical bonds between the atoms in the specimen is not expected to be large. Therefore, in most cases it is enough for a phantom generator to model only the contribution from the nuclei. As an example, for crystals about 95–99% of the total contribution to the interaction potential is from the nuclei [44, p. 8 and 428].

The potential accounting for the nuclei is positive and decreases rapidly with the distance from the nucleus. For tissue water, the positions of the ions and atoms are not known and therefore the contribution from the nuclei cannot be computed exactly. However, there are two approaches to address this issue: (i) Find the optimal positions of water and ion atoms by performing molecular dynamics simulation and then compute the potential by using tabulated potentials as for the case of the macromolecules. (ii) Compute the average value of the potential given the density of the tissue water. Note that the latter averaging approach is significantly less computationally expensive. Using it for the ions does, however, require one to perform the averaging bearing in mind that the distributions of the ions are described by the Boltzmann distribution.

Yet another issue relates to inelastic scattering. The quantum state of both the incident electron and the specimen change in an inelastic collision between them. Hence, the interaction Hamiltonian is inevitably time dependent. Mathematically it is always possible to separate the interaction Hamiltonian into a time dependent and a time-independent part. The interpretation is that the time dependent part models interactions involving an exchange of energy between the incident high-energy electron and the specimen. In that sense, it models inelastic scattering. The time-independent part will therefore account for the elastic scattering. For natural reasons, simulating time dependent scattering is very complex. One can, however, make a simplified treatment whereby inelastic scattering is considered as an "absorption effect" since the flux of elastically scattered electrons is reduced due to inelastic scattering. This "absorption effect" is modeled by introducing an imaginary part, the absorption (optical) potential, to the scattering potential. A rigorous derivation from quantum mechanics is quite involved and depends on the type of inelastic scattering; see, for example, [44,17].

In conclusion, it is clear that devising an accurate phantom generator is far from straightforward and requires using a number of carefully chosen approximations whose validity must be checked against the EM imaging modality one seeks to simulate.

## 10.7.4 Simulation of Image Formation

The model for image formation depends to a large extent on the type of EM imaging modality one seeks to simulate, and the type of specimens whose EM images are to be simulated. In general, it is, however, fair to claim that the task of simulation naturally divides into simulating

(1)  emission of electrons
(2)  electron–specimen interaction
(3)  electron optical elements
(4)  detector

In this review, we focus on simulating TEM images of native skin, i.e., of an unstained biological specimen. A full derivation of models relevant for simulating this type of imaging studies is outside the scope of this review, so here we confine ourselves to presenting a very brief outline. The interested reader is referred to [45–47] for a more detailed exposition.

The starting point is to assume that we have perfect coherent imaging, i.e., the incoming electron wave is a monochromatic plane wave (coherent illumination) and electrons only scatter elastically. This assumption alone takes care of the issue of simulating the emission of electrons, since we simply assume incoming electrons are plane waves. The scattering properties of the specimen are in this case given by the electrostatic potential and the electron–specimen interaction is modeled by the scalar Schrödinger equation. Adding a description of the effects of the optics and detector, both modeled as convolutions, completes the picture.

Inelastic scattering and incoherent illumination, however, introduces partial incoherence, so the basic assumption of perfect coherent imaging must be relaxed. The incoherence that stems from inelastic scattering is accounted for within the coherent framework by introducing an imaginary part to the scattering potential; see the above discussion related to the phantom generator. Next, the incoherence that stems from incoherent illumination is modeled by modifying the convolution kernel that describes the effect of the optics.

The above provides a fairly complete model for image formation in a TEM. An issue is, however, related to simulating the electron–specimen interaction. The wave equation of the scattered electron is given as a solution to the scalar Schrödinger equation. Numerically solving this partial differential equation is, however, extremely challenging even for very small regions. To give an idea of the computational complexity, consider the task of simulating the scattering of a 300 keV electron against a specimen occupying a cubic region 50 nm in size. The size of the region translates into 25,000 wavelengths, so using any finite difference/element method is entirely out of the question.

The *multi-slice method* assumes that the wave function of the scattered electron is only highly oscillating along the beam direction. This makes sense if the incident electron has high energy and does not change significantly on the scale of its wavelength along that direction. Under this assumption, one can simulate the electron–specimen interaction in a computationally feasible manner.

Another commonly used method is based on the *projection assumption*. This is derived as follows. First, as shown in [45], taking the first order Born approximation enables one to explicitly express the wave function of the scattered electron in terms of the propagation operator acting on the scattering potential. Next, the propagation operator can be replaced by its high-energy limit as the wave number tends to infinity. This yields a model for the electron–specimen interaction that is based on projecting the scattering potential of the specimen.

Finally, it should be underlined, however, that both the multi-slice and projection methods dot not really model inelastic scattering. The multi-slice has the advantage that it properly accounts for the positioning of the specimen along the optical axis and allows for multiple forward scattering. The projection assumption assumes single forward scattering and does not account for the positioning of the specimen along the optical axis.

## 10.8 Future Perspective

In order to formulate a more general model of horny layer permeability, the molecular structure and physicochemical properties of the keratin-filled cells as well as of the interface between cells and fat matrix, must be taken into account along with the extracellular lipid matrix. Structure determination of complex 3D molecular assemblies, such as the corneocyte keratin filament network and the corneocyte cell envelope, will likely be more challenging than structure determination of the two-dimensionally organized (layered) lipid matrix [7]. We, therefore, outline potential future improvements of present technology that may aid achievement of our goal.

## 10.8.1　3D Reconstruction for ET

To better account for a priori information in the regularization is a key issue to get more *reliable* 3D reconstruction. Iterative methods, such as ART and SIRT, have traditionally been more efficient for large-scale problems, whereas variational methods offer the most flexible framework for reconstruction. Thanks to the rapid development in hardware, the latter can nowadays also be used for large-scale reconstruction problems, such as those arising in 3D tomography. Future progress in 3D reconstruction will therefore probably be related to development and maturation of variational methods, such as COMET [36–37] or TV regularization.

## 10.8.2　Regularization Functionals

In many reconstruction problems, it is desirable to preserve edges while reducing oscillatory behavior and background clutter. Another property is the ability to recover slowly varying grayscale regions.

The above are all examples of regularity properties that a solution to the 3D reconstruction problem should possess. The variational methods mentioned before (Section 10.6.7) enforce such a priori regularity through the appropriate regularization functional. As an example, TV-regularization (1-norm of the gradient magnitude) suppresses oscillatory behavior and background clutter while preserving edges, but has a tendency to ignore slowly varying regions (stair-casing). The 2-norm will instead blur edges but capture slowly varying regions. For ET in life sciences, it turns out that using a -norm of the gradient magnitude in between 1 and 2 gives better results than using the 1- or 2-norm. In this context, one can also consider Besov type of norms [48] that are known to better handle stair-casing while reducing background clutter. Yet another approach is to vary the value of the -norm. Near an edge, one would like the 1-norm, and away from an edge one would like to approach the 2-norm. The characterization of visible edges in [42–43] can here be combined with TV-type of regularization for handling both anisotropic resolution and reducing the stair-casing phenomena.

One can also consider combining variational methods with Bregman iterates for obtaining better resolution, e.g., the Bregman-TV method [49] is better at addressing the issue of stair-casing without impairing upon the ability to preserve edges.

Finally, one can also consider designing dictionaries for compression of 3D ET volumes. Such dictionaries can then be used in a sparsity promoting variational method. Dictionary design does, however, require a good training set from which one can then construct learned and/or analytic dictionaries. For ET this translates into having access to a good phantom generator [50].

### 10.8.3   Noise Model and Regularization Parameter

Both iterative and variational methods need a notion of discrepancy in data space to quantify how well a reconstruction fits measured data. Ideally this notion is derived from the log-likelihood of the random variable representing the noise component of data. In ET, data is more appropriately modeled as a Poisson distributed random variable, leading to a data discrepancy notion that differs from the 2-norm [51].

Another open area is to devise practically usable methods for choosing the regularization parameter when data is extremely noisy. Standard methods, such as Morozov discrepancy principle and the L-curve, do not work in this setting and generalized cross-validation is computationally unfeasible. One approach specifically suitable for ET in life sciences is presented in [52].

### 10.8.4   Simultaneous Reconstruction and Image Processing

Another development is related to combining the reconstruction step with the 3D image analysis/processing steps, such as segmentation. Today, these two are performed independently of each other. However, for noisy data it turns out that it is better to do reconstruction and image analysis/processing in one step.

Part of this is already achieved within the variational methods by the appropriate choice of regularization functional. One can, however, choose the latter in a way that directly relates to specific image processing tasks. One example from ET is given in [53] where the Mumford-Shah method is combined with the characterization of visible edges [42] for simultaneous reconstruction and segmentation in ET.

Another approach for 3D reconstruction is shape-based regularization, where one seeks to account for shape-based à priori information. Variational regularization with a spatial shape prior is applied to ET in [54]. There, the benefit of using shape based prior knowledge is clearly demonstrated even in cases where shape information is available only on a small subset of the 3D volume. A more sophisticated approach is to use variational regularization where the regularization functional is based on shape metrics from the large-displacement-diffeomorphic mapping framework [55–56].

## 10.8.5 Statistical Regularization

In its original deterministic formulation (classical regularization), the output of a regularization method is a *single* reconstruction and the only randomness is in the noise associated with measurements. On the other hand, in statistical regularization, *all* quantities related to the problem are modeled as random variables. The output is *not* a single reconstruction but a *probability distribution of reconstructions* [57–58].

For ET, the above translates into reconstructing all possible 3D structures and their probabilities instead of a single 3D structure. From a practical point of view, a user cannot easily visualize a set of 3D reconstructions, so one typically uses an estimator to pick out a single one. The added benefit, however, is that one also has the possibility to estimate the uncertainty in that reconstruction. Statistical regularization, and Bayesian regularization in particular, also offers a unified framework for accounting for a variety of a priori assumptions that could be of interest, e.g., the ability to include a docking procedure (i.e., to assume that a sub-volume in the reconstruction docks well with a given PDB-template). Another benefit is the ability to handle nuisance parameters that are handled in an ad hoc manner in classical regularization.

The challenge associated with Bayesian regularization in imaging is that of handling the computational complexity. Imaging problems, such as those in ET, lead to large-scale computational problems, so clever computational approaches are needed when using Bayesian regularization. This is especially the case for priors that seek to enforce sparsity since they involve optimizing quantities that are computationally difficult to handle (-norms, TV-semi norms or Besov norms that are non-differentiable). There has, however, been tremendous progress in this area and large-scale 3D reconstruction problems can nowadays be handled in a computationally feasible manner; see [59] for an example from 3D medical imaging. These reconstruction techniques are, however, yet to be applied to ET.

### 10.8.6 EM Simulation

The biggest, and yet not properly addressed, challenge in EM simulation is to model inelastic scattering. This is perhaps less of an issue when simulating unstained thin biological specimens like vitreous sections of skin, but if one seeks to properly simulate thicker or stained specimens, then one needs to include more accurate modeling of inelastic scattering.

A more important, but less scientifically exciting need, is to make TEM simulation methods more available to the wider scientific community. This requires further development in terms of interface design and calibration protocols. This applies especially to the phantom generator. Equipped with a more accurate model for the interaction potential, a phantom generator can also be used for docking; see, for example, the TexMol/VolRover software suite [60].

Another line of development is to look into models for electron–specimen interaction that have the potential of providing a common framework for simulation that would cover a wide range of EM imaging modalities. Proper software libraries for simulation of passage of particles through matter can be based on Monte Carlo methods, so with appropriate cross sections, a variety of physical phenomena can be included into the simulation. Examples relevant for EM are simulation of transmitted electrons (both elastic and inelastic), secondary electrons, back-scattered electrons, and emission of characteristic X-rays. Furthermore, charged particle optical elements (e.g., phase plates and stigmators), energy filters and detector characteristics can be simulated with high-level accuracy.

## References


1. Brody I (1966). Intercellular space in normal human *stratum corneum*, *Nature*, **209**, 472–476.

2. Breathnach AS, Goodman T, Stolinski C, and Gross M (1973). Freeze fracture replication of cells of *stratum corneum* of human epidermis, *J Anat*, **114**, 65–81.

3. Elias PM and Friend DS (1975). The permeability barrier in mammalian epidermis, *J Cell Biol*, **65**, 180–191.

4. Wertz P and Norlén L (2003). "Confidence intervals" for the "true" lipid composition of the human skin barrier, in *Skin, Hair and Nails: Structure and Function* (Forslind B and Lindberg M, eds), Marcel Dekker, New York, pp. 85–106.

5. Masukawa Y, Narita H, Sato H, Naoe A, Kondo N, Sugai Y, Oba T, Homma R, Ishikawa J, Takagi Y, and Kitahara T (2009). Comprehensive quantification of ceramide species in human *stratum corneum*, *J Lipid Res*, **50**, 1708–1719.

6. Norlén L, Öktem O, and Skoglund U (2009). Molecular cryo-electron tomography of vitreous tissue sections: current challenges, *J Microsc*, **235**, 293–307.

7. Iwai I, Han H, den Hollander L, Svensson S, Öfverstedt L-G, Anwar J, Brewer J, Bloksgaard Mølgaard M, Laloeuf A, Nosek D, Masich S, Bagatolli L, Skoglund U, and Norlén L (2012). The human skin barrier is organized as stacked bilayers of fully-extended ceramides with cholesterol molecules associated with the ceramide sphingoid moiety, *J Invest Dermatol*, **132**, 2215–2225.

8. Norlén L (2012). Skin Lipids, in *Encyclopedia of Biophysics* (Roberts GCK, ed.), Springer-Verlag, Berlin Heidelberg, 5, pp. 2368–2373.

9. Swartzendruber DC, Wertz PW, Kitko DJ, Madison KC, and Downing DT (1989). Molecular models of the intercellular lipid lamellae in mammalian *stratum corneum*, *J Invest Dermatol*, **92**, 251–257.

10. Forslind B (1994). A domain mosaic model of the skin barrier, *Acta Derm Venereol* (*Stockh*), **74**, 1–6.

11. Bouwstra JA, Dubbelaar FER, Gooris GS, and Ponec M (2000). The lipid organisation in the skin barrier, *Acta Derm Venerol Suppl* (*Stockh*), **208**, 23–30.

12. Hill JR and Wertz PW (2003). Molecular models of the intercellular lipid lamellae from epidermal *stratum corneum*, *Biochim Biophys Acta*, **1616**(2), 121–126.

13. McIntosh TJ (2003). Organization of skin *stratum corneum* extracellular lamellae: diffraction evidence for asymmetric distribution of cholesterol, *Biophys J*, **85**, 1675–1681.

14. Schröter A, Kessner D, Kiselev MA, Hauss T, Dante S, and Neubert RHH (2009). Basic nanostructure of *stratum corneum* lipid matrices based on ceramides [EOS] and [AP]: a neutron diffraction study, *Biophys J*, **97**, 1–11.

15. Studer D, Michel M, Wohlvend M, Hunziker EB, and Buschmann M (1995). Vitrification of articular cartilage by high-pressure freezing, *J Microsc*, **179**, 321–332.

16. Al-Amoudi A, Norlén L, and Dubochet J (2004). Cryo-electron microscopy of vitreous sections of native biological cells and tissues, *J Struct Biol*, **148**(1), 131–135.

17. Rullgård H, Öfverstedt L-G, Masich S, Daneholt B, and Öktem O (2011). Simulation of transmission electron microscope images of biological specimens, *J Microsc*, **243**(3), 234–256.

18. Gilbert PFC (1972). Iterative methods for the three-dimensional reconstruction of an object from projections, *J Theor Biol*, **36**, 105–117.

19. Bracewell RN and Riddle AC (1967). Inversion of fan-beam scans in radion astronomy, *Astrophys J*, **150**, 427–434.

20. Engl HW, Hanke M, and Neubauer A (eds) (1996). *Regularization of Inverse Problems*, Kluwer Academic Publishers, Dordrecht.

21. De Rosier DJ and Klug A (1968). Reconstruction of three dimensional structures from electron micrographs, *Nature*, **217**, 130–134.

22. Vainshtein BK (1970). Finding the structure of objects from projections, *Kristallograftya*, **15**(5), 894–902, Translated in *Soviet Physics-Crystallography*, **15**, 781–787.

23. Hoppe W, Langer R, Knesch G, and Poppe C (1968). Protein-Kristallstrukturanalyse mit Elektronenstrahlen, *Naturwissenschaften*, **55**, 333–336.

24. Herman GT (ed) (1980). *Image Reconstruction from Projections: The Fundamentals of Computerized Tomography*, Academic Press, New York.

25. Frangakis AS and Hegerl R (2001). Noise reduction in electron tomographic reconstructions using nonlinear anisotropic diffusion, *J Struct Biol*, **135**, 239–250.

26. Narasimha R, Aganj I, Borgnia M, Sapiro G, McLaughlin S, Milne J, and Subramaniam S (2006). From gigabytes to bytes: Automated denoising and feature identification in electron tomograms of intact bacterial cells, *IMA Preprint Series 2145*, Mineapolis.

27. Frangakis AS and Hegerl R (2006). Segmentation of three-dimensional electron tomographic images, in *Electron Tomography. Methods for Three-Dimensional Visualization of Structures in the Cell* (Frank J, ed.), Springer Verlag, 2nd edition, New York, pp. 353–370.

28. van der Heide P, Xu X-P, Marsh BJ, Hanein D, and Volkmann N (2007). Efficient automatic noise reduction of electron tomographic reconstructions based on iterative median filtering, *J Struct Biol*, **158**, 196–204.

29. Kaczmarz S (1937). Angenäherte Auflösung von Systemen linearer Gleichungen, *Bull Int Acad Pol Sci Lett, Cl Sci Math Nat, A Sci Math*, **35**, 355–357.

30. Landweber L (1951). An iteration formula for Fredholm integral equations of the first kind, *Am J Math*, **73**, 615–624.

31. Gordon R, Bender R, and Herman GT (1970). Algebraic reconstruction techniques (ART) for three-dimensional electron microscopy and X-ray photography, *J Theor Biol*, **29**, 471–481.

32. Carazo J-M, Herman GT, Sorzano COS, and Marabini R (2006). Algorithms for three-dimensional reconstruction from the imperfect projection data provided by electron microscopy, in *Electron Tomography: Methods for Three-Dimensional Visualization of Structures in the Cell* (Frank J, ed), Springer Verlag, 2nd edition, New York, pp. 217–243.

33. Schoenmakers R, Perquin RA, Fliervoet TF, and Voorhout W (2005). High resolution, high throughput electron tomography reconstruction, *Microsc Microanal*, **11**(suppl 2), 312–313.

34. Voorhout W, De Haas F, Frederik P, Schoenmakers R, Busing W, and Hubert D (2006). An optimized solution for cryo-electron tomography, *Microsc Microanal*, **12**, 1110–1111.

35. Furuie SS, Herman GT, Narayan TK, Kinahan PE, Karp JS, Lewitt RM, and Matej S (1994). A methodology for testing for statistically significant differences between fully 2D PET reconstruction algorithms, *Phys Med Biol*, **39**, 341–354.

36. Skoglund U, Öfverstedt L-G, Burnett RM, and Bricogne G (1996). Maximum-entropy three-dimensional reconstruction with deconvolution of the contrast transfer function: a test application with Adenovirus, *J Struct Biol*, **117**, 173–188.

37. Rullgård H, Öktem O, and Skoglund U (2007). A component-wise iterated relative entropy regularization method with updated prior and regularization parameter, *Inverse Probl*, **23**, 2121–2139.

38. Carazo JM, Sorzano COS, Reitzel E, Schröder R, and Marabini R (1999). Discrete tomography in electron microscopy, in *Discrete Tomography: Foundations, Algorithms and Applications* (Herman GT and Kuba A, eds), Birkhäuser, Boston, pp. 405–416.

39. Liao HY and Herman GT (2006). A method for reconstructing label images from a few projections, as motivated by electron microscopy, *Ann Oper Res*, **148**, 117–132.

40. Aganj I, Bartesaghi A, Borgnia M, Liao HY, Sapiro G, and Subramaniam S (2006). Regularization for inverting the Radon transform with wedge consideration, *IMA Preprint Series 2144*, Mineapolis.

41. Lawrence A, Bouwer JC, Perkins GA, and Ellisman MH (2006). Transform-based backprojection for volume reconstruction of large format electron microscope tilt series, *J Struct Biol*, **154**, 144–167.

42. Quinto ET and Öktem O (2008). Local tomography in electron microscopy, *SIAM J Appl Math*, **68**(5), 1282–1303.

43. Quinto ET, Skoglund U, and Oktem O. (2009). Electron lambda-tomography, *Proc Natl Acad Sci USA*, **106**(51), 21842–21847.

44. Peng L-M, Dudarev SL, and Whelan MJ (eds) (2004). *High-Energy Electron Diffraction and Microscopy, Monographs on the Physics and Chemistry of Materials, volume 61*, Oxford University Press, USA.

45. Fanelli F and Öktem O (2008). Electron tomography: A short overview with an emphasis on the absorption potential model for the forward problem, *Inverse Probl*, **24**, 013001.1-013001.51.

46. Hawkes PW and Kasper E (eds) (1994). *Principles of Electron Optics, Volume 3, Wave Optics*, Academic Press, San Diego.

47. Reimer L (ed) (2008). *Transmission Electron Microscopy, volume 36, Springer series in optical sciences*, Springer Verlag, 5th edition, New York.

48. Lassas L, Saksman E, and Siltanen S (2009). Discretization invariant Bayesian inversion and Besov space priors, *Inverse Probl Imag*, **3**, 87–122.

49. Burger M and Osher S (2004). Convergence rates of convex variational regularization, *Inverse Probl*, **20**, 1411–1421.

50. Elad M (ed) (2010). *Sparse and Redundant Representations: From Theory to Applications in Signal and Image Processing*, Springer Verlag, New York.

51. Burger M and Osher S (2004). Convergence rates of convex variational regularization, *Inverse Probl*, **20**, 1411–1421.

52. Rullgård H (2008). A new principle for choosing regularization parameter in certain inverse problems, arxiv:0803.3713v2, http://arxiv.org/abs/0803.3713.

53. Klann E (2011). A Mumford-Shah-like method for limited data tomography with an application to electron tomography, *SIAM J Imaging Sci*, **4**(4), 1029–1048.

54. Gopinath A, Xu G, Ress D, Öktem O, Subramaniam S, and Bajaj C (2012). Shape based regularization of electron tomography reconstruction, *IEEE T Med Imaging*, **31**(12), 2241–2252.

55. Younes L (2010). *Shapes and Diffeomorphisms, Applied Mathematical Sciences, volume 171*, Springer Verlag, Berlin Heidelberg.

56. Grenander U and Miller M (2007). *Pattern Theory: From Representation to Inference*, Oxford Studies in Modern European Culture, Oxford University Press, USA.

57. Evans SN and Stark PB (2002). Inverse problems as statistics, *Inverse Probl*, **18**, 55–97.

58. Kaipio J and Somersalo E (eds) (2005). *Statistical and Computational Inverse Problems, Applied Mathematical Sciences, volume 160*, Springer Verlag, Berlin Heidelberg.

59. Kolehmainen V, Siltanen S, Jarvenpaa S, Kaipio JP, Koistinen P, Lassas M, Pirttila J, and Somersalo J (2013). Statistical inversion for medical X-ray tomography with few radiographs II: Application to dental radiology, *Phys Med Biol*, **48**, 1465–1490.

60. Bajaj C, Djeu P, Siddavanahalli V, and Thane A (2004). TexMol: Interactive Visual Exploration of Large Flexible Multi-component Molecular Complexes, in *Proceedings of the Annual IEEE Visualization Conference*, IEEE Computer Society Press, Austin, pp. 243–250.

# Part 4

# Skin Fluids and Components

# Chapter 11

# Water Diffusion through *Stratum Corneum*

Bob Imhof[a] and Perry Xiao[b]

[a]*Biox Systems Ltd, Technopark Building,*
*90 London Road, London SE1 6LN, England*
[b]*London South Bank University,*
*London SE1 0AA, England*

bob@biox.biz

## 11.1    Introduction

The epidermal barrier resides in the *stratum corneum* (SC) and is essential to life. It protects from dehydration, poisoning and microbial attack. However, the SC is not an impenetrable barrier. Free water from the viable tissues (VT) continually diffuses through the SC, evaporating from the SC surface. This is known as TransEpidermal Water Loss (TEWL). TEWL is important because it can be used to quantify the barrier property of the SC. TEWL measurement by evaporimetry is well-established, non-invasive and widely used for this purpose.

The aim of the model presented in this chapter is to provide a means to understand how skin interacts with the air in contact with it and how this interaction affects the steady-state SC

*Computational Biophysics of the Skin*
Edited by Bernard Querleux

properties of hydration and TEWL. The model represents in vivo skin, but can also be adapted to represent ex vivo or in vitro constructs that mimic in vivo skin, i.e. dry on top, wet underneath. The air-side uses a fluid dynamic representation of ambient air, but this can be adapted to represent the microclimate inside the measurement chambers of evaporimeters used for TEWL measurement, for example. The model can also be used to calculate changes following SC perturbations such as tape stripping. However, the model is restricted to steady-state properties—dynamic processes require a different approach. Also, this is a physics-based mathematical model, incapable of representing biological changes that undoubtedly accompany physical changes.

The physical aspects of the model presented in this chapter are similar to those assumed by Miller et al. [1]. They used a finite difference method to calculate the dependence of steady-state TEWL on ambient humidity for the case of an open-chamber evaporimeter. As in the present work, a sorption isotherm was used as a boundary condition at the SC/air interface.

## 11.2  Assumptions and Approximations

Given the complexity of bio-systems, any practical physics-based model will rely heavily on assumptions and approximations. The global ones used in this model are listed here, the more specific ones are presented within the context in which they arise:

(1)  simplified skin structure of SC atop a substrate of VT
(2)  structureless and uniform SC of constant thickness and diffusion coefficient
(3)  steady-state conditions only
(4)  one-dimensional diffusion only
(5)  water is condensed within the tissues and evaporates from the SC surface
(6)  the SC/air interaction is calculated from the sorption isotherm
(7)  free water only; water binding effects are subsumed into an effective diffusion coefficient

(8) the temperature of the air immediately adjacent to the SC surface is equal to the SC surface temperature

Temperature is an important variable, but not everywhere. Physical properties such as diffusion coefficient and layer thickness depend only weakly on temperature and this is ignored. But air temperature is important, because it affects relative humidity.

Of course, these assumptions and approximations can be modified to make the model more realistic. Effects such as SC swelling, temperature-dependent sorption and hydration-dependent diffusion coefficient can readily be included. However, this chapter is about the approach rather than the detail.

## 11.3  Notation and Abbreviations

The main symbols used in the calculations and the abbreviations used in the text are defined in Table 11.1. SI units are used in all equations, but calculated results are converted to common units for presentation purposes. Note that it is common practice to express relative humidity (RH) as a percentage, whereas SI uses fractional RH. Absolute humidity (vapour density) is preferred to vapour pressure to maintain consistency of treatment for vapour and condensed water.

**Table 11.1**  Summary of notation and abbreviations

| Notation | | |
| --- | --- | --- |
| **Symbol** | **Unit** | **Definition** |
| $\theta$ | °C | Temperature |
| $\chi$ | SI | Relative humidity ($\chi$ = 0–1 for RH = 0–100%) |
| $h$ | $kgm^{-3}$ | Absolute humidity (vapour density) |
| $c$ | $kgm^{-3}$ | Concentration of condensed water |
| $J$ | $kgm^{-2}s^{-1}$ | Flux density |
| $L$ | m | Thickness |
| $D$ | $m^2s^{-1}$ | Mass diffusion coefficient |

*(Continued)*

**Table 11.1** (*Continued*)

|  | Abbreviations |  |
| --- | --- | --- |
| **Abbreviation** | **Unit** | **Definition** |
| SI |  | International System of Units (Système international d'unités) |
| SC |  | *Stratum corneum* |
| VT |  | Viable tissues |
| RH | % | Relative humidity |
| TEWL | $gm^{-2}h^{-1}$ | TransEpidermal water loss |
| SSWL | $gm^{-2}$ | Skin surface water loss |

## 11.4 Components of the Model

The model consists of seven components: two skin-side regions, two air-side regions and three boundaries, as illustrated in Fig. 11.1.

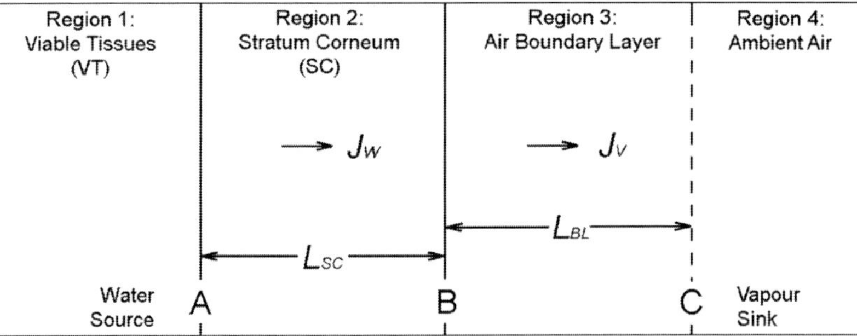


**Figure 11.1** Components of the model consisting of two skin-side regions, two air-side regions and three boundaries. Note that the TEWL flux density $J_W$ changes to a water vapor flux density $J_V$ at the SC/air interface.

### 11.4.1 Skin-Side Properties

The skin is represented by two regions, namely a VT substrate with a SC layer on top. Their main properties are as follows:

**Region 1: Viable Tissues**

The intercellular fluid of the VT is assumed to be the source of water for TEWL. Its water concentration $c_{VT}$ is taken as constant, maintaining a constant hydration of the base of the SC, irrespective of the magnitude of the TEWL flux. The temperature of this region does not feature in the model.

**Region 2: *Stratum Corneum***

The SC is treated as a structureless and uniform layer of thickness $L_{SC}$. Its low diffusion coefficient for water, $D_{SC}$, is the reason why it is an effective barrier to water loss. Depending on the TEWL flux, the water concentration within the SC decreases linearly towards the surface, in accordance with Fick's first law of diffusion. Only the temperature of the SC surface is important in the model.

## 11.4.2 Air-Side Properties

The air is also represented by two regions based on established boundary layer concepts of fluid dynamics [2,3]. Their main properties are as follows:

**Region 3: Air Boundary Layer**

The air adjacent to the SC is still irrespective of any air movements in the ambient air beyond, because of air viscosity and frictional forces at the SC/air interface. The thickness of this boundary layer, $L_{BL}$, depends on air movements in complex ways, including velocity, turbulence, the size, shape and orientation of the object, etc. Wheldon and Monteith [3] give equations for estimating boundary layer thickness for the human body in both forced and natural convection conditions. Representing the volar forearm as a cylinder of ~8 cm diameter, these give a typical value for normal indoor conditions of $L_{BL} \sim 3$ mm, with values as large as $L_{BL} \sim 7$ mm possible in still conditions. These values are not stable and are perturbed by minor air movements, normal body movements and breathing. Within the boundary layer, diffusion is assumed to be the only transport mechanism for water vapour and heat. The temperature of the air at the SC surface is assumed to be equal to the SC surface temperature. This is important because RH is temperature-dependent.

### Region 4: Ambient Air

The ambient air beyond the boundary layer is assumed to be the sink for the water vapour flux. Its RH and temperature are taken as constant, irrespective of the magnitude of the TEWL flux or the thickness of the diffusion boundary layer.

## 11.4.3  Boundary Properties

The four regions described above are delimited by three boundaries. Their properties are assumed to be as follows:

### Boundary A between Regions 1 and 2

This is the boundary between the VT and the SC. It is characterised by an abrupt change of water diffusion coefficient, from an effectively infinite value within the VT to a finite and generally low value, $D_{SC}$, within the SC. Water concentration is assumed to be continuous across this boundary.

### Boundary B between Regions 2 and 3

This is the boundary between the SC and the adjacent air, where there is a discontinuous change from condensed water to water vapour. Equilibrium conditions are assumed to hold at this boundary, where the relationship between SC surface hydration and RH in the immediately adjacent air is assumed to be determined by the sorption isotherm; see Section 11.5. The TEWL flux changes to water vapour flux across this boundary.

### Boundary C between Regions 3 and 4

This boundary marks the transition between the still-air microclimate within the boundary layer and ambient conditions of RH, temperature and air movement. It is characterised by an abrupt change from diffusion transport within the boundary layer to the steady sink conditions of ambient air.

## 11.5   SC/Air Interaction

It is well known that keratinised tissues such as SC are hygroscopic, with properties such as hydration, elasticity, diffusion coefficient and swelling changing in response to changes of humidity in the adjacent air [4]. Water–keratin interactions are commonly characterised as sorption isotherms that relate equilibrium water uptake of isolated in vitro samples to the RH of the surrounding air. Of course, such isotherms are bulk properties of in vitro samples and it may not be correct to assume that they can be used to characterise in vivo SC. However, Blank et al. [5] argued that it is reasonable to expect that the outside cell layer of in vivo SC will have a similar hydration to that of a piece of in vitro SC exposed to the same conditions of temperature and humidity. The cell layers below the surface will additionally be hydrated from the VT, with a hydration gradient consistent with TEWL. On this basis, the sorption isotherm of in vitro SC can be used as a boundary condition that must be satisfied in vivo under steady-state conditions.

The present calculations use a parametric representation of the sorption isotherm of an in vitro sample of SC reported by Lévêque [4] and illustrated in Fig. 11.2.

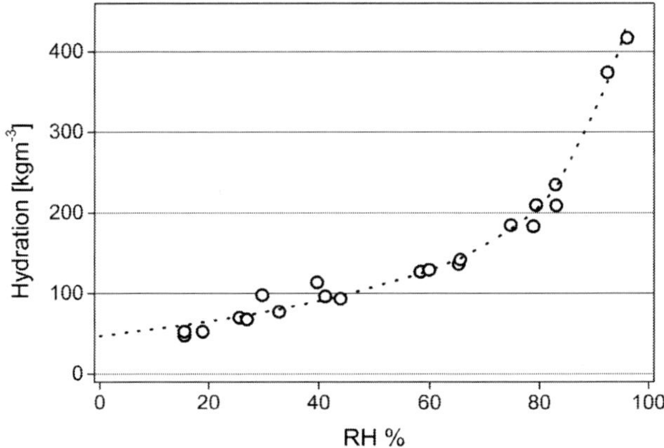


**Figure 11.2**   Sorption isotherm for excised SC. The points are from [4], the dotted line is a least-squares parameterization.

Note the following when using a sorption isotherm as a boundary condition of the model:

(1) The sorption properties of SC vary with individual, site, skin health and time. The present work uses just one sorption isotherm in the model calculations.

(2) The sorption properties of SC also change with temperature, but this is not taken into account in the present work.

(3) There is hysteresis in the relationship between hydration and RH. Hydration values measured from low to high RH (absorption isotherm) are lower than those measured from high to low RH (desorption isotherm). This effect is not taken into account in the present work.

(4) The parametric representation used in the calculation does not go to zero water content at zero RH. This is deliberate. Zero water content can only be achieved by deep dehydration (elevated temperatures, vacuum) that is inapplicable to in vivo SC.

(5) There can be significant differences between SC surface RH and ambient RH, because the temperature of the air in contact with the SC is generally higher than ambient temperature. This has the effect of shifting the onset of the steeply rising part of the sorption isotherm to higher values of ambient RH than is commonly assumed.

## 11.6   Calculations

The approach is to calculate skin-side TEWL flux and air-side water vapour flux densities separately before combining them in a self-consistent way.

### 11.6.1   Skin-Side Calculation

The skin-side calculation uses Fick's first law to relate the TEWL flux density, $J_W$, to the above-defined quantities, as illustrated in Fig. 11.3.

Thus,

$$J_W = D_{SC} \frac{c_A - c_B}{L_{SC}} \tag{11.1}$$

The concentration $c_A$ at Boundary A and the SC thickness $L_{SC}$ are typically treated as known user inputs.

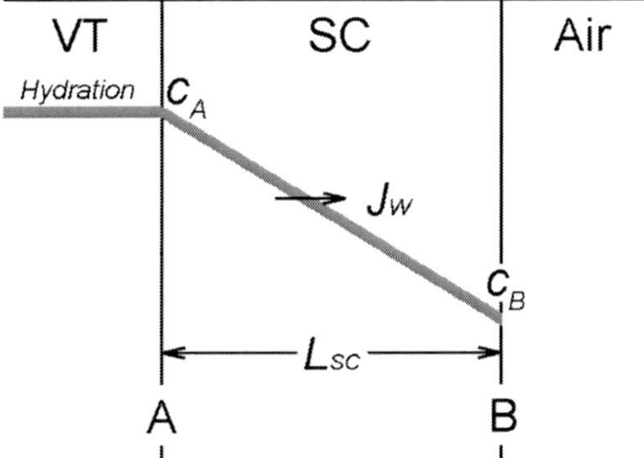

**Figure 11.3**   Diagram to illustrate the skin-side calculation.

## 11.6.2   Air-Side Calculation

The air-side calculation similarly uses Fick's first law to relate the water vapour flux density, $J_V$, to the above-defined quantities, as illustrated in Fig. 11.4.

Thus,

$$J_V = D_{VA} \frac{h_B - h_C}{L_{BL}} \tag{11.2}$$

The ambient temperature $\theta_C$ and humidity $h_C$ (at Boundary C), the air temperature $\theta_B$ at the SC surface (at Boundary B) and the boundary layer thickness $L_{BL}$ are typically treated as user inputs.

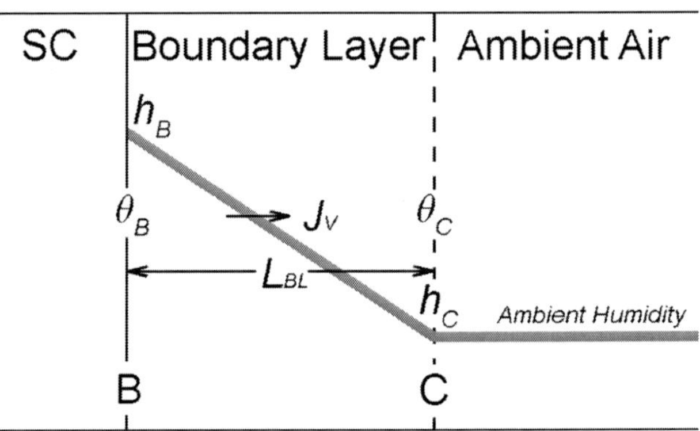

**Figure 11.4**   Diagram to illustrate the air-side calculation.

### 11.6.3   Combined Model Calculation

The calculations for the combined model bring the skin-side and air-side calculations together. Two boundary conditions must be satisfied at the SC/air interface. These are

(1)  **Flux Continuity.** The TEWL flux density $J_W$ on the skin-side must be equal to the water vapour flux density $J_V$ on the air side.

(2)  **Sorption.** SC surface hydration $c_B$ must be consistent with the humidity $h_B$ of the immediately adjacent air in accordance with the sorption isotherm.

The use of the sorption boundary condition requires conversion between absolute and relative humidity, which is done using

$$\chi = \frac{h(\theta)}{h_{\text{sat}}(\theta)}, \tag{11.3}$$

where the absolute humidity at saturation $h_{\text{sat}}$ is calculated using the Lowe polynomial [6] together with the ideal gas law.

## 11.7   Results and Discussion

In this section, we present a number of specific calculations to illustrate how the model can be used and adapted. The calculations require a one-parameter iteration to find solutions that satisfy the SC/air boundary conditions. The method of iteration used was adapted from a gradient-search non-linear least-squares algorithm. The iterated parameter is either $J_W$ or $D_{SC}$, depending on the purpose of the calculation. In Table 11.2 for example, $D_{SC}$ was iterated in order to determine its value when $J_W = 10$ gm$^{-2}$h$^{-1}$. In a subsequent calculation, this value of $D_{SC}$ may be used as a constant in order to explore changes of $J_W$ with parameters such as ambient temperature or RH.

Unless otherwise stated, the calculations presented in this section use parameter values from Table 11.2, which are typical of volar forearm SC in a normal indoor environment. Note that common units are used in the table and text, but SI units are used in the equations.

**Table 11.2**   Typical parameters values used in the calculations

| Parameters of Skin | | | |
|---|---|---|---|
| **Symbol** | **Value** | **Unit** | **Description** |
| $J_W$ | 10 | $\text{gm}^{-2}\text{h}^{-1}$ | TEWL flux density |
| $L_{SC}$ | 15 | µm | SC thickness |
| $c_A$ | 700 | $\text{kgm}^{-3}$ | Water concentration at the base of the SC |
| **Parameters of Air** | | | |
| **Symbol** | **Value** | **Unit** | **Description** |
| $L_{BL}$ | 5 | mm | Boundary layer thickness |
| $\theta_B$ | 30 | °C | Air temperature at the SC surface |
| $\theta_C$ | 20 | °C | Ambient air temperature |
| $\text{RH}_C$ | 50 | % | Ambient RH |
| $D_{VA}$ | $2.42 \times 10^{-5}$ | $\text{m}^2\text{s}^{-1}$ | Diffusion coefficient for water vapour in air |
| **Calculated Quantities** | | | |
| **Symbol** | **Value** | **Unit** | **Description** |
| $D_{SC}$ | $6.7 \times 10^{-14}$ | $\text{m}^2\text{s}^{-1}$ | SC Diffusion coefficient for water (for $J_W = 10\ \text{gm}^{-2}\text{h}^{-1}$) |
| $c_B$ | 76.4 | $\text{kgm}^{-3}$ | Water concentration at the SC surface |
| $(c_A + c_B)/2$ | 389 | $\text{kgm}^{-3}$ | Mean SC hydration |
| $\text{RH}_B$ | 30 | % | Microclimate RH immediately adjacent to the SC surface |

The calculated quantities in Table 11.2 conform with reasonable expectations, except maybe for a microclimate RH of 30% immediately adjacent to the SC surface, which is substantially lower than ambient RH. This is a direct consequence of the higher than ambient temperature of the air immediately adjacent to the SC surface, as noted in Section 11.5. Another quantity of interest is the mean hydration of the SC. With a linear concentration gradient, this is simply calculated as the mean of the base and surface hydration values $(c_A + c_B)/2$.

## 11.7.1   Normal Volar Forearm SC Barrier Property

For these calculations, $D_{SC}$ was held constant while changes of TEWL with ambient RH or SC surface temperature were explored.

The model predicts a weak, monotonically decreasing TEWL with increasing ambient RH, contradicting experimental evidence of an opposite trend [7]. According to the model, an increased RH leads to an increased SC surface hydration via the sorption isotherm. This leads to a decreased water concentration change across the SC and hence a decreased TEWL.

The model also predicts a weak, monotonically increasing TEWL with increasing SC surface temperature, typically by ~0.3% per °C. The cause of this increase is the decrease of SC surface RH with temperature. This is much less than the ~7% per °C TEWL increase reported by Halkier-Sorensen et al. [8], which, however, may have medical rather than physical origin. If it were physical in origin, then this could have come from temperature dependences of SC sorption and diffusion coefficient, which are neglected in these calculations

## 11.7.2 Normal Volar Forearm SC Surface Hydration

For these calculations, $D_{SC}$ was held constant while changes of SC surface hydration with ambient RH and temperature were explored. In the curves presented in Fig. 11.5, the sorption isotherm is the main influence, modified by the lowered RH of the warmer than ambient air immediately adjacent to the SC surface. Of lesser influence are the values of water vapour flux density and boundary layer thickness, both tending to increase the RH immediately adjacent to the SC surface.

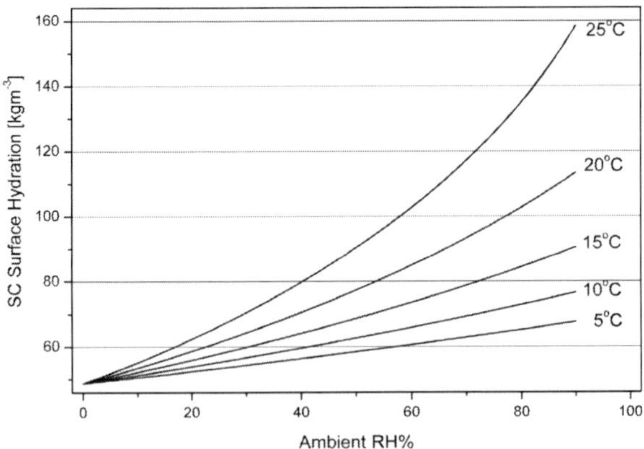


**Figure 11.5** Dependence of SC surface hydration on ambient RH and temperature.

### 11.7.3   Effect of Tape Stripping

Tape stripping of the SC [9] is a minimally invasive technique for studying SC properties in pharmaceutical, medical, cosmetic and other research. Of interest are the properties of the stripped SC and the quantity and composition of the material removed by the tapes. The model can be used to calculate steady-state TEWL and hydration and relate these to the thickness of SC removed by the tapes.

The tape stripping process is modelled in three stages as follows:

**Stage 1** is before stripping, when the SC surface, at point 1 in Fig. 11.6, is in equilibrium with the ambient environment. Surface hydration, hydration gradient & TEWL values are all stable.

**Stage 2** is stripping, where a thickness $\Delta L_{SC}$ of SC is removed quasi instantaneously by the tape or tapes. Immediately after stripping, the hydration gradient within the remaining SC is unaltered, because a gradient change would require a redistribution of water throughout the SC by the relatively slow mechanism of diffusion. Therefore, the surface hydration immediatley after stripping is elevated by an amount that can be calculated from this gradient and $\Delta L_{SC}$, as indicated by point 2 in Fig. 11.6. The excess surface hydration leads to an increased humidity $h_B$ in the immediately adjacent air via the sorption isotherm which, according to Eq. 11.2 leads to an increased water vapour flux $J_V$. However, since the hydration gradient within the SC is unaltered, $J_W$ (TEWL) must, according to Eq. 11.1 be unaltered. Therefore, the increased water loss into the adjacent air is SSWL, not TEWL. In this non-equilibrium state immediately after stripping, $J_V$ is higher than $J_W$—the SC is losing excess water by evaporation.

**Stage 3** is acclimatisation, where the new SC surface returns to equilibrium with the adjacent air. The SC/air boundary conditions cause the surface hydration to decrease to a new equilibrium value denoted by point 3 in Fig. 11.6. This is lower than the non-equilibrium value at point 2, but higher than the pre-stripping value at point 1. Water within the remaining SC re-distributes by diffusion in response to this hydration change at the surface, to establish a new and steeper linear hydration gradient. The steeper hydration gradient leads to an increased TEWL. The SSWL of Stage 2 decays to zero as the excess hydration is depleted. When fully acclimatised, $J_V$ and $J_W$ are again equal.

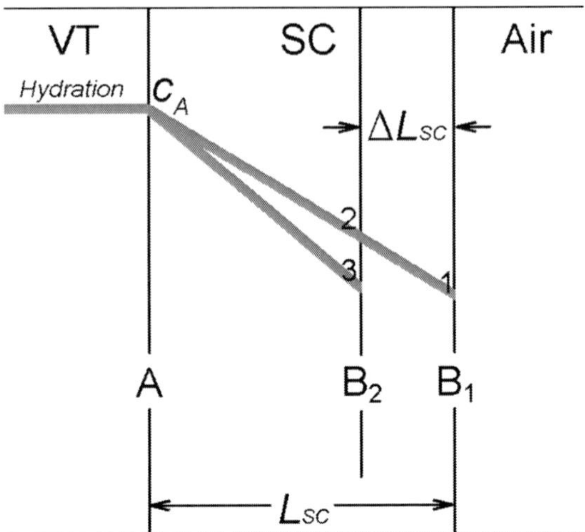


**Figure 11.6** Model of the tape stripping process.

The dynamic changes during Stage 3 are outwith the scope of this model, although it would be useful to be able to calculate the rate at which the SC acclimatises to a new steady state after perturbation. A rough value can be calculated from $\Delta t$, the characteristic time constant of diffusion [2]

$$\Delta t = \frac{(L_{SC} - \Delta L_{SC})^2}{\pi D_{SC}} \tag{11.4}$$

which works out to $\Delta t \sim 15$ min for Table 11.2 values with $\Delta L_{SC}$ = 2 μm. Acclimatisation before measurement is therefore important.

For the calculations below, $D_{SC}$ was held constant while changes of hydration, hydration gradient and TEWL during tape stripping were explored.

In Fig. 11.7, the black lines are equilibrium hydration gradients within the remaining SC as layers are removed 1 μm at a time. The black points are equilibrium surface hydration, with their locus indicated by the dotted line. The open circles are non-equilibrium surface hydration immediately after stripping.

The change of steady-state TEWL during stripping is illustrated in Fig. 11.8, where the reciprocal of TEWL is plotted against thickness of SC removed.

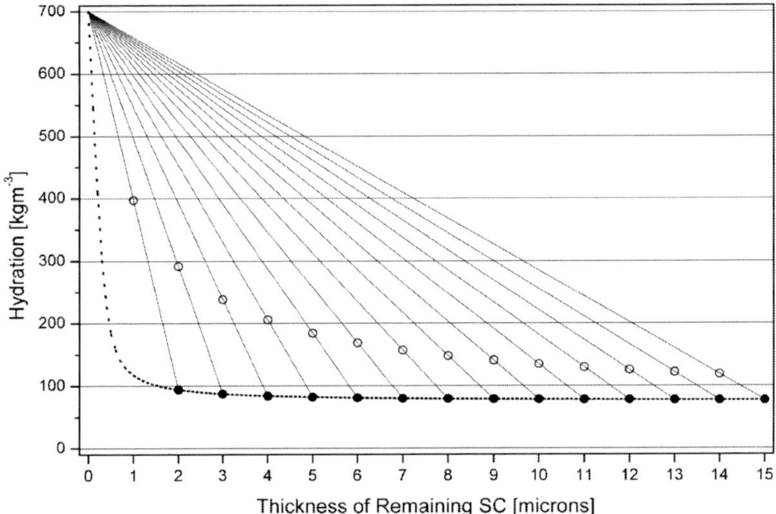



**Figure 11.7**  Changes of SC Hydration and hydration gradient during tape stripping, as layers are removed 1 μm at a time.

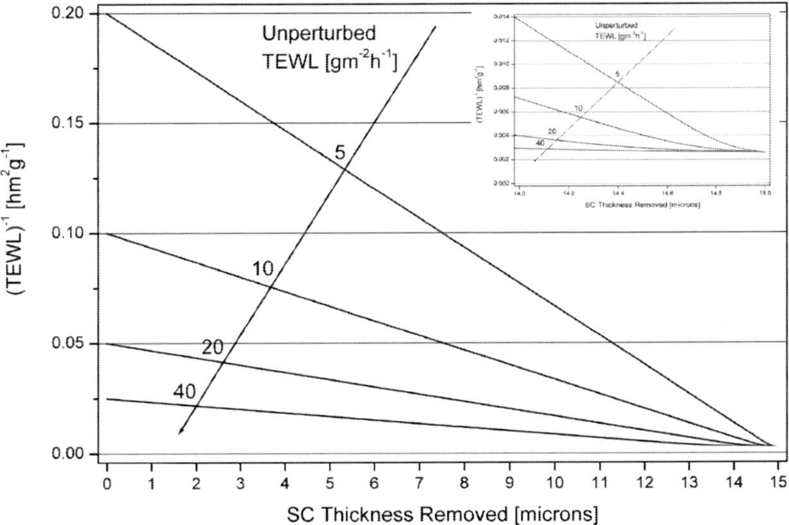



**Figure 11.8**  Near-linear change of $(TEWL)^{-1}$ as SC is removed by tape stripping for a range of unperturbed TEWL values. The insert shows deviations from linearity as the final 1 μm of SC is removed.

The remarkable linearity of the $(TEWL)^{-1}$ lines with thickness removed has been used by Kalia et al. to measure SC thickness [10]. There are three main differences between the model they used and the one presented here, as follows:

(1) Model [10] does not take SC/air interactions into account, approximating SC surface hydration to $c_B = 0$ under all conditions. The deviations of the $(TEWL)^{-1}$ lines from linearity shown in Fig. 11.8, or their dependence on ambient conditions, are therefore not predicted.

(2) Model [10] assumes that TEWL can increase without limit, with $(TEWL)^{-1} = 0$ for fully stripped skin. Of course, TEWL is not an appropriate descriptor in this limit, where microclimate rather than the SC barrier controls the water loss. In the model presented here, SC/air interaction is taken into account and the water loss of fully stripped skin approximates more realistically to a typical barrier-free evaporation rate.

(3) Model [10] assumes that water transport through the SC is restricted to the lipid matrix with only ~6% of the free water of the VT partitioning into it. This has the effect of increasing by a factor ~10 the diffusion coefficient in Eq. 11.1 for the same SC thickness and TEWL. This does not affect steady-state properties, but reduces the characteristic time constant of diffusion, $\Delta t$ of Eq. 11.4 by the same factor. The estimated acclimatisation time then works out to ~1.8 min for the typical values in Table 11.2. This is a fundamental difference that is amenable to experimental verification.

Despite these differences, the linear relationship between SC thickness removed and $(TEWL)^{-1}$ provides a useful means for measuring SC thickness in a minimally invasive way. Thickness values calculated by the two models agree closely, within ~1% for a wide range of conditions. Of course, this conclusion may change with more realistic models, where SC swelling and hydration-dependent diffusion rates are taken into account, for example.

## 11.8 Further Developments

The model presented in this chapter can be developed further to include the effects of hydration-dependent swelling and diffusion, and temperature-dependent sorption.

SC swelling can be assumed to be additive in a first approximation, where the volume of hydrated SC is given by the sum of the volumes of dry SC and water of hydration. With this assumption,

$$\frac{\Delta L}{L_{\mathrm{DRY}}} = \frac{c}{3(\rho_{\mathrm{W}} - c)},$$

(11.5)

where $\Delta L$ is the hydration-dependent swelling, $L_{\mathrm{DRY}}$ is the thickness of dry SC and $\rho_{\mathrm{W}}$ is the density of water. The above result assumes that the swelling is isotropic. If in-plane swelling is constrained, swelling becomes unidirectional (in thickness only) when the thickness change would be three times larger.

Our starting point for hydration-dependent diffusion is the work of Wu on fetal hog periderm [11] and in vivo volar forearm [12], from which they proposed the following representation:

$$D_{\mathrm{SC}}(c) = D_{\mathrm{SC}}(0)(1 + k_1 c^{k_2}),$$

(11.6)

where $D_{\mathrm{SC}}(0)$, is the diffusion coefficient of dry SC and the constants $k_1$ and $k_2$ work out to $8.26 \times 10^7$ and 0.69, respectively.

Both effects can be incorporated into the model by dividing the SC into a number of layers. For the first layer, the hydration of the surface adjoining the VT is known. Use this value to calculate the layer's thickness and diffusion coefficient. These values, together with an assumed TEWL value are then used to calculate the hydration of the opposite face of the layer, which is also the hydration of the adjoining face of the next layer. And so on to calculate the total thickness of the SC and SC surface hydration. The assumed value of TEWL is then adjusted iteratively until the SC/air boundary conditions are satisfied. First indications from these calculations are disappointing—the model still fails to reverse the trend of monotonically decreasing TEWL with increasing ambient RH. But this is outwith the scope of this chapter.

## 11.9 Conclusions

The aim of the model presented in this chapter is to provide a means to understand how physical variables such as temperature and humidity affect the steady-state SC properties of hydration and TEWL. The approach is capable of further development, to include effects such as hydration-dependent diffusion and swelling, and temperature-dependent sorption, which have thus far been neglected. Comparisons of model predictions with experimental data can then be used to understand to what extent an observed property is physical rather than biological in nature. Another direction for further development is to model dynamic effects such as the rate of return to steady-state after a perturbation.

## References


1. Miller DL, Brown AM, and Artz EJ (1981). Indirect measures of transepidermal water loss, in *Bioengineering and the Skin* (Marks R and Payne PA, eds), MTP Press, Lancaster, pp. 161–171.

2. Çengel YA (ed) (1998). *Heat Transfer: A Practical Approach*, McGraw Hill, Boston.

3. Wheldon AE and Monteith JL (1980). Performance of a skin evaporimeter, *Med Biol Comput*, **18**, 201–205.

4. Lévêque J-L (1994). Water–keratin interactions, in *Bioengineering of the Skin: Water and the Stratum Corneum* (Elsner P, Berardesca E and Maibach HI, eds), CRC Press, Boca Raton, pp. 13–22.

5. Blank IH, Moloney J, Emslie AG, Simon I, and Apt C (1984). The diffusion of water across the *stratum corneum* as a function of its water content, *J Invest Dermatol*, **82**, 188–194.

6. Lowe PR (1997). An approximating polynomial for the computation of saturation vapour pressure, *J Appl Meteorol*, **16**, 100–103.

7. Egawa M, Oguri M, Kuwahara T, and Takahashi M (2002). Effect of exposure of human skin to a dry environment, *Skin Res Technol*, **8**, 212–218.

8. Halkier-Sorensen L, Thestrup-Pedersen K, and Maibach HI (1993). Equation for conversion of transepidermal water loss (TEWL) to a common reference temperature: what is the slope? *Contact Dermatitis*, **29**, 280–281.

9. Pinkus H (1951). Examination of the epidermis by the strip method of removing horny layers, *J Invest Dermatol*, **16**, 383–386.

10. Kalia YN, Pirot F, and Guy RH (1996). Homogeneous transport in a heterogeneous membrane: water diffusion across the human *stratum corneum* in vivo, *Biophys J*, **71**, 2692–2700.

11. Wu M-S (1983). Determination of concentration-dependent water diffusivity in a keratinous membrane, *J Pharm Sci*, **72**, 1421–1423.

12. Wu MS (1983). Water diffusivity and water concentration profile in human *stratum corneum* from transepidermal water loss measurement, *J Soc Cosmet Chem*, **34**, 191–196.

# Chapter 12

# Accurate Multiscale Skin Model Suitable for Determining the Sensitivity and Specificity of Changes of Skin Components


Jürg Fröhlich,[a] Sonja Huclova,[a] Christian Beyer,[a] and Daniel Erni[b]

[a]*Group for Electromagnetics in Medicine and Biology,*
*Institute of Electromagnetic Fields (IEF), ETH Zurich,*
*Gloriastrasse 35, CH-8092 Zurich, Switzerland*
[b]*General and Theoretical Electrical Engineering (ATE), Faculty of Engineering,*
*University of Duisburg-Essen, and CENIDE–Center for Nanointegration*
*Duisburg-Essen, D-47048 Duisburg, Germany*

juergfr@ethz.ch


In this chapter, we provide an overview of our own research carried out on the modeling of human skin in the framework of projects for assessing the suitability of transcutaneous monitoring of specific physiological changes, the measurement of dielectric changes in cell suspensions and by impedance flow cytometry. Different kinds of models of human skin are compared and applied to scenarios where a sensor is placed on top of human skin represented by a complex heterogeneous and partly anisotropic multilayer structure. These models are based on a rigorous analysis of all components present in human skin at different length scales. The aim was to identify the


*Computational Biophysics of the Skin*
Edited by Bernard Querleux
Copyright © 2014 Pan Stanford Publishing Pte. Ltd.
ISBN  978-981-4463-84-3 (Hardcover),  978-981-4463-85-0 (eBook)
www.panstanford.com

relevant features and structures that have to be taken into account in order to reliably reproduce measured dielectric spectroscopy data in the frequency range from MHz up to the virtually few GHz. Focusing on the relevant dispersion-dominated frequency region of 1–100 MHz models, including very different levels of details, are developed: First, a model including sublayers obtained from two-phase mixtures, second, including three-phase mixtures of cell-like core–shell ellipsoids and finally, including multiphase mixtures obtained from numerical models of single cells with flexible shapes using a surface parameterization based on superquadrics. All skin models are numerically evaluated using the finite element method (FEM) where the frequency response is retrieved from a fringing field sensor on top of the multilayer system serving as an impedance probe. Using these models, the achievable sensitivity and specificity are evaluated. Furthermore, measurements with a planar sensor probing skin in vivo were carried out. The validity of the models was tested by measuring the spectral response of the skin before and after removing the *stratum corneum*, which stands for the uppermost skin layer, and therefore for the most influential one. It was found that at least a three-phase mixture (with the constituents extracellular medium, cell membrane, and cytoplasm) is required to qualitatively reproduce the measured frequency response of the truncated skin model if any a priori knowledge of the underlying material dispersion (e.g., a Cole–Cole fit to measured data) is lacking. Consequently, microstructural features of tissue are an essential part of any accurate skin model in the MHz region.

## 12.1  Introduction

In clinical practice, there is a trend toward non-invasive diagnostics, mainly in order to reduce the infection risk and enabling continuous monitoring but also to increase patient comfort. Dielectric spectroscopy and electric impedance spectroscopy are already used for inspection of cervical squamous tissue (since the cell shape is subsequently modified with advancing precancerous stage) [3], skin cancer [4], skin irritations [5], ischemia detection [6], measurement of edema in irritant-exposed skin [7], monitoring of in vitro tissue engineering [8], or tumor characterization [9]. On the microscopic or cellular scale, specific techniques based on dielectric spectroscopy such as impedance flow cytometry, dielectrophoresis, and electrorotation [10–15] are employed for the characterization or investigation of specific features of single cells or cell arrangements. Medical applications such as electro-cardiography, electroencephalography, and communication along and in the human body as well as some new methods for non-invasive diagnostics include the application of electromagnetic fields. A particular application that seems to be feasible is the analysis of blood parameters through monitoring variations of dielectric properties caused by physiological changes [16,71].

Common to all of the mentioned medical applications or biological analysis techniques is the coupling of electromagnetic waves, electric or magnetic fields as well as currents and electric potentials to the human body, cell cultures or cell suspensions.

Non-invasive diagnostics require a unique correlation between observed quantities and variations of geometrical and constitutional parameters representing cells or tissues. In order to fulfill this criterion knowledge about the relation between changes in cellular features and their manifestation in the dielectric spectra as well as a sensitive experimental setup are indispensable. Especially for the development of instrumentation for single-cell monitoring, the probe geometry and the specific measurement configuration also become highly relevant. In these cases, numerical modeling of the specific sensor-tissue configurations is key to identifying the relevant parameters.

Additionally transcutaneous measurements face similar challenges as experienced when applying electrodes on the skin in other medical applications such as EEG, EMG, etc. The skin itself is a lossy, layered heterogeneous tissue, whereby the sublayers possess very distinct material compositions and therefore distinct dielectric properties. In addition to the skin structure itself the electrode–skin interface affect dielectric measurements. Facing the mentioned issues numerical modeling turns out to become increasingly challenging. In order to be able to extract any desired parameter—not to mention the associated parameter variations—from measured data extremely accurate solutions of the forward problem (i.e., the electromagnetic tissue simulation) are needed.

Skin is one of the most complex and dynamic organs of the human body consisting of many different features and structures influencing behavior and material properties. In addition to this complexity, the skin also features temporal variations in thickness and constituents. Some of these changes occur on a daily time scale and others on a scale of hours or minutes.

Here, a stationary setting is assumed and the multiscale modeling of skin is approached by first dividing skin tissue into different layers according to their different bulk properties. On another scale, the bulk dielectric properties of the different layers are determined by mixing formulas or full wave simulations. In Fig. 12.1, the different features contained in human skin are illustrated and a display of the characteristic length scales of these features is listed in Table 12.1. Within such a regime, it is most important to be able to distinguish between the normal variations of the changes exhibited by the dynamics of the skin parameters and the systematic changes that might be used as a diagnostic target. In this respect, it is of primary importance to assess the achievable sensitivity of a given sensor geometry or sensing principle together with its specificity, i.e., the unambiguous relation between the changes in target quantity and the associated specific feature of the measured signal. This can be achieved by carrying out large-scale measurement campaigns in the framework of clinical trials collecting various physiological data together with numerical simulations leading to the identification of certain functional dependencies. Especially with respect to numerical simulation a typical average scenario should be defined as starting point or rather as reference. Based on this average scenario, the necessary features to be included for the frequency range of interest can be determined, i.e., potential influences of different sub-structures can be extracted. The range of variations can also be numerically estimated by altering the parameters in the model within a physiologically and anatomically realistic range. This way the expected uncertainties and signal variations introduced by the different single aspects can be estimated and also common mode effects such as changes in certain features contributing to similar changes in the measured signal can also be identified. However, it has to be pointed out that with this kind of static approach not all of the possible side effects can be incorporated. The quality of the model has to be checked by appropriate experimental means. In the case of human tissue most of the tests cannot be carried out non-invasively. Therefore, determining an appropriate method for validation is a key component in the process of tissue modeling.

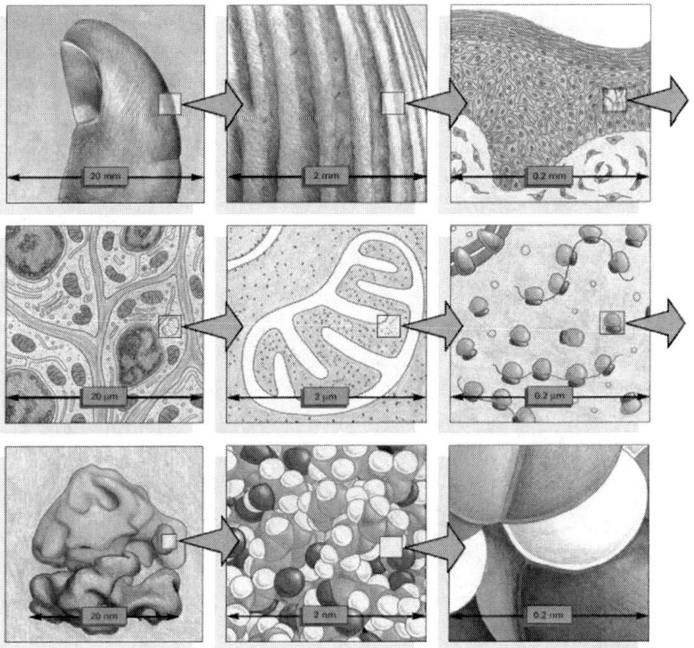

**Figure 12.1**  Schematics of different scales of features present in human skin (*source*: http://www.ncbi.nlm.nih.gov/books/NBK26880/ figure/A1716/?report=objectonly).

**Table 12.1**  Size ranges of different features

| Feature | Size |
| --- | --- |
| Tissue structure | 100 µm-1 mm |
| Cells | 1–100 µm |
| Organelles | 100 nm-1 µm |
| Proteins/macromolecules | 10–100 nm |
| Molecules | 1–10 nm |

In this review, an overview of our work during the last five years on modeling of human skin is given. Starting from various modeling issues regarding the effective dielectric properties of materials containing diverse types of biological cells, the focus is then shifted toward the development and the validation of a multilayer tissue model consisting of different structural features. This leads to an accurate multiscale approach where the effective dielectric properties are derived by an iterative mixing approach. For a detailed description of all approaches and a more extensive discussion of the results we refer to [1] and [2].

## 12.2 Brief Review on Skin Morphology and Composition for Modeling

In order to properly decide which features are actually necessary to be included in an appropriate skin model, detailed knowledge of the skin morphology is required. Therefore, a brief literature review on skin anatomy as sketched in Fig. 12.2 is given in the following.

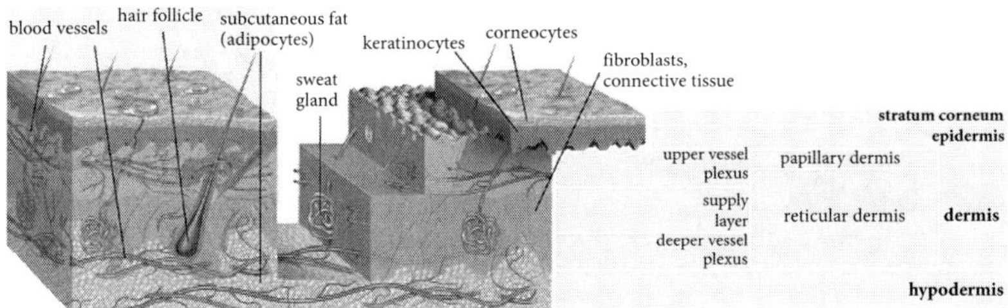


**Figure 12.2** Structure of the skin containing the sub-structures and different cell types. Adapted from [1].

From the modeling perspective, the human skin morphology consists of structures on several spatial scales. On the sub-microscopic and microscopic levels, there are macromolecules, organelles, and cells. Although most types of cells share the same basic structure consisting of extracellular medium, phospholipid cell membrane and cytoplasm, the composition of the generally aqueous extracellular medium and cytoplasm varies and is, on macroscopic scale, reflected by its effective dielectric properties. On this scale, the skin is divided into three layers that are mainly distinguished by their water content. On a scale in the order of a few 100 μm, blood vessels form a network contributing a different type of morphology to the apparent layer structure of skin tissue.

Starting from the outmost layer, the *stratum corneum* (SC) contains flat hexagonally shaped corneocytes embedded in a lipid matrix forming a so-called "bricks-and-mortar" structure [18–20]. The diameter of a corneocyte is 40 μm and the height 0.8 μm [21]. The intercellular distance is approximately 0.1 μm yielding a cellular volume fraction $\varphi$ for SC of $\varphi_{SC}$ = 0.85. The cytoplasm contains ceramides, free fatty acids, cholesterol, proteins (keratin), and water. In contrast to most other cells, the corneocyte does not contain a nucleus. The extracellular matrix, i.e., the "mortar," mainly consists of lipids and proteins and very little bound water (less than a monolayer). The total water volume fraction in the SC is 0.15–0.25, while 90% of the water is contained within the corneocyte [22,23]. By definition, the SC belongs to the epidermis, but due to the high lipid and protein and low water content, it differs significantly from the lower-lying epidermal layers and is here therefore considered separately.

The SC thickness depends on the body site but exhibits only little interindividual variations among healthy subjects. On the dorsal site of the upper arm, where our multiscale model will be validated, the SC is approximately 20 μm thick [18–20,24].

The living epidermis (E) mainly consists of keratinocytes. The cuboidal to columnar epidermal cells are gap-connected and occupy a volume fraction of 0.83 [25]. The overall water volume fraction in the dermis of 0.7 is equally distributed among intra- and extracellular space [26]. The epidermis is approximately 0.1–0.2 mm thick [27].

The transition zone between epidermis and dermis (D), the so-called dermo-epidermal junction is not planar but forms papillae with a depth of 50 μm. The papillary dermis (PD) occupies the upper 10% of the dermis and consists of a dense collagen network [28] and blood ($\varphi_{blood}$ = 0.04 [29]). The major part of the dermis, the reticular dermis (RD) consists of irregular connective tissue, lymphatic vessels, nerves, blood vessels, stromal cells such as fibroblasts and other cellular components, e.g., macrophages or plasma cells. The capillaries in the approximately 200 μm-long dermal papillae are oriented perpendicular to the skin surface, while the upper vessel plexus (UVP) is a dense vascular network parallel to the skin surface ($d_{UVP}$ = 80 μm, $\varphi_{blood,UVP}$ = 0.3).

The sparsely distributed blood vessels of the supply layer (SL) ($d_{SL}$ = 1.3 mm, $\varphi_{blood,SL}$ = 0.04) are also perpendicular to the skin surface. The lowest layer is again a dense vascular network parallel to the skin surface, the deeper vessel plexus (DVP) ($d_{DVP}$ = 100 μm,

$\varphi_{blood,DVP}$ = 0.1) [27]. The cellular volume fraction in the dermis is much smaller than in the epidermis [30]. The stellar-shaped fibroblasts form a continuous network making a determination of the proper cell boundaries rather difficult.

According to [31] the "body" of the cell has an approximate diameter of 5–10 μm, the extensions called *stellae* (4–6 per cell) are approximately 70 μm long. The collagen fibers are aligned parallel to the skin surface. Collagen is a major component embedded in the dermal matrix ($\varphi_{collagen,dry}$ = 0.17 [32]). A thick collagen bundle can reach 2–15 μm in diameter. In addition to collagen and elastin the extracellular space is mainly composed of glycosaminoglycans, gelatin and sugars embedded in water.

The hypodermis (HYP) mainly consists of white fat cells, the adipocytes building the subcutaneous fat. White adipocytes are spherically shaped with a mean cell diameter of 82.6 μm [33]. The intracellular fat forms a spherical droplet pushing the cytoplasm, including nucleus, toward the cell membrane. The volume fraction of the lipid droplet within the cytoplasm is $\varphi_{fat,intracellular}$ = 0.9 [34], the aqueous phase volume fraction is therefore only 0.1. The HYP thickness is subject to large intra- and interindividual variations.

Finally, muscular tissue (M) consisting of tightly packed narrow cigar-shaped cells is situated beneath the HYP. Muscle cells are oriented with their long axis parallel to the long axis of the humerus (upper arm bone).

Other features such as hair follicles, sweat ducts, and sebaceous glands cross the entire skin down to the HYP and are mentioned for completeness.

As can be seen from these observations, the skin contains many different features causing different dielectric contrasts and current paths that lead to a behavior that is hardly predictable in full detail. It is also obvious that a numerical model representing all those textures is barely achievable. Therefore, approaching a hierarchical multiscale model via successive inclusion of an increasing number of details seems to be the most realistic measure to face human skin complexity. However, the work carried out here should be considered only as a preliminary step in order to identify the features and parameters that have to be included in a model in order to achieve a sufficient accuracy for estimating the behavior of a skin-sensor configuration.

## 12.3 Dielectric Properties of Constituents in Human Skin

To date, no comprehensive (continuous) set of the dielectric material parameters for the skin layers—*stratum corneum*, epidermis, dermis, and hypodermis—is available in the frequency range from 1 MHz up to 100 MHz. In [64,65] the dielectric properties of the uppermost layer, the SC, have been assessed within a differential analysis relying on in vivo measurements of skin with and without this top layer. Coaxial probes of different sizes were employed in order to distinguish the SC, epidermis/dermis and hypodermis (subcutaneous fat), providing permittivity estimations for these layers, however, only at single frequencies [65]. Powdered native SC was also measured with a coaxial probe using the time domain reflectometry (TDR) method by [66], including an identification and quantification of two relaxation processes in the microwave regime. In vivo skin measurements as well as measurements of blood, infiltrated and non-infiltrated fat were performed in [36], also providing Cole–Cole relaxation models for all measured materials. In [67], human skin was measured in vivo, including a Cole–Cole fit too. As observed in [68] the Cole–Cole fits are a popular and useful tool in order to describe dielectric spectra of aggregate tissue in general. However, an unambiguous physical and physiological interpretation of the obtained Cole–Cole parameters remains difficult, because the impact of the numerous morphological and dielectric parameters as well as their variations has only partially been assessed so far.

Depending on the probe geometry, the effective dielectric parameters of layered skin tissue are usually a combination of the (effective) dielectric properties of the sublayers. In order to resolve the dielectric behavior at different depths within the skin, sensors with multiple planar electrodes can be employed.

However, the assessment of exact (effective) dielectric parameters of single skin layers or even of the single constituents of skin remains an open task. More accurate dielectric parameters would allow for better models on different scales, and, though, for solving the ambitious forward problem considered here.

## 12.4  Features of the Dielectric Spectrum

Up to the lower gigahertz region, the dielectric spectrum of cell suspensions, tissue or a single cell exhibits three main dispersion mechanisms: the electrode polarization due to diffusion of counter ions through the electrical double-layer is referred to as α-dispersion. Below 1 MHz, capacitive charging/short-circuiting of the poorly conductive cell membrane leads to the β-dispersion between 1 to 10 MHz. The dipolar relaxation of free water molecules above 1 GHz causes the γ-dispersion. In suspensions additionally a weak dispersion above 100 MHz originating from relaxation of small dipolar segments of biomolecules (e.g., proteins) and bound water can be observed [35]. This is then referred to as δ-dispersion. In the megahertz region, the β-dispersion yields the dominant spectral signature. The different regions of the dielectric spectrum together with the corresponding relaxation mechanisms are depicted in Figs. 12.3 and 12.4.

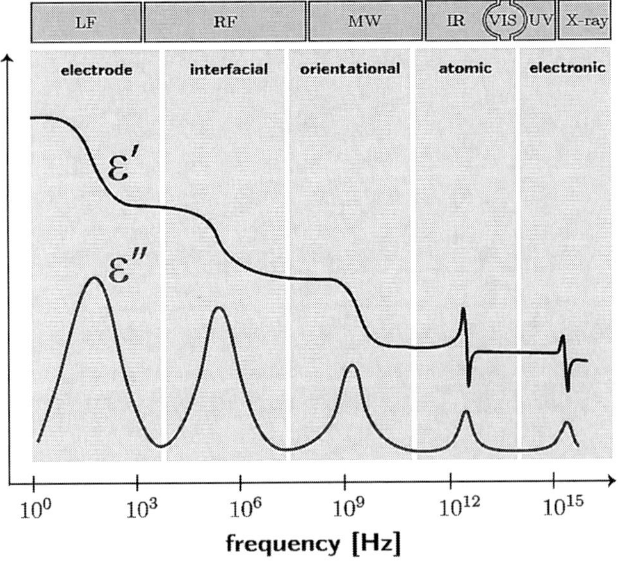


**Figure 12.3**  A generic spectrum of the complex permittivity, i.e., the dielectric function, for materials with distinct dispersive contributions from different polarization and resonance phenomena.

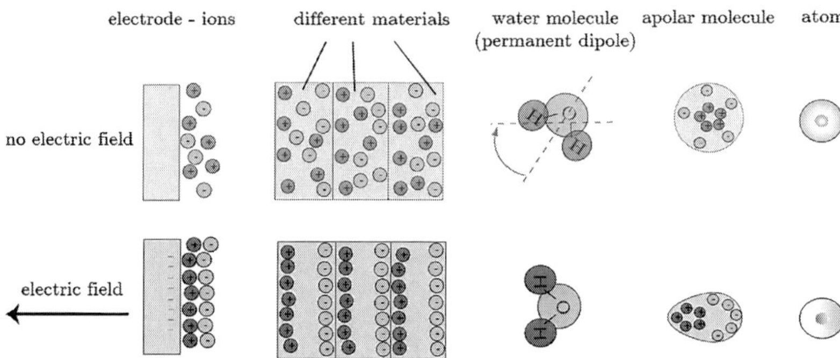


**Figure 12.4** Polarization mechanisms causing relaxations and resonances in the dielectric spectrum shown in Fig. 12.3.

A very straightforward and thus popular way to describe the spectral dispersion of cell suspensions or tissue from 1 Hz up to several GHz is to fit Cole–Cole or Cole–Cole-type relaxation models to measurement data [36–38]. Such relaxation models can be represented—similar to the Maxwell-Wagner model for membrane polarization—as equivalent circuits [39] because the dimensions involved are far below the wavelength. However, using this kind of representation even in the presence of pronounced differences among tissue types the attribution of features of the dispersion spectrum to specific microstructures in the tissue is difficult and hardly practical. For heterogeneous mixtures representing tissue, very different combinations of dielectric and geometric parameters can generate the same aggregate spectral behavior of the effective dielectric parameters. The dominant feature in the dielectric spectra especially in the megahertz range is the β-dispersion caused by the interfacial polarization at the cell membrane. Besides the expected changes in the microstructure, variations of cellular volume fraction, dielectric properties of intra- and extracellular medium (e.g., ion concentration, the presence of organelles) or cell shape have a measurable impact on the dispersion of the effective permittivity. In order to uniquely correlate cellular features to corresponding spectral signatures within the dielectric function a sophisticated model of cell suspensions or tissue textures is required.

## 12.5 Numerical and Semi-Analytical Modeling of Single Biological Cells and Cell Suspensions

The first step toward a dielectric multiscale model representing the main features of human skin is to find an appropriate representation for a single tissue or a suspension containing biological cells. This can be approached by using mixing formulas developed for the calculation of the effective dielectric properties of heterogeneous materials. Other approaches are the modeling of biological tissues as a composite structure including simple microscopic features such as spheres or ellipsoids. Finally full numerical models of three dimensional biological cells can be used together with a method to approximate a matrix of cells (i.e., the microstructure) representing a tissue. The different approaches are summarized in the following.

### 12.5.1 Modeling Effective Dielectric Properties Using Mixing Formulas

In the literature dealing with heterogeneous multiphase composites there exists a variety of mixing formulas each tailored to corresponding class of microstructures. The principal features and limitations of mixing formulas for tissue modeling are summarized in the following paragraphs. A comprehensive overview on the different formulas and detailed descriptions can be found in [40].

#### 12.5.1.1 Maxwell–Garnett

The effective permittivity of a suspension containing spherical particles can be described by the Maxwell–Garnett (MG) formula. Spherical particles (or inclusions) are introduced into a host material. If the particles are far enough from each other (dilute suspension with a low volume fraction $\varphi < 0.1$), then the effective parameters derived from the MG formula hold for the entire medium. The concept can be extended to a confocal multishelled ellipsoidal, and even to a cylindrical inclusion, since we are by definition in the quasi-static regime, where such core–shell particle can always be replaced by a homogeneous particle with a corresponding (effective) permittivity. As long as the coordinate system is such that the Laplace equation $\nabla^2\phi = 0$ where $\phi$ denotes the electric potential, is separable in the various regions of the problem the general form of the MG formula provides an exact solution for the effective permittivity [40].

### 12.5.1.2 Hanai–Bruggeman

Another description of the effective properties of a two-phase mixture is given by the Bruggeman formula (BR) [41]. Contrary to most other schemes, Bruggeman's mixing formula is symmetric with respect to the interchange of inclusion and host material. This formula applies if one has to deal with concentrated particle suspensions or systems where the interactions between induced dipoles of particles have to be taken into account. Bruggeman approached this rather difficult task with his effective medium theory. The initially low volume fraction is gradually increased by an infinitesimal addition of particles [42]. When a small amount of particles of $\varepsilon_i$ is added to the particle suspension, which is regarded as an effective medium, the Hanai–Bruggeman (HB) formula delivers an expression for $\varepsilon_{\text{eff}}$ of randomly oriented inclusions. The HB formula for two phases is said to provide excellent agreement with experiments for volume fractions up to 0.8 for colloidal suspensions containing homogeneous spherical particles [43].

### 12.5.1.3 Landau–Lifshitz–Looyenga

The Landau–Lifshitz–Looyenga formula (LLL) was independently developed by Landau and Lifshitz [44] and Looyenga [45], respectively, using different approaches. In contrary to the MG or HB, the LLL formula does not take the geometry of the inclusion into account. In case of multiphase particles (e.g., core–shell ellipsoids) the effective permittivity of the particle is calculated according to the MG or HB formulas. LLL is a special case of Lichtenecker's formula [40].

Similarly to the MG, the LLL formula does not take any interparticle interactions into account, therefore one would expect a validity limit around a volume fraction of $< 0.1$. However, it was shown in various experiments that for certain biphasic mixtures with statistically distributed particle size the LLL formula provides good agreement for almost any particle volume fraction [46].

## 12.5.2 Spectral Density Function Approach

Another analytical method for modeling various kinds of shapes is the spectral decomposition method or spectral density function approach developed in [47]. This method is based on the separation of geometry and material properties. The spectral density method is relatively fast, since it does not require any discretization of the geometry. However, it was shown that the geometrical contributions to the pure dielectric response of a composite can be separated from the material properties if and only if the dielectric properties of the constituents are known [48]. In practice, experimental data is used to determine the spectral density function [49]. This procedure belongs to the class of the so-called ill-posed problems and a correct solution is possible only with the use of proper stabilization techniques [50]. Mention may be also made of the work based on an expansion of the modified spectral density function in terms of Legendre polynomials where the reconstruction of the spectral density function relies on Padé approximation derived from a constrained minimization problem. A further approach is based on the Monte Carlo integration in conjunction with a constrained least-squares algorithm [51]. The spectral density approach has been applied to the calculation of effective dielectric properties of cells in [49,50,52,53]. Depending on the choice/determination of the spectral density function it is possible to extract a binary mixture equation, such as the MG [54] or the LLL formula [48].

A notable drawback of the approach is the fact that the analytical description gets very cumbersome with increasing complexity of the shape of the inclusion [55] and increasing number of phases—a situation clearly occurring in biological tissue.

## 12.5.3 Three-Dimensional Modeling

The principal approach presented in [17] consists of implicitly representing the cell suspension as a periodic assembly of unit cells, each containing a single model of a biological cell. The unit cell—with a volume that relates to the included cell volume according to the volume fraction—is consecutively exposed to an external homogeneous electric field in all three spatial directions, which correspond to the principal axes of the dielectric tensor to be extracted. In this particular configuration, the field exposure is provided by two opposite electrodes rendering the enclosed unit cell as the proper volume of an idealized parallel-plate capacitor. In the following, the derived dielectric tensor can be used in order to describe the bulk material in an either micro- or macroscopic model, rendering this description an effective anisotropic material representation.

An application of this idea was presented in [56] for the dielectric spectroscopy of the human skin in the MHz region, employing a fringing-field sensor. The skin is subdivided into three layers parallel to the skin surface, while each layer is described as a suspension of a defined cell type. For all three cell types the effective dielectric properties of a suspension of aligned single-shelled ellipsoidal particles are analytically calculated using the MG formula. The obtained (effective) dielectric tensor is then inserted into a macroscopic multilayer model of the skin.

This first approach provided already promising results, when successfully approximating the spectral response of the retrieved sensor signals. However, in order to improve the reproduction and in particular the explanation power of the measured data a more sophisticated cell model than obtained by the MG formula is required.

In order to assess the range of observable deviations due to certain changes in cellular properties, numerical models of realistically shaped biological cells become indispensable. First of all, this includes the development of an efficient modeling framework allowing for quantification of small changes in the overall morphology, including particularly the cellular volume fraction and the cell shape. One of the key aspects of accurate three-dimensional single cell modeling comprises three important issues, namely how, at which frequency, and with what magnitude the dielectric function is actually influenced by the shape variations. Before realizing a measurement setup this knowledge is advantageous in order to optimize the sensitivity and specificity to the target quantity. Due to the availability of increased computational power and in particular larger working memory, it becomes feasible to numerically investigate three-dimensional models of single cells and larger arrangements of cells where high aspect ratios occur if the cell membrane and eventually other small features are included.

## 12.5.4   Modeling of Tissue as a Composite Material

In order to solve the resulting systems of equations in a reasonable time the complexity of the tissue models has to be kept within a certain range of degrees of freedom. One technical approach therefore is to consider suspensions and tissues as a kind of composite material. A composite can be generalized as a heterogeneous arrangement of two or more materials with different properties combined together. This mixture may provide a combination of properties that cannot be attained with the original materials. Two scales characterize the material, the microscopic scale describing the heterogeneities and the macroscopic scale describing the global behavior of the composite. If the microstructure is partly unknown only bounds for the effective permittivity matrix can be derived. A mathematical assessment of generalized bounds in dielectric mixing is discussed in detail in [57].

If the wavelength within all involved materials is much larger than the dominant length scales in the heterogeneous arrangement, the composite can be represented as a multi component regular metamaterial structure that can be reduced to so-called unit cells. And conversely the unit cells, when periodically continued in all directions, will result in a bulk metamaterial supporting the same volume fractions as the heterogeneous composite. It is worth mentioning that this regularization to a periodic representation may fail if the (randomized) morphology of the composite is non-trivially entangled. In this case, the unit cell may be replaced by a representative microstructure with a volume that conforms to the corresponding correlation length scales of the underlying morphology, which have again to be significantly smaller than the wavelength in order to be admitted to a quasi-static analysis. Coming back to the periodic representation the unit cell as such can be computed using periodic boundary conditions and the dielectric properties can therefore be extracted from a significantly reduced model. The resulting dielectric properties can then be considered as an approximate representation the real composite material. Figure 12.5 displays the basic principle how to extract a unit cell from a bulk material consisting of regularly arranged inclusions in a background material.

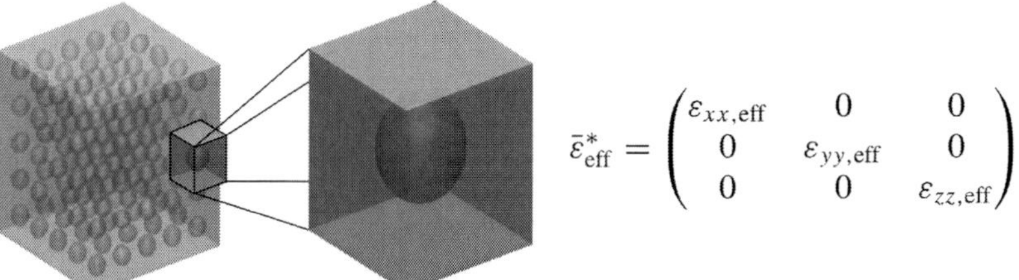

$$\bar{\varepsilon}^*_{\text{eff}} = \begin{pmatrix} \varepsilon_{xx,\text{eff}} & 0 & 0 \\ 0 & \varepsilon_{yy,\text{eff}} & 0 \\ 0 & 0 & \varepsilon_{zz,\text{eff}} \end{pmatrix}$$

**Figure 12.5** Determination of the effective dielectric tensor: Mixing scheme for composite materials modeled as a regular array of inclusions in a background material.

In the framework of the unit cell approach, different kinds of inclusions in a host material are computed. The underlying electromagnetic analysis is then carried out in the quasi-static limit where only the electric potential $\phi$ (cf. Eq. 12.1) has to be evaluated.

$$\nabla \cdot \left( \varepsilon^* \nabla \frac{\partial}{\partial t} \phi \right) = 0 \tag{12.1}$$

Referring to the aforementioned idealized capacitor setup the solution of the quasi-static analysis will then provide the input admittance of the unit cell. The effective dielectric parameters can be directly extracted. If a whole tissue—which is represented by a multilayer material structure—is analyzed by a probe setup, the admittance of the probe has to be taken into account too. This procedure is scrutinized in [58]. The next paragraph summarized the results of a comprehensive study assessing the dependence of the effective dielectric properties on various cell shapes.

## 12.6 Modeling Effective Dielectric Properties of Materials Containing Diverse Types of Biological Cells

In [17] a methodological framework was developed for the accurate analysis of tissue, including an algorithm for the generation of different biological cells with realistic cell shapes. The dielectric properties of the corresponding unit cells were calculated within the aforementioned capacitor setup using the finite element code provided by the simulation platform COMSOL multiphysics [59]. The FEM relies on a unstructured discretization mesh that is best suited to handle the large aspect ratios present in cellular structures with thin or small features such as a membrane and/or organelles.

One of the innovations of our modeling approach is to approximate the proper cell boundary using highly flexible parameterized shape representations based on the so-called superformula, which is closely related to the superquadrics and was actually first applied in plant taxonomy [60]. This method also allows for generating non-axisymmetric shapes such as box-shaped cells and complex shapes representing echonocytes featuring thorn-like structures on the surface of the cell membrane. Equipped with such detailed cell models our numerical analysis is now ready to resolve characteristic features in the tensorial effective dielectric function stemming from different cell morphologies as well as from potential pathogenetic alterations. A successful but cursory validation of the numerical model was carried out for spherical inclusions at a low volume fraction aiming at a direct comparison with the analytical Maxwell–Garnett and the Hanai–Bruggeman mixing formulas. Please note that the term "cursory" just refers to the fact that a comprehensive numerical model is actually not supposed to be validated against an approximate mixing formula.

Figure 12.6 depicts the flow diagram of the modeling procedure to calculate the effective dielectric properties of an inclusion in a background material. First, the cell shape is mimicked by a proper selection of the parameters for the superformula. Then the surface can be extracted and a correspondingly small offset is introduced in order to generate the membrane. The resulting structure is then discretized by different means and meshing strategies depending on the software used. In our case a finite element model of the cell in the capacitor setup is generated and the complex effective dielectric tensor is computed. In Fig. 12.7, various numerical models encompassing realistic cell shapes of different cell types are listed. Depending on the specific cell shape, different mesh resolutions can be deduced being then correspondingly applied.

In Fig. 12.8 the spectral response of the effective dielectric properties of a box-shaped cell is compared to the spectrum derived by applying the MG and HB mixing formula for two different volume fractions.

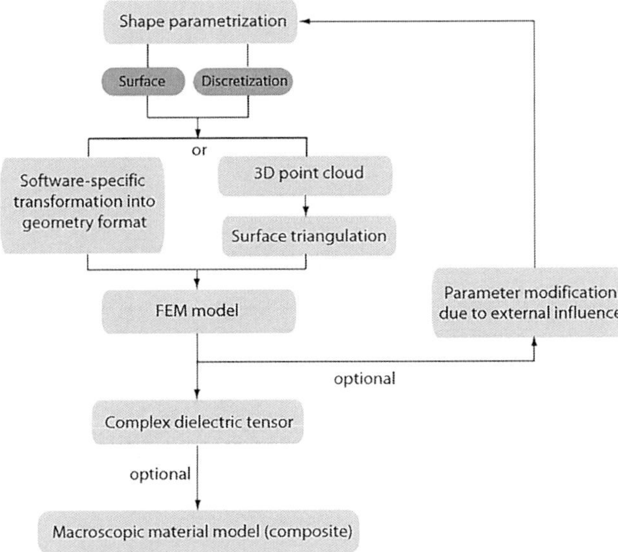



**Figure 12.6** Flow diagram of cell shape generation and computation of the dielectric tensor of the composite's effective material properties.

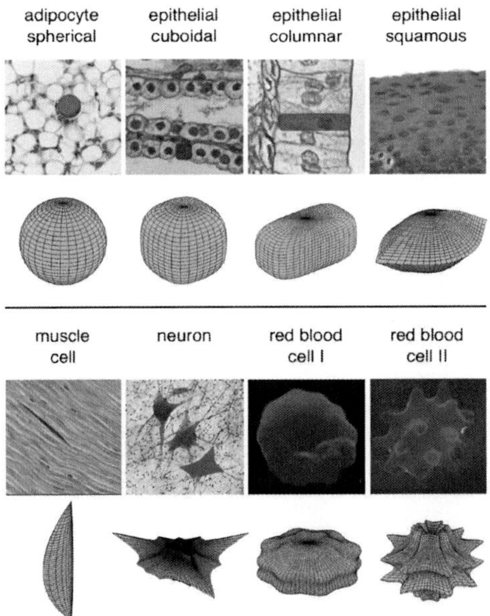



**Figure 12.7** Different numerical models representing different cell types.

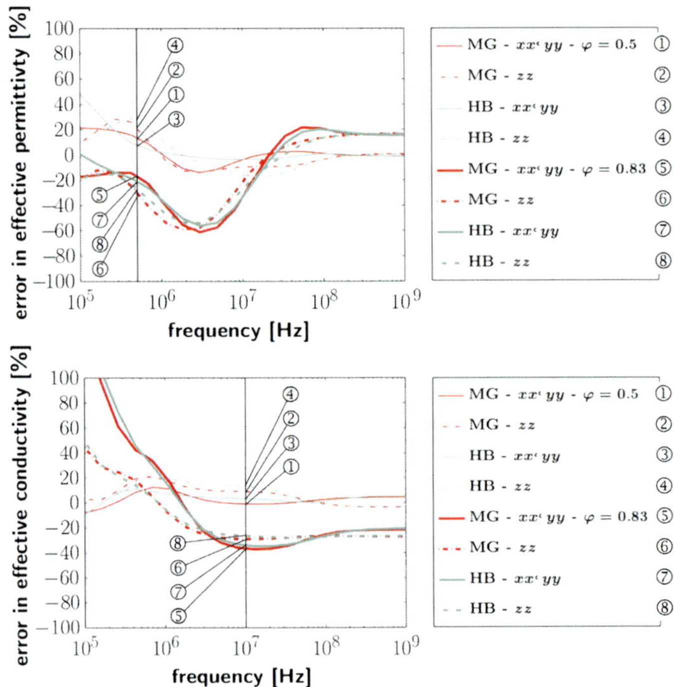

**Figure 12.8** Difference between the numerically retrieved complex effective dielectric function for box-shaped cells versus the results derived by applying the corresponding model of the MG and HB mixing formula. The results are shown for two volume fractions, i.e., 0.5 and 0.83. Adapted from [1].

The results clearly indicate that the use of the mixing formula is restricted to a certain frequency range depending on the shape and the volume fraction of the cell-background arrangement. For certain frequency ranges the deviation of the numerical model compared to the mixing formula can reach up to 65% for the effective dielectric constant and up to more than 100% for the effective conductivity. This has to be taken into account when applying mixing formulas to determine the effective dielectric properties of composites containing inclusions with a more complex shape. It may also hamper the unique interpretation of measured results in dielectric spectroscopy if small changes in cellular features are of diagnostic interest, namely when the changes caused by these cellular features are masked by the differences introduced by the cell shape or by changes thereof.

## 12.6.1 Conclusions on Modeling Effective Dielectric Properties of Materials Containing Diverse Types of Biological Cells

Using the presented framework for cell shape rendering, the influence of various shape variations and volume fractions on the effective dielectric function was explored between 100 kHz and 1 GHz. The quantification of the cell shape's influence was introduced via the relative deviation between non-spherical and spherical cell responses. Our results suggest that below 1 MHz the effective dielectric properties of different cell shapes at different volume fractions significantly deviate from the spherical case. Furthermore, three different cell shapes were compared with a simple but popular equivalent circuit (EC) representation (serial connection) of the membrane layer using scaled thicknesses to exploit the changing influence of the cell membrane. The absolute values for the effective dielectric parameters of such EC models are significantly larger than for the single-cell models but the spectral signatures remain comparable.

Concerning measurability, it can be stated that the changes are pronounced in the upper kHz range but potentially masked by electrode polarization effects. Above the occurrence of electrode polarization, starting from low MHz frequencies the magnitude of the deviations due to shape changes is smaller and would therefore require a higher sensitivity of the measurement setup.

As the superformula (SF) has proven to be a suitable parameterization method for non-axisymmetric shaped biological cells, it becomes also applicable for testing functional dependencies between environmental changes (concentration of a species, pressure, temperature, etc.). As an example, the shape of the red blood cell (RBC) strongly depends on the electrolyte concentration in the blood plasma. Although the SF cannot approximate completely asymmetrical shapes this drawback could be compensated by additional "deformation" functions acting on the various "supershapes." Furthermore, multiplying the SF with other functions or another SF would also extend the variety of possible cell shapes [61]. An interesting alternative surface parameterization technique based on smooth facet selection was recently proposed by Vogelgesang [69].

Followed by finite element simulations of the dielectric function of the mentioned cell models, the overall method turned out to be very flexible for single cell and tissue modeling, required for the design of noninvasive spectroscopic tools. However, in order to establish an efficient and reliable macroscopic tissue model the influence of other aspects such as ion channels, proteins and organelles have to be investigated as well, especially for frequencies above 50 MHz. More detailed and accurate tissue models could significantly improve non-invasive dielectric sensing instruments. On the microscopic scale the developed models are also applicable for the analysis of the local distribution of applied electromagnetic fields. This particular realm has become a highly active research field in bioelectromagnetics dealing with the microscopic exploration of potential non-thermal effects.

## 12.7 Numerical and Semi-Analytical Modeling of Multilayer Systems

In [58] and [62], the skin is modeled as a multilayer system. Figure 12.9 shows an MR image of the human skin taken at the dorsal upper-left arm and the derived layered model based on the assessed thickness. There, the different layers of epidermis, dermis, hypodermis and muscle are clearly distinguishable. The model of the human skin employed in the following is based on this multilayer structure. The uppermost layer of the epidermis, the SC, lies below the resolution limit of the MR image in Fig. 12.3a. The SC has a thickness of around 20 μm and consists of dead cells containing approximately 20% water. The SC builds the first layer of the human skin model. Although composed of different microstructures, the epidermis (thickness of 100–200 μm) and dermis (thickness of 1–1.2 mm) are similar regarding the water content, i.e., between 60% and 70%. Therefore, they can be combined in one epidermis/dermis (E/D) layer, constituting the second layer. The hypodermis (HYP) is mainly composed of subcutaneous fat with about 20% of water and forms the third layer. The muscle tissue below the HYP layer is not considered in the skin model, as discussed in Section 12.9. The resulting three-layer model is shown in Fig. 12.3b. The thicknesses of the layers are $d_1 = 20$ μm, $d_2 = 1$ mm and $d_3 = 2$ cm.

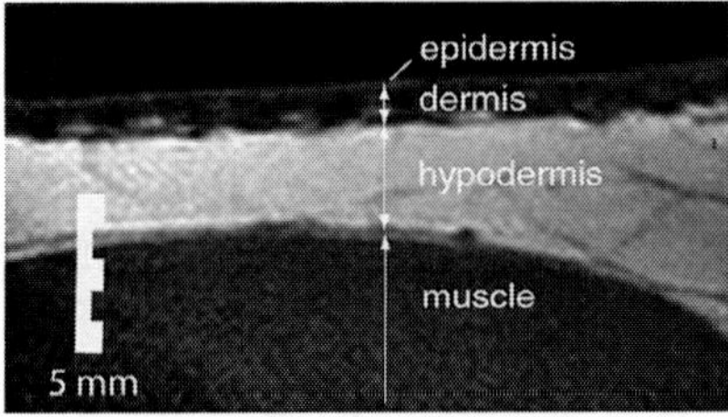


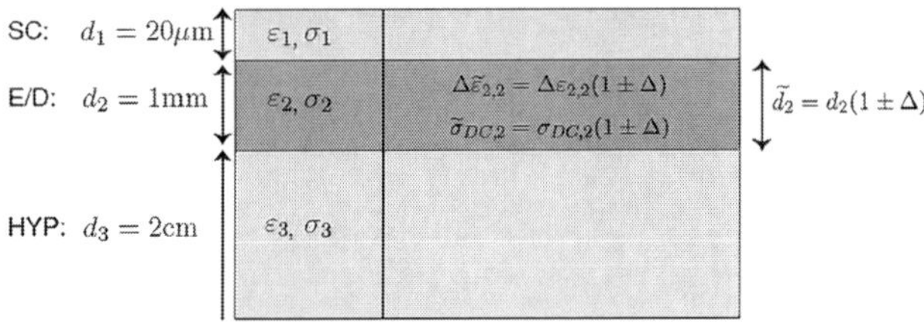


**Figure 12.9** Sensitivity and specificity analysis: MR image and corresponding layer model of the skin.

The experimentally determined dispersive dielectric characteristics of biological tissues are commonly approximated by a Cole–Cole model as already described. In the three-layer skin model, each layer labeled with the index $i$ is represented by a complex (effective) relative permittivity $\varepsilon^{*}_{r,i}$ that is made up by the following Cole–Cole model:

$$\varepsilon^{*}_{r,i} = \varepsilon_{\infty,i} + \sum_{n} \frac{\Delta\varepsilon_{n,i}}{1 + (j\omega\tau_{n,i})^{(1-\alpha_{n,i})}} + \frac{\sigma_{DC,i}}{j\omega\varepsilon_0}, \tag{12.2}$$

where $\varepsilon_\infty$ denotes the optical limit of the permittivity, and $\varepsilon_0$ the vacuum permittivity, $\omega = 2\pi f$ the angular frequency, $n$ the number labeling the corresponding dispersions contribution, $\Delta\varepsilon_{n,i}$ the $n$-th permittivity increment, $\tau_{n,i}$ the $n$-th relaxation time, $\alpha_{n,i}$ the $n$-th broadening parameter, and $\sigma_{DC,i}$ the static conductivity, all in the layer with index $i$.

In [62] the material parameters of "untreated *stratum corneum*" published in [63] are used for SC. To our best knowledge, there are no material parameters available for the isolated epidermis/dermis. In the dermis, blood vessels are non-uniformly distributed and make up roughly 30% of its volume. A large part of the remaining epidermis/dermis (E/D) components are cells exhibiting similar water content and dielectric characteristics as blood in terms of β-dispersion. Thus, dispersive dielectric parameters of blood [36] were considered to be an appropriate approximation of the epidermis/dermis layer. The subcutaneous tissue, the hypodermis (HYP), is modeled by "infiltrated fat" as given in [36]. This model served as a basis to assess the sensitivity of certain sensor geometries to changes in the E/D layer described in Section 12.9. Note that the model consists of three planar layers not taking the geometry of the proper interface into account. Therefore, the influence of the exact geometry of the interface, especially between SC and E/D is not taken into account. In the low frequency limit, where effective material descriptions reign, such hetero-interface can be accurately modeled just by introducing an additional thin homogeneous layer of corresponding permittivity [70].

If more details are taken into account a more complex multilayer model can be derived starting from the basic constituents, while setting up an iterative mixing scheme that encompasses subsequent scales of the morphology, including different layers and other structures. In Fig. 12.10 an extended skin model is shown that is further explained in Section 12.8.

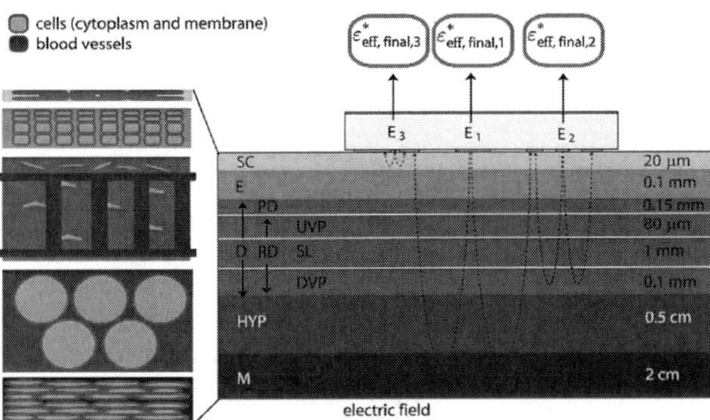


**Figure 12.10** 2D cross-sectional sketch of the layered skin model consisting of *stratum corneum* (SC), epidermis (E), dermis (D), hypodermis (HYP) and muscle (M). In the basic model denoted as MGW in [58] the epidermis and dermis are concatenated to one single layer denoted as (E/D). In the most refined model the dermis is subdivided into papillary dermis (PD) and reticular dermis (RD), whereas the latter contains the upper vessel plexus (UVP), the supply layer (SL) and the deeper vessel plexus (DVP). A sketch of the microstructure of the skin layers is given on the left.

## 12.8 Multiscale Approach

In order to take different features ranging from microscopic to macroscopic into account a highly detailed multiscale approach was developed as reported in [58]. The schematic of the formal procedure is depicted in Fig. 12.11. Starting from initial dielectric parameters and a corresponding geometry mixing is achieved by analytical or semi-analytical methods or within the framework of a fully numerical structure model. If anisotropy has to be taken into account the resulting effective dielectric parameter of the bulk property turns out to be a tensorial quantity instead of a single scalar. If the mixture is part of a configuration on a larger scale the result can be introduced into the next step of the formal procedure and iterated until the final scale is reached.

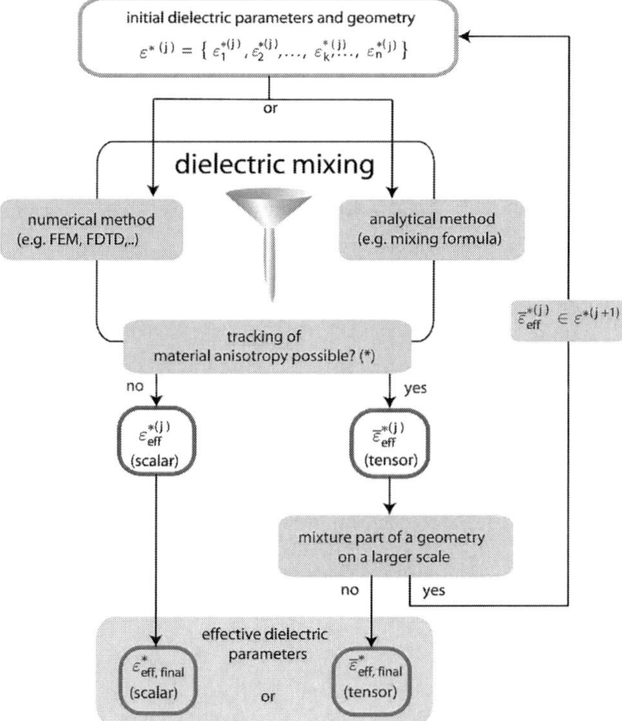


**Figure 12.11** Schematic of the dielectric homogenization procedure for a material with (quasi-) periodic structures on one or more scales.

The first model consists of modeling the different skin layers as two-phase mixtures. Biological tissue in general is mainly made up of an aqueous phase (extracellular liquid, cytoplasm) and a lipid phase (cell membrane, intra- and extracellular lipids) being significantly distinct from a dielectric point of view.

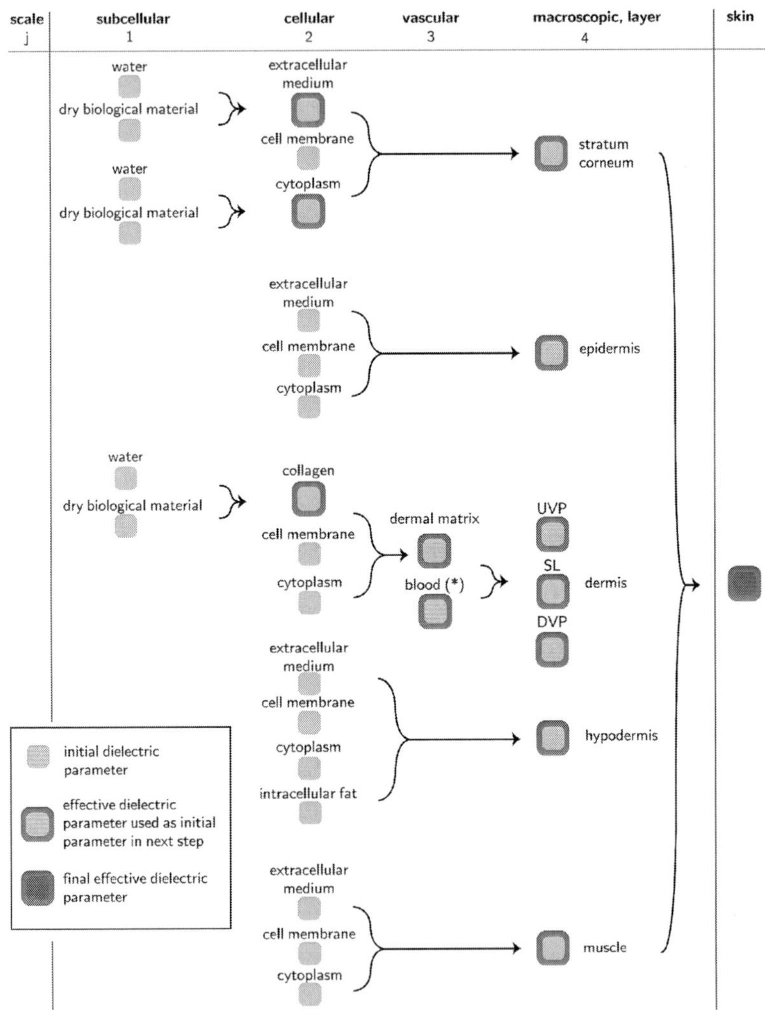



**Figure 12.12** Mixing steps for multiscale model of human skin starting from the basic constituents up to the different scales of the skin tissue. Abbreviations for dermis subdivision: upper vessel plexus (UVP), supply layer (SL) and deeper vessel plexus (DVP). Adapted from [1].

In Fig. 12.12, the different scales of the multiscale approach for human skin are depicted. First, the different constituents on the subcellular scale are combined into the appropriate cellular structures of the different layers. For the dermis the cellular structures are combined with the dermal matrix and blood representing the vascular structures. On the macroscopic scale the different layers, *stratum corneum*, epidermis, dermis, hypodermis and muscle can be combined to the bulk properties of skin. The way of combining the different layers depends on the operating frequency range of the specific application. For applications where the wavelength within all layers is much larger than the thickness of the layers the different layers can be combined into bulk effective dielectric properties of the skin. As the geometry of the probe generates a non-uniform field distribution the resulting measurement value could be interpreted as a weighted average of the different layers' dielectric properties with the electric field as distribution function. For these cases a calibrated sensor has to be used in order to assess subtle changes in the dielectric properties. Depending on the specific tissue model different bulk materials can be generated representing different parts of the human skin. This of course is also applicable to any other kind of layered composite structure occurring in the area of, for instance, polycrystalline materials for solar cells, nanocomposites in photonic applications or airborne remote sensing. The aim of the work presented in [58] was the development of a reliable computationally efficient numerical model for the dielectric behavior of the skin in the MHz region. The focus was on the required degree of complexity in order to reconstruct and interpret measured dielectric data of the skin. Therefore, different multiscale models having different degrees of complexity were set up based on the corresponding shape of the cells, volume fraction and material composition.

The second model further refines the initial subdivision into three layers. In this model a first attempt to incorporate microstructural information into the different skin layers is undertaken by approximating single tissue cells by shelled ellipsoids. The cell dimensions, volume fractions and material compositions were estimated based on literature values. Although the water content in both the epidermis and the dermis is comparable, a unified morphological description of these two layers turned out to be difficult. The structural properties even suggest subdividing at least the dermis into sublayers. The cellular volume in the dermis is so small that the influence of the cell shapes on the dielectric properties will become negligible compared to the influence of the collagen network or the orientation of blood vessels. Consequently, the epidermis/dermis (E/D) layer is partitioned into the joint layer consisting of epidermis and papillary dermis layer (PD), the upper vessel plexus layer (UVP), the supply layer and the deeper vessel plexus (DVP). The dimensions of the layers and the parameters for blood volume fractions were set according to literature values. The different layers were modeled using different analytical models or using Cole–Cole parameters obtained from reported measurements.

The third model relies on partly numerically calculated multiphasic mixtures. The aim of this model was to include additional features that are expected to have an influence on the dielectric function at the macroscale. As elucidated in Section 12.5.3 and in accordance with the approach developed in [17], the single cells were placed in a parallel-plate capacitor-like simulation domain filled with extracellular medium. To obtain the diagonal dielectric tensor the model was altered according to all three spatial directions representing the principal axes, i.e., the electric field was subsequently applied in the $x$-, $y$- and $z$-directions using appropriate boundary conditions. The single cell shapes were generated utilizing the correspondingly parameterized "superformula." A detailed description of the different models is given in [58].

## 12.9   Sensitivity and Specificity Analysis

Sensitivity and specificity are the key parameters for any detection or sensing technique characterizing its suitability for the target application. In the case of transcutaneous monitoring of physiological variations in the dermis layer the changes are expected to manifest themselves as changes in conductivity and/or permittivity. Therefore, the amount of change observable in the bulk dielectric properties caused by a certain variation of the conductivity and/or permittivity has to be evaluated in the framework of the multilayer model. Considering all changes in the bulk dielectric properties caused by variations in the dermis layer's conductivity and/or permittivity the specificity is evaluated regarding one specific feature, e.g., diagnostic parameter. The specificity of the target feature is evaluated in terms of uniqueness of its change and for example the corresponding response in the changes in bulk dielectric properties for the case of transcutaneous measurements applying a sensor on the skin. In general the specificity can be given in terms of a change in the target parameters and its measurable counterpart on the same or larger scale.

If a unique correlation between the different variations and the characteristics in the bulk dielectric properties can be identified featuring a high sensitivity the analyzed method is highly suited for the target application. However, if the specifity is not guaranteed, i.e., different variations cause the same changes in the measured signal, additional means have to be taken in order to achieve a unique correlation between the target quantity and the measured signal.

In [62], the sensitivity and specificity of different sensor geometries applied to the detection of dielectric changes inside a multilayered structure is investigated. The focus is on providing a reliable base for sensing physiological changes in the human skin, i.e., in the epidermal and dermal layers. The correlation between changes of the human skin's effective permittivity and changes of dielectric parameters and layer thickness of the epidermal and dermal layers is assessed using the numerical multiscale approach for the skin tissue in conjunction with a corresponding representation of the senor topology. This includes fringing-field probes placed directly on the multilayer structure presented in Section 12.7. The resulting dielectric function in the range from 100 kHz up to 100 MHz for different layer parameters and sensor geometries are used for a sensitivity and specificity analysis of the underlying multilayer system.

First, employing a coaxial probe, a sensitivity analysis is carried out for specific variations of the parameters of the epidermal and dermal (E/D) layers. Figure 12.13 shows an example of the relative deviations in effective permittivity and conductivity caused by changes in the E/D layer with respect to the unchanged reference system.

Second, the specificity of this system is then analyzed based on the roots and corresponding sign changes of the computed dielectric function and respective their first and second derivatives. The transferability of the derived results is shown by comparing the resulting dielectric functions retrieved by coplanar probe and a scaled coaxial probe. Additionally, a comparison of the sensitivity of a coaxial probe and an interdigitated probe as a function of electrode separation was performed. It was found that the sensitivity for detecting changes of dielectric properties in the epidermal and dermal layers strongly depends on the operating frequency.

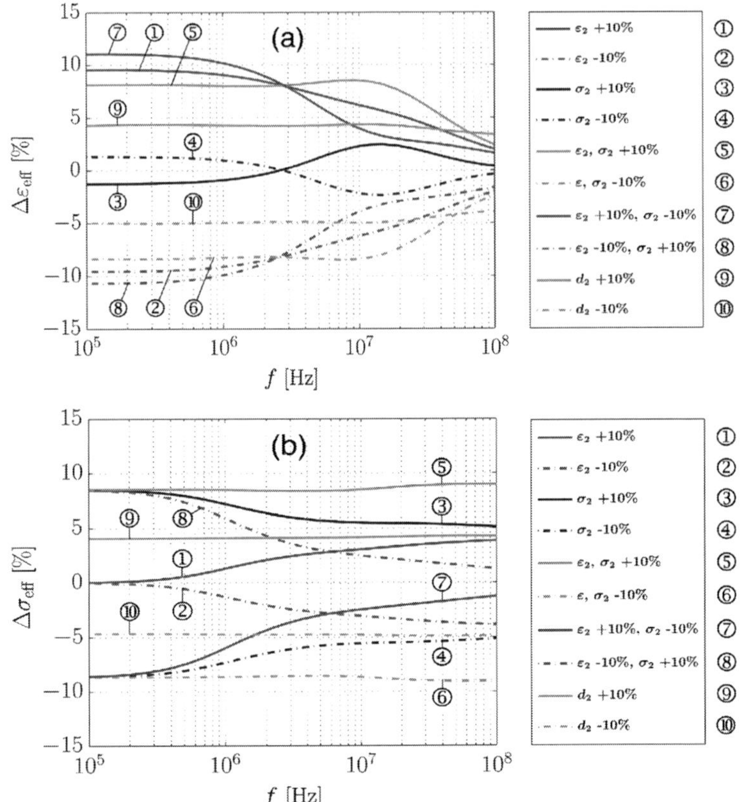

Figure 12.13 Example of the relative deviations in effective permittivity (a) and conductivity (b) due to changes in the E/D layer indicated with respect to the reference three-layer system under a coaxial probe. Adapted from [1].

Based on an analysis of the dielectric spectra, changes in the effective dielectric parameters can in principle be uniquely assigned to specific changes in permittivity and conductivity within the E/D layer. However, in practice, measurement uncertainties may degrade the observed performance of the system. This is then subject to signal processing, which might apply appropriate methods to reconstruct the signal content even for highly noisy biosignals. In [72], the sensitivity analysis for two different experimental systems for differential dielectric spectroscopy is evaluated. The first system features cells in suspension above 10 planar interdigitated microelectrodes measuring differences in dielectric properties. The second system is an implementation of an impedance microfluidic cytometer and allows for single cell analysis. By numerical simulations, including models of single cells the uncertainties caused by variations in shape, membrane thickness and position of the cells relative to the electrode configurations were assessed. Based on such simulations the necessary number of repetitions of experiments and the required minimal number of cells can be determined in order to end up with a sufficient statistical power. By evaluating the effects of certain changes in cellular features on the measured signal, the specificity of such systems can also be assessed.

## 12.10 Application to Human Skin

Different multilayer skin models as described in Section 12.8, were investigated in [58]. First, with sublayers obtained from two-phase mixtures, second, three-phase mixtures of shelled cell-like ellipsoids and finally, multiphase mixtures obtained from full numerical models with single cell shapes from a flexible surface parameterization method. All these different models of the layered skin were numerically evaluated within a FEM simulation of the overall configuration having a probe on top of the multilayer system serving as a fringing-field probe. Furthermore, measurements with the sensor probing skin in vivo were performed.

The validity of the different models was tested by removing the uppermost skin layer, i.e., the *stratum corneum* (SC). These dielectric measurements were carried out in the frequency range from 5 MHz up to 100 MHz using the multi-electrode sensor as depicted in Fig. 12.14 connected to a vector network analyzer (VNA). The sensor includes three electrodes having different gap widths. The wider the gap between driven and ground electrode the larger the penetration depth of the electric field into the tissue material. The setup was calibrated in air and deionized water with known static conductivity. Measurements were carried out at the upper arm of volunteers. This particular location was chosen because of its accessibility and relative homogeneity of the tissue layers parallel to the sensor surface (as determined by MRI imaging [see Fig. 12.9]) compared to other body parts. On the upper arm, the sensor could be easily tightly attached, which is crucial to reduce artifacts caused by movements and potential changes in the layer between the skin and the sensor.

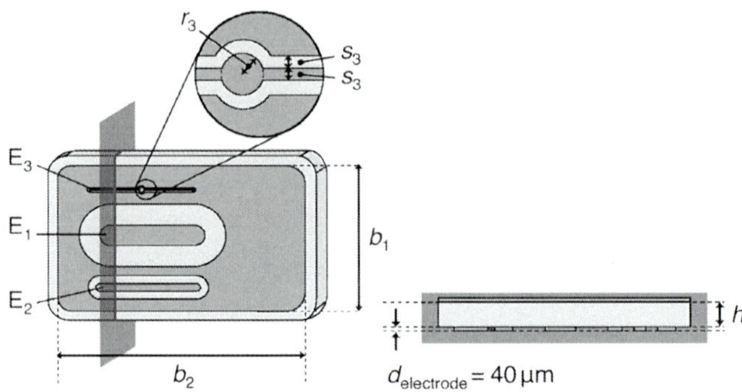

**Figure 12.14** Geometry of the sensor electrodes used for the measurements on the upper arm. The sensor is a prototype that is now integrated into a monitoring platform (www.biovotion.com).

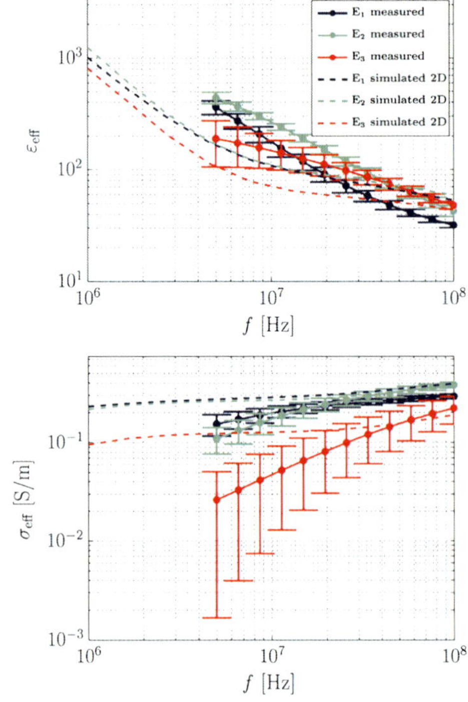



**Figure 12.15** Comparison of measured values versus simulated results for the case of the untreated dry skin. The curves show the relative dielectric constant (left) and the conductivity (right) for the three different electrodes E1 (large gap), E2 (medium gap) and E3 (small gap). Adapted from [1].

After measuring untreated, dry skin the *stratum corneum* was removed by consecutive stripping with adhesive tape. After each stripping the admittance was measured. The procedure was repeated about 40 times. All measurements were carried out at room temperature.

Both Figs. 12.15 and 12.16 depict the measured values in comparison to the simulated results using the third numerical multilayer skin model (cf. Section 12.8) for the two cases with untreated dry skin and the removed SC. The measured values are represented as mean values of four measurements on the same subject together with the standard deviation.

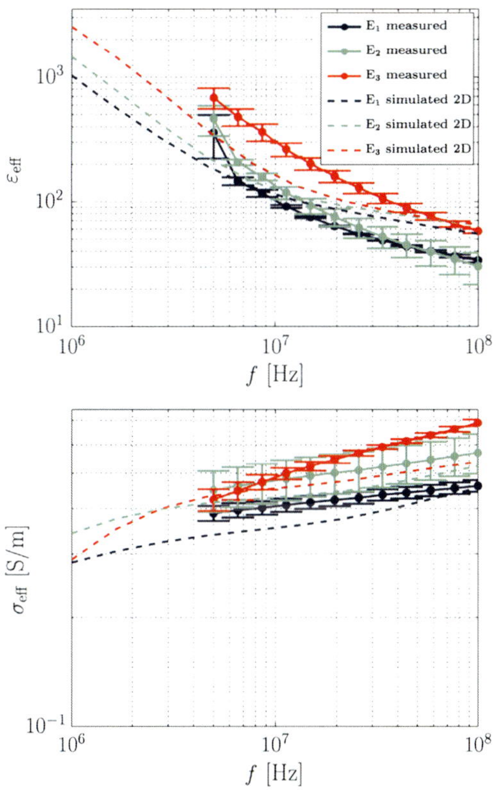

**Figure 12.16** Comparison of measured values versus simulated results for the case of the removed *Stratum Corneum*. The curves show the relative dielectric constant (left) and the conductivity (right) for the three different electrodes E1 (large gap), E2 (medium gap) and E3 (small gap). Adapted from [1].

### 12.10.1 A Preliminary Résumé on Appropriate Models for Tissue Monitoring

The presented results underpin the need for a dielectric multiscale model of human skin in the frequency range from 1 to 100 MHz. The model with the biphasic water mixtures fails to reproduce the skin's dielectric properties after removal of the SC. The latter model type characterized only by the water content of each layer as the relevant parameter is only applicable above 400 MHz as reported previously.

Below 100 MHz at least the basic structures of tissue (cells) have to be taken into account in order to correctly reproduce the spectral signature. Here, core–shell particles in conjunction with MG- or HB-mixing are already capable to recover the correct trends in the dielectric function. Nevertheless, the numerical model with realistic cell shapes (grasped by the "superformula") resulting in anisotropic effective dielectric properties for each skin layer has proven to provide the best results. The removal of the SC as a validation criterion for the need of an at least three-phase mixtures containing realistic cell shapes was successfully demonstrated. The presented analysis together with the validation suggests that our multiscale model is prone to adaptation to other tissues with different cell morphologies and material composition. A further refinement of the fully evolved skin model is expected to include perfusion, mass transport and aging on the micro scale adding potential temporal variations and, hence, different time scales to the multiscale model hierarchy.

## 12.11 Conclusions

A flexible framework for the modeling of dielectric parameters of biological tissue was successfully established using mixing formulas and accurate numerical models within a multiscale approach. The skin model was experimentally validated while comparing simulations and measurements of a fringing-field sensor configuration. Moreover, prosperously using the removal of the *stratum corneum* in model and experiment as an additional validation criterion underpinned the suggested modeling method.

To the best of our knowledge the presented model is the only one which is entirely based on the microstructure encompassing morphology and material composition without any fitting of parameters to measured data, and may be therefore claimed as amongst the most comprehensive and most accurate skin models available at this stage.

Focusing on the distinct microstructure it was shown that for frequencies up to few 100 MHz shape and volume fraction of cells strongly influence the dielectric spectra of biological bulk materials such as cell suspensions and tissues. Above 100 MHz shape and volume fraction lose their importance and the principal characteristic in effective material properties is determined by the volume fractions of the different constituents only. This somehow counter-intuitive observation owes mainly to the relative dominance of the cell shape dependent $\beta$-dispersion and less to the scale relation of the wavelength with respect to the cell dimensions and other feature sizes. In other words for dielectric modeling of biological tissue below 100 MHz cell shape and cellular volume fraction has still to be well represented in the model—in particular when aiming at anisotropies in the tissue's effective material representation. Mixing formulas can always serve as a first approximation, but for more realistic scenarios only numerical simulations offer the required flexibility and accuracy. A limitation is the actual cell shape generation in the employed software. To remedy this deficiency the model could be easily extended in a further refinement when even more general types of surface parameterization techniques [69] are utilized.

As some tissues exhibit a layered substructure on the macro- or sub-macroscopic scale the uniqueness of effective properties as well as the sensitivity in the latter to parameter variations was investigated. Generally, such type of reconstruction defines an ill-posed problem. Only if the range of unknowns is sufficiently small one can potentially assign the origin of a certain change with respect to a reference scenario in the effective parameters to a distinct parameter variation in a specific layer.

The multiscale concept was successfully validated by measurements on human skin resulting in a good agreement regarding the spectral characteristics of the (effective) dielectric properties. Before calling our comprehensive multiscale approach an electromagnetic ab initio model, further research is strictly mandatory in order to improve the accuracy of the model and to validate it for other tissues. This is also required in order to apply the model for numerical design and optimization of sensor geometries for successfully tracking down specific physiological parameters with high sensitivity. Furthermore, the experimental setup for validation measurements on human skin has to be re-designed focusing on reproducibility and the capturing of effects on measured data due to environmental and temporal changes present in any living object.

## References


1. Huclova S (2011). Modeling of Cell Suspensions and Biological Tissue for Computational Electromagnetics, Diss. ETH No. 19863, ETH Zurich, (DOI: 10.3929/ethz-a-006711951).

2. Beyer C (2013). Investigation of possible interactions of electromagnetic fields with proteins and cells, Diss. ETH No. 21405, ETH Zurich, (DOI: 10.3929/ethz-a-006256581).

3. Walker DC, Brown BH, Smallwood RH, Hose DR, and Jones DM (2002). Modeled current distribution in cervical squamous tissue, *Physiol Meas*, **23**, 159–168.

4. Åberg P, Geladi P, Nicander I, Hansson J, Holmgren U, and Ollmar S (2005). Non-invasive and microinvasive electrical impedance spectra of skin cancer—a comparison between two techniques, *Skin Res Technol*, **11**, 281–286.

5. Ferreira DM, Silva CS, and Souza MN (2007). Electrical impedance model for evaluation of skin irritation in rabbits and humans, *Skin Res Technol*, **13**, 259–267.

6. Marzec E and Warchol W (2005). Dielectric properties of a protein-water system in selected animal tissues, *Bioelectrochemistry*, **65**, 89–94.

7. Miettinen M, Mönkkönen J, Lahtinen MR, Nuutinen J, and Lahtinen T (2006). Measurement of oedema in irritant-exposed skin by a dielectric technique, *Skin Res Technol*, **12**, 235–240.

8. Bagnaninchi P-O, Dikeakos M, Veres T, and Tabrizian M (2004). Complex permittivity measurement as a new noninvasive tool for monitoring *in vitro* tissue engineering and cell signature through the detection of cell proliferation, differentiation, and pre-tissue formation, *IEEE Trans Nanobiosci*, **3**, 243–250.

9. Skourou C, Rohr A, Hoopes PJ, and Paulsen KD (2007). In vivo EIS characterization of tumour tissue properties is dominated by excess extracellular fluid, *Phys Med Biol*, **52**, 347–363.

10. Hakoda M, Hachisu T, Wakizaka Y, Mii S, and Kitajima N (2005). Development of a method to analyze single cell activity by using dielectrophoretic levitation, *Biotechnol Prog*, **21**, 1748–1753.

11. Yang J, Huang Y, Wang X, Wang XB, Becker FF, and Gascoyne PRC (1999). Dielectric properties of human leukocyte subpopulations determined by electrorotation as a cell separation criterion, *Biophys J*, **76**, 3307–3314.

12. Morgan H, Sun T, Holmes D, Gawad S, and Green NG (2007). Single cell dielectric spectroscopy, *J Phys D Appl Phys*, **40**, 61–70.

13. Debuisson D, Treizebré A, Houssin T, Leclerc E, Bartès-Biesel D, Legrand D, Mazurier J, Arscott S, Bocquet B, and Senez V (2008). Nanoscale devices for online dielectric spectroscopy of biological cells, *Physiol Meas*, **29**, S213–S225.

14. Sun T, Gawad S, Green NG, and Morgan H (2007). Dielectric spectroscopy of single cells: time domain analysis using Maxwell's mixture equation, *J Phys D Appl Phys*, **40**, 1–8.

15. Gimsa J, Müller T, Schnelle T, and Fuhr G (1996). Dielectric spectroscopy of single human erythrocytes at physiological ionic strength: dispersion of the cytoplasm, *Biophys J*, **71**,495–506.

16. Talary MS, Dewarrat F, Huber D, and Caduff A (2007). In vivo life sign application of dielectric spectroscopy and non-invasive glucose monitoring, *J Non-Cryst Solids*, **353**, 4515–4517.

17. Huclova S, Erni D, and Fröhlich J (2010). Modelling effective dielectric properties of materials containing diverse types of biological cells, *J Phys D Appl Phys*, **43**, 365405.

18. Chrit L, Bastien P, Sockalingum GD, Batisse D, Leroy F, Manfait M, and Hadjur C (2006). An in vivo randomized study of human skin moisturization by a new confocal raman fiber-optic microprobe: assessment of a glycerol-based hydration cream, *Skin Pharmacol Physiol*, **19**, 207–215.

19. Wertz PW (2005). *Stratum corneum* lipids and water, *Exogenous Dermatol*, **3**, 53–56.

20. Chen L, Lian G, and Han L (2008). Use of 'bricks and mortar' model to predict transdermal permeation: model development and initial validation, *Ind Eng Chem Res*, **47**, 6465–6472.

21. Kashibuchi N, Hirai Y, O'Goshi K, and Tagami H (2002). Three-dimensional analyses of individual corneocytes with atomic force

microscope; morphological changes related to age, location and to the pathologic skin conditions, *Skin Res Technol*, **8**, 203–211.

22. Potts RO and Francoeur ML (1991). The influence of *stratum corneum* morphology on water permeability, *J Invest Dermatol*, **96**, 495–499.

23. Bouwstra JA, de Graaff A, Gooris GS, Nijsse J, Wiechers JW, and van Aelst AC (2003). Water distribution and related morphology in human *stratum corneum* at different hydration levels, *J Invest Dermatol*, **120**, 750–758.

24. Nakagawa N, Sakai S, Matsumoto M, Yamada K, Nagano M, Yuki T, Sumida Y, and Uchiwa H (2004). Relationship between nmf (lactate and potassium) content and the physical properties of the *stratum corneum* in healthy subjects, *J Invest Dermatol*, **122**, 755–763.

25. Klein-Szanto AJP (1977). Clear and dark basal keratinocytes in human epidermis, *J Cutan Pathol*, **4**, 275–280.

26. Lee AJ, King JR, and Rogers TG (1996). A multiple-pathway model for the diffusion of drugs in skin, *Math Med Biol*, **13**, 127–150.

27. Mogensen M, Morsy HA, Thrane L, and Jemec GBE (2008). Morphology and epidermal thickness of normal skin imaged by optical coherence tomography, *Dermatology*, **217**, 14–20.

28. Prum RO and Torres RH (2004). Structural colouration of mammalian skin: convergent evolution of coherently scattering dermal collagen arrays, *J Exp Biol*, **207**, 2157–2172.

29. Meglinski IV and Matcher SJ (2002). Quantitative assessment of skin layers absorption and skin reflectance spectra simulation in the visible and near-infrared spectral regions, *Physiol Meas*, **23**, 741–753.

30. Tamura T, Tenhunen M, Lahtinen T, Repo T, and Schwan HP (1994). Modeling of the dielectric properties of normal and irradiated skin, *Phys Med Biol*, **39**, 927–936.

31. Novotny GE and Gnoth C (1991). Variability of fibroblast morphology in vivo: a silver impregnation study on human digital dermis and subcutis, *J Anat*, **177**, 195–207.

32. Silver FH, Freeman JW, and DeVore D (2001). Viscoelastic properties of human skin and processed dermis, *Skin Res Technol*, **7**, 18–23.

33. Després JP, Savard R, Tremblay A, and Bouchard C (1983). Adipocyte diameter and lipolytic activity in marathon runners: relationship with body fatness, *Eur J Appl Physiol Occup Physiol*, **51**, 223–230.

34. Gomillion CT and Burg KJL (2006). Stem cells and adipose tissue engineering, *Biomaterials*, **27**, 6052–6063.

35. Gabriel C (2006). Dielectric properties of biological materials, in *Handbook of Biological Effects of Electromagnetic Fields* (Barnes FS and Greenebaum B, eds), Taylor and Francis, London, pp. 52–94.

36. Gabriel S, Lau RW, and Gabriel C (1996). The dielectric properties of biological tissues: III. Parametric models for the dielectric spectrum of tissues, *Phys Med Biol*, **41**, 2271–2293.

37. Raicu V, Kitagawa N, and Irimajiri A (2000). A quantitative approach to the dielectric properties of the skin, *Phys Med Biol*, **45**, L1–L4.

38. Tamura T, Tenhunen M, Lahtinen T, Repo T, and Schwan HP (1994). Modeling of the dielectric properties of normal and irradiated skin, *Phys Med Biol*, **39**, 927–936.

39. Morgan H, Sun T, Holmes D, Gawad S, and Green NG (2007). Single cell dielectric spectroscopy, *J Phys D: Appl Phys*, **40**, 61–70.

40. Sihvola AH (ed) (1999). *Electromagnetic Mixing Formulas and Applications*, The Institution of Electrical Engineers, London.

41. Bruggeman DAG (1937). Berechnung verschiedener physikalischer Konstanten von heterogenen Substanzen. III. Die elastischen Konstanten der quasiisotropen mischkörper aus isotropen substanzen, *Annalen der Physik*, **421**(2), 160–178.

42. Hanai T (1960). Theory of the dielectric dispersion due to the interfacial polarization and its application to emulsions, *Colloid Polym Sci*, **171**(1), 23–31.

43. Asami K (2002). Characterization of heterogeneous systems by dielectric spectroscopy, *Prog Polym Sci*, **27**, 1617–1659.

44. Landau LD, Lifshitz EM, and Pitaevskii LP (eds) (1960). Course of theoretical physics, in *Electrodynamics of Continuous Media*, vol. 8, Pergamon Press, Oxford.

45. Looyenga H (1965). Dielectric constants of heterogeneous mixtures, *Physica*, **31**(3), 401–406.

46. Dube D (1970). Study of Landau–Lifshitz–Looyenga's formula for dielectric correlation between powder and bulk, *J Phys D Appl Phys*, **3**, 1648.

47. Milton G (2002). *The Theory of Composites*, Cambridge University Press, Cambridge.

48. Tuncer E (2010). Geometrical description in binary composites and spectral density representation, *Materials*, **3**, 585–613.

49. Lei J, Wan JTK, Yu KW, and Sun H (2001). First-principle approach to dielectric behaviour of nonspherical cell suspensions, *Phys Rev E*, **64**, 012 903-1–012 903-4.

50. Goncharenko AV and Chang Y-C (2009). Effective dielectric properties of biological cells: Generalization of the spectral density function approach, *J Phys Chem B*, **113**, 9924–9931.

51. Tuncer E (2005). Extracting the spectral density function of a binary composite without a priori assumptions, *Phys Rev B*, **71**(1), 012101.

52. Gheorghiu E, Balut C, and Gheorghiu M (2002). Dielectric behaviour of gap junction connected cells: A microscopic approach, *Phys Med Biol*, **47**, 341–348.

53. Prodan C and Prodan E (1999). The dielectric behaviour of living cell suspensions, *J Phys D Appl Phys*, **32**, 335–343.

54. Tuncer E (2005). The Landau-Lifshitz/Looyenga dielectric mixture expression and its self-similar fractal nature, arXiv:cond-mat/0503750.

55. Goncharenko A (2004). Spectral density function approach to homogenization of binary mixtures, *Chem Phys Lett*, **400**(4–6) 462–468.

56. Huclova S, Fröhlich J, Falco L, Dewarrat F, Talary MS, and Vahldieck R (2009). *Validation of Skin Models in the MHz Region*, paper presented at the 31st *IEEE Eng Med Biol Soc Conf*, Minneapolis.

57. Engström C (2006). *Effective Properties of Heterogeneous Materials with Applications in Electromagnetics*, Ph.D. dissertation, Lund.

58. Huclova S, Erni D, and Fröhlich J (2012). Modeling and validation of dielectric properties of human skin in the MHz region focusing on skin layer morphology and material composition, *J Phys D Appl Phys*, **45**, 025301.

59. Finite-Element simulation platform COMSOL Multiphysics. http://www.comsol.com.

60. Gielis J (2003). A generic geometric transformation that unifies a wide range of natural and abstract shapes, *Am J Botany*, **90**, 333–338.

61. Gielis J, Beirinckx B, and Bastiaens E (2003). *Superquadrics with Rational and Irrational Symmetry*, paper presented at the 8th ACM Symposium on Solid Modeling SM'03, Seattle.

62. Huclova S, Baumann D, Talary MS, and Fröhlich J (2011). Sensitivity and specificity analysis of fringing-field dielectric spectroscopy applied to a multi-layer system modeling human skin, *Phys Med Biol*, **56**, 7777–7793.

63. Naito S, Hoshi M, and Yagihara S (1998). Microwave dielectric analysis of human *stratum corneum* in vivo, *Biochim Biophys Acta*, **1381**, 293–304.

64. Martinsen ØG, Grimnes S, and Sveen O (1997). Dielectric properties of some keratinised tissues: I. *Stratum corneum* and nail in situ, *Med Biol Eng Comput*, **35**, 172–176.

65. Alanen E, Lahtinen T, and Nuutinen J (1999). Measurement of dielectric properties of subcutaneous fat with open-ended coaxial probes, *Phys Med Biol*, **43**, 475–485.

66. Naito S, Hoshi M, and Yagihara S (1998). Microwave dielectric analysis of human *stratum corneum* in vivo, *Biochim Biophys Acta*, **1381**, 293–304.

67. Raicu V, Kitagawa N, and Irimajiri A (2000). A quantitative approach to the dielectric properties of the skin, *Phys Med Biol*, **45**, L1–L4.

68. Tatara T and Tsuzaki K (2000). Derivation of extracellular fluid volume fraction and equivalent dielectric constant of the cell membrane from dielectric properties of the human body: II. A preliminary study for tracking the progression of surgical tissue injury, *Med Biol Eng Comput*, **38**, 384–389.

69. Vogelgesang R (2011). Global surface parametrization by smooth facet selection, *J Comput Theor Nanosci*, **8**(8), 1631–1638.

70. Zhang D (2011). Photonic Heterostructures. Diploma thesis, Fachgebiet Allgemeine und Theoretische Elektrotechnik (ATE), Universität Duisburg-Essen.

71. Colella L, Beyer C, Fröhlich J, Talary M, Renaud P (2012). Microelectrode-based dielectric spectroscopy of glucose effect on erythrocytes, *Bioelectrochemistry*, **85**, 14–20.

72. Beyer C, Krawczyk K, Colella L, and Fröhlich J (2012). *Sensitivity of Dielectric Spectroscopy of Erythrocyte Suspensions with different glucose concentrations*, paper presented at the 7th International Workshop on Biological Effects of Electromagnetic fields, Valletta, Malta. (DOI: 10.3929/ethz-a-007634790).

# Chapter 13

# Model-Based Quantification of Skin Microcirculatory Perfusion

Ingemar Fredriksson,[a,b] Marcus Larsson,[a] and Tomas Strömberg[a]

[a]*Department of Biomedical Engineering, Linköping University, 581 85 Linköping, Sweden*
[b]*Perimed AB, Datavägen 9A, 175 43 Järfälla, Sweden*

ingemar.fredriksson@liu.se

During the past decades, new tools, such as magnetic resonance imaging and Doppler ultrasound imaging, have been rapidly taken into clinical practice for studying the flow dynamics of the macro-circulation. Meanwhile, techniques for quantifying the microcirculation have struggled to become clinically accepted. This includes the use of laser Doppler flowmetry (LDF), an optical technique that is capable of monitoring either spatial or temporal changes in the microcirculation by analyzing the backscattered Doppler-shifted light from a laser-illuminated tissue. Until now, LDF has only been capable of producing non-absolute relative measures, which has limited its clinical acceptance. With a model-based analysis approach, as presented here, this can be overcome, and objective diagnosis of the microcirculation may finally be a part of everyday clinical praxis. The most important advantages with the proposed method are that a quantitative perfusion estimate (% RBC × mm/s) can be extracted and that this measure can be resolved into different speed regions.

*Computational Biophysics of the Skin*

Edited by Bernard Querleux

Copyright © 2014 Pan Stanford Publishing Pte. Ltd.

ISBN 978-981-4463-84-3 (Hardcover), 978-981-4463-85-0 (eBook)

www.panstanford.com

## 13.1 Introduction

The microcirculation includes the capillaries, arterioles, venules, and shunting vessels (arteriovenous anastomosis), the most peripheral part of the vascular tree [1]. In the skin, each of the different compartments has a different anatomy and function. The most superficial layer, the epidermis, is avascular, while the dermal papilla hosts the capillaries that are mainly responsible for the exchange of oxygen and metabolites with its surrounding tissue. Therefore, the blood perfusion through the capillaries is frequently referred to as the nutritive blood flow. The deeper dermal structures contain arterioles, venules, and shunting vessels. The main role of these vessels is to feed and drain the capillary network through the adjustment of their peripheral resistance and permeability and to promote the maintenance of an adequate body temperature by dissipating heat to the environment through the regulation of shunting vessel blood flow.

In other organs, the oxygen transport/nutritive blood flow may start already in the arterioles and not be predominantly in the capillaries. There are longitudinal oxygen gradients in the microcirculation from the larger arterioles down to the capillaries. These gradients depend on the metabolic demands of the tissue in relationship to the microcirculatory blood flow level [2]. In the brain, metabolism lowers tissue oxygen concentration, causing large oxygen diffusion gradients. However, blood flow is large to compensate for this, resulting in intravascular longitudinal oxygen gradients that are relatively small. In resting muscle, metabolic oxygen demand is low, but blood flow is also low resulting in intravascular oxygen gradients that are much larger than in brain vessels.

Since the 1970s, laser Doppler flowmetry has been used to assess the microcirculatory blood perfusion, i.e., the concentration of red blood cells (RBCs) times their average speed [3]. The technique utilizes the Doppler shift that occurs when light is scattered by moving RBCs. These Doppler shifts can indirectly be detected by analyzing the temporal fluctuations found in speckle patterns formed by backscattered light from a laser-illuminated tissue. In conventional LDF, a perfusion measure is generated by calculating the first order moment of the power spectrum of the detected speckle fluctuations. This perfusion measure will scale to both the amount and speed of the moving RBCs in the examined tissue. However, it also strongly depends on other factors such as the geometrical and optical properties of the tissue and is thus given in arbitrary units [4].

This chapter presents a model-based analysis approach that circumvents several inherent weaknesses of conventional LDF. The core of this approach is an individually adaptive mathematical/ bio-optical tissue model that is based on numerous photon propagation simulations for a range of physiologically relevant properties. By tuning the free model parameters, LDF spectra that mimic real measurements can be produced. When the modeled and measured spectra match, output data, given in physiologically relevant units, are obtained from the tissue model. This includes tissue fraction of RBC and perfusion values in absolute units (% RBC and % RBC × mm/s). Information about the speed distribution of these estimates can also be extracted.

We have previously presented a similar method [5] but without the important vessel packaging effect. In tissue, RBCs are located in the blood vessels and are not homogeneously distributed. It has previously been reported that this affects the magnitude of light absorption, which can be accounted for by including a factor depending on the average vessel diameter [6–8]. In LDF, the vessel packaging leads to changes in the shift distribution as the following: (1) consecutive Doppler shifts tend to be caused by RBCs moving with similar velocities; (2) photons that reaches a blood vessel will have a higher degree of multiple Doppler shifts; and (3) the degree of shifted photons will decrease when blood is non-homogeneously distributed. A recently presented method that combines LDF and white light diffuse reflectance spectroscopy includes these vessel packaging effects [9].

A related technique that can decompose the Doppler power spectrum into a speed distribution has been presented by Adam Liebert et al. [10]. Although their method decomposes the spectrum into speeds in mm/s, i.e., the RBC concentration at each speed, the absolute magnitude still remains in arbitrary units. A major limitation of their method is that it assumes that the detected light is Doppler shifted only once. In tissue, already for a homogeneously distributed blood concentration as low as 0.1%, about 2/3 of the detected Doppler-shifted light is shifted more than once [11]. Taking the vessel packaging effect into account, an even smaller amount of the Doppler-shifted light is single shifted. Hence, it is important that high levels of multiple shifted light are treated appropriately.

## 13.2  Model Description

The adaptive bio-optical model is governed by both geometrical and optical properties, as well as the speed distribution of moving RBCs. It is important to include a minimal but sufficient number of free parameters. Minimal in order to avoid overfitting and raising conditions when optimizing the model, sufficient in order to be able to find a solution that fits measured spectra well. A model, valid at 780 nm, could, for example, be defined by

- fix probe parameters
    - source–detector separation: 1.2 mm
    - fiber radius: 0.1 mm
    - numerical aperture: 0.37
- fix parameters of the static tissue
    - skin tissue with 80 µm epidermis above infinitely deep dermis
    - scattering coefficient 10 mm$^{-1}$
    - Henyey–Greenstein scattering phase function with anisotropy factor $g = 0.8$
    - absorption coefficient epidermis 0.6 mm$^{-1}$
    - absorption coefficient dermis 0 mm$^{-1}$
    - refractive index 1.4
- fix blood and blood vessels parameters
    - blood hematocrit of 42%
    - average blood vessel diameter of 40 µm
    - scattering coefficient 222 mm$^{-1}$
    - Gegenbauer kernel phase function with parameters $\alpha_{Gk} = 1.0$, $g_{Gk} = 0.948$ ($g = 0.991$)
    - absorption coefficient 0.5 mm$^{-1}$
    - refractive index 1.4
- free blood parameters
    - speed distribution of moving red blood cells
    - amount of moving red blood cells

With Monte Carlo simulations, it is possible to describe photon propagation through tissue for a given set of parameters. In this context, this is referred to as the *forward problem* (Section 13.3). However, when trying to find which model that best fits the measured data, the *inverse problem* (Section 13.4) needs to be solved, which is a computationally demanding non-linear iterative optimization problem. Hence, it is not feasible to use time-consuming Monte Carlo simulations directly in the optimization algorithm. This is solved by using photon path length distributions from pre-simulated data, where the effect of absorption and the speed distribution can be added in a post-processing step, when calculating the Doppler power spectra in the optimization algorithm. To accurately account for multiple layers, the path length in each layer should be stored for all detected photons in the simulation in order to generate path length distributions. The path length distributions for the model above are given in Fig. 13.1.

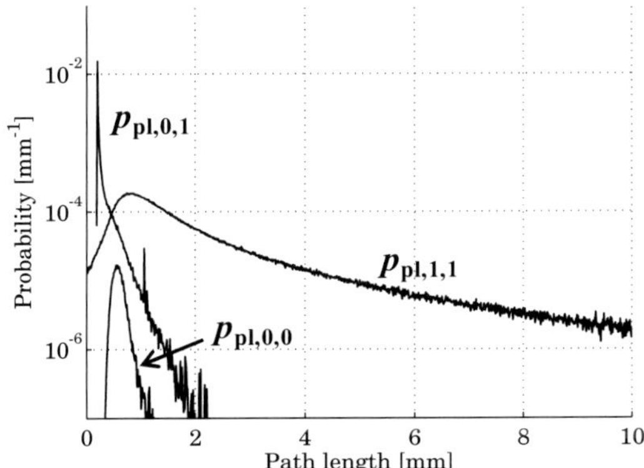


**Figure 13.1**  Example of simulated path length distributions of photons that have propagated either only the top layer ($p_{\mathrm{pl},0,0}$) or both layers ($p_{\mathrm{pl},0,1}$ and $p_{\mathrm{pl},1,1}$).

The above-mentioned model is a minimal free parameter model where only the speed distribution and amount of RBCs are variable. More complex models are discussed in Section 13.7.

## 13.3  Forward Calculation

A flowchart for the calculation of modeled LDF spectra is shown in Fig. 13.2. The details are given in the following subsections. The minimal model given in Section 13.2 is used in this example, but the description is valid for models with an arbitrary number of layers.

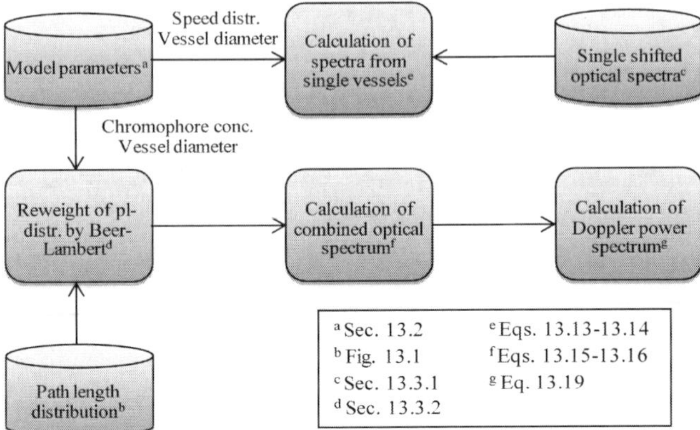


**Figure 13.2** Flowchart of forward calculation of the Doppler power spectrum.

## 13.3.1 Analytic Calculation of Single Shifted Spectrum

A Doppler shift arises when light is scattered an angle $\theta$ by an RBC moving with velocity (speed and direction) $\mathbf{v}$ (see Fig. 13.3). The single shifted optical Doppler spectrum is the probability density function (PDF) of all possible frequency shifts. Given a Gegenbauer kernel scattering phase function [12] with $\alpha_{Gk} = 1$, this PDF can be calculated analytically by assuming an isotropic relationship between the direction of the incoming light and the direction of the moving RBC.

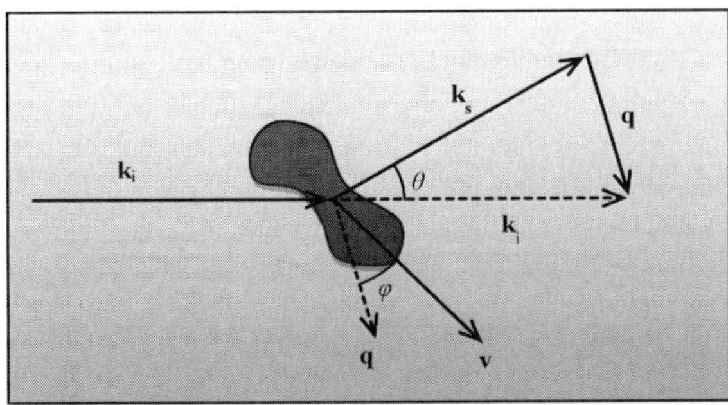


**Figure 13.3** Single Doppler shift with all relevant vectors and angles identified.

The Doppler frequency shift $f$ occurring when light is scattered an angle $\theta$ by an RBC moving with velocity $\mathbf{v}$ can be expressed by

$$f = \mathbf{v}\cdot\mathbf{q} = \frac{2nv}{\lambda}\sin\left(\frac{\theta}{2}\right)\cos\varphi$$
$$= \frac{2nv}{\lambda}\sqrt{\frac{1-\cos\theta}{2}}\cos\varphi = \begin{bmatrix} \mu = \cos\theta \\ \xi = \cos\varphi \end{bmatrix} \tag{13.1}$$
$$= \frac{2nv}{\lambda}\sqrt{\frac{1-\mu}{2}}\xi,$$

where $v = |\mathbf{v}|$, $\mathbf{q}$ is the difference between the wave vectors $\mathbf{k}_i$ and $\mathbf{k}_s$ of the incident and scattered light wave, respectively, $\lambda$ is the laser wavelength, $n$ is the refractive index of the medium, $\theta$ is the scattering angle and $\varphi$ is the angle between $\mathbf{v}$ and $\mathbf{q}$. The single shifted optical Doppler spectrum $y_{0,1}(f)$ for a given set of $v$, $\lambda$, and $n$ can thus be calculated by considering the probability distributions of the angles $\theta$ and $\varphi$. Specifically, for each $f$ given by those $\mu$ and $\xi$ fulfilling

$$\sqrt{\frac{1-\mu}{2}}\xi = \underbrace{\frac{f\lambda}{2nv}}_{A} \quad\Rightarrow\quad \sqrt{\frac{1-\mu}{2}} = x \text{ and } \xi = \frac{A}{x}. \tag{13.2}$$

Hence, $x$ is limited to $[A, 1]$, that is $\mu \in [-1, 1-2A^2]$. The probability of $\mu$ is given by the scattering phase function of blood and the probability of $\xi$ can be assumed to be rectangular distributed between 0 and 1 for positive frequency shifts. The PDF for $\xi = A/x$ is given by

$$y_\xi(x) = \frac{A}{x}. \tag{13.3}$$

The PDF for $\mu$ is given by the scattering phase function (Gegenbauer kernel [12]) which for $\alpha = 1$ is

$$y_\mu(\mu) = \frac{K}{(1+g_{Gk}^2 - 2g_{Gk}\mu)^2}, \tag{13.4}$$

where

$$K = \frac{g_{Gk}(1-g_{Gk}^2)^2}{2((1+g_{Gk})^2 - (1-g_{Gk})^2)}. \tag{13.5}$$

The PDF $y_{0,1}(f)$ is thus given by

$$y_{0,1}(f) = \frac{1}{f}\int_{-1}^{\mu_0} p_\mu(\mu) y_\xi\left(\sqrt{\frac{1-\mu}{2}}\right)d\mu$$

$$= \left[B = \frac{(1-g_{Gk})^2}{4g_{Gk}}\right] = \frac{K\lambda}{8nvg_{Gk}^2}\int_A^1 \frac{1}{(B+x^2)^2}dx$$

$$= \underbrace{\frac{K\lambda}{2nvg_{Gk}(1-g_{Gk})^2}}_{a}\left(\underbrace{\frac{1}{1+B}+\frac{1}{\sqrt{B}}\arctan\frac{1}{\sqrt{B}}}_{b}-\underbrace{\frac{x}{A^2+B}}_{c(f)}-\underbrace{\frac{1}{\sqrt{B}}\arctan\frac{A}{\sqrt{B}}}_{d(f)}\right). \qquad (13.6)$$

The discrete PDF for a frequency bin $f_i$ to $f_{i+1}$ is given by

$$y_{0,1}(f_i) = a\int_{f_i}^{f_{i+1}}(b-c(f)-d(f))\mathrm{d}f$$

$$= \frac{K\lambda}{2nvg_{Gk}(1-g_{Gk})^2}\left[f\left(\frac{1}{1+B}+\frac{1}{\sqrt{B}}\left(\arctan\frac{1}{\sqrt{B}}-\arctan\frac{\lambda f}{2nv\sqrt{B}}\right)\right)\right]_{f_i}^{f_{i+1}}. \qquad (13.7)$$

Note that this expression is only valid for a Gegenbauer kernel phase function with $\alpha_{Gk} = 1$. Note also that the expression is only valid for positive frequency shifts, but the shape is identical (mirrored) for negative frequency shifts.

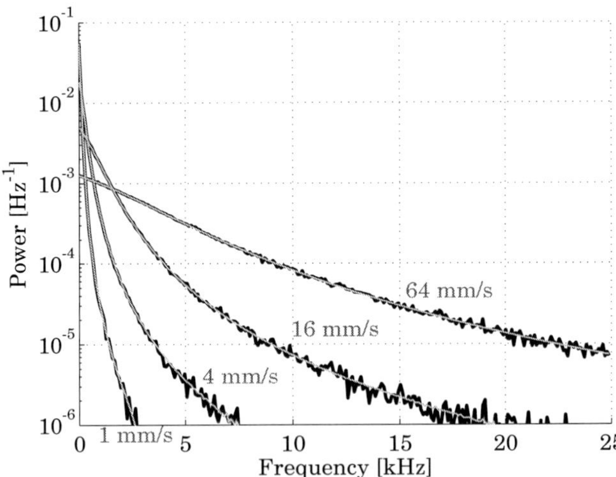


**Figure 13.4** Comparison between simulated (thick black line) and analytically calculated (thin gray line) single shifted optical Doppler spectra for speeds 1.0, 4.0, 16, and 64 mm/s, respectively.

A comparison of an analytically calculated single shifted Doppler spectrum and a simulated spectrum is given in Fig. 13.4. The simulated spectra were generated by randomly sampling the angle $\varphi$ from a uniform distribution and the scattering angle $\theta$ from the scattering phase function for speeds 1.0, 4.0, 16, and 64 mm/s, respectively. A histogram was then generated by calculating Eq. 13.1 for $10^6$ photons.

## 13.3.2 Absorption Effects

Before combining single shifted spectra into the resulting Doppler power spectrum, the path length distributions (see Fig. 13.1) have to be modified due to light absorption. This is done by applying Beer–Lamberts law [13].

The total detected intensity $I_{0,n}$ for photons reaching layer $n$, is given by

$$I_{0,n} = \sum_d p_{\mathrm{pl},m,n}(d),\tag{13.8}$$

where $I_{0,n}$ is independent of $m \leq n$, $p_{\mathrm{pl},m,n}(d)$ is the path length distribution for the photon path length $d$ of photons in tissue layer $m$ that penetrated at most to layer $n$. The path length distributions are then normalized to unity $p'_{\mathrm{pl},m,n}(d) = p_{\mathrm{pl},m,n}(d)/I_{0,n}$. The absorption effect is introduced in the path length distributions for all path lengths $d$ by using Beer–Lamberts law:

$$p''_{\mathrm{pl},m,n}(d) = p'_{\mathrm{pl},m,n}(d)\exp(-d\mu_{\mathrm{a},m}c_{\mathrm{vp}}),\tag{13.9}$$

where $\mu_{\mathrm{a},m}$ is the absorption coefficient of layer $m$, which is calculated as the sum of the absorption coefficients weighted with the chromophore concentrations in that layer. In tissue, RBCs are however located in the blood vessels and not homogeneously distributed. To accurately account for this vessel packaging effect, the absorption coefficient of blood should be modified with a factor $c_{\mathrm{vp}}$ [6–8]:

$$c_{\mathrm{vp}} = \frac{1-\exp(-D\mu_{\mathrm{a,blood}})}{D\mu_{\mathrm{a,blood}}},\tag{13.10}$$

where $D$ is the average vessel diameter. It can be realized that $c_{\mathrm{vp}} \rightarrow 1$ when $D \rightarrow 0$ or $\mu_{\mathrm{a,blood}} \rightarrow 0$.

The detected intensity for all photons that propagated down to layer $n$ and back is now given by

$$I_n = I_{0,n} \prod_{m=1}^{n} \sum_{j} p''_{\text{pl},m,n}(d_j),$$

(13.11)

and the total detected intensity $I$ can then simply be calculated as the sum of the $I_n$:s as follows:

$$I = \sum_n I_n.$$

(13.12)

### 13.3.3 Calculation of Doppler Power Spectrum

In [5], it is described how Doppler power spectra can be calculated using shift distributions that are based on the path length distributions. Here, an extension of that theory is presented where the vessel packaging effect is taken into account in two steps: first, the optical Doppler spectra resulting from passing through one single vessel is modeled; second, all Doppler shifts are summarized by modeling the number of vessels the light passes through. This is a small but important difference from [5]. A mathematical description of this is given in Eqs. 13.13–13.19.

Consider a single shifted optical Doppler spectrum originating from a certain evenly distributed speed distribution between 0 and $2v$ mm/s, $y_{1,v}(f)$ (i.e., the distribution in a vessel with a laminar flow of average velocity $v$). The optical Doppler spectrum for any number of shifts is given by cross correlating the single shifted optical Doppler spectrum as

$$y_{s,v}(f) = y_{s-1,v}(f) * y_{1,v}(f).$$

(13.13)

The non-Doppler-shifted spectrum, $y_{0,v}(f)$, equals Dirac's delta function. Since $y_{s,v}(f)$ can be assumed to be symmetric around $f = 0$ (equal amount of positive and negative Doppler shifts), the cross correlation is equal to a convolution. Fourier transforming ($\mathcal{F}\{\cdot\}$) the optical Doppler spectrum results in $Y_v(\gamma) \equiv \mathcal{F}\{y_{1,v}(f)\}$ and thus $\mathcal{F}\{y_{s,v}(f)\} = Y_v^s(\gamma)$ (i.e., $Y_v(\gamma)$ to the power of $s$), which is a more convenient form.

Assume a vessel with diameter $D$ with a parabolic flow profile with mean speed $v$. When light passes perpendicular through the center axis of that vessel, the number of times the light will be

Doppler-shifted is described by a Poisson distribution with expectation value $\hat{n}_{\text{shifts}} = D\mu_{s,\text{blood}}$ (neglecting a slightly increased path length due to scattering). The light will thus on average be Doppler-shifted $\hat{n}_{\text{shifts}}$ times when passing the vessel, under the assumption that the average path length through the vessel is $D$ (some will propagate a shorter way through the periphery of the vessel and some will propagate a longer way through the vessel with a rather oblique angle). The Fourier transformed optical Doppler spectrum from a single vessel is then given by

$$Y_{\text{vessel},v}(\gamma) = \sum_s Y_v^s(\gamma) p_{\text{Po}}(s;\hat{n}_{\text{shifts}}), \tag{13.14}$$

where $p_{\text{Po}}(s;\hat{n}_{\text{shifts}})$ denotes the probability of $s$ shifts given by the Poisson distribution with $\hat{n}_{\text{shifts}}$. Summarizing these Fourier transformed optical Doppler spectra over the whole distribution of vessels with various flow speeds in the model results in

$$Y_{\text{vessel}}(\gamma) = \sum_j p_{v,j} Y_{\text{vessel},v_j}(\gamma), \tag{13.15}$$

where $p_{v,j}$ denotes the fraction of blood moving with speed $v_j$.

For each path length $d_j$ in a layer, the distribution of the number of vessels that are traversed can be assumed to follow a Poisson distribution with parameter $\hat{n}_{\text{vessels}} = d_j f_{\text{blood},n}/D$. Thus, the distribution of traversed vessels can be calculated from the normalized, absorption modified, path length distribution $p'''_{\text{pl},m,n}(d) = p''_{\text{pl},m,n}(d)/\Sigma_j p''_{\text{pl},m,n}(d_j)$ by

$$p_{\text{vessel},m,n}(s) = \sum_j p'''_{\text{pl},m,n}(d_j) p_{\text{Po}}(s;\hat{n}_{\text{vessels}}). \tag{13.16}$$

This can be compared to the shift distribution $p_{\text{shifts},m,n}$ given by Eq. 13.5 in ref. [5].

The Fourier transformed optical Doppler-shifted spectrum for light that has passed several vessels for all photons in layer $m$ that have been propagating down to layer $n$ can then be calculated as

$$Y_{\text{ms},m,n}(\gamma) = \sum_{v=0}^{V} p_{\text{vessel},m,n}(v) Y_{\text{vessel},m,n}^v(\gamma), \tag{13.17}$$

where $V$ is the maximum number of vessels that the light has passed through.

The next step is to summarize the multiple shifted optical Doppler spectra from all layers by cross correlating them, i.e., calculating the product in the Fourier domain:

$$Y_{\mathrm{ml}}(\gamma) = \sum_{n=1}^{N} I'_n \prod_{m=1}^{n} Y_{\mathrm{ms},m,n}(\gamma), \tag{13.18}$$

where $I'_n = I_n / \sum_m I_m$ and $N$ is the index of the deepest dermis layer (this step is only needed for models with more than one layer containing blood). Finally, the Doppler power spectrum $Y_\mathrm{D}(f)$ is calculated as

$$Y_\mathrm{D}(f) = \mathcal{F}^{-1}\{Y_{\mathrm{ml}}^2(\gamma)\}. \tag{13.19}$$

## 13.4 Inverse Problem

When solving the inverse problem, 10 speed parameters, $p_{v,j}$ ($j \in [0, ..., 9]$) are optimized to fit measured LDF spectra. Each of the 10 speed parameters consists of speeds between 0 and $2v$, where $v$ is the average speed of each speed parameter, $v \in 10^{[-5/6, -3/6, ..., 13/6]}$ mm/s (i.e., between about 0.15 and 150 mm/s). The optimization problem is given by

$$\min_{\mathbf{p}_v} F_{\mathrm{obj,LDF}}(\mathbf{p}_v) \text{ subject to } p_{v,j} \geq 0, \sum_j p_{v,j} \leq 1, j \in [0,9], \tag{13.20}$$

where $\mathbf{p}_v = [p_{v,0}, ..., p_{v,9}]^T$ and the objective function is given by

$$F_{\mathrm{obj,LDF}}(\mathbf{p}_v) = \left\| F_{\mathrm{diff}}(\mathbf{p}_v) \right\|_2^2. \tag{13.21}$$

The inner part, $F_{\mathrm{diff}}(\mathbf{p}_v)$, of the objective function is given by $F_{\mathrm{diff}}(\mathbf{p}_v) = [\mathbf{W}(F_{\mathrm{M1,model}}(\mathbf{p}_v) - fF_{\mathrm{M1,meas}})]$, where $\mathbf{W}$ is a diagonal weight matrix. Here, $F_{\mathrm{M1,model}}(\mathbf{p}_v)$ is given by

$$F_{\mathrm{M1,model}}(\mathbf{p}_v)\begin{bmatrix} \int_{f_0}^{f_1} f y_{\mathrm{D,model}}(f, \mathbf{p}_v)\,df \\[2ex] \int_{f_{i_{\max}-1}}^{f_{i_{\max}}} f y_{\mathrm{D,model}}(f, \mathbf{p}_v)\,df \\[2ex] \int_{f_0}^{f_{i_{\max}}} f y_{\mathrm{D,model}}(f, \mathbf{p}_v)\,df \end{bmatrix}, \tag{13.22}$$

where $f_i = (f_\varepsilon + i\Delta f)^2$, $f_\varepsilon$ is a low frequency above 0, and $y_{D,model}(f, \mathbf{p}_v)$ is the Doppler power spectrum calculated from the model. In analogy, $F_{M1,meas}$ is given by replacing $y_{D,model}(f, \mathbf{p}_v)$ with $y_{D,meas}(f)$ in Eq. 13.22. Note that the last element of the vectors $F_{M1,meas}$ and $F_{M1,model}$ equals the conventional perfusion estimate, i.e., the first order moment of the Doppler power spectrum. The other elements represent the first order moment in certain frequency intervals.

The 10 speed parameters $p_{v,j}$ affect $f_{M1,model}(\mathbf{p}_v)$ approximately linearly:

$$F_{M1,model}(\mathbf{p}_v) + \mathbf{J}(\mathbf{p}_v)\boldsymbol{\delta} = F_{M1,model}(\mathbf{p}_v + \boldsymbol{\delta}) + \boldsymbol{\varepsilon}, \qquad (13.23)$$

where $\mathbf{J}(\mathbf{p}_v)$ denotes the Jacobian matrix, i.e., the derivative of each element in $F_{M1,model}(\mathbf{p}_v)$ with respect to $\mathbf{p}_v$ for each element in $\mathbf{p}_v$. Furthermore, $\boldsymbol{\delta}$ is a change in $\mathbf{p}_v$, and $\boldsymbol{\varepsilon}$ is the deviation from the linear approximation. Based on this, the optimization problem is solved by iterating the following steps:

(1) Choose an initial $\mathbf{p}_v$.
(2) Calculate $f_{M1,model}(\mathbf{p}_v)$.
(3) Calculate the Jacobian at $\mathbf{p}_v$ (using finite differences).
(4) Use constrained regression for finding $\boldsymbol{\delta}$, which approximately solves the optimization problem.
(5) Calculate $F_{M1,model}(\mathbf{p}_v + \boldsymbol{\delta})$.
(6) Calculate $\boldsymbol{\varepsilon}$ from Eq. 13.23.
(7) If $\boldsymbol{\varepsilon}$ is small enough, STOP.
(8) Else, use Broyden's update to estimate the Jacobian at $\mathbf{p}_v + \boldsymbol{\delta}$
(9) Iterate from 4.

This iterative procedure is based on a special case of Broyden's quasi-Newton method, with a full step size (i.e., no line search) in each iteration [14]. The full step size is possible due to the close to linear behavior of $F_{M1,model}(\mathbf{p}_v)$. Broyden's update is an approximate update of the Jacobian over the step $\boldsymbol{\delta}$:

$$\hat{\mathbf{J}}(\mathbf{p}_v + \boldsymbol{\delta}) = \hat{\mathbf{J}}(\mathbf{p}_v) + \frac{(F_{M1,model}(\mathbf{p}_v + \boldsymbol{\delta}) - F_{M1,model}(\mathbf{p}_v) - \mathbf{J}(\mathbf{p}_v)\boldsymbol{\delta})\boldsymbol{\delta}^T}{\boldsymbol{\delta}\boldsymbol{\delta}^T}$$
$$(13.24)$$

In the proposed algorithm, the time-consuming part is to calculate the spectra from the model, which is done once in step 2, 10 times in step 3, and once in step 5. Since only step 5 is iterated among the computationally expensive steps, this optimization is potentially very fast, which is also the case in practice as it converges on average in about four iterations from a randomly generated initial $\mathbf{p}_v$.

## 13.5 Accuracy and Sensitivity

The model given in Section 13.2 was used on 50 simulated Doppler power spectra from complex models containing individual blood vessels with varying speed (parabolic speed profiles), diameter, orientation, and blood oxygenation. Since the "true" perfusion in these models is known, they can be used to evaluate the accuracy of the model-based LDF method. In order for this evaluation to be representative, the model parameters were randomly chosen to cover normal skin variations according to Table 13.1.

**Table 13.1** Skin model parameters for the simulations

|  | **Mean** | **Min** | **Max** | **Std** |
| --- | --- | --- | --- | --- |
| Number of vessels [–] | 285 | 160 | 670 | 125 |
| Vessel diameter [µm] | 21 ± 5 | 6.2 ± 0.1 | 115 ± 60 | 16 ± 7 |
| Vessel speed$^*$ [mm/s] | 3.2 ± 1.2 | 0 | 102 ± 36 | 11 ± 3 |
| Blood oxygenation [%] | 45 ± 10 | 17 ± 14 | 100 | 25 ± 4 |
| Epidermis thickness [µm] | 80 | 10 | 218 | 42 |
| Epidermis $\mu_a$ [mm$^{-1}$] | 0.56 | 0.02 | 2.2 | 0.46 |
| Epidermis $\mu_s'$ [mm$^{-1}$] | 2.9 | 1.4 | 5.0 | 0.7 |
| Dermis $\mu_s'$ [mm$^{-1}$] | 2.0 | 1.2 | 2.9 | 0.4 |

$^*$Mean speed in parabolic flow profile. Smaller vessels have lower speed in general.

The relative root mean square (RMS) deviation between estimated and true perfusion ($[\langle((perf_{est} - perf_{true})/perf_{true})^2\rangle]^{1/2}$) in the sampling volume was 24%. For convenience, the perfusion estimate was resolved into three different speed regions, based on the estimated speed distribution: 0–1 mm/s, 1–10 mm/s, and above 10 mm/s. For the speed-resolved perfusion values the RMS deviation relative to the total perfusion ($[\langle((perf_{v,est} - perf_{v,true})/perf_{tot,true})^2\rangle]^{1/2}$) was 4.6, 11, and 22%, for speed regions 0–1, 1–10, and >10 mm/s, respectively. The estimated perfusion values are plotted against the true values for each of the 50 simulations in Fig. 13.5. For comparison, the conventional perfusion estimate, normalized to the average estimated modeled perfusion for values below 0.2% RBC × mm/s, is also plotted in Fig. 13.5a. The nonlinear behavior [4] of the conventional perfusion estimate becomes clear for high perfusion values. The spectral fit for two of the simulations is shown in Fig. 13.6.

The sensitivity of the method to some parameters that are constant in the model presented in Section 13.2 is shown in Fig. 13.7. In addition to the parameters shown in that figure, the effect of changing the oxygen saturation of blood between 0% and 100%, corresponding to an absorption coefficient for blood between 0.58 and 0.39 mm$^{-1}$ at 780 nm, was also tested. The maximum difference among these 50 models was less than 5%.

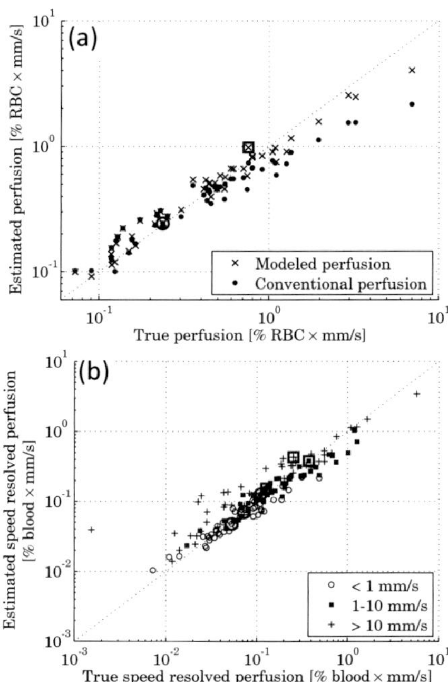


**Figure 13.5** Estimated perfusion as a function of true perfusion in the sampling volume for the 50 simulated skin models. (a) Total modeled perfusion, conventional perfusion; (b) Speed-resolved perfusion. Examples of spectral fits for the marked points are found in Fig. 13.6.

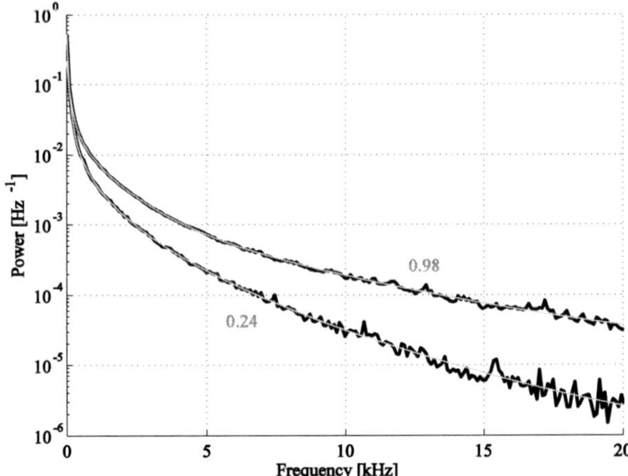

**Figure 13.6** Two examples of spectral fit for total perfusion 0.24% RBC × mm/s (marked with circles in Fig. 13.5) and total perfusion 0.98% RBC × mm/s (marked with square in Fig. 13.5). Thick (noisy) spectra are simulated, and thin spectra are modeled spectra.

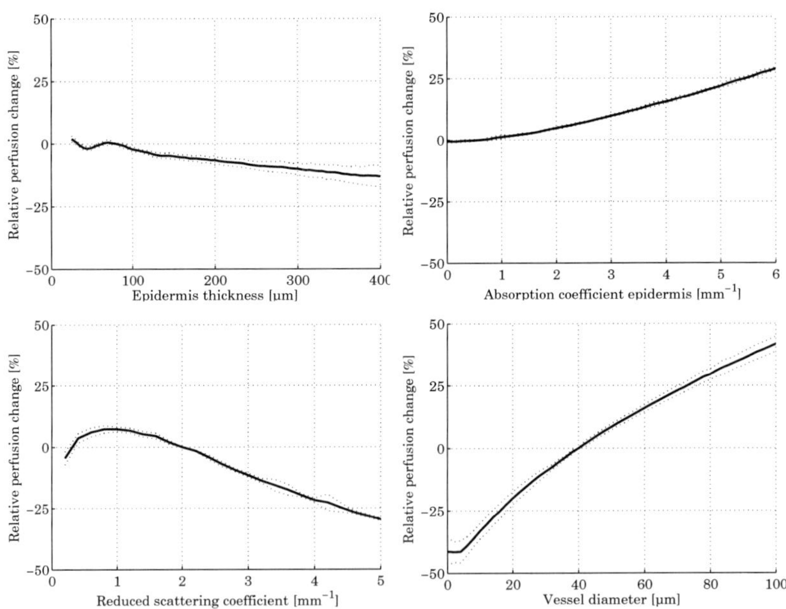

**Figure 13.7** Average (solid lines) ± one standard deviation (dotted lines) change in estimated perfusion as a function of values on four fix model parameters, for the 50 simulated models.

## 13.6   In vivo Example

An example from a heat provocation on the dorsal side of the foot of a healthy volunteer (32-year-old male, fair skin) is shown in Fig. 13.8. The total perfusion increased 11 times from the baseline during the first five minutes to the last five minutes of the provocation. The increase in the low speed region was 5.8 times, in the middle 26 times, and for speeds above 10 mm/s the increase was 7.7 times. Examples of the spectral fit at 5 min, i.e., just before the start of the provocation, and at 25 min are shown in Fig. 13.9.

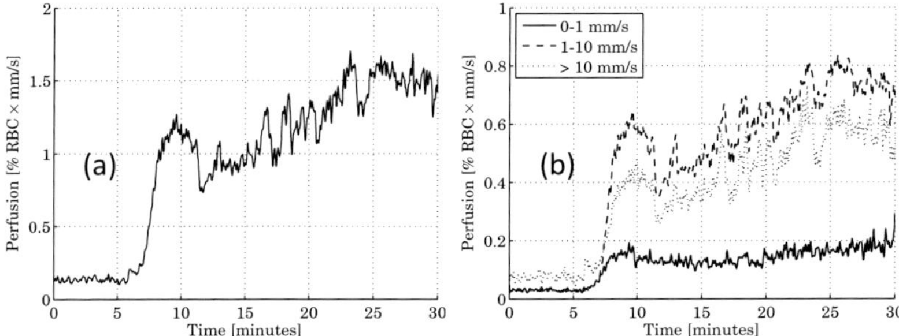


**Figure 13.8**   Heat provocation starting at 5 min (a) Total perfusion. (b) Speed resolved perfusion.

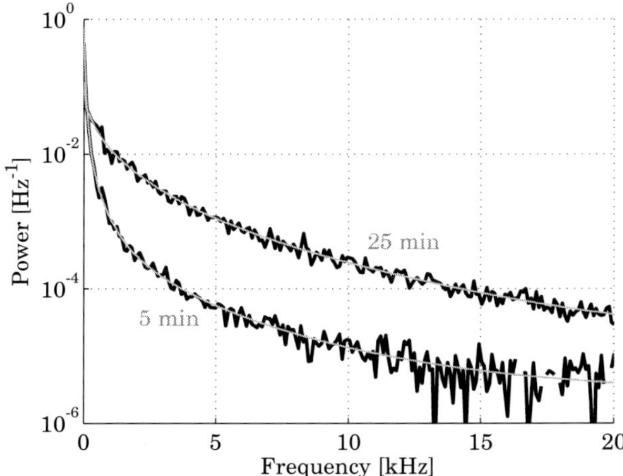


**Figure 13.9**   Examples of spectral fit of modeled spectra (thin line) and measured spectra (thick line) at two time points during a heat provocation (5 min = baseline; 25 min = maximal dilatation).

## 13.7 Discussion and Perspectives

### 13.7.1 Weaknesses and Strengths

Compared to the conventional perfusion, the perfusion estimate from this model-based approach has a number of obvious advantages. First of all, the perfusion can be expressed in a quantitative unit ($\% RBC \times mm/s$). It also lacks the inherent non-linearity to the concentration of moving blood cells that the conventional perfusion estimate suffers from. The most important advantage of the proposed method is probably the ability of differentiating different speeds, an ability that may prove very valuable in clinical settings when studying the capillary activity [15]. Another advantage is the ability to predict the sampling volume using the model [16]. We have chosen to calculate the output data from a volume representative to the sampling volume.

When using the simplified model with fix values on, for example, optical properties described in Section 13.2, the modeled perfusion estimate suffers to some extent from the same weaknesses as the conventional perfusion estimate, i.e., being sensitive to some of these parameters according to Fig. 13.7. That can also be observed in Fig. 13.5a where the deviations from the true perfusion values are similar for the modeled and the conventional perfusion values (except for the non-linearity in the conventional perfusion value). However, a priori knowledge about these parameters can easily be included in the model in order to minimize this effect (see Section 13.7.3).

Compared to conventional LDF, the model-based method is far more computational demanding. First of all, the forward problem is significantly more demanding than calculating the first moment of the Doppler power spectrum, and second, an iterative process that requires multiple calculations of the forward problem is needed to solve the inverse problem. Nevertheless, using an ordinary laptop (dual core 2.5 GHz CPU) with a basic CUDA-enabled GPU (NVIDIA Quadro NVS 160M, 1 multiprocessor with 8 cores), allows for analyzing up to 10 measured spectra per second, and by using a GPU found in a standard stationary computer, hundreds of measured spectra can be analyzed per second. This is possible by utilizing hyper-parallel computing with CUDA when solving the forward problem, which is possible since most calculations are done in the

Fourier domain (see Section 13.3.3). Also, the use of Broyden's update for the Jacobian when solving the inverse problem drastically reduces the number of times the forward problem has to be calculated (see Section 13.4).

## 13.7.2  Calibration

The calibration process is central for the model-based analysis. In conventional LDF, the calculated perfusion signal is calibrated to a controlled motility standard. An improved calibration procedure has been developed to be used with the model-based method, which compensates for any frequency characteristics of the measurement system (including filter characteristics) and absolute calibrates the Doppler power spectrum [11]. Although the new calibration routine is somewhat more demanding from a computational point of view, it is easier to perform in practice as the requirements of the motility standard used are lower. In fact, any scattering liquid, for example, milk, can be used with the same result. This is possible since it is the total energy of the Doppler power spectrum that is calibrated, not the first moment which is dependent on the size and number of Doppler shifts. All light is Doppler shifted due to Brownian motion in any scattering liquid, and the total energy is therefore independent of the liquid used. Thus, the improved calibration procedure is also advantageous for conventional LDF.

## 13.7.3  Extensions

By using more than one source–detector separation, additional model parameters can be determined and should thus be variable or free in the model (for example, the thickness of the epidermis layer). More layers with different speed distributions could also be added. Such an extension may improve the accuracy of the estimated perfusion and it may also add valuable clinical information.

The model is, from a bio-optical point of view, general and easily extendable by, for example, adding additional chromophores and wavelengths. Thus, only with small modifications, other bio-optical measurement modalities may be added to further improve the parameter estimation accuracy and/or enabling other clinically relevant parameters to be determined. For example, by incorporating white light diffuse reflectance spectroscopy

(DRS), model parameters such as epidermis thickness, scattering coefficient (wavelength dependent), total RBC tissue fraction, RBC oxygen saturation and average vessel diameter can be free in the model and fitted to DRS spectra. The same pre-simulated path length distributions can be used where the absorption effect is added for each wavelength according to Section 13.3.2. We have already described this type of model-based DRS [13]. By integrating LDF and DRS into the same measurement probe and analysis model, the sensitivity to the parameters described in Fig. 13.7, could be minimized. At the same time, some of these parameters, especially the oxygen saturation, are clinically interesting themselves.

## 13.7.4 Clinical Impact

A first study indicating the potential clinical impact of model-based LDF has already been presented [15]. For the first time we observed, using this technique, that increased blood flow during local heating is a process involving non-nutritive vessels and that diabetes patients have a reduced nutritive but increased AV-shunt flow at baseline.

These findings were made possible due to the differentiation of the flow into different flow speed regions. This is probably the most important ability of the model-based approach compared to the conventional approach. One reason that LDF has not yet gained widespread clinical acceptance is that it is non-quantitative in its nature which makes it hard to interpret and to compare results with other techniques, between individuals and between different LDF measurement systems. The model-based approach eliminates this limitation as well.

The clinical need for a robust method to measure the microcircular blood flow is evidently high, especially for diagnosing microvascular changes in one of the fastest growing diseases in the world — diabetes mellitus. Lower limb ischemia resulting in peripheral artery disease (PAD) often leads to leg and foot ulcers and is a common complication in diabetes. Only in the United States, there are about 4 million diabetes patients who suffer from these ulcers [17] and up to 1/4 of these ulcers eventually lead to an amputation [18]. In the inter-society consensus document about PAD [18], the importance of evaluating the microcirculation in these patients in order to give the correct diagnosis and proper treatment is clearly emphasized. However, this is often not done in the clinical practice. One reason for this is the lack of methods that allow measurements to be done in physiologically relevant units.

## 13.8 Conclusions

A model-based approach may be used to drastically increase the amount and quality of information that can be extracted from LDF measurements. The most important advantages are that a quantitative perfusion estimate (% RBC × mm/s) can be attained and that this measure can be resolved into different speed regions. The approach also makes it possible to reveal the sampling volume and, by adding multiple source–detector separations, a depth resolved perfusion may be extracted. The model presented in this chapter may relatively easily be extended to be valid also for other bio-optical measurement modalities, such as DRS, which would add more clinical relevant parameters and improve the accuracy of the estimated perfusion quantities.

### Acknowledgments

This work was financed by VINNOVA through the Research& Grow program (VINNOVA D. no. 2011-03074), and also by Nova-MedTech, supported by the European Union Regional Development Fund.

### References

1. Rhodin JAG (1981). Anatomy of the microcirculation, in *Microcirculation: Current Physiologic, Medical and Surgical Concepts* (Effros RM, Schmid-Schoenbein H, and Dietzel J, eds), Academic Press, New York, pp. 11–17.

2. Tsai AG, Johnson PC, and Intaglietta M (2003). Oxygen gradients in the microcirculation, *Physiol Rev*, **83**(3), 933–963.

3. Riva C, Ross B, and Benedek GB (1972). Laser Doppler measurements of blood flow in capillary tubes and retinal arteries, *Invest Ophthalmol Visual Sci*, **11**(11), 936–944.

4. Fredriksson I, Larsson M, and Strömberg T (2012). Laser Doppler Flowmetry, in *Microcirculation Imaging* (Leahy MJ, ed), Wiley-Blackwell, Weinheim, pp. 67–86.

5. Fredriksson I, Larsson M, and Strömberg T (2010). Model-based quantitative laser Doppler flowmetry in skin, *J Biomed Opt*, **15**(5), 057002.

6. Svaasand L, Fiskerstrand E, Kopstad G, Norvang LT, Svaasand EK, Nelson JS, and Berns MW (1995). Therapeutic response during pulsed laser treatment of port-wine stains: Dependence on vessel diameter and depth in dermis, *Laser Med Sci*, **10**(4), 235–243.

7. van Veen RLP, Verkruysse W, and Sterenborg HJCM (2002). Diffuse-reflectance spectroscopy from 500 to 1060 nm by correction for inhomogeneously distributed absorbers, *Opt Lett*, **27**(4), 246–248.

8. Fredriksson I, Larsson M, and Strömberg T (2011). Accuracy of vessel diameter estimated from a vessel packaging compensation in diffuse reflectance spectroscopy, *Proc SPIE*, **8087**, 80871M.

9. Fredriksson I, Burdakov O, Larsson M, and Strömberg T (2013). Inverse Monte Carlo in a multilayered tissue model—merging diffuse reflectance spectroscopy and laser Doppler flowmetry, *J Biomed Opt*, **18**(12), p. 127004–127004.

10. Liebert A, Wojtkiewicz S, and Maniewski R (2012). Toward assessment of speed distribution of red blood cells, in *Microcirculation Imaging* (Leahy MJ, ed); Wiley-Blackwell, Weinheim, 87–112.

11. Fredriksson I, Larsson M, Salomonsson F, and Strömberg T (2011). Improved calibration procedure for laser Doppler perfusion monitors, in *Optical Diagnostics and Sensing XI: Toward Point-of-Care Diagnostics; and Design and Performance Validation of Phantoms Used in Conjunction with Optical Measurement of Tissue III* (Nordstrom RG and Coté GL, eds), *Proc SPIE*, 7906, San Francisco, 790602.

12. Reynolds LO and McCormick NJ (1980). Approximate two-parameter phase function for light scattering, *J Opt Soc Am*, **70**(10), 1206–1212.

13. Fredriksson I, Larsson M, and Strömberg T (2012). Inverse Monte Carlo method in a multilayered tissue model for diffuse reflectance spectroscopy, *J Biomed Opt*, **17**(4), 047004-12.

14. Nocedal JA and Wright SJ (eds) (2006). *Numerical Optimization*. 2nd ed, Springer Verlag, New York.

15. Fredriksson I, Larsson M, Nyström FH, Länne T, Östgren CJ, and Strömberg T (2010). Reduced arteriovenous shunting capacity after

local heating and redistribution of baseline skin blood flow in type 2 diabetes assessed with velocity-resolved quantitative laser Doppler flowmetry, *Diabetes*, **59**(7), 1578–1584.

16. Fredriksson I, Larsson M, and Strömberg T (2009). Measurement depth and volume in laser Doppler flowmetry, *Microvasc Res*, **78**(1), 4–13.

17. (2010). *Diabetic Foot Ulcers, Peripheral Artery Disease and Critical Limb Ischemia*. The Sage Group, http://thesagegroup.us/pages/reports/dfu-statistics.php.

18. Norgren L, Hiatt WR, Dormandy JA, Nehler MR, Harris KA, Fowkes FG, TASC II Working Group, Bell K, Caporusso J, Durand-Zaleski I, Komori K, Lammer J, Liapis C, Novo S, Razavi M, Robbs J, Schaper N, Shigematsu H, Sapoval M, White C, White J, Clement D, Creager M, Jaff M, Mohler E 3rd, Rutherford RB, Sheehan P, Sillesen H, and Rosenfield K (2007). Inter-society consensus for the management of peripheral arterial disease (TASC II), *Eur J Vasc Endovasc Surg*, **33**(1) (Supplement 1), S1–S75.

# PART 5

# SKIN HOMEOSTASIS

# Chapter 14

# Graphical Multi-Scale Modeling of Epidermal Homeostasis with EPISIM

Thomas Sütterlin[a,b] and Niels Grabe[a,b]

[a]Department of Medical Oncology, National Center for Tumor Diseases,
University Hospital Heidelberg,
Im Neuenheimer Feld 267 Heidelberg, D-69120, Germany
[b]Hamamatsu Tissue Imaging and Analysis Center, BioQuant, Heidelberg University,
Im Neuenheimer Feld 267 Heidelberg, D-69120, Germany

niels.grabe@bioquant.uni-heidelberg.de

## 14.1    Introduction

The investigation of epidermal homeostasis and differentiation is ideal for developing systems biological models linking the molecular to the cellular and further on to the tissue level. There to a certain extent literature on in silico models of human epidermis and of course more of epithelia in general. Early models date back to the 1980s when epidermal tissue formation has been simulated with vertical stacks of flattened tetrakaidecahedral cells [1,2]. Mitrani used a lattice-based model to show that upward migration of keratinocytes within the epidermis is a passively driven process. Passive migration results from the extrusion of basal cells due to forces exerted by dividing cells [3]. The first spatial simulation of an epidermis using a lattice-free (off-lattice) model was

*Computational Biophysics of the Skin*

Edited by Bernard Querleux

Copyright © 2014 Pan Stanford Publishing Pte. Ltd.

ISBN  978-981-4463-84-3 (Hardcover),  978-981-4463-85-0 (eBook)

www.panstanford.com

developed in 1995. This mode mainly focused on cell proliferation and differentiation [4]. More recently, off-lattice models of epithelial monolayers [5,6] and three-dimensional epithelial cell populations [7] were developed. In 2005, Grabe et al. presented a two-dimensional model of human epidermis that includes not only cell proliferation and differentiation but also the essential process of epidermal barrier formation [8]. Moreover, the transepidermal water flux and the associated flow of $Ca^{2+}$ ions leading to the characteristic transepidermal $Ca^{2+}$ gradient was part of this model. Terminal differentiation is controlled by this $Ca^{2+}$ gradient. Simulation showed a horizontally layered in silico tissue morphology as a result of the $Ca^{2+}$ differentiation program. An application with clinical relevance of this human epidermal homeostasis model was developed by reproducing main pathological characteristics of psoriatic skin [9]. One of the first three-dimensional epidermal homeostasis models also considering in silico melanoma development was published in the same year [10]. Finally, Adra et al. presented a multi-scaled three-dimensional in silico model of human epidermis linking keratinocyte behavior and transforming growth factor (TGF-β1) signaling [11].

Multi-scale models are characterized by bridging the sub-cellular, the cellular, and sometimes even the tissue modeling level by semantically linking models on these distinct levels. Undeniably, only such multi-scaled models are able to comprehensively represent biological reality. Whereas the majority of published systems biological models still focus exclusively on the subcellular level, multi-scale models become increasingly frequent. Large research consortia such as the German Virtual Liver Network [12] or the European Human Brain Project [13] set out to build highly complex multi-scaled models linking even the tissue with the organ level. Building highly complex and at the same time reusable and extendable multi-scale in silico models requires a sound software technology base. User-friendly software tools to build, simulate, analyze, archive, and publicly provide multi-scale models will be more and more crucial.

The majority of the currently available software tools target modeling on the subcellular level (e.g., Cytoscape is a well-known software for modeling, integrating and analyzing qualitative large-scale biomolecular interaction networks). The software CellDesigner allows graphical quantitative modeling of biochemical reaction and gene-regulatory networks without a spatial resolution [14]. COPASI is a widely used tool for the simulation and the analysis of biochemical networks [15]. Virtual Cell can be used for modeling biochemical processes with spatial resolution [16]. These software tools and more than 200 other software packages support the systems biology markup language (SBML) which is the most commonly used standard for mainly quantitative subcellular models [17]. This standard allows exchanging models built with different software tools. The database BioModels provides a huge variety of SBML-based models for download. Some software tools, such as CellDesigner and VirtualCell, already allow direct importing of complete ready-to-run SBML-based models from BioModels. Providing read-to-run models in a standardized format is a very promising technological approach and avoids tedious and error prone model reproduction from literature. This way of publishing and reusing of models is groundbreaking for the future of in silico modeling.

Unfortunately, there is not a commonly supported standard for cell-based tissue models or for multi-scale models linking the subcellular to the cellular modeling level. The availability of dedicated software tools for building single or even multi-scale cell-based tissue models is very limited. Modeling and simulation frameworks such as Chaste [18] require extensive programming skills and can therefore hardly be used by scientists with a rather biological background. Currently, there is no ready-to-use and easy-to-install software tool that fully hides the technical complexity of realizing multi-scaled models. An exception is the software CompuCell3D [19,20]. It enables to directly reference and simulate SBML-based models within a multi-cellular tissue simulation which is based on the Glazier–Graner–Hogeweg Model [21]. However, CompuCell3D models are manually built and configured with Python scripts and extensible mark-up language (XML)-files. This, in turn, requires dedicated knowledge of these computer science-related concepts. To our knowledge, there is no intuitive and user-friendly software tool semantically linking and integrating models on different scales to a multi-cellular tissue model without any kind of coding.

To this end, we developed a modular multi-scale model architecture for cell-based tissue models. Based on the modular architecture, we built the ready-to-use software platform EPISIM for graphical cell behavioral modeling and multi-agent–based tissue simulation [22,23]. This software allows graphically building Cell behavioral models (CBMs) in the form of process diagrams. These CBMs can be semantically linked to imported SBML-based subcellular models. By this, cellular states like proliferation and differentiation can be flexibly coupled to biochemical or gene-regulatory networks. EPISIM automatically generates highly efficient executable code based on both, the graphical CBMs and the imported SBML-based models. This executable coded model version can be dynamically loaded by EPISIM's simulation environment performing a multi-scale agent-based tissue simulation.

We used EPISIM to graphically implement our model of epidermal homeostasis [8]. Semantically self-contained model aspects like cell cycle, cell differentiation, or epidermal barrier formation are modeled in form of hierarchically connected graphical cell behavioral sub-models. The cell cycle sub-model is semantically linked with the imported SBML based version of Tysons cell cycle model available in BioModels database. The resulting graphical multi-scale CBM is dynamically linked to a 2D and a 3D center-based biomechanical model provided by our simulation environment. Finally, a 2D as well as a 3D multi-scale simulation of epidermal homeostasis is conducted and simulation results are compared.

## 14.2   Methods and Software Technologies

Our graphical multi-scale modeling and simulation platform EPISIM is composed of the following ready to use software tools: (i) the graphical modeling system EPISIM Modeller and (ii) the simulation environment EPISIM Simulator. The EPISIM Modeller was built using the open source rich client platform Eclipse. Eclipse is based on the Equinox framework developed by the Open Services Gateway initiative (OSGi). This allows Eclipse to be dynamically extended by plug-ins. EPISIM Modeller is subdivided into four individual components, each one representing a set of Eclipse plug-ins: (i) Variable-Sheet Editor, (ii) Graphical Model Editor (GME), (iii) Function Library, and (iv) SBML Model Editor (SBME). We applied a model-driven software development approach to build these components. Each component was designed with a Unified Modeling Language (UML) based meta-model. The components' meta-models in turn are instances of the meta-meta model Ecore of the Eclipse Modeling Framework (EMF). The EMF code generator is able to derive source code from Ecore-instances. The java-classes resulting from this code generation process are the data model components of EPISIM Modeller. For implementing the GEF components, the in this way generated java-classes are deployed using the Graphical Editing Framework (GEF). In general, the GEF is used to implement a component which is able to graphically create and manipulate instances of a given data model [24,25].

Graphical CBMs built with the GME are stored in the XML-Metadata-Interchange (XMI) format, which is an open standard of the Object Management Group (OMG). For EPISIM we implemented a code generator to generate optimized Java source code out of the XMI-files. This source code is then translated into java byte code using Oracles java compiler. Graphical CBMs are automatically validated by a parser realized with the open source Java Compiler Compiler (JavaCC). The parser generator JavaCC allows generating a LL(k)-parser on the basis of a given grammar [26]. The translated executable CBMs control an agent's behavior in a multi-agent simulation. Thereby each cell of a multi-cellular simulation is represented by an individual agent. We developed a graphical multi-agent–based simulation environment EPISIM Simulator to execute and thereby simulate the translated CBMs in a multi-cellular tissue context. EPISIM Simulator is built on top of George Mason University's multi-agent simulation framework MASON (Multi Agent Simulation Of Neighborhoods) [27].

To enable multi-scale cell behavioral modeling, the EPISIM Modeller allows importing quantitative subcellular models that are based on the SBML (SBML) standard. Systems biology markup language model files are imported using the library JSBML offering purely Java based data structures for reading, writing and manipulating SBML files [28]. All species, reactions, and parameters are stored in a separate XMI-file. This file represents the input for the SBME while the original SBML file remains unchanged. We integrated COPASI (Complex Pathway Simulator) as a plug-in for EPISIM Simulator. COPASI is used for deterministic time course simulations (LSODA solver) of imported SBML models [15].

## 14.3 EPISIM Multi-Scale Modeling & Simulation Platform

The EPISIM platform offers two ready-to-use software tools with an easy to handle out of the box installation routine [22,23]. EPISIM targets a community without extensive computational skills. Hence, the major objective behind the development of EPISIM is to abstract away from the technical complexity of building multi-scaled biological models and simulations respectively. EPISIM Modeller allows graphical modeling of cellular behavior in a multi-cellular context. The graphical CBMs are automatically translated into highly efficient executable code that in turn can be loaded by the simulation environment EPISIM Simulator. The simulation environment performs a multi-agent–based tissue simulation where each cell is represented by an individual agent. An agent's and thereby a cell's behavior is controlled by the loaded CBM.

The EPISIM platform is freely available on the website of the Hamamatsu TIGA Center: http://www.tiga.uni-hd.de.

### 14.3.1 EPISIM Multi-Scale Model Architecture

Each spatio-temporal multi-cellular tissue simulation conducted with EPISIM has the same underlying multi-scaled model architecture (Fig. 14.1). An EPISIM cell-based in silico tissue model consists at least of a graphical CBM and a Biomechanical Model (BM). Optionally, quantitative subcellular models that are based on the systems biology markup language (SBML) [17] can be imported with EPISIM Modeller and semantically integrated in a CBM. The BM comprises all spatial and biophysical cellular aspects of an EPISIM based model such as cell size and shape, cell growth, cell migration as well as cell–cell adhesion. The CBM, in turn, reflects processes that lead to the general cellular states: proliferation, differentiation and cell-death. Moreover, a CBM includes cell–cell communication as well as secretion and absorption of molecules. CBM and BM are linked with a Model Connector Component (MCC). EPISIM Simulator offers BMs for 2D as well as 3D tissue simulations. It is up to the modeler to link a graphical CBM to one of these models by importing the according MCC with EPISIM Modeller. All input and output parameters of a BM can then be referenced and modified within a CBM and by that semantically integrated into processes resulting in a particular cellular state. The MCC enables the bi-directional data flow between BM and CBM during simulation.

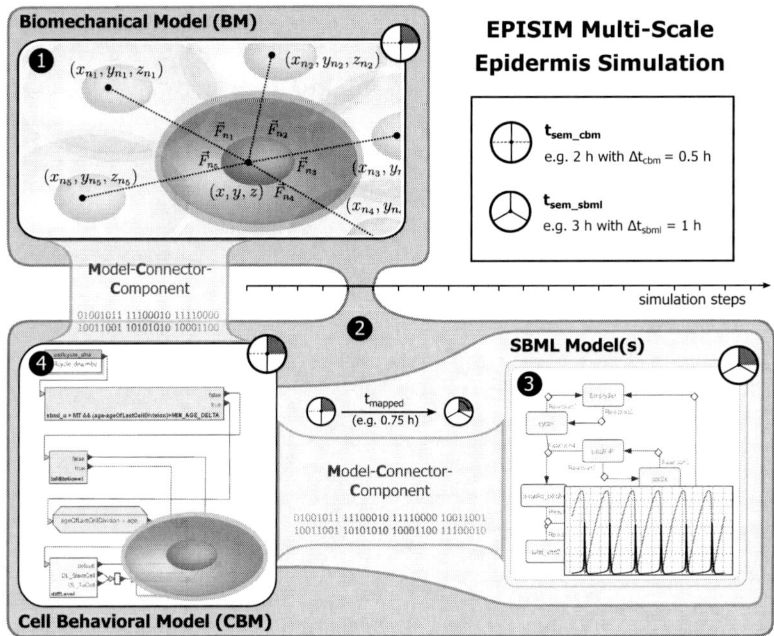


**Figure 14.1** EPISIM multi-scale cell-based tissue model architecture.

Tools like CellDesigner can be used to build subcellular SBML based models mainly reflecting gene-regulatory or biochemical reaction networks [29]. There is also a number of publicly available models that can be loaded from databases like BioModels [30]. An arbitrary number of SBML models can be imported with EPISIM Modeller and semantically integrated in the CBM. A MCC for each imported SBML model is automatically generated, when a CBM is translated into executable code. This MCCs are similar to the one connecting BM and CBM. The MCC enables accessing an SBML model's species, parameters, and reaction fluxes. In addition, an SBML model MCC realizes a couple of other functionalities which have been described in detail earlier [23]. We here focus on the automatic time scale mapping between CBM and a particular SBML model during simulation as this mapping done by the MCC needs a modeler's parameterization.

As depicted in Fig. 14.1 CBM and BM have the same time scale, which is the clock frequency of the multi-cellular tissue simulation. The simulation clock causes the assumption of an atomic time step for a CBM as well as a BM here denoted $\Delta t_{cbm}$. This atomic time step is not explicitly defined. Moreover, it is a result of the chosen values for the BM and CBM parameters. The SBML model's simulation time $\Delta t_{smbl}$ denotes the model's time-unit (e.g., hours). The mapped time $t_{mapped}$ then corresponds to the time interval a particular SBML model is simulated within each tissue simulation step $\Delta t_{cbm}$. The modeler hast to determine semantically equivalent time periods $t_{sem\_cbm}$ in the CBM and $t_{sem\_smbl}$ in the SBML model. Such time periods can be the cell cycle time in the CBM and the time in the semantically linked SBML-based cell cycle model (Section 14.4.2.1).

$$t_{mapped} = \frac{\Delta t_{cbm} \times t_{sem\_sbml}}{\Delta t_{sbml} \times t_{sem\_cbm}} \tag{14.1}$$

During time course simulation of an SBML model, $n_{points}$ time points subdividing $t_{mapped}$ are calculated. The time interval $\Delta t_{point}$ between two such time points is

$$\Delta t_{point} = \frac{t_{mapped}}{n_{points}} \tag{14.2}$$

The value of $\Delta t_{point}$ influences the accuracy a SBML model's numerical time course simulation. While too large values lead to incorrect simulation results, too small values cause an unnecessary increase of computation time without improving the simulation accuracy. An optimal value for $n_{points}$ has to be determined depending on the kinetics underlying a particular SBML model. The values for $t_{mapped}$ (*No Of Time Units Per Simstep*) and $n_{points}$ (*No Of Points Per CBM Simstep*) have to be individually set in EPISIM Modeller for each imported SBML model.

### 14.3.2 EPISIM Modeller: The Graphical Modeling System

EPISIM Modeller enables building multi-scaled graphical CBMs for multi-cellular tissue simulations. As illustrated in Fig. 14.2, EPISIM Modeller has four major components: (i) the Variable-Sheet Editor,

(ii) the Graphical Model Editor (GME), (iii) the Function Library, and (iv) SBML Model Editor (SBME).

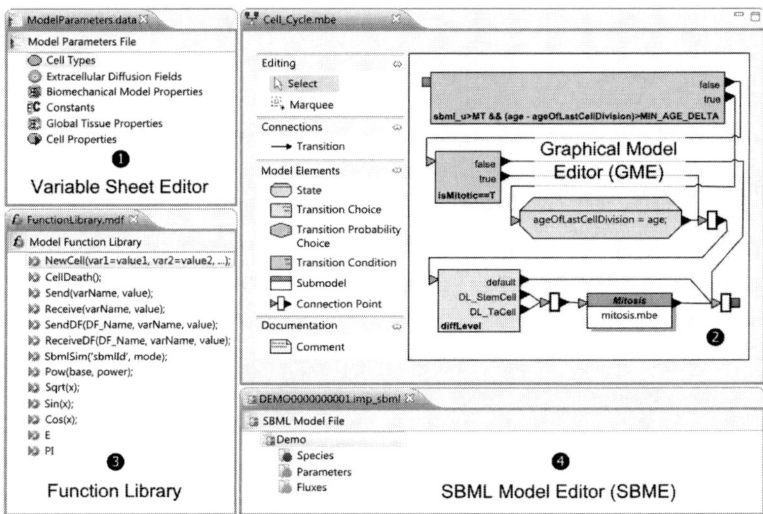


**Figure 14.2** EPISIM Modeller with major components: (1) Variable-Sheet Editor, (2) Graphical Model Editor, (3) Function Library and (4) SBML Model Editor.

There are six different types of model parameters that can be defined and administered using the Variable-Sheet Editor:

(1) *Cell Types*: Each cell in a tissue simulation is assigned a unique cell type. Optionally, such a cell type can comprise multiple differentiation stages. The definition of two distinct cell types would be sensible for keratinocytes and fibroblasts whereas spinosum and granulosum cells would rather be defined as two differentiation stages assigned to cell type "keratinocyte."

(2) *Extracellular Diffusion Fields*: Each tissue simulation can contain an arbitrary number of user defined extracellular diffusion fields simulating chemokine milieus. Cells can secrete to or absorb from these fields. The diffusion and the decay of chemokines are simulated numerically during the simulation of the graphical CBMs based on the chosen field parameterization.

(3) *Biomechanical Model Properties*: Input and output values of the BM that is linked to the CBM are called biomechanical

model properties. Such a property can define read-only or read-write access. In case of read-only access (e.g., cell location coordinates), the value of a biomechanical model property is restricted to one directional referencing. The access type is defined in the BM's MCC.

(4) *Constants*: A model parameter defined as constant never changes its value during simulation (e.g., Mitotic Threshold *MT*).

(5) *Global Tissue Properties*: These variables hold values of global properties that are the same for all cells in the simulated tissue. Contrary to "constants," the value of global tissue properties can be modified interactively in EPISIM Simulator prior to or during tissue simulation.

(6) *Cell Properties*: This kind of variable reflects anything that is individual each cell such as the intracellular concentration of a molecule, the activation of a signaling pathway or the presence of a particular receptor. During simulation each cell occupies these variables with individual values, thus realizing a personal state for each cell. A maximum and/or a minimum value can optionally be defined for cell properties. These values can be referenced by concatenating the suffixes "_min" or "_max" to a cell property's name. EPISIM Simulator ensures that the simulated cell property values lie within the range given by the maximum and minimum value.

The GME is used to interactively build graphical CBMs in form of process diagrams. The model elements of this graphical modeling language (GML) are described in detail in Table 14.1. The GML can be utilized to build purely deterministic, purely stochastic but also hybrid CBMs. Branching within a model can be done based on Boolean expressions, mathematical relations, variable values and finally based on probabilities. Sub-models allow realizing a hierarchical model structure where each sub-model realizes a self-contained biological function.

The Function Library contains commands for cell division, cell death, cell–cell communication, intercellular molecule exchange and the secretion or absorption of molecules to and from an extracellular diffusion field. The command *Send*(*varName, value*) can be used to distribute an amount "*value*" of cell property "*varName*" among all adjacent cells. *Receive*(*varName, value*) realizes the inverse process.

The command *CellDeath()* causes a cell's removal from the tissue simulation reflecting apoptosis. On the contrary, *NewCell(...)* leads to cell division and includes a new cell in the simulation. The initial parameterization of the new cell's properties can be done in the parentheses.

**Table 14.1**  Model elements for the specification of graphical cell behavioral models

| Model element | Symbol | Description |
|---|---|---|
| State | 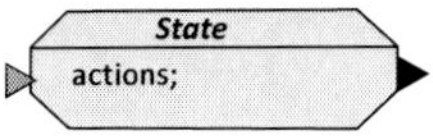 | In a state element a set of "actions strings" can be defined which are sequentially executed at runtime. Action strings may be assignments of values to cell properties or calls of predefined functions for cell division, cell–cell communication, etc. |
| Transition choice | 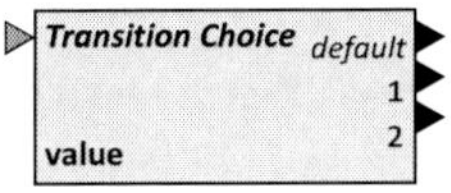 | Transition choices allow to branch to multiple paths in a model in dependence of a mathematical expression or a value. Output ports can be defined for all expected results or values. The path connected to the "default output port" is followed if the value of the evaluated variable matches none of the defined output ports. |
| Transition probability choice | 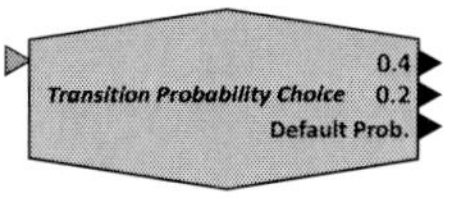 | Transition probability choices allow to branch to multiple paths based on given rates assigned to a particular output port. An unlimited number of output ports can be defined. A "Default Prob." port can be added as a default path to be followed if none of the other output ports was chosen by the random experiment underlying this model element. |

*(Continued)*

**Table 14.1** (*Continued*)

| Model element | Symbol | Description |
|---|---|---|
| Transition condition | Transition Condition / condition / false / true | Transition conditions allow to branch to two distinct paths in a model in dependence of a Boolean expression being either true or false. |
| Sub-model | Submodel / submodel.mbe | Sub-models allow implementing a hierarchical CBM structure. The overall CBM can be physically distributed over different model files. Semantically, each file realizes a certain self-contained functional CBM. The number of sub-models is unlimited. |
| Connection point |  | In case multiple transitions shall lead to a single common model element, a connection point has to be used to join the incoming edges. |
| Edge |  | Edges connect two model elements using their input port and output port (symbolized by triangles), respectively. |
| Comment | This is an explanation of the model. | Textual descriptions or explanations of model semantics can be added as a comment. |

The SBML Model Editor (SBME) allows to access an imported SBML based quantitative model. A model's reactions (also called fluxes), species and parameters can be directly dragged and dropped to any model element in the GME where a particular value should be referenced. Moreover, the value of parameters and species can be modified within the model element "state." This enables semantic interleaving of the subcellular and cellular modeling scale. Furthermore, SBME allows defining the values $t_{\mathrm{mapped}}$ and $n_{\mathrm{points}}$ for an SBML model (see Section 14.3.1).

Each CBM is automatically validated before it is translated into executable code. This validation comprises model completeness, variable uniqueness, syntactical correctness and assignment correctness [22]. After successful validation, the EPISIM code generator translates the graphical CBM into highly efficient executable Java code, which is optimized in terms of computational performance. Furthermore, an MCC is generated for each imported SBML model. The MCCs, the original SBML model files as well as the translated CBM are stored in a single file called model archive.

### 14.3.3  EPISIM Simulator: The Multi-Agent–Based Simulation Environment

The graphical simulation environment EPISIM simulator allows conducting a multi-agent–based tissue simulation based on a loaded model archive built with EPISIM Modeller. In a multi-agent–based simulation each cell is represented by an individual agent [31] whose interaction with neighboring agents is controlled by the CBM and the linked BM. Each agent and each cell respectively holds its own CBM and accordingly its own BM instance. The individual model instances represent the individual states of the simulated cells. A single tissue simulation step comprises

(1)  simulation of the defined extracellular diffusion fields
(2)  simulation of the cells in random order in three substeps:
    (a)  simulation of the biomechanical model instance
    (b)  simulation of the imported subcellular SBML-based models
    (c)  simulation of the CBM instance based on the results of steps (a) and (b)
(3)  update of the data monitoring components

For each imported SBML model that has been semantically integrated in the CBM, the EPISIM Simulator runs an individual time course simulation for each cell using COPASI. This means $n \times m$ time course simulations at simulation step $t$ for $n$ simulated cells and $m$ imported SBML models. Thereby a SBML model's MCC administers the time course simulation states and the data flow between EPISIM Simulator and COPASI.

EPISIM Simulator has three main components (Fig. 14.3): (i) the tissue visualization window, (ii) the tissue simulation controller, and (iii) the data monitoring unit. A tissue simulation can be interactively started, stopped, and paused with the tissue simulation controller. Moreover, the controller allows storing tissue simulation snapshots (TSSs) at any time. A TSS represents the tissue simulation state at a particular simulation step. Tissue simulation snapshots can be used to archive or exchange simulation results. The EPISIM Simulator can load such a TSS and fully resume a tissue simulation based on this input. The data monitoring unit allows defining and generating data monitoring components (DMCs) in form of charts (Fig. 14.3) for real-time visualization of the simulation outcome. Moreover, a DMC can be a data export to write pre-processed simulation results to comma-separated files for further evaluation with third party tools.

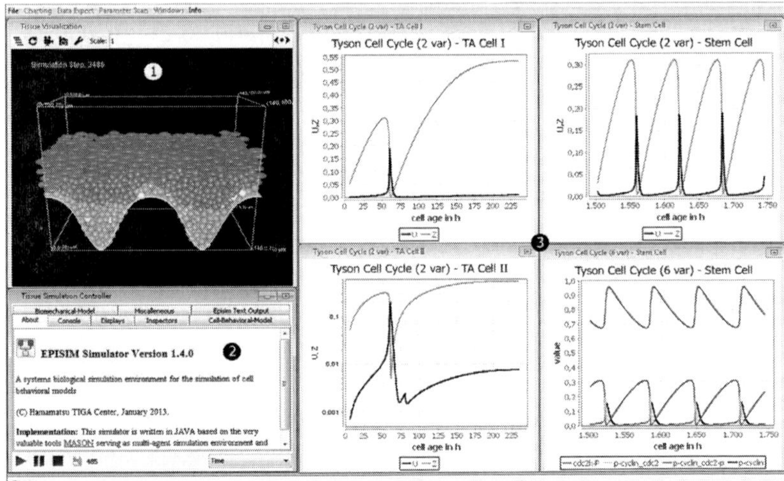

**Figure 14.3**   EPISIM Simulator with (1) tissue visualization window, (2) tissue simulation controller, and (3) data monitoring unit.

## 14.4   Model of Human Epidermal Homeostasis

We realized a multi-scale model of human epidermal homeostasis demonstrating the capabilities of our modeling and simulation platform EPISIM. We used EPISIM Modeller to realize a graphical CBM for keratinocytes in human epidermis. This graphical CBM can be dynamically linked to a 2D as well as a 3D cell-center-based biomechanical model (BM) offered by the EPISIM Simulator. Both, the CBM in conjunction with the BM, represent the model of human epidermal homeostasis. This paragraph will first describe the 2D as well as the 3D BM. Subsequently, the graphical CBM for keratinocytes is introduced. The model simulation results for a 2D and 3D in silico epidermis are subject of Section 14.4.3.

## 14.4.1 Cell-Center-Based Biomechanical Model

EPISIM Simulator offers a 2D as well as a 3D cell-center based BM for multi-cellular simulations. As elucidated in paragraph 14.3.1, a BM comprises all biophysical and spatial cellular properties such as cell morphology in terms of size and shape, active or passive cell migration or cell–cell adhesion. The BM being part of the epidermis model is an off-lattice, center-based model thus allowing cells to move freely in space. Cells are modeled by discrete objects and all occurring forces act on a cell's center of mass is therefore named center-based [32,33]. In such a BM a cell's spatial representation is commonly either a circle or a sphere [5,7,10,11,34] or an ellipse or ellipsoid [35,36]. Based on the 2D BM of Grabe et al. [8] using circular cells, we developed an extended BM assuming an elliptical cell shape in 2D and a ellipsoidal cell shape in 3D. As illustrated in Fig. 14.4 the BM equilibrates the distance between a cell $c$ and its neighboring cells $c_{n_i}$. Figure 14.4 shows the optimal equilibration between two consecutive simulation steps. The equilibration that is performed for all cells in the tissue simulation leads to passive

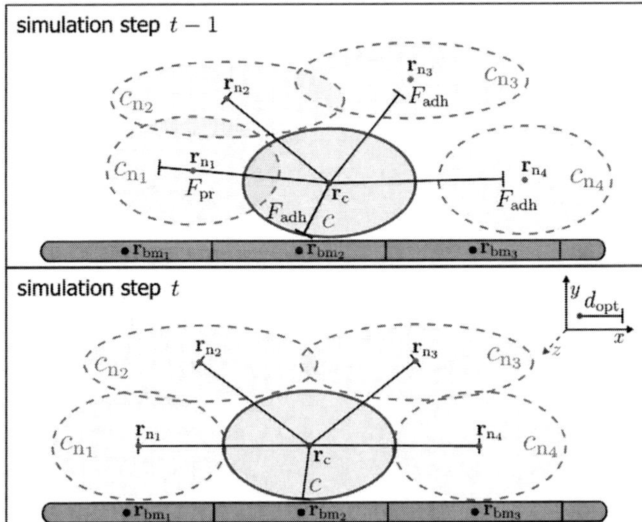


**Figure 14.4** Cell-center-based biomechanical model. A cell $c$ balances the distance to all neighboring cells and the basal membrane, respectively. The balancing involves intercellular pressure $F_{pr}$ as well as cell-cell adhesion $F_{adh}$.

migration. The cell distance equilibrium is continuously perturbed by proliferating cells whose daughter cells exert pressure on their cellular environment. Besides intercellular pressure (e.g., between cell $c$ and cell $c_{n_1}$), the distance equilibration involves the calculation cell–cell adhesion (see cells $c_{n_3}$ and $c_{n_4}$) and finally adhesion to the basal membrane. A cell's position corresponds to its center of mass $\mathbf{r}$. To calculate adhesion to the basal membrane, the membrane is discretized into sections of equal length with section centers $\mathbf{r}_{\text{bm}_i}$.

### 14.4.1.1 Optimal distance calculation

The optimal distance between two elliptical or ellipsoidal neighboring cells is needed to calculate whether or not these cells exert adhesive or pressure force on each other. An ellipse or an ellipsoid is given by

$$E \equiv (\mathbf{x} - \mathbf{r})^T M^2 (\mathbf{x} - \mathbf{r}) = 1 \tag{14.3}$$

$$\text{with } M = \begin{pmatrix} \dfrac{1}{a} & 0 \\ 0 & \dfrac{1}{b} \end{pmatrix} \text{ in 2D and } M = \begin{pmatrix} \dfrac{1}{a} & 0 & 0 \\ 0 & \dfrac{1}{b} & 0 \\ 0 & 0 & \dfrac{1}{c} \end{pmatrix} \text{ in 3D} \tag{14.4}$$

The semi-major axis of the ellipse is $a$. Accordingly the semi-minor-axis is denoted by $b$. Finally, the semi-principal axes of the ellipsoid are $a$, $b$, and $c$. An ellipse's or ellipsoid's axes are aligned with the axes of the used Cartesian coordinate system. The calculation of the optimal distance (Fig. 14.5) between two ellipses as well as two ellipsoids is done in three steps:

(1) determination of the line $L$ through cell centers (of mass) $\mathbf{r}_c$ and $\mathbf{r}_n$ with direction vector $\mathbf{v}_{cn}$ (and inverted direction vector $\mathbf{v}_{nc}$)

(2) calculation of the intersection points between this line $L$ with the ellipses or ellipsoids

(3) summation of the line segment length between a cell's center and the according intersection point ($|\text{seg}_c|$ and $|\text{seg}_n|$)

Consequently, the optimal distance between two ellipsoidal cells located at $\mathbf{r}_c$ and $\mathbf{r}_n$ is

$$d_{opt}\left(\mathbf{r}_c,\mathbf{r}_n\right)=\underbrace{\left\|\frac{\hat{\mathbf{v}}_{cn}}{\sqrt{\left(\dfrac{\hat{v}_{cn_1}^2}{a_c^2}+\dfrac{\hat{v}_{cn_2}^2}{b_c^2}+\dfrac{\hat{v}_{cn_3}^2}{c_c^2}\right)}}\right\|_2}_{|seg_c|}+\underbrace{\left\|\frac{\hat{\mathbf{v}}_{nc}}{\sqrt{\left(\dfrac{\hat{v}_{nc_1}^2}{a_n^2}+\dfrac{\hat{v}_{nc_2}^2}{b_n^2}+\dfrac{\hat{v}_{nc_3}^2}{c_n^2}\right)}}\right\|_2}_{|seg_n|} \tag{14.5}$$

with

$$\hat{\mathbf{v}}_{cn}=\frac{\left(\mathbf{r}_n-\mathbf{r}_c\right)}{\|\mathbf{r}_n-\mathbf{r}_c\|_2};\ \hat{\mathbf{v}}_{nc}=\frac{\left(\mathbf{r}_c-\mathbf{r}_n\right)}{\|\mathbf{r}_c-\mathbf{r}_n\|_2}, \tag{14.6}$$

Accordingly, the optimal distance between an ellipsoidal cell located at $\mathbf{r}_c$ and the closest basal membrane segment with center $\mathbf{r}_{bm}$ is

$$d_{opt}\left(\mathbf{r}_c,\mathbf{r}_{bm}\right)=\left\|\frac{\hat{\mathbf{v}}_{c\_bm}}{\sqrt{\left(\dfrac{\hat{v}_{c\_bm_1}^2}{a_c^2}+\dfrac{\hat{v}_{c\_bm_2}^2}{b_c^2}+\dfrac{\hat{v}_{c\_bm_3}^2}{c_c^2}\right)}}\right\|_2, \tag{14.7}$$

$$\hat{\mathbf{v}}_{c\_bm}=\frac{\left(\mathbf{r}_{bm}-\mathbf{r}_c\right)}{\left\|\mathbf{r}_{bm}-\mathbf{r}_c\right\|_2}$$

The optimal distance between two elliptical cells and between an elliptical cell and a basal membrane segment is analogously calculated.

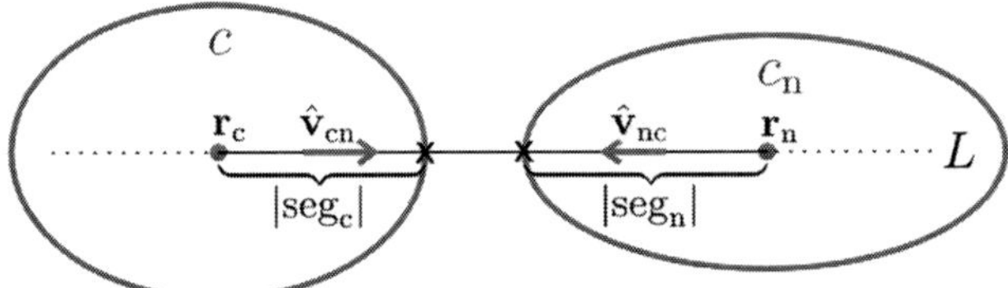


**Figure 14.5** Optimal distance calculation.

### 14.4.1.2 Cell migration based on intercellular pressure, cell–cell adhesion, and basal membrane adhesion

Intercellular pressure $F_{pr}(\mathbf{r}_c, \mathbf{r}_n)$ between overlapping cells is determined by the ratio between optimal distance and the actual Euclidean distance:

$$F_{pr}(\mathbf{r}_c, \mathbf{r}_n) = \begin{cases} \dfrac{\delta_{ol} \cdot d_{opt}(\mathbf{r}_c, \mathbf{r}_n)}{\|\mathbf{r}_c - \mathbf{r}_n\|_2} & \text{if} \quad \mathbf{r}_c \neq \mathbf{r}_n \\ 0 & \text{else} \end{cases} \tag{14.8}$$

The factor $\delta_{ol}$ $(0 < \delta_{ol} \leq 1)$ modulates the tolerated overlap between two adjacent cells and by that a cell's compressibility.

Cell–cell adhesion and the underlying force $F_{adh}(\mathbf{r}_c, \mathbf{r}_n)$ between two adjacent cells are calculated as follows:

$$F_{adh}(\mathbf{r}_c, \mathbf{r}_n) = \begin{cases} \dfrac{d_{opt}(\mathbf{r}_c, \mathbf{r}_n)}{\|\mathbf{r}_c - \mathbf{r}_n\|_2} & \text{if} \quad \mathbf{r}_c \neq \mathbf{r}_n \wedge \|\mathbf{r}_c - \mathbf{r}_n\|_2 < \delta_{adh} \cdot d_{opt}(\mathbf{r}_c, \mathbf{r}_n) \\ 0 & \text{else} \end{cases}$$

$$\tag{14.9}$$

Cell–cell adhesion is limited to those cells whose distance is below $\delta_{adh} \cdot d_{opt}(\mathbf{r}_c, \mathbf{r}_n)$. Both, intercellular pressure and cell–cell adhesion are finally used to calculate a cell movement vector which the result of the interaction of two adjacent cells:

$$\mathbf{m}(\mathbf{r}_c, \mathbf{r}_n) = \begin{cases} (F_{pr}(\mathbf{r}_c, \mathbf{r}_n) - 1)\mathbf{v}_{nc} & \text{if} \quad F_{pr}(\mathbf{r}_c, \mathbf{r}_n) > 1 \\ -{}^{adh}k_{cn}(1 - F_{adh}(\mathbf{r}_c, \mathbf{r}_n))\mathbf{v}_{nc} & \text{if} \quad \begin{array}{l} F_{pr}(\mathbf{r}_c, \mathbf{r}_n) < 1 \\ \wedge F_{adh}(\mathbf{r}_c, \mathbf{r}_n) > 0 \end{array} \\ 0 & \text{else} \end{cases} \tag{14.10}$$

The adhesion coefficient ${}^{adh}k_{cn}$ can be interpreted as linear spring constant, which scales the strength of the adhesive force between two cells. The adhesion coefficient is the BM parameter that allows considering different types of cell–cell junctions with individual mechanical properties. The adhesion to the basal membrane is analogously determined. The pressure $F_{pr}(\mathbf{r}_c, \mathbf{r}_{bm})$, the adhesive force $F_{adh}(\mathbf{r}_c, \mathbf{r}_{bm})$ as well as the movement vector $\mathbf{m}(\mathbf{r}_c, \mathbf{r}_{bm})$ are calculated according to Eqs. (14.8)–(14.10) based on the optimal distance $d_{opt}(\mathbf{r}_c, \mathbf{r}_{bm})$ resulting from Eq. (14.7). The final cell position and by that the migration of cell $c$ is determined using the sum of all movement vectors $\mathbf{m}(\mathbf{r}_c, \mathbf{r}_n)$ calculated for each adjacent cell—as well as the movement vector of the closest basal membrane segment $\mathbf{m}(\mathbf{r}_c, \mathbf{r}_{bm})$.

## 14.4.2 Keratinocyte Cell Behavioral Model

We used EPISIM Modeller and its graphical cell behavioral modeling language to build a multi-scale CBM for keratinocytes in human epidermis based on the works of Grabe et al. [8]. Figure 14.6 shows the main graphical CBM of the keratinocyte model being composed of the main model itself and the three sub-models: (i) *Cell Cycle*, (ii) *Diff.(usion)Waterflux* and (iii) *Differentiation*. These sub-models are addressed in detail in Sections 14.4.2.1–14.4.2.3. In the overall model, we distinguish the following "differentiation stages" for keratinocytes:

- *Stem cell*: A fixed number of immortal stem cells (*DL_StemCell*) are placed on the basal membrane. Stem cells are dominantly located at the bottom of the rete ridges [37]. Hence, seeding of stem cells within a rete ridge is restricted to positions below an adjustable minimal depth threshold (default: 2 %).
- *Transit amplifying (TA) cell*: Stem cells spawn TA cells (*DL_TaCell*) which in turn spawn spinosum cells in a first fraction of their lifetime (see Section 14.4.2.4). TA cells differentiate to spinosum cells after the initial proliferative phase (see Section 14.4.2.2).
- *Spinosum cell*: We distinguish early (*DL_EarlySpiCell*) and late spinosum cells (*DL_LateSpiCell*) forming the stratum spinosum [38].
- *Granulosum cell*: Granulosum cells (*DL_GranuCell*) build the outermost cell layer in our in silico epidermis model.

Throughout the whole keratinocyte model, we assume the real-time interval $\Delta t_{cbm}$ of 0.5 h per simulation step. All keratinocytes except stem cells have a limited lifespan of 1000 h (*age_max*). Keratinocytes exceeding this age die. This is reflected by the call of the function *CellDeath()* causing the removal of a cell from the simulation (Fig. 14.6 (1a–c)).

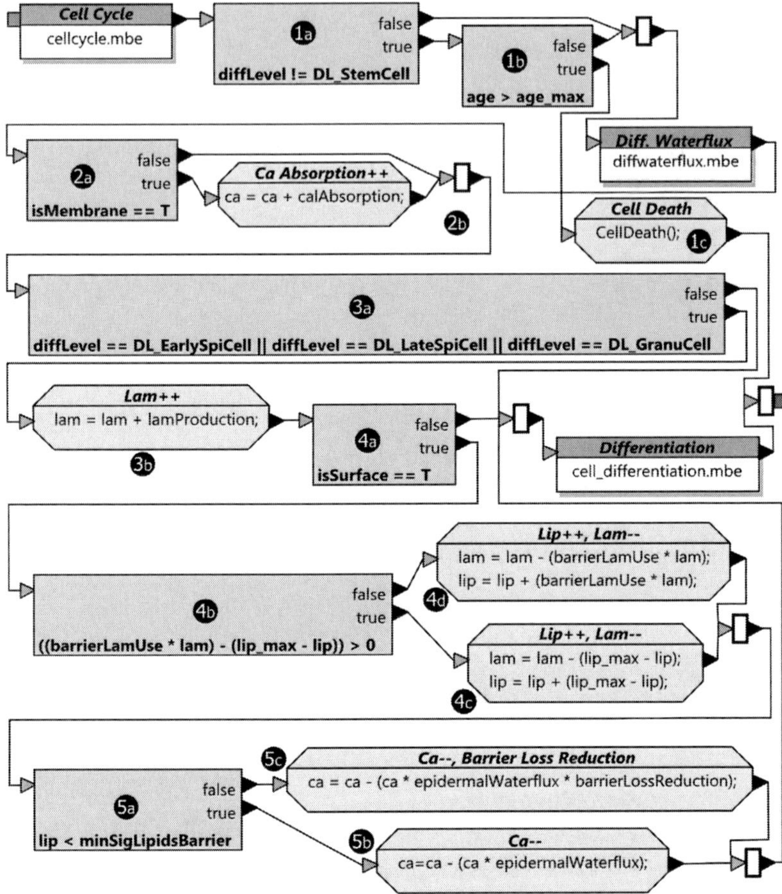


**Figure 14.6** Keratinocyte cell behavioral model: main graphical CBM.

Healthy human epidermis shows a characteristic gradient of $Ca^{2+}$ ions with relatively low $Ca^{2+}$ levels in the basal and spinous layers, and high $Ca^{2+}$ levels in the granular layer. Finally, the $Ca^{2+}$ level sharply decreases in the *stratum corneum*. The $Ca^{2+}$ ion gradient is one of the important regulators of keratinocyte differentiation and by that of epidermal barrier formation [39]. As the bulk of free $Ca^{2+}$ in the epidermis is located in intracellular stores such as the Golgi and the endoplasmic reticulum [40], we consider only intracellular $Ca^{2+}$ in our model. We defined that keratinocytes being in contact with the basal membrane (Fig. 14.6 (2a)) take up $Ca^{2+}$ ions with a rate of 4 mg/kg/h (*calAbsorption*, Fig. 14.6 (2b)). The $Ca^{2+}$ flux within the epidermis is part of sub-model *Diff. Waterflux* (see Section 14.4.2.2).

Spinosum and granulosum cells synthesize lamellar bodies [41] with a rate of 20 units/h (*lamProduction*, Fig. 14.6 (3a, b)). According to the brick-and-mortar model [42,43] the epidermal barrier is composed of dead corneocytes as the bricks and the lipid mixture of lamellar bodies as the mortar. Air-exposed cells in the outermost cell layer of the in silico epidermis therefore convert lamellar bodies into lipids with rate of 50% (*barrierLamUse*) reflecting lamellar body secretion in the stratum granulosum (Fig. 14.6 (4a–d)). We defined a lamellar body saturation and respectively a lipid saturation (*lip_max*) of 150 units. There is a constant loss of $Ca^{2+}$ ions as long as the epidermal barrier is not intact. The $Ca^{2+}$ loss is then relative to the transepidermal water flux (*epidermalWaterflux* = 0.06) and water loss respectively [44]. Once there are enough lipids (*minSigLipidsBarrier* = 130 units) present around the surface cells, the loss of $Ca^{2+}$ is reduced to 3% (*barrierLossReduction*) of the water flux (Fig. 14.6 (5a–c)). This is the case when the in silico epidermis is homeostatic and the epidermal barrier was fully developed.

### 14.4.2.1  Multi-scale cell cycle model

Tysons well-known subcellular cell cycle model [45] is the basis for our cell cycle model on the cellular level. We obtained Tysons two-variable cell cycle model from BioModels database [30]. The model file in SBML-format was imported with EPISIM Modeller and the model's readout (*sbml_u*) was semantically integrated in the graphical model (Fig. 14.7). Tysons mathematical model of cdc2 and cyclin interaction exhibits three modes: (i) steady state with high maturation promoting factor (MPF) activity, (ii) spontaneous oscillator and (iii) excitable steady state of low MPF activity. Mode (ii) corresponds in our model with cell division cycles in stem and TA cells. Mode (i) is associated with no longer proliferating but differentiated spinosum and granulosum cells (see Section 14.4.2.2). The concentration of active MPF relative to cdc2 is represented by SBML model species *sbml_u*. Cell division is triggered by high active MPF concentrations exceeding mitotic threshold (*MT* = 0.125, Fig. 14.7 (1)). We defined a minimum time interval between two cell divisions (*MIN_AGE_DELTA* = 25, Fig. 14.7 (2)) in order to avoid multiple cell divisions in consecutive simulation steps. For this purpose, a cell's age at cell division is stored in the cell property *ageOfLastCellDivision* (Fig. 14.7 (4)).

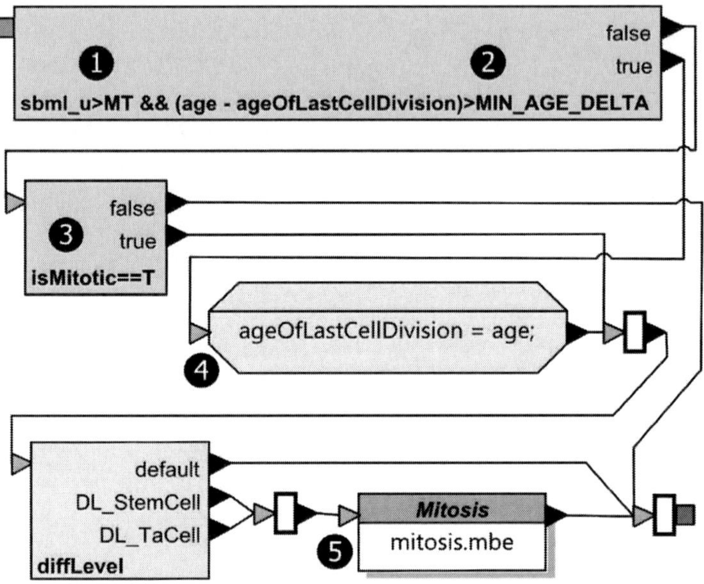


**Figure 14.7**  Multi-scale cell cycle model.

The link between active MPF levels and cell divisions is at the same time a semantic link between the subcellular and the cell behavioral modeling level, making the overall cell cycle model multi-scaled. Due to contact inhibition, a proliferating cell might go into cell cycle arrest. This indicates too high cell densities in a cell's microenvironment. In such a case, cell division is delayed and *isMitotic* is set to true (*T*) in the mitosis sub-model (Fig. 14.7 (5)). The value of *isMitotic* triggers cell division in one of the following simulation steps (Fig. 14.7 (3)).

Tyson's model yields an active MPF concentration peak every 35 time units using the default parameterization of BioModels database. The time units are interpreted as hours ($\Delta t_{\text{sbml}}$ = 1 h) in our model. With this model kinetics threshold MT is reached every 34.2 h. The keratinocyte cell cycle time is assumed to be 60 h [46, 47]. With atomic CBM time interval $\Delta t_{\text{cbm}}$ = 0.5 h, $t_{\text{sem\_sbml}}$ = 34.2 h and accordingly $t_{sem\_cbm}$ = 60 h, the mapped time $t_{mapped}$ is 0.285 h for Tyson's model. We set $n_{points}$ = 1 as the resulting $\Delta t_{point}$ is 0.285 h being sufficiently small for an accurate time course simulation.

### 14.4.2.2 Multi-scale cell differentiation model

The cell differentiation sub-model depicted in Fig. 14.8 shows how sub-cellular model behavior can be linked to the cell states "proliferating" and "differentiating." TA cells undergo a limited number of cell cycles before they finally differentiate to early spinosum cells [48]. In our model TA cells proliferate in the first 10% of their life time (*maxBirthAgeFrac*, Fig. 14.8 (1)). The intracellular $Ca^{2+}$ concentration of all simulated keratinocytes constitutes the

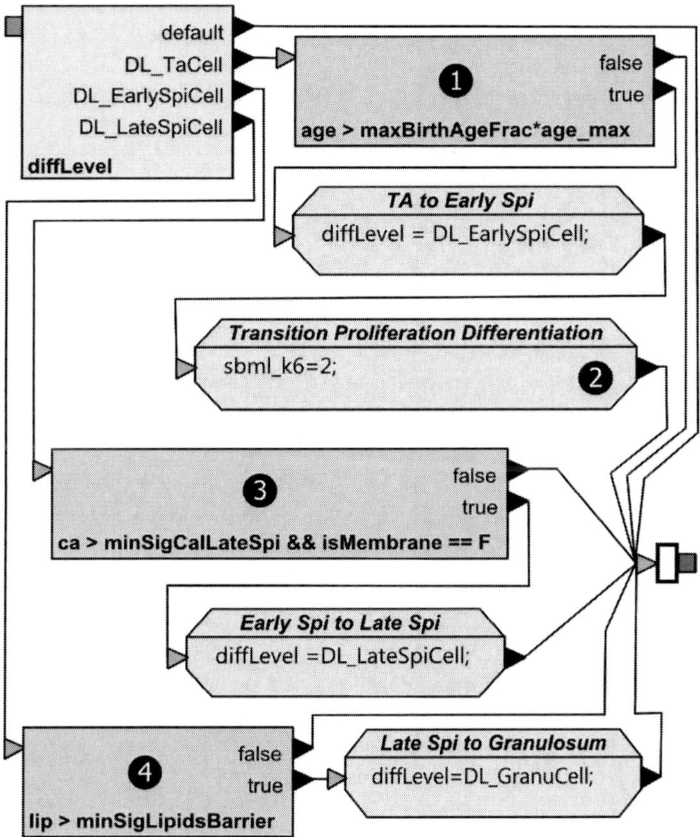


**Figure 14.8** Cell differentiation model.

vertical epidermal $Ca^{2+}$ gradient. This gradient in turn directly influences cell differentiation [39]. Accordingly, early spinosum cells become late spinosum cells based on their intracellular $Ca^{2+}$ level (Fig. 14.8 (3)). The according threshold *minSigCalLateSpi* is 250 mg/kg. Spinosum cells finally differentiate to granulosum cells based on the lipid concentration (*minSigLipidsBarrier* = 130 units) in the outermost layers of the tissue (Fig. 14.8 (4)). TA cell differentiation to early spinosum cells represents a cell state transition from proliferation to differentiation. As described in Section 14.4.2.1, Tyson's cell cycle model exhibits three modes. The model's parameter *k6* (named *sbml_k6* after import) allows switching between these modes. By setting *sbml_k6* = 2 (Fig. 14.8 (2)), the model behavior changes from oscillation to steady state on a low active MPF level. As cell division is triggered by high active MPF concentrations, cells in the spinous and the granular layer never divide.

### 14.4.2.3   Transepidermal water flux and diffusion model

The transepidermal water flux has been identified as a directed passive molecular transport mechanism. It has been shown that disruption of the epidermal barrier causes an increased water flux. This in turn results in a sudden local loss of ion concentrations in the respective tissue area [49, 50]. As depicted in Fig. 14.9, we modeled transport of $Ca^{2+}$ ions and lamellar bodies relative to the transepidermal waterflux (*epidermalWaterflux* = 0.06). If a cell has neighboring cells, in the first step there is a diffusive undirected transport of $Ca^{2+}$ ions with diffusion rate *epidermalDiffusion* of 1.0E-4 (Fig. 14.9 (1, 2)). In the second step, $Ca^{2+}$ ions and lamellar bodies are requested from the neighboring (and at the same time vertically lower located) cells based on their intracellular concentrations *n_ca* and *n_lam* (Fig. 14.9 (3, 4)).

The value of a neighboring cell property can be referenced by adding the prefix "*n_*." The number of adjacent neighboring cells varies from simulation step to simulation step due to the off-lattice BM that is linked to the keratinocyte CBM. The number of neighboring cells is an output value of the BM being stored in the biomechanical property *numberOfNeighbours*. It is not neces-sary to explicitly define a loop for the iteration over all neighbor-ing cells for referencing all the different neighboring cell property values. Moreover, a loop is automatically induced starting at the graphical model element where a neighboring cell property value was referenced for the first time. This loop includes all succeeding model elements until the last element of the model file (see yellow highlighted area in Fig. 14.9). Within this automatic loop, the call of the predefined function *Receive(varName, value)* allows to request an amount of *value* of cell property *varName* from a particular neighboring cell. The requested amount of, for example, *n_ca*epidermalWaterflux* is then added to the own value of the respective cell property (e.g., *ca*).

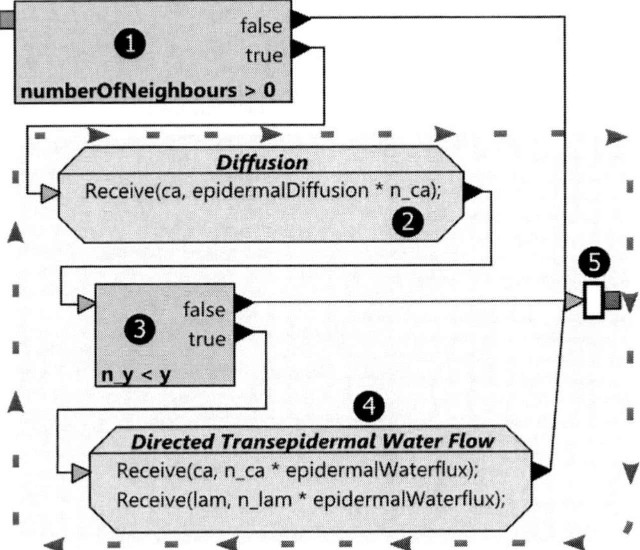


**Figure 14.9**  Transepidermal water flux and diffusion model.

### 14.4.2.4  Mitosis model

The mitosis sub-model is entered when cell division is triggered in the cell cycle sub-model (Section 14.4.2.1). As shown in the graphical model in Fig. 14.10 (1), there is an initial check for collisions with neighboring cells. The BM output value *hasCollision* is set to *true* (*T*) in case of too high cell densities in a cell's microenvironment. In such a case, cell division is delayed to one of the following simulation steps. This cell cycle arrest is expressed by assigning the value *true* to cell property *isMitotic* (Fig. 14.10 (2)). The epidermal proliferative compartment comprises stem cells and TA cells (Fig. 14.10 (3)) with asymmetric cells division. Stem cells spawn TA cells which in turn spawn early spinosum cells. TA cells only proliferate in the first

10% of their lifetime (*maxBirthAgeFrac*, see Section 14.4.2.2). A daughter cell can be introduced in the simulation by calling the function *NewCell*. Cell properties of the new cell can be explicitly initialized between the parentheses (Fig. 14.10 (4)). The intracellular $Ca^{2+}$ is equally distributed among mother and daughter cell.

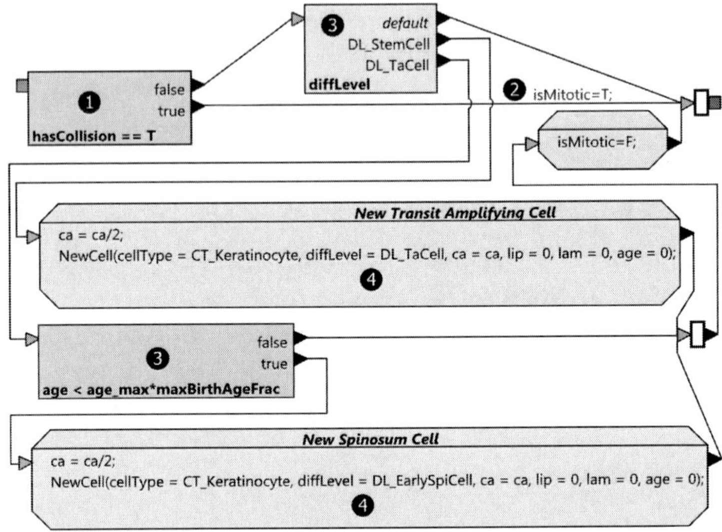



**Figure 14.10** Mitosis model with asymmetric cell division.

## 14.4.3 Multi-Scale Epidermis Simulation Results

We linked the graphical keratinocyte CBM introduced in Section 14.4.2 to the 2D and the 3D version of the cell-center-based BM described in Section 14.4.1 using EPISIM Modeller's MCC model linkage mechanism (Section 14.3.1). We then automatically translated the graphical keratinocyte model linked to the 2D BM and the same graphical CBM linked to the 3D BM into executable code with the EPISIM code generator. By that we obtained two model archives for the simulation of a 2D and a 3D in silico epidermis. We subsequently conducted a multi-scale 2D and 3D tissue simulation based on these model archives with the multi-agent-based EPISIM Simulator. 10,000 simulation steps corresponding to 5,000 h real time were simulated for each setup.

With the evaluation of the simulation results, we tackle the following four questions:

(1) What is the simulation outcome of the semantic interplay of Tyson's subcellular cell cycle model and the cell-based differentiation model (see Section 14.4.3.1)?

(2) Do both, the 2D and the 3D in silico epidermis, show the same horizontally layered tissue morphology in homeostasis (see Section 14.4.3.2)?

(3) How do the $Ca^{2+}$ gradient controlling keratinocyte differentiation and the barrier formation represented by the lipid gradient compare in 2D and 3D (see Section 14.4.3.3)?

(4) Do both simulation setups yield the same epidermal tissue kinetics (see Section 14.4.3.4)?

Answering these questions moreover tackles the more general question whether or not it is possible to use the EPISIM modeling approach to build modular, reusable and at the same time multi-scaled graphical CBMs, which can be deployed in different spatial and biomechanical setups.

### 14.4.3.1  Multi-scale cell cycle simulation

The SBML-based version of Tyson's two-variable cell cycle model was semantically integrated in the cell cycle sub-model (see Section 14.4.2.1) and the cell differentiation model (see Section 14.4.2.2) of the graphical keratinocyte CBM. We embedded COPASI [15] in our multi-agent–based EPISIM Simulator to numerically calculate a time course simulation for each imported SBML-based model for every single cell in a particular tissue simulation. EPISIM Simulator allows generating charts to monitor single cells that meet a user defined condition. We used this charting facility to generate charts for visualization of the time course simulation of Tyson's model in stem cells and TA cells (Fig. 14.3 (3)). We used $t_{\mathrm{mapped}} = 0.285$ to map the imported cell cycle model's time scale to the time scale of our epidermis model. In stem cells we observed oscillating model behavior with active MPF ($U$) peaks every 60 h. Cell division was triggered each time when the subcellular SBML model species U exceeded mitotic threshold $MT = 0.125$. Hence, the subcellular SBML-based model successfully controlled cell division in stem and TA cells with a cell cycle time of 60 h. There is a transition from cell state proliferation to differentiation in our cell differentiation model. This transition can be observed in TA cells and is semantically linked to a change from oscillating to steady-state model behavior on the subcellular modeling level (Fig. 14.3 (3)). After one cell division, a TA cell differentiates to an early spinosum cell, which no longer proliferates because of the steady state of Tyson's model on a low active MPF level.

### 14.4.3.2 Homeostatic epidermal in silico tissue morphology

The simulation of the keratinocyte CBM and the linked BM on an undulated basal membrane yields a horizontally layered in silico epidermis. This is the case in the 2D and the 3D simulation as depicted in Figs. 14.11a,b. Compared to the undulation of the basal membrane the simulation is able to generate a rather flat epidermal surface once homeostasis is achieved. Stem cells have fixed positions on the basal membrane. TA cells can be found close to the stem cells. The three main visible cell layers from bottom to top are early spinosum cells, late spinosum cells, and granulosum cells. The vertical thickness of the 2D as well as the 3D homeostatic in silico epidermis ranges from 60 to 70 µm. This corresponds to the 60 µm (15 µm SD) mean thickness of the nucleated part of the epidermis found in punch biopsies [51]. No significant differences between the 2D and the 3D in silico tissue morphology have been detected.

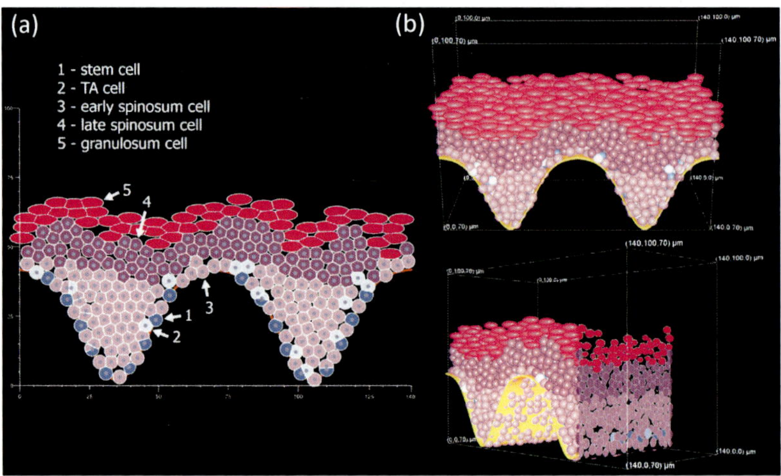


**Figure 14.11** Horizontally layered in silico epidermis in 2D and 3D simulation.

### 14.4.3.3   Transepidermal $Ca^{2+}$ gradient and barrier formation

We took a cell sample in a strip of 10 µm width in the middle of the left rete ridge in the simulated homeostatic epidermis (Figs. 14.12a,b). This cell sample was used to determine the transepidermal $Ca^{2+}$ gradient having the same shape in 2D and 3D epidermis simulation (Figs. 14.12c,d). Intracellular $Ca^{2+}$ levels significantly increase in cells located between 30 and 40 µm on the $y$-axis. The maximum $Ca^{2+}$ level is reached at 40 µm. This corresponds to the border between the early and late spinosum cell layer (Figs. 14.11a,b) and illustrates the regulation of cell differentiation by the $Ca^{2+}$ gradient. The $Ca^{2+}$ distribution reflected by this vertical gradient corresponds to the in vivo situation [44,50] and to simulation results of dedicated epidermal $Ca^{2+}$ profile models [52,53]. Concerning the relative cell numbers, we find that in the 3D simulation around

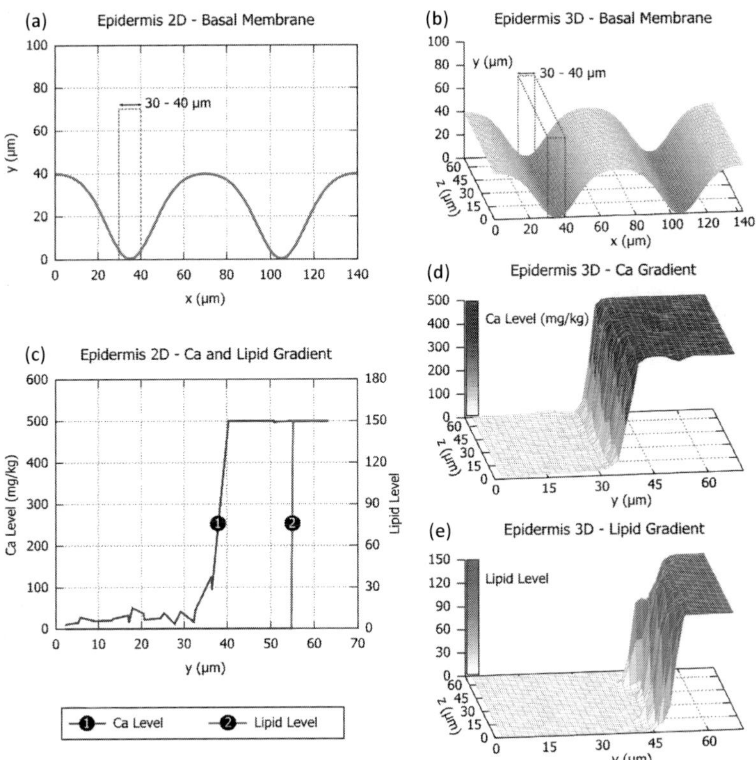

**Figure 14.12**   $Ca^{2+}$ and lipid gradient in the 2D and the 3D in silico epidermis.

10% more cells are in direct contact with the basal membrane, which can be explained by the third degree of freedom of cell movement in the 3D BM. These basal cells take up $Ca^{2+}$ ions with a rate *calAbsorption* = 4 mg/kg/h. This rate was reduced to 3.5 mg/kg/h in the 3D in silico epidermis simulation accommodating the increased number of basal cells.

The lipid gradient has the same shape in the 2D as well as the 3D in silico epidermis (Fig. 14.12 (c), (e)). A high lipid concentration is in our model equivalent with the epidermal barrier against water and $Ca^{2+}$ ion loss. The maximum lipid level is reached between 50 and 60 µm corresponding to the lower border of the stratum granulosum in the homeostatic in silico epidermis (Fig. 14.11 (a), (b)).

### 14.4.3.4 Epidermal tissue kinetics

We calculated tissue kinetic parameters turnover time and growth fraction for the 2D and the 3D in silico epidermis. The turnover time is the time needed for full renewal of the tissue [54]. It corresponds to the ratio between the total number of cells in the tissue and the proliferation rate (i.e., new cells per hour). The turnover time for nucleated in vivo epidermis is between 672 h and 1080 h [55]. The growth fraction is defined as the proportion of proliferating basal cells and has been determined to be not larger than 20% of the whole cell population [56]. The turnover time and the growth fraction were calculated every 100 simulation steps. Mean values and standard deviations were determined based on the calculated values for the tissue kinetic parameters (based on the values from simulation step $x$ to 10,000). The results are shown in charts (a) and (b) in Fig. 14.13. Both the 2D and the 3D in silico epidermis have turnover times close to 700 h. The growth fraction in the 3D simulation is a little lower as there are more basal cells. However, both growth fraction values are below 20%. There is no significant difference between the relative cell numbers in the 2D and the 3D simulation when just the "differentiation stage" of the cell is considered (Figs. 14.13c,d). As stated earlier, we find around 10% more basal cells in the 3D simulation.

The turnover time as well as the growth fraction is stable from simulation step 3,000 in both 2D and 3D. This is also the case for the relative cell numbers. Both together gives rise to the assumption that the in silico epidermis is homeostatic from simulation step 3,000. However, an in-depth investigation of the lipid gradient development showed that the shape of the gradient stays stable from simulation step 4,000. For this reason, we defined simulation step 4,000 (2,000 h) to be the point of time when the 2D as well as the 3D in silico epidermis is in homeostasis.

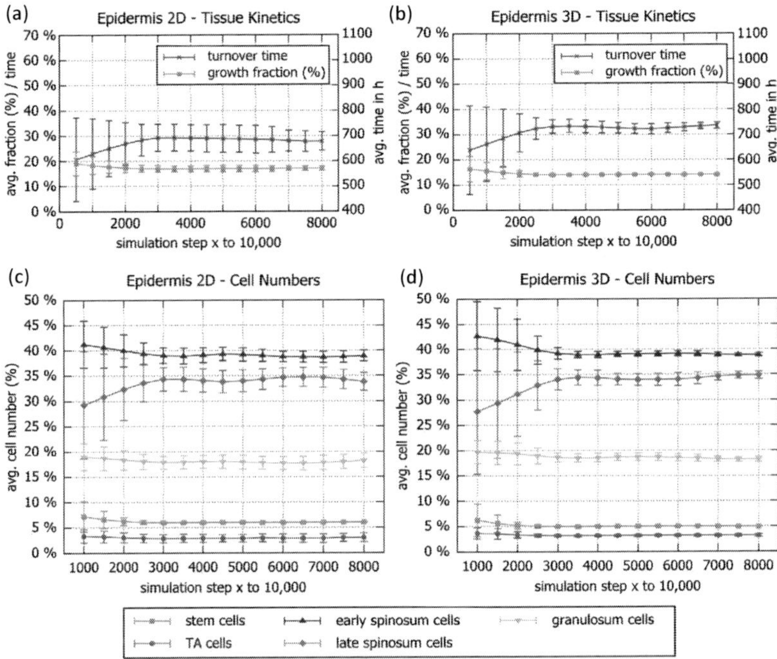

**Figure 14.13** Comparison of epidermal tissue kinetics and relative cell numbers.

## 14.5　Discussion and Conclusion

With the EPISIM platform, we developed and introduced the first entirely graphical multi-scale cell behavioral modeling and simulation software. Using the systems biological model standard SBML, it semantically links the sub-cellular and the cellular level in tissue simulations. EPISIM is a ready-to-use, out-of-the-box software solution in contrast to dedicated simulation software development frameworks like Chaste [57] or FLAME [58]. In terms of flexibility and generality, out-of-the-box computer programs with a graphical user interface can hardly compete with software development frameworks. Nevertheless, the EPISIM platform or parts of it can be either transferred or reused within other simulation environments. EPISIM Modeller could be linked to CompuCell3D as the graphical CBMs are not directly translated into EPISIM Simulator specific Java code. A programming language independent representation is generated in an intermediate step. This representation is the input for our code generator, which uses transformation style sheets to generate specific executable code. These style sheets can be easily exchanged in order to produce any kind of output format.

The EPISIM model architecture uses automatically generated model connector components (MCCs) to semantically link graphical CBMs with SBML-based mechanistic subcellular models and bio-mechanical models (BMs) respectively. Reusable and dynamically extendable tissue model entities can be realized with this modular multi-scale architecture. While cellular behavior and subcellular models can be graphically modeled with EPISIM Modeller and tools like CellDesigner [14], the biomechanical models are still a hard coded part of the EPISIM Simulator. To make the integration of novel BMs as easy as possible, EPISIM Simulator offers a BM plug-in inter-face. The realization of a new BM method simply has to implement a given Java interface. The MCC, used to link a graphical CBM to the novel BM, can be automatically generated. Moreover, besides the BM introduced in Section 14.4.1 a lattice-based 2D and 3D BM consider-ing passive as well as active cell migration is already available.

We demonstrated the power of our EPISIM model architecture as well as of our software platform by realizing a graphical multi-scaled keratinocyte CBM. The graphical cell-based cell cycle model semantically integrated Tysons subcellular cell cycle model [45]. Cell division was triggered by high active MPF concentrations during simulation. The different time scales were successfully mapped by the generated MCC. The cell differentiation model controlled the behavior of Tyson's model by switching from oscillating to steady state mode. This bidirectional semantic link between the subcellular and the cellular modeling level was technically realized by the generated MCC. Furthermore, one and the same graphical keratinocyte CBM was linked to a 2D and a 3D cell-center-based off-lattice BM. Simulation of the keratinocyte CBM in a 2D and a 3D spatial setup yielded no significant differences in terms of tissue morphology, transepidermal $Ca^{2+}$ gradient, relative cell numbers, tissue kinetics and barrier formation. This can be seen as a proof of concept that our modular model architecture allows building loosely coupled model entities that can by dynamically combined to either 2D or 3D multi-scale tissue simulations.

The in silico multi-scale model of human epidermal homeostasis reproduced a horizontally layered 2D and 3D epidermis with a stable lipid barrier and a physiological $Ca^{2+}$ gradient controlling terminal cell differentiation. The homeostatic in silico epidermis shows characteristic thickness, turnover time and growth fraction in 2D as well as in 3D. Indisputably our model is to a large extent simplifying complex epidermal processes. For instance, only passive movement of keratinocytes is considered. This model assumption is shared with other skin in silico models [10,11]. Moreover, our model only considers intracellular $Ca^{2+}$. A continuum tissue model of human epidermis which also includes extracellular $Ca^{2+}$ was recently published [53]. However, such continuum models cannot be reproduced with EPISIM as we rely on a multi-agent-based tissue modeling approach that considers cells as individual spatial objects.

The EPISIM platform and the graphical keratinocyte CBM can be seen as a model base for developing increasingly holistic in silico epidermis models. The platform as well as the model is publicly available. The keratinocyte CBM can be extended without having extensive skills in computer science. With the up to now unique approach of graphical cell behavioral modeling, EPISIM hides to a large extend the technical complexity of modeling and simulating cellular behavior in a tissue context. We think that the separation of technical complexity and systems biological model complexity is crucial for building highly complex models. This is a lesson learned from the field of software engineering where graphical model-driven architectures are nowadays used to build and generate highly complex systems in an analogous way. In order to come up with more realistic and consequently more complex biological models it is inevitable to rely on an existing, ready-to-use model base. It is a waste of scientific resources to reproduce existing models over and over again from literature. Public databases such as BioModels already provide complete ready-to-run SBML-based subcellular models [59]. With EPISIM we established a link to this large and up to now unexploited potential for building multi-scale models in a multi-cellular context. EPISIM motivates the development subcellular models with a focus on functional and behavioral change of cells and their integration into a multi-cellular tissue simulation. In conclusion, we expect that developing and utilizing graphical multi-scale modeling and simulation software platforms like EPISIM is the only way of successfully dealing with the increasing biological model complexity.

## 14.6  Outlook

A current application of our EPISIM platform and especially of the biomechanical model (BM) introduced in Section 14.4.1 is an in silico reepithelialization model of acute cutaneous wounds. In our experimental setup we used commercially obtainable epidermal full thickness cultures to construct a reproducible in vitro wound model. Using this in vitro model we studied cell migration during wound reepithelialization. These investigations unraveled a collective cell migration mechanism we denote as the extending shield mechanism (ESM). The ESM challenges the three commonly known mechanisms that have been proposed earlier: the leap-frog [60], the tractor-tread [61], and the Usui-model [62].

We used whole slide imaging for large-scale histological evaluation of our in vitro wound model. One day post wounding we observed an Extending Epidermal Tongue (EET) in form of two cell layers at the wound margin and one cell layer at the tongue's leading edge. Four to five days post wounding, the whole wound was fully covered by keratinocytes forming a neo-epidermis which had a thickness of about three cell layers near the wound margin and one cell layer at the center of the wound. The neo-epidermis thickened and formed a multi-layered epithelium from day 4 to day 10. Finally, we showed that collective cell migration supplies cells to the edge of the EET. There they become subsequently lifted and connected to the extending shield of the neo-epidermis. This results in an incremental reconstruction of a multi-layered epithelium.

We modeled and simulated the ESM in 2D as well as in 3D with the EPISIM platform. We built a novel keratinocyte CBM with a cell differentiation program that controls the strength of cell–cell adhesion. Thereby, we were able to generate a differentiation dependent adhesion profile for individual cells using our cell-center-based BM. We were able to reproduce in silico the ESM observed in the in vitro wound model (Fig. 14.14). The in silico reepithelialization phases thereby nicely correspond to histological sections of the in vitro reepithelialization phases of the cutaneous wound.

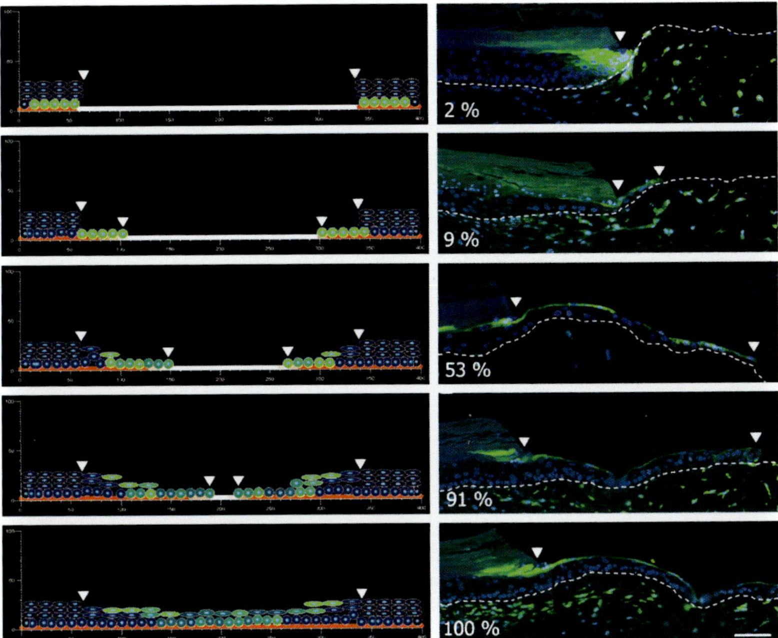


**Figure 14.14** In silico and in vitro reepithelialization model for acute cutaneous wounds with different degrees of wound closure. Cells adjacent to the wound margin were stained with a green fluorescent dye in the in vitro model. This allowed spatial dynamic tracking of cell migration during reepithelialization.

## References


1. Honda H, Morita T, and Tanabe A (1979). Establishment of epidermal cell columns in mammalian skin: computer simulation, *J Theor Biol*, **81**(4), 745–759.

2. Honda H and Oshibe S (1984). A computer simulation of cell stacking for even thickness in mammalian epidermis, *J Theor Biol*, **111**(4), 625–633.

3. Mitrani E (1983). Is upward basal cell movement independent of mitosis in the normal epidermis? *Br J Dermatol*, **109**(6), 635–642.

4. Stekel D, Rashbass J, and Williams ED (1995). A computer graphic simulation of squamous epithelium, *J Theor Biol*, **175**(3), 283–293.

5. Walker DC, Southgate J, Hill G, Holcombe M, Hose DR, Wood SM, Mac Neil S, and Smallwood RH (2004). The epitheliome: agent-based modelling of the social behaviour of cells, *Bio Systems*, **76**(1–3), 89–100.

6. Walker DC, Hill G, Wood SM, Smallwood RH, and Southgate J (2004). Agent-based computational modeling of wounded epithelial cell monolayers, *IEEE Trans Nanobiosci*, **3**(3), 153–163.

7. Galle J, Loeffler M, and Drasdo D (2005). Modeling the effect of deregulated proliferation and apoptosis on the growth dynamics of epithelial cell populations in vitro, *Biophys J*, **88**(1), 62–75.

8. Grabe N and Neuber K (2005). A multicellular systems biology model predicts epidermal morphology, kinetics and $Ca^{2+}$ flow, *Bioinformatics*, **21**(17), 3541–3547.

9. Grabe N and Neuber K (2007). Simulating psoriasis by altering transit amplifying cells, *Bioinformatics*, **23**(11), 1309–1312.

10. Schaller G and Meyer-Hermann M (2007). A modelling approach towards epidermal homoeostasis control, *J Theor Biol*, **247**(3), 554–573.

11. Adra S, Sun T, MacNeil S, Holcombe M, and Smallwood R (2010). Development of a three dimensional multiscale computational model of the human epidermis, *PLoS ONE*, **5**(1), e8511.

12. VLN (2013). Virtual Liver Network [online]. Available from: http://www.virtual-liver.de/[Accessed 30 May 2013].

13. HBP (2013). The Human Brain Project [online]. Available from: http://www.humanbrainproject.eu/[Accessed 30 May 2013].

14. Funahashi A, Morohashi M, Kitano H, and Tanimura N (2003). CellDesigner: a process diagram editor for gene-regulatory and biochemical networks, *Biosilico*, **1**(5), 159–162.

15. Hoops S, Sahle S, Gauges R, Lee C, Pahle J, Simus N, Singhal M, Xu L, Mendes P, and Kummer U (2006). Copasi—a Complex Pathway Simulator, *Bioinformatics*, **22**(24), 3067–3074.

16. Schaff J, Fink CC, Slepchenko B, Carson JH, and Loew LM (1997). A general computational framework for modeling cellular structure and function, *Biophys J*, **73**(3), 1135–1146.

17. Hucka M, Finney A, Sauro HM, Bolouri H, Doyle JC, Kitano H, Arkin AP, Bornstein BJ, Bray D, Cornish-Bowden A, Cuellar AA, Dronov S, Gilles ED, Ginkel M, Gor V, Goryanin II, Hedley WJ, Hodgman TC, Hofmeyr

J-H, Hunter PJ, Juty NS, Kasberger JL, Kremling A, Kummer U, Le Novère N, Loew LM, Lucio D, Mendes P, Minch E, Mjolsness ED, Nakayama Y, Nelson MR, Nielsen PF, Sakurada T, Schaff JC, Shapiro BE, Shimizu TS, Spence HD, Stelling J, Takahashi K, Tomita M, Wagner J, and Wang J (2003). The systems biology markup language (SBML): a medium for representation and exchange of biochemical network models, *Bioinformatics*, **19**(4), 524–531.

18. Pitt-Francis J, Bernabeu MO, Cooper J, Garny A, Momtahan L, Osborne J, Pathmanathan P, Rodriguez B, Whiteley JP, and Gavaghan DJ (2008). Chaste: using agile programming techniques to develop computational biology software, *Philos Transact A Math Phys Eng Sci*, **366**(1878), 3111–3136.

19. Swat MH, Hester SD, Balter AI, Heiland RW, Zaitlen BL, and Glazier JA (2009). Multicell simulations of development and disease using the CompuCell3D simulation environment, *Methods Mol Biol*, **500**, 361–428.

20. Andasari V, Roper RT, Swat MH, and Chaplain MAJ (2012). Integrating intracellular dynamics using CompuCell3D and Bionetsolver: applications to multiscale modelling of cancer cell growth and invasion, *PLoS ONE*, **7**(3), e33726.

21. Graner F and Glazier JA (1992). Simulation of biological cell sorting using a two-dimensional extended Potts model, *Phys Rev Lett*, **69**(13), 2013–2016.

22. Sütterlin T, Huber S, Dickhaus H, and Grabe N (2009). Modeling multicellular behavior in epidermal tissue homeostasis via finite state machines in multi-agent systems, *Bioinformatics*, **25**(16), 2057–2063.

23. Sütterlin T, Kolb C, Dickhaus H, Jäger D, and Grabe N (2013). Bridging the scales: semantic integration of quantitative SBML in graphical multi-cellular models and simulations with EPISIM and COPASI, *Bioinformatics*, **29**(2), 223–229.

24. Gamma E and Beck K (eds) (2004). *Contributing To Eclipse: Principles, Patterns, And Plug-Ins*, 1st ed., Addison-Wesley, Amsterdam.

25. Moore B, Dean D, Gerber A, Wagenknecht G, and Vanderheyden P (eds) (2004). *Eclipse Development Using the Graphical Editing Framework and the Eclipse Modeling Framework*, 1st ed., Reasearch Triangle Park, Durham.

26. Copeland T (ed) (2007). *Generating Parsers with JavaCC,* 2nd ed., Centennial Books, Alexandria.

27. Luke S. (2005). MASON: A Multiagent Simulation Environment, *Simulation*, **81**(7), 517–527.

28. Dräger A, Rodriguez N, Dumousseau M, Dörr A, Wrzodek C, Le Novère N, Zell A, and Hucka M (2011). JSBML: a flexible Java library for working with SBML, *Bioinformatics*, **27**(15), 2167–2168.

29. Kitano H, Funahashi A, Matsuoka Y, and Oda K (2005). Using process diagrams for the graphical representation of biological networks, *Nat Biotechnol*, **23**(8), 961–966.

30. Le Novère N, Bornstein B, Broicher A, Courtot M, Donizelli M, Dharuri H, Li L, Sauro H, Schilstra M, Shapiro B, Snoep JL, and Hucka M (2006). BioModels database: a free, centralized database of curated, published, quantitative kinetic models of biochemical and cellular systems, *Nucleic Acids Res*, **34**(Database issue), D689–D691.

31. Merelli E, Armano G, Cannata N, Corradini F, D'Inverno M, Doms A, Lord P, Martin A, Milanesi L, Möller S, Schroeder M, and Luck M (2007). Agents in bioinformatics, computational and systems biology, *Brief Bioinformatics*, **8**(1), 45–59.

32. Drasdo D (2007). Center-based single-cell models: an approach to multi-cellular organization based on a conceptual analogy to colloidal particles, in *Single-Cell-Based Models in Biology and Medicine* (Anderson AA, Chaplain MJ and Rejniak K, eds.), Birkhäuser Basel, Basel, pp. 171–196.

33. Dallon J (2007). Models with lattice-free center-based cells interacting with continuum environment variables, in *Single-Cell-Based Models in Biology and Medicine* (Anderson AA, Chaplain MJ, and Rejniak K, eds.), Birkhäuser Basel, Basel, pp. 197–219.

34. Höhme S, Brulport M, Bauer A, Bedawy E, Schormann W, Hermes M, Puppe V, Gebhardt R, Zellmer S, Schwarz M, Bockamp E, Timmel T, Hengstler JG, and Drasdo D (2010). Prediction and validation of cell alignment along microvessels as order principle to restore tissue architecture in liver regeneration, *Proc Natl Acad Sci U.S.A.*, **107**(23), 10371–10376.

35. Dallon J and Othmer H (2004). How cellular movement determines the collective force generated by the Dictyostelium discoideum slug, *J Theor Biol*, **231**(2), 203–222.

36. Palsson E and Othmer H (2000). A model for individual and collective cell movement in Dictyostelium discoideum, *Proc Natl Acad Sci U.S.A.*, **97**(19), 10448–10453.

37. Webb A, Li A, and Kaur P (2004). Location and phenotype of human adult keratinocyte stem cells of the skin, *Differentiation*, **72**(8), 387–395.

38. Fuchs E and Byrne C (1994). The epidermis: rising to the surface, *Curr Opin Genet Dev*, **4**(5), 725–736.

39. Elias PM, Ahn SK, Denda M, Brown BE, Crumrine D, Kimutai LK, Kömüves L, Lee SH, and Feingold KR (2002). Modulations in epidermal calcium regulate the expression of differentiation-specific markers, *J Invest Dermatol*, **119**(5), 1128–1136.

40. Celli A, Sanchez S, Behne M, Hazlett T, Gratton E, and Mauro T (2010). The epidermal $Ca^{2+}$ gradient: measurement using the phasor representation of fluorescent lifetime imaging, *Biophys J*, **98**(5), 911–921.

41. Odland GF and Holbrook K (1981). The lamellar granules of epidermis, *Curr Probl Dermatol*, **9**, 29–49.

42. Elias PM (2004). The epidermal permeability barrier: from the early days at Harvard to emerging concepts, *J Invest Dermatol*, **122**(2), xxxvi–xxxix.

43. Elias PM (1983). Epidermal lipids, barrier function, and desquamation, *J Invest Dermatol*, **80**(1 Suppl), 44s–49s.

44. Mauro T, Bench G, Sidderas-Haddad E, Feingold K, Elias PM, and Cullander C (1998). Acute barrier perturbation abolishes the $Ca^{2+}$ and $K^+$ gradients in murine epidermis: quantitative measurement using PIXE, *J Invest Dermatol*, **111**(6), 1198–1201.

45. Tyson JJ (1991). Modeling the cell division cycle: cdc2 and cyclin interactions, *Proc Natl Acad Sci U.S.A.*, **88**(16), 7328–7332.

46. Dover R and Potten CS (1983). Cell cycle kinetics of cultured human epidermal keratinocytes, *J Invest Dermatol*, **80**(5), 423–429.

47. Castelijns FA, Ezendam J, Latijnhouwers MA, Van Vlijmen-Willems IM, Zeeuwin PL, Gerritsen MJ, Van de Kerkhof PC, and Van Erp PE (1998). Epidermal cell kinetics by combining in situ hybridization and immunohistochemistry, *Histochem J*, **30**(12), 869–877.

48. Potten CS (1981). Cell replacement in epidermis (keratopoiesis) via discrete units of proliferation, *Int Rev Cytol*, **69**, 271–318.

49. Grubauer G, Elias PM, and Feingold KR (1989). Transepidermal water loss: the signal for recovery of barrier structure and function, *J Lipid Res*, **30**(3), 323–333.

50. Elias P, Ahn S, Brown B, Crumrine D, and Feingold KR (2002). Origin of the epidermal calcium gradient: regulation by barrier status and role of active vs passive mechanisms, *J Invest Dermatol*, **119**(6), 1269–1274.

51. Bauer J, Bahmer FA, Wörl J, Neuhuber W, Schuler G, and Fartasch M (2001). A strikingly constant ratio exists between Langerhans cells and other epidermal cells in human skin. A stereologic study using the optical disector method and the confocal laser scanning microscope, *J Invest Dermatol*, **116**(2), 313–318.

52. Cornelissen LH, Oomens CWJ, Huyghe JM, and Baaijens FPT (2007). Mechanisms that play a role in the maintenance of the calcium gradient in the epidermis, *Skin Res Technol*, **13**(4), 369–376.

53. Adams MP, Mallet DG, and Pettet GJ (2012). Active regulation of the epidermal calcium profile, *J Theor Biol*, **301**, 112–121.

54. Iizuka H, Ishida-Yamamoto A, and Honda H (1996). Epidermal remodelling in psoriasis, *Br J Dermatol*, **135**(3), 433–438.

55. Hoath SB and Leahy DG (2003). The organization of human epidermis: functional epidermal units and phi proportionality, *J Invest Dermatol*, **121**(6), 1440–1446.

56. Heenen M, Thiriar S, Noël J-C and Galand P (1998). Ki-67 immunostaining of normal human epidermis: comparison with $^3$H-thymidine labelling and PCNA immunostaining, *Dermatology*, **197**(2), 123–126.

57. Pitt-Francis J, Pathmanathan P, Bernabeu MO, Bordas R, Cooper J, Fletcher AG, Mirams GR, Murray P, Osborne JM, Walter A, Chapman SJ, Garny A, van Leeuwen IMM, Maini PK, Rodríguez B, Waters SL, Whiteley JP, Byrne HM, and Gavaghan DJ (2009). Chaste: A test-driven approach to software development for biological modelling, *Comput Phys Commun*, **180**(12), 2452–2471.

58. Sun T, McMinn P, Coakley S, Holcombe M, Smallwood R, and Macneil S (2007). An integrated systems biology approach to understanding the rules of keratinocyte colony formation, *J R Soc Interface*, **4**(17), 1077–1092.

59. Hucka M and Le Novère N (2010). Software that goes with the flow in systems biology, *BMC Biol*, **8**, 140.

60. Krawczyk WS (1971). A pattern of epidermal cell migration during wound healing, *J Cell Biol*, **49**(2), 247–263.

61. Radice GP (1980). The spreading of epithelial cells during wound closure in Xenopus larvae, *Dev Biol*, **76**(1), 26–46.

62. Usui ML, Underwood RA, Mansbridge JN, Muffley LA, Carter WG, and Olerud JE (2005). Morphological evidence for the role of suprabasal keratinocytes in wound reepithelialization, *Wound Repair Regen*, **13**(5), 468–479.

# Chapter 15

# Heuristic Modelling Applied to Epidermal Homeostasis

François Iris,[a] Manuel Gea,[a] Paul-Henri Lampe,[a] and Bernard Querleux[b]

[a]*Bio-Modeling Systems, 3 Rue de l'Arrivée, Paris, 75015, France*
[b]*L'Oréal Research and Innovation, Aulnay-sous-bois, France*

francois.iris@bmsystems.net

Besides its key physiological functions as a stable, waterproof barrier adapted to withstand a variety of physical, chemical, and biological insults, the epidermis also plays major psychological and social roles, in particular with respect to appearance and social acceptance as well as non-verbal communication. However, its strategic location at the direct interface between the external and internal environments makes the epidermis particularly prone to a wide variety of disorders that can compromise both its physiological and psychological functions, sometimes dramatically so. Hence, understanding epidermal homeostasis has long been highly desirable for a wide variety of therapeutic and cosmetic applications. However, to be productively achieved, such an understanding must be undertaken from a holistic basis, which, in turn, requires a systems-based analytical approach (systems biology). But the task entails more difficulties than might appear at first sight. Even if reduced to

*Computational Biophysics of the Skin*
Edited by Bernard Querleux
Copyright © 2014 Pan Stanford Publishing Pte. Ltd.
ISBN 978-981-4463-84-3 (Hardcover), 978-981-4463-85-0 (eBook)
www.panstanford.com

its simplest possible representation (dermal–epidermal junction + stratified keratinocytes undergoing terminal differentiation + melanocytes that may or not be synthesizing melanin and transferring melanosomes to keratinocytes), the variety of biological processes and regulatory mechanisms intimately involved is daunting and, in their vast majority, cannot be reduced to, let alone be manipulated through, gene-based interaction networks, thereby precluding classical systems approaches.

This chapter provides an overview of the problems that must be solved and describes the logic and working principles behind a systems-based approach that has proven its efficacy in various medical and biological fields. The closing sections are devoted to a brief demonstration of how this approach can be implemented by proposing a detailed analytical reconstruction of the mechanisms that could sustain a still largely obscure aspect of epidermal homeostasis.

## 15.1 Introduction

Skin, the largest organ of the human body, structurally consists of three compartments, which differ in function, structure, and embryological origin. The outer compartment, or epidermis, is formed by a non-vascularized epithelium of ectodermal origin [15]. The underlying thicker compartment, the dermis, consists of fibroblasts embedded in connective tissue. It is vascularized and originates from the mesoderm. Epidermis and dermis are separated by a complex basement membrane, the dermal–epidermal junction (DEJ), which results from interactions and cross-talks between fibroblasts and keratinocytes [18]. The DEJ tightly binds the epidermis to the dermis and provides an adhesive and dynamic interface. It determines the polarity of basal keratinocytes, the spatial organization of keratinocytes and epidermal architecture. Epidermal stratification proceeds with the proliferating keratinocytes remaining attached to the basement membrane and the daughter cells migrating towards the upper layers [20]. The DEJ constitutes the intermediate anchorage zone for the anchoring filaments originating from the epidermis and the anchoring fibrils stemming from the fibrillar dermis. The DEJ also plays key regulatory role in the segregation and delivery of growth factors, cytokines and signalling effectors of dermal and vascular origins to basal and supra-basal keratinocytes as well as to melanocytes and resident immunological components [22].

Beneath the dermis resides a subcutaneous loose connective tissue, the hypodermis or subcutis, which binds the skin to underlying structures (muscular fascia). Hair follicles, sweat glands and sebaceous glands are of epithelial origin and are almost systemic appendages of the skin.

## 15.2 Structural and Functional Characteristics of the Epidermis

Structurally, the epidermis is characterized by a highly deceptive apparent simplicity. Yet, the epidermis, detects, integrates, and responds to a wide range of external factors. It also has immunological functions and provides some protection against ultraviolet radiation via induced or constitutive pigmentation. These functions are met by its particular histological organization, a multi-stratified squamous epithelium, generated by the keratinocytes through a tightly regulated differentiation process, called epidermal terminal differentiation or keratinization [23]. Most of the relevant information relative to epidermal stratified structures is given in previous chapters as well as below, and only a brief overview concerning the role of skin appendages, which play a considerable role in overall epidermal homeostasis, will be provided in this section.

One characteristic feature of the human skin is the apparent absence hair (pili) on most of the body surface. Nevertheless, most of the skin actually bears hair, which, in most areas, are short, thin and lightly pigmented. Only palms and soles, phalanges and sides of fingers, toes and parts of the external genitalia are truly hairless. Each hair follicle is associated with a sebaceous gland, forming a pilo-sebaceous unit. The lipid secretion of sebaceous glands (sebum) shows antibacterial and antifungal activity thereby selecting a resident lipophilic flora. It also contains proteases [24].

Two types of sweat glands are also present in human skin, distinguished by (i) their secretory mechanisms into eccrine (merocrine) and apocrine sweat, (ii) the composition of excreted sweat, and (iii) their structures, where the apocrine duct, contrarily to that of eccrine glands, admix within the pilo-sebaceous canal, i.e., with sebum.

Eccrine sweat glands are of paramount importance for the regulation of body temperature and epidermal homeostasis. About 3,000,000 eccrine sweat glands are distributed all over the body, with the exception of parts of external genitalia. They empty directly onto the skin surface excreting a watery eccrine sweat, as well as a mucin-like secretion which contain antimicrobial peptides, including cathelicidin and dermcidin [25] as well as a wide range of proteolytic enzymes, known as kallikrein-related peptidases (KLK), which govern an orchestrated proteolytic cascade that regulates corneocyte shedding, epidermal antimicrobial peptides activation, maintenance of the pH and calcium gradients inherent to the *stratum corneum* while playing a key role in epidermal repair process [26]. Interference with sweat gland functions compromises skin barrier integrity, leading to aberrant KLK cascade activities. All these events are involved in skin diseases such as psoriasis vulgaris, atopic dermatitis and Netherton syndrome (skin covered by fine, translucent scales) [27,28].

Apocrine sweat glands are stimulated by sexual hormones and are not fully developed or functional before puberty [29]. Apocrine sweat is, at least in mammals other than humans, of importance for sexual attraction.

In addition, the epidermis contains resident immunological mediators, and in particular radio-resistant hematopoietic precursors cells (RRLCs), also found in hair follicles, together with a type of dendritic cells known as Langerhans cells. These resident precursor and dendritic cells constitute the first line of epidermal defence following surface infection or induction of the keratinocytes inflammasome in response to irritants or allergens [30].

While most of the skin sensory receptors (Merkel discs, Krause end bulbs, Meissner and Pacinian corpuscles, Ruffini endings, etc.) are located in the dermis, the epidermis is nevertheless rich in sensory nerve termini [31], endowing the skin with an important role as a peripheral neuro-endocrine-immune organ tightly net-worked to central regulatory systems [32,33]. Epidermal and dermal cells produce and respond to classical stress neurotransmitters, neuropeptides, and hormones. Their production is stimulated by ultraviolet radiations (UVR), biological factors (infectious and non-infectious), and various other physical and chemical agents. Local biologically active components include cytokines, amines (catecholamines, histamine, serotonin, etc.), melatonin, acetylocholine, neuropeptides, including pituitary (proopiomelanocortin [POMC]-derived ACTH, β-endorphin, MSH peptides), thyroid-stimulating hormone and hypothalamic hormones (corticotropin-releasing factor and related urocortins, thyroid-releasing hormone), as well as enkephalins and dynorphins, thyroid hormones, steroids (glucocorticoids, mineralocorticoids, sex hormones, 7-δ steroids), secosteroids, opioids, and endocannabinoids. The production of these molecules is hierarchical, organized along the classical neuroendocrine axes such as hypothalamic-pituitary-adrenal axis (HPA), hypothalamic-thyroid axis (HPT), serotoninergic, melatoninergic, catecholaminergic, cholinergic, steroid/secosteroidogenic, opioid, and endocannbinoid systems [34]. These local neuroendocrine networks can maximally restrict or exacerbate the effects of noxious environmental agents, thereby impacting local and consequently global homeostasis.

Finally, cutaneous microcirculation has a unique anatomical arrangement that accommodates different, and sometimes conflicting, functions (See Part 4).

In the epidermis, pO2 is strongly affected by both skin surface and internal conditions. Under normal conditions, pO2 in the mid-layers of the epidermis (upper spinous and granular layers) is very close to, if not below, critical oxygen partial pressure [35] and cells in these regions are under constant threat of oxygen starvation when fluctuations in blood circulation occur.

Besides its key physiological functions, the epidermis, and mostly its derived *stratum corneum*, also plays major psychological and social roles with respect to appearance and social acceptance as well as non-verbal communication. However, its localization at the direct interface between the external and internal environments makes it particularly prone to a wide variety of disorders that can compromise both its physiological and psychological functions. In this context, sex steroids play very significant roles. They modulate epidermal and dermal thickness as well as immune system function, and changes in these hormonal levels with aging and/or disease processes alter skin surface pH, quality of wound healing, and propensity to develop autoimmune disease, thereby significantly influencing potential for infection and other pathological conditions [36]. Furthermore, with increasing age, the concentrations of important circulating hormones, including growth hormone and sex-related steroids, decrease continuously. As a result, physiologic processes are negatively influenced, giving rise to age-associated disorders [37].

Hence, a better understanding of epidermal homeostasis has long been highly desirable for a wide variety of therapeutic and cosmetologic applications.

However, to be productively achieved, a deeper understanding of epidermal homeostasis cannot rely upon in-depth analyses of individual components. This would not only mask a large part of the cross-talks that actually constitute the homeostatic machinery in this tissue, but would also prevent apprehending the associated feed-forward and feed-back dynamics which do maintain homeostatic equilibrium.

There are thus few options other than approaching the problem from a holistic basis, which, in turn, requires a systems-based analytical approach (systems biology).

The epidermis presents a heterogeneous structure. According to ethnic background and anatomical location, the epidermis indeed offers very substantial phenotypic differences, not merely in terms of pigmentation but also in terms of structural characteristics [38–43]. Furthermore, like all organs, the epidermis is subject to the effects of ageing which, themselves, may be modulated by behavioural or occupational parameters such as sun exposure (intensity and frequency), regular contacts with irritant materials or substances, etc. [44,45].

It therefore appears that with respect to the epidermis, "homeostasis" becomes an eminently context-dependent concept. Hence, modelling the homeostatic mechanisms through which, in a given context, epidermal integrity and appearance may be preserved or manipulated, appears best approached from a relativistic standpoint.

However, the task is fought with many more difficulties than might appear at first sight.

## 15.3 Problems Imposed by Enormous Variety of Mechanisms to Be Considered

Even if reduced to its simplest possible representation (dermal–epidermal junction [DEJ] + stratified keratinocytes undergoing terminal differentiation + melanocytes that may or not be actively synthesizing melanin and transferring melanosomes to keratinocytes), the variety of biological processes and regulatory mechanisms intimately involved is daunting.

A brief overview of the main biological processes that must be addressed might provide a realistic appreciation of the difficulties to overcome.

## 15.3.1 Considerations Addressing the DEJ

The homeostasis of the DEJ involves contributions from both dermal fibroblasts and germinal keratinocytes [46]. The DEJ is structured as a two-layered compartment. The upper layer, the *lamina lucida*, appears as a clear gelatinous structure whereas the lower layer, the *lamina densa*, shows a fibrous organization. Hemidesmosomes at the ventral side of basal keratinocytes are connected to anchoring filaments which traverse the *lamina lucida* ($\approx$40–50 nm) and connect with anchoring fibrils originating from the *lamina densa* ($\approx$70 nm), either ending in the anchoring plaques or looping back to the *lamina densa*. Anchoring fibrils often entrap dermal collagen fibrils, thus ensuring the connection between the anchoring complex and the dermal extracellular matrix (Fig. 15.1). In vivo, the initiation of DEJ requires nidogen-1 and 2, produced by fibroblasts [47].

Dystonin, collagen type XVII$\alpha$1, and integrins $\alpha$1$\beta$1, $\alpha$2$\beta$1, $\alpha$3$\beta$1, and $\alpha$6$\beta$4 are constitutively produced by keratinocytes, whereas fibroblasts are responsible for deposition of uncein, laminins 5, 6 and 10/11 as well as nidogen-1 and 2 [48]. Types IV and type VII collagen and glycosaminoglycans (GAGs), such as perlecan, chondroitin, dermatan and hyaluronic acid, are produced by both keratinocytes and fibroblasts. These can be further stimulated by growth factors such as EGF, KGF and GM-CSF. Deficiency in keratinocytes of integrin-linked kinase (ILK), a cytoplasmic pseudo-kinase that functions within the integrin signalling pathway, leads to epidermal hyperplasia, impaired keratinocyte differentiation and a discontinuous DEJ [49]. Thus, modelling DEJ functional regulation necessarily requires that signalling responses in keratinocytes be taken into account. Both keratinocytes and fibroblasts have considerable GAGs synthesis capabilities. As a result of their high water-holding capability, GAGs control skin volume and elasticity. But more importantly, in the DEJ, their patterns of sulphate substitution confer to GAGs differential affinities for cytokines, growth factors, and

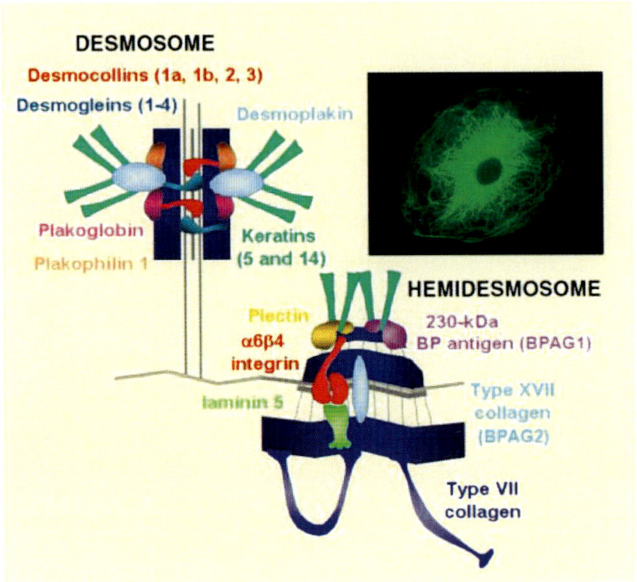



**Figure 15.1** Structure of desmosomes and hemidesmosomes, the attachment complexes at the cell-cell and DEJ interface, respectively. The keratin intermediate filament network is visualized by immunofluorescence on the upper right corner. In basal keratinocytes of the epidermis, keratins 5 and 14 form the network which attaches to desmoplakin in desmosomes and to plectin in hemidesmosomes. Critical protein-protein interactions of the desmosomal and hemidesmosomal components are required for physiologic integrity of the basal layer of epidermis and its attachment to the underlying matrix or to adjacent keratinocytes. Genetic or immunologic perturbations in the hemidesmosome and/or desmosome network structures result in skin fragility (modified from [177]).

morphogens at the cellular-DEJ interface [50]. This complex interplay between peptides and glycans influences their availability to neighbouring cells and their diffusion through tissue, thereby modulating cellular responses [51]. Perlecan of epidermal origin (but not that originating from dermal fibroblasts) functions as a reservoir for soluble factors (FGF1 to 9, EGF, VEGF, PDGF, GM-CSF, NGF, HGF, etc.) involved in the survival and differentiation of keratinocytes and melanocytes [52], as well as in the function of resident and incoming components of the immune system [53]. Furthermore, GAGs of relatively low abundance, such as fibromodulin, a small leucine-rich proteoglycan produced by keratinocytes that has a central role in the maintenance of collagen fibrils structure and in regulation of TGF-β biological activity, can have a pivotal role in the stratification process [54].

In response to chronic UVB exposure (inducing photoageing), keratinocytes produce heparanase and proteases such as urokinase-type plasminogen activator (uPA) and matrix metalloproteinases (MMPs). Heparanase degrades perlecan, leading to loss of heparan sulphates at the DEJ, resulting in uncontrolled diffusion of heparan sulphate-binding cytokines (FGFG2, FGF7, VEGF, etc.) out of the DEJ [55]. This, in turn, results in

- Cutaneous changes, such as epidermal hyperplasia, angiogenesis, lymphangiogenesis and wrinkling [56];
- Reduced keratinocyte expression of differentiation-related genes and up-regulation of degradation-enzyme-related genes [57];
- Formation of hyper-pigmented solar lentiginese [58].

Concurrently, uPA, MMP2 and MMP9 degrade laminins, thereby disorganizing the DEJ architecture, leading to impairment of DEJ assembly and subsequently to lower keratinocyte adhesion and defective epidermal differentiation [59].

Hence, any possible model of epidermal homeostasis must necessarily integrate the context-associated events that will affect DEJ structures and functions together with related physiological consequences upon overlaying components.

## 15.3.2 Considerations Addressing Keratinocyte Stratification and Differentiation

Epidermal stratification involves a differentiation-process concurrently associated with both keratinocytes migration and turnover. Failure to properly control these mechanisms gives rise to severe skin disorders such as psoriasis [60]. Furthermore, the epidermis ranks among the most dynamic of human tissues, continuously self-regenerating and responding to cutaneous insults. Keratinocytes journey from the basal compartment upwards to the cornified layers in a process which, at each step, is paralleled by key re-organizations of adhesive junctions and their associated cytoskeletal elements.

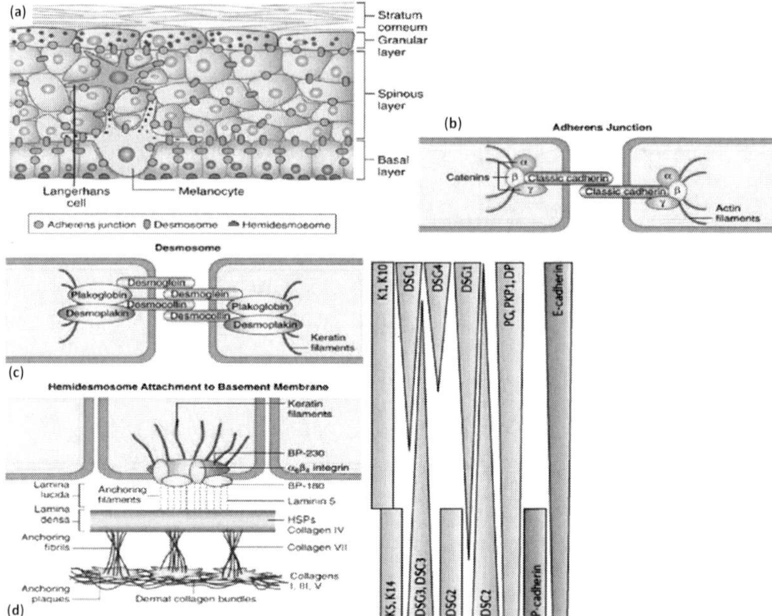


**Figure 15.2** The characteristics of epidermal architecture. The epidermis is composed of stratified cell layers, which undergo programmed differentiation to allow for constant renewal of the skin. (a) Four main layers, i.e. the *stratum basale*, the *stratum spinosum*, the *stratum granulosum* and the *stratum corneum*, are illustrated. The basal, proliferating cell layer of the epidermis remains in contact with the dermis through hemidesmosomes and integrin-based adhesions, both of which provide connections to the underlying extracellular matrix (ECM). During keratinocyte differentiation, a unique cytoarchitecture is elaborated in each of the four layers that comprise specific cytoskeleton and cell junction types, including adherent junctions (b), desmosomes (c) and hemi-desmosomes (d). The differentiation-dependent changes in the composition and organization of epidermal cytoarchitecture help to drive tissue morphogenesis while supporting the specific functions of each layer, from the regenerative capacity of the *stratum basale* to the assembly of the cornified envelope and the sloughing of terminally differentiated cells from the *stratum corneum*. The graded distribution of specific cytoskeletal and junction components (blue and green wedges on the right), including specific keratins (Ks), desmogleins (DSGs) and cadherins, is crucial in driving morphogenesis. DP: desmoplakin; DSC: desmocollin; E-cadherin: epithelial cadherin; P-cadherin: placental cadherin; PG: plakoglobin; PKP1: plakophilin 1 (Modified from [4]).

Basal keratinocytes are anchored to each other through desmosomes and tight junctions and to the DEJ through hemi-desmosomes (Figs. 15.1 and 15.2). In basal keratinocytes, keratins 5 and 14 form the network which attaches to desmoplakin in desmosomes and to plectin in hemi-desmosomes (Fig. 15.2). Critical protein–protein interactions of desmosomal and hemi-desmosomal components are required for the physiologic integrity of the epidermis basal layer and its attachment to the underlying DEJ or to adjacent keratinocytes. Genetic or immunologic perturbations in hemi-desmosome and/or desmosome structures result in skin fragility [61]. Desmosomes must be disassembled and later re-assembled in an orderly manner to allow keratinocyte migration and differentiation (Fig. 15.2). Although tight junctions are crucial in preventing excessive water loss, their remodelling also has an active role in antigen sampling. These re-organizations not only involve regulation of gene expression but also intracellular protein degradation mechanisms, cell-surface protease trafficking as well as secretion of proteolytic enzymes and protease inhibitors. Furthermore, the complex cytoarchitectural elements involved are far from being passive scaffolds. They actively cooperate with numerous signalling, transcriptional and translational pathways to establish cell and tissue polarity, control differentiation and regulate cutaneous responses to environmental insults and pathogens.

Stratification-associated alterations in integrin and cadherin-based adhesions are important for balancing proliferation and differentiation [62]. Under normal circumstances, mitogenic signalling from epidermal growth factor receptor (EGFR) to mitogen-activated protein kinase (MAPK) pathways is limited to basal keratinocytes, which abundantly express integrins [63]. Crosstalk of integrins with receptor tyrosine kinases (RTKs) regulates proliferation [64].

The proper construction of corneodesmosomes makes an essential contribution to skin barrier, but their timely breakdown is crucial for maintaining normal epidermal turnover. Terminally differentiating keratinocytes, the enucleated squamous corneocytes, assemble a complex of cross-linked proteins and lipids at their periphery called the cornified cell envelope [CE], involving the participation of at least 20 proteins [65] which organize extracellular lipids into orderly lamellae. Corneocytes are sloughed from the surface, and continually replaced by inner cells. Although the corneocytes are incapable of synthesizing new proteins, their extracellular environment is an active hub for metabolic activities regulating various skin barrier functions [24].

The *stratum corneum* (SC) of human skin normally shows a slightly acidic pH [66]. This so-called "acid mantle" partly originates from three endogenous mechanisms that are operative in the outer epidermis, namely (1) the secretory phospholipase A2 (sPLA2)-mediated generation of extracellular free fatty acids (FFA) from phospholipids [67], (2) the activity of a sodium–proton exchanger, type 1 (NHE1) [68], which localizes to membrane domains of the outer granular layer [69] and (3) the outer epidermal generation of trans-urocanic acid from filaggrin proteolysis [70].

Possibly linked to an antimicrobial function [71], this acidic pH regulates at least two other epidermal functions, that is, permeability barrier homeostasis and SC integrity/cohesion (the converse of desquamation) [72]. This latter function is dependent upon acidic pH-mediated inhibition of kallikrein serine proteases (SPs), which display neutral-to-alkaline pH optima [73]. When the pH-induced increase in SP activity is sustained, the conversion of pro-IL-1$\beta$ into active cytokine increases, which could initiate inflammation [74]. Key lipid-processing enzymes ($\beta$-glucocerebrosidase [$\beta$-GlcCer'ase] and acidic sphingomyelinase [aSMase]) and constitutive proteins of corneodesmosomes are degraded while the protease-activated receptor-2 (PAR-2) is activated, inhibiting lamellar body (LB) secretion [75].

Hence, any model of epidermal homeostasis must necessarily integrate the context-associated events that will affect keratinocyte stratification and differentiation. This necessarily implicates signalling cross-regulations, intracellular and extracellular receptors trafficking, cytoskeleton and cell junctions dynamics, scaffold proteins and signalling platforms trafficking, endocytosis and exocytosis regulation, ionic and pH gradients modulation, redox and energy-dependent mechanisms, peptide-mediated regulatory cascades. In brief, a plethora of associated mechanisms which cannot be merely reduced to gene-based interaction networks.

### 15.3.3 Considerations Addressing Pigmentation

Human skin pigmentation shows a strong positive correlation with UVR intensity, suggesting that variation in human skin colour is, at least partially, due to adaptation via natural selection. Pigmentation of skin, hair and eyes primarily depends upon melanocytes, a very minor population of cells dedicated to the synthesis and distribution of the pigmented biopolymer melanin(s).

Melanocytes are found interspersed between keratinocytes in the germinal layer of the epidermis and in hair follicles [76]. There are typically between 1000 and 2000 melanocytes per square millimetre of human epidermis [257], corresponding to 5%–10% of the cells in the basal layer.

Melanocytes are derived from precursor cells originating from the neural crest, the melanoblasts, during embryological development. In human skin, melanocytes are located at the dermal/epidermal border in a rather regular pattern. Each melanocyte at the basal layer of the epidermis is functionally connected to underlying dermal fibroblasts and to keratinocytes in the overlying epidermis. These three types of cell are highly interactive and communicate with each other via secreted factors and their receptors and via cell/cell contacts to regulate the pigmenting function and ultimately phenotyping the skin.

Epidermal melanocytes occur at an approximate ratio of 1:10 among basal keratinocytes. They distribute the melanin they produce to about 36 overlying supra-basal keratinocytes [271] via their elongated dendrites and cell/cell contacts, except in the palmo-plantar epidermis where, irrespective of ethnic pigmentation characteristics, melanocytes are maintained in an inactive state [93]. Mature melanocytes are eventually shed through the *stratum corneum*. Unlike keratinocytes, melanocytes are not anchored to the DEJ via hemidesmosomes. In resting skin, melanocytes are attached to the DEJ via multiple adhesion mechanisms, including integrin–laminin and DDR1–collagen IV binding [76].

Melanocyte dendrites also establish multiple contacts with keratinocytes. Once adhesion to keratinocytes is established (E-cadherin), keratinocytes control melanocyte growth and expression of cell surface receptors through five major mechanisms: (1) regulation of receptors important for communication with keratinocytes such as E-cadherin, P-cadherin, and desmoglein, which is achieved through growth factors such as hepatocyte growth factor (HGF), platelet-derived growth factor (PDGF), and endothelin-1 (EDN1) produced by fibroblasts or keratinocytes; (2) regulation of receptors and signalling molecules important for melanocyte–fibroblast interactions, such as N-cadherin, Mel-CAM, and zonula occludens (ZO) protein-1; (3) regulation of morphogens, such as Notch receptors and their ligands; (4) anchorage to the basement membrane through cell–matrix adhesion molecules (integrins), and (5) secretion of metalloproteases [77–78]. Whereas melanocytes and stem cell keratinocytes in the basal layer of the epidermis are very stable populations that slowly proliferate under normal circumstances, keratinocytes in the upper layers of the epidermis proliferate somewhat more rapidly. Thus it is not the melanin(s) within melanocytes but the pigments accumulated in the outermost layers that mainly give skin its characteristic colour.

### 15.3.3.1  Genetic aspects

Whether constitutive or facultative, the basic processes involved in the production of eumelanin (brown to black) and pheomelanin (yellow to red) and the melanosomes within which they are synthesized and packed, are comparable. Melanin synthesis involves a bipartite process in which structural proteins are exported from the endoplasmic reticulum and fuse with melanosome-specific regulatory glycoproteins released in coated vesicles from the Golgi apparatus and are subsequently sorted and exported to the pre-melanosome via complex and tightly controlled mechanisms. Melanosomes, which are closely related to lysosomes and are within the family of lysosome-related organelles (LROs), require a number of specific enzymatic and structural proteins to mature and become competent to produce melanin.

As melanosomes mature and their constituent proteins are delivered, the organelles themselves become cargos carried by various molecular motors from the perinuclear area where they were elaborated to the cell periphery, after which they are transferred to neighbouring keratinocytes.

The amounts and type(s) of melanin produced depend on the function of melanogenic enzymes, the availability of substrates (phenylalanine and/or tyrosine and cysteine), the pH conditions within the melanosomes, the presence and state of co-factors and, naturally, on the complex mechanisms of melanosome biogenesis and melanosome transfer to keratinocytes.

Over 125 distinct genes are currently known to regulate pigmentation either directly or indirectly. Many of these affect developmental processes critical to melanoblasts, others regulate the differentiation, survival, etc. of melanocytes, while others regulate processes affecting the biogenesis or function of melanosomes (see below) [79–80]. Single nucleotide polymorphism (SNP) in TYR, TYRP1, OCA2 (P-protein, unknown functions), SLC45A2 (MATP, no currently known function), SLC24A4 (NCKX4), SLC24A5 (NCKX5, involved in both melanosome biogenesis and control of intra-melanosomal environment through unknown mechanisms), and TPCN2 are all of direct relevance to the processes of melanosome genesis and melanin synthesis. SNPs which affect MC1R, ASIP, KITLG, HERC2, FoxP2 and IRF4 functions address multi-cellular signal transduction and protein homeostasis mechanisms.

While SLC45A2 (MATP) plays a key role in determining normal skin pigmentation, polymorphisms in ASIP and OCA2 appear to play a shared role in shaping light and dark pigmentation across the world. On the other hand, SLC24A5, MATP, and TYR have a predominant role in the evolution of light skin in Europeans but not in East Asians [80]. It is to be noted that the functions of proteins encoded by several genes tightly linked with pigmentation phenotypes remain entirely unknown and mutations in any of these typically lead to inherited pigmentary disorders which may differentially affect skin and hair.

A particularly striking example of this is represented by OA1. This G-protein coupled receptor (GPR 143), which functions through unknown mechanisms, is inserted in the melanosomal membrane, the receptor side facing the melanosome lumen. Its intra-melanosomal ligand appears to be L-DOPA (an early intermediate in melanin biosynthesis). While loss-of-function mutations in OA1 lead to severe eye and hair depigmentation, they have no effects at all upon skin pigmentation. The reason(s) for this remain a mystery.

### 15.3.3.2 Biochemical and structural aspects

Detectable levels of pheomelanin are found in human skin regardless of ethnicities, colour, and skin type. The fairest (European, Chinese and Mexican) skin types have approximately half as much epidermal melanin as the darkest (African and Indian) skin types. Furthermore, the composition of melanin in these lighter skin types is comparatively more enriched with lightly coloured, alkali-soluble pheomelanin components (up to three-fold) [81]. However, eumelanin is always the major constituent of epidermal melanin, and skin colour appears to be determined more by the amount than by the nature of melanins produced [82]. The biochemistry of melanogenesis requires pulses of pH regulation, from acidic to allow supply of substrate and essential co-factors, to near-neutral to allow melanin production, as well as cyclic hydrogen peroxide generation to sustain melanogenesis and regulate the oxidative environment within the melanosome. The mechanisms governing melanosomal pH and cysteine supply through GSH degradation (itself linked to melanosomal oxidative potential) act as regulators of eumelanine/pheomelanin production, thereby ultimately defining skin colour [83–84].

Cutaneous pigmentation is the outcome of two events: the synthesis of melanin by melanocytes and the transfer of melanosomes to surrounding keratinocytes. Indeed, differences in size, number and aggregation patterns of melanosomes, and not the number of melanocytes, correlate with skin colour and with ethnic origin [85].

Melanosome biogenesis proceeds through four different stages.

- Stage I melanosomes are vesicles derived from early endo-somal membranes [86] which contain the amyloid protein Pmel17 [87] and MART-1 which forms a complex with Pmel17 and affects its distribution, stability, processing and sorting through a Rab7-dependent pathway [88].

- As the stage I melanosome matures, Pmel17 forms lumenal fibrillar striations that characterize stage II melanosomes [89] through a process requiring proteases [90]. A partial clathrin coat is seen on stage I melanosomes, and this might be involved in sorting proteins into intra-lumenal vesicles (ILVs) of vacuolar endosomes [91]. Endosomal ILVs form in all cells; in melanocytes, however, the presence of Pmel17 gives rise to the structurally important intra-lumenal fibrils that characterize stage II melanosomes.

- The resulting pre-melanosomes mature to stage III and IV organelles after the delivery of melanogenic enzymes Tyr and Tyrp1 from other early endosomes via vesicular transport and fusion [92]. The melanogenic enzymes follow delivery pathways that are distinct from those used by Pmel17. Again, the endosomal system is important at such stage. Tyr and Tyrp1 are thought to traffic preferentially to melanosomes from early endosomes. They are present in tubular endosomal domains that are distinct from the regions occupied by

Pmel17. Tyr and Tyrp1-positive endosomal membranes have buds coated with the adaptor proteins AP1 or AP3 [93]. BLOC1 and 2 are also implicated in the regulation of endosome to melanosome transport [94]. These widely expressed protein complexes are particularly important in the formation of lysosome-related organelles. Similar to AP1 and AP3, BLOC1 has been localized to tubular regions on early endosomes.

Once these proteins have been imported into the maturing melanosomes, melanin is synthesized and deposited onto the Pmel17 striation fibrils (stage III melanosome), eventually giving rise to stage IV melanosome, which appears opaque in electron microscopy [95–96].

Structurally, the biosynthesis of melanosomes involves mechanisms controlling both the endosome and autophagosome biogenesis pathways. The endosome-associated mechanisms appear to control protein trafficking while those associated with autophagosomes control melanosomal membrane constitution, particularly with respect to lipids composition.

In melanocytes, vesicles containing melanosomal proteins bud from the endoplasmic reticulum (ER). These vesicles are then moved forward along microtubules to the cis-Golgi by dynein/dynactin. In the Golgi, the spectrin mesh stabilizes the different arriving vesicles and continues the anterograde transport. The presence of actin filaments at both ends of the Golgi cisternae provide support for this compartment and probably interact with spectrin. At the trans-Golgi network (TGN), sorting vesicles containing spectrin-like mosaics are delivered to downstream compartments in conjunction with other motor and budding systems.

The new vesicle is then directed to stage I melanosomes. The presence of dyneins in stage I and II melanosomes appears to favour their accumulation in the central area of the cell, thereby facilitating delivery of incoming melanosomal components-loaded vesicles. The spectrin-like mosaics in early melanosomes may help to stabilize the organelle and interact with either spectrin-adaptor proteins or actin filaments [97]. In late melanosomes, the presence of kinesins promotes the transport of these organelles to the cell periphery using microtubules (MT). Stage IV melanosomes are transferred to actin filaments for secretion. The lack of spectrin in the plasma membrane is the major structural difference between un-pigmented and pigmented cells.

The transition from MT-dominant transport to actin-dominant transport mainly occurs during dynein-driven motion. This decreases minus-end motion, favouring dispersion. Here, increased levels of cAMP will not increase the formation of the melanophilin/Rab27/myosin transporter complex itself but it will increase its binding to actin [98].

Thus, since MT-dependent transport can go in both directions, it cannot totally account, *per se*, for the net accumulation of melanosomes in melanocyte dendrites [99]. It is likely that the interactions between melanosomes and the actomyosin system prevent the net return of melanosomes to the cell centre. Immature melanosomes are linked to the MT system via Rab7 and dynactin [100,101], while mature melanosomes recruit myosin Va via the Rab27a/melanophilin (SLAC2a) complex and are linked to actin. This complex is dysregulated in the heritable disease Griscelli syndrome and some related animal models [102].

Thus, melanosomes are simultaneously linked to MTs and actin during dispersion, with continuous competition between these two systems. It is apparently a second Rab27A effector, the synaptotagmin-related protein SLP2a, which controls melanosome distribution in the cell periphery [103].

### 15.3.3.3 Melanosome trafficking and degradation

Four main sequential, MyoX-driven events are apparent:

- MyoX-driven melanocyte filopodia formation and elongation (e.g. by anticapping activity of Mena/VASP; [104]);
- Adhesion of melanocytes filopodia to keratinocytes membrane via integrins, [105];
- MyoX-associated motor force at the filopodial tip helps insert filopodia into the keratinocyte plasma membrane [106]; and
- MyoX-driven phagocytic force in keratinocytes causes melanocyte filopodia (containing melanosomes) to be taken up by keratinocytes.
- Here, MyoX provides a molecular link between PI3K and pseudopod extension during phagocytosis, while PAR-2, expressed on keratinocytes but not on melanocytes, when activated by trypsin or the peptide agonist LIGR, induces melanosme uptake by keratinocytes [107,108].

In addition, PAR-2 also affects skin pigmentation by stimulation of melanocyte dendricity through a series of interconnected mechanisms.

In keratinocytes, PAR-2 activation stimulates the release of PGE2 and PGF2α which then act as paracrine factors that stimulate melanocyte dendricity. Here, PAR-2 activation appears to trigger specific up-regulation of mPGES-1 (microsomal prostaglandin E synthase 1) that is dependent on prostanoids precursors formed via the MEK/ERK/cPLA2/PTGS1 pathway [109].

After transfer, melanin is transported to the apical face of the keratinocyte nucleus, an appropriate location for protecting DNA against UVR-induced damage.

Within keratinocytes, melanosomes are transported between the cell centre and the cell periphery along microtubules via the action of the motor proteins kinesin and dynein [110]. Beneath the plasma membrane, melanosomes undergo short-range movements along the sub-lemmal actin network via association with the motor protein myosin Va, which attaches to melanosomes through interaction with melanophilin and Rab27a. But melanosomes are also transferred amongst keratinocytes and a sequence of events similar to that described above could operate for melanosome transfer at this level.

Numerous growth factors and hormones, together with their multiple receptors, are implicated in melanogenesis and melanocyte dendrite formation, including EDN1, SCF, bFGF, PGE2, ACTH and α-MSH [111,112], many of which are induced by sunlight [113]. In addition, cAMP induces the formation of dendrites in melanocytes, implicating the potential role of PKA-mediated intracellular signalling cascades [114]. In this context, activation of PAR-2 leads to serine protease secretion by keratinocytes, creating a positive feedback loop [115]. PAR-2 signals up-regulate Rho activity and, conversely, inactivation of Rho, or its downstream effector Rho kinase, abolishes PAR-2-stimulated phagocytosis [116].

While dark skin (DS; phototype V/VI) melanosomes are approximately 0.8 μm in diameter, light-skin (LS; phototype I/II) melanosomes are significantly smaller in size. The pattern and distribution of melanosomes in the cytoplasm of keratinocytes also differ between LS and DS.

Melanosomes in keratinocytes of LS are often distributed in membrane-bound clusters of approximately four to eight melanosomes, while they are predominantly individually dispersed in keratinocytes of DS. This distinct pattern of melanosome distribution within the keratinocytes appears to be governed by the keratinocytes milieu itself [117,118].

Skin type also appears to regulate the pattern of melanosome degradation. As keratinocytes undergo terminal differentiation, melanosomes are completely degraded in the upper skin layers of LS, resulting in corneocytes devoid of melanosomes whereas some melanosomes are present unaltered in the desquamating corneocytes of DS. Within 48 hours following uptake, LS keratinocytes show accelerated loss of melanosome as compared to DS keratinocytes. Overall, DS biopsies show retention of melanosomes throughout the epidermis, with melanosomes still apparent in the upper skin layers, including the stratum granulosum (SG) and *stratum corneum* (SC). In contrast, LS biopsies lack melanosomes in SG and SC while some melanosomes are present in SB and fewer in SS, suggesting a differential processing of melanosomes between fair and dark skins [119].

To date, the mechanisms associated with melanosome degradation remain obscure, particularly those giving rise to differential degradation processes between light and dark skin types.

Hence, any possible model of epidermal homeostasis aiming to address pigmentation aspects must necessarily integrate the context-associated events that will affect melanogenesis, melanosome transfer and degradation during keratinocytes stratification and differentiation. This necessarily implicates signalling cross-regulations, scaffold proteins and signalling platforms dynamics, intracellular vesicles trafficking and transport dynamics, ionic and pH gradients modulation, redox biochemistry and a plethora of associated mechanisms which cannot be reduced to interaction networks.

### 15.3.4 Signalling and Epidermal Homeostasis

The melanocyte–keratinocyte complexes quickly respond to a wide range of environmental stimuli, in paracrine as well as autocrine manners.

Following UVR exposure, the expression of POMC, the precursor of MSHs and ACTH, and melanocortin 1 receptor (MC1-R), TYR and TYRP1, protein kinase C (PKC), and other signalling factors are increased in melanocytes [120].

On the other hand, it is known that UVR stimulates the production of endothelin-1 (ET-1/EDN1) and POMC by keratinocytes and these factors can then act in a paracrine manner to stimulate melanocyte function. In addition to keratinocytes, fibroblasts, and resident dendritic cells in the skin produce cytokines, growth factors, and inflammatory mediators that can affect keratinocyte growth and differentiation, melanin production and/or melanin transfer to keratinocytes by melanocytes as well as DEJ structure and composition. Growth factors affect not only the size and pigmentation of melanocytes but their shape, dendricity, adhesion to matrix proteins, and mobility as well.

At least nine signalling networks cooperatively regulate epidermal homeostasis and pigmentation.

α-MSH, ACTH, basic fibroblast growth factor (bFGF/FGF-2), nerve growth factor (NGF), endothelins (EDN1-3), granulocyte-macrophage colony-stimulating factor (GM-CSF), steel factor (SCF), and leukemia inhibitory factor (LIF) are keratinocyte-derived. Dickkopf 1 (DKK1), keratinocyte growth factor (KGF/FGF-7) and hepatocyte growth factor (HGF) are fibroblast-derived factors. All are involved in the regulation of the proliferation and/or differentiation of melanocytes and keratinocytes, some acting through receptor-mediated signalling pathways. However, in the epidermis, the melanocortin signalling pathway (α-MSH-MC1R) does not couple eumelanin with pheomelanin synthesis, unlike in hair follicles. Even by shared signalling pathways, hair and skin melanocytes are regulated quite independently [121,122].

α-MSH and ACTH are produced in and released by keratinocytes and are involved in regulating melanogenesis and/or melanocyte dendrite formation [123,124]. α-MSH and ACTH bind to a melanocyte-specific receptor, MC1R [125], which activates adenylate cyclase through Gαs protein, which then elevates cyclic AMP (cAMP) [126]. cAMP exerts its effect in part through protein kinase A (PKA) [127], which phosphorylates and activates the cAMP response element binding protein (CREB) that binds to the cAMP response element (CRE) present in the M promoter of the microphthalmia-associated transcription factor (MITF) gene.

However, in cells, PKA is present in the form of an inactive tetrameric holoenzyme composed of two regulatory and two catalytic subunits. cAMP causes the dissociation of the inactive holoenzyme into a dimer of regulatory subunits bound to four cAMP and two free monomeric catalytic subunits which then phosphorylate a diverse set of proteins, including the transcription factor CREB, ion channels and metabolic enzymes. PKA is localized to specific sites near these substrates within cells by scaffolding proteins known as "A kinase anchoring proteins" (AKAPs). Four different regulatory subunits (PKARIα and RIβ, PKARIIα and RIIβ) and three catalytic subunits (PKACα, Cβ and Cγ) have been identified in humans. Clearly, the signalling outcome depends upon the catalytic isoforms present at the time. Increase in MITF-M expression induces up-regulation of TYR, TYRP1, and DCT [128,129], which leads to melanin synthesis.

Keratinocytes produce and release NGF, while normal human melanocytes express the NGF receptors TrkA-TrkB [130] and also the NT-3 (TRK-C) receptor [131]. NGF signalling regulates melanogenesis and/or dendritogenesis in melanocytes [131]. NGF expression is up-regulated by UVR, suggesting another paracrine influence of keratinocytes on melanocytes with relevance to the tanning response.

EDN1 is a 21 amino acid peptide with vasoactive properties synthesized and secreted by keratinocytes, particularly following exposure to UVR [132]. In human melanocytes, the overall effect of EDN1 is the increase in MC1R mRNA level, regardless of melanin content, and the enhancement in melanocyte dendricity, melanosome migration and melanization [133–134]. Binding of EDN1 to its G protein-coupled receptor (EDNRB) on melanocytes activates a cascade of signalling pathways, resulting in mobilization of intracellular calcium, activation of PKC, elevation of cAMP levels, and activation of mitogen-activated protein kinase (MAPK) [135].

UVR stimulates keratinocytes to produce EDN1 and also induces interleukin-1 (IL-1) production in these cells. IL-1 is known to induce EDN1 in keratinocytes in an autocrine manner. Therefore, it has been suggested that these intracellular events in keratinocytes lead to increased TYR mRNA, protein, and enzymatic activity in neighbouring melanocytes together with an increase in melanosome number [136].

Prostaglandins (PG) E2 and PGF2α are produced and released from human keratinocytes following stimulation of proteinase-activated receptor 2 (PAR-2). PGE2 and PGF2α stimulate dendritogenesis in human epidermal melanocytes in culture [137] through EP1, EP3, and FP receptors. Their influence on melanocyte dendricity has been suggested to be cAMP-independent and may be mediated through phospholipase C (PLC) [137]. The signalling mechanisms mediated by the GPCR EP2 receptor contribute to keratinocyte proliferation through two different pathways. A G-protein-independent pathway involving the formation of a GPCR-β-arrestin-Src signalling complex which promotes EGFR activation, and a G-protein-dependent pathway which activates PKA, increases cAMP levels, inhibits GSK3β while activating CREB together with Akt, ERK1/2, and STAT3 signalling [138].

FGF-2 and SCF/KitL are expressed by keratinocytes [139,140]. These secreted factors are involved in regulating the proliferation and melanogenesis/dendritogenesis of human epidermal melano-cytes in normal skin and/or in UV-A/UV-B-irradiated skin [133]. FGF-2 up regulates MC1R mRNA level in human melanocytes with high melanin contents but not in those with low melanin contents [134].

Binding of keratinocyte produced GM-CSF to its specific receptor, GM-CSFR [141], activates the MAPK signal transducers [142] and members of the "activator of transcription" family (STAT-1, STAT-3, and STAT-5) [143,144], inducing up-regulation of proteins required for the proliferation of melanocytes and the expression of TYR, TYRP1, and DCT as well. GM-CSF is also a key activator of Langerhans cells, the main antigen-presenting cells in the epidermis [145]. This establishes a clear link between keratinocyte responses to UVR and inflammation [125].

Hepatocyte growth factor (HGF) is a fibroblast-derived protein that affects the growth, motility, and differentiation of epithelial cells including epidermal keratinocytes and melanocytes. On the cell surface, the HGF receptor (MET) forms a complex with E-cadherin, desmoglein 1 and plakoglobin, which then regulates intercellular adhesion [146]. HGF signalling induces

(i) sustained activation of the Ras-MAPK pathway which mediates HGF-induced scattering and proliferation signals (modulated via different BAG1 isoforms [147]), and leads to branching morphogenesis [148] and melanocyte proliferation [149];

(ii) the JAK-JNK-STAT3 pathway, through a SH2 domain [150], which, together with sustained MAPK activation, is necessary for HGF-induced branching morphogenesis [148];

(iii) the PI3K pathway, that can act either downstream of Ras or can be directly recruited [151], the activation of which is associated with cell motility through remodelling of adhesion to the extracellular matrix (e.g. down regulation of E-cadherin and desmoglein 1 in melanocytes), which contributes to adhesion between melanocytes and keratinocytes [146] as well as with cytoskeletal reorganization, through RAC1 and PAK, and survival signalling through activation of AKT [152];

(iv) the Wnt-β-catenin pathway, in which β-catenin translocates into the nucleus following MET activation [153] and frizzled-related protein (Frzb/FRP3), a secreted antagonist of the Wnt receptor system (Frizzled : LRP5/6), inhibits Met signalling [154]; and

(v) the Notch pathway, through transcriptional activation of Delta ligand [155].

In the PI3K-mediated pathway, Akt is recruited to the plasma membrane by virtue of its interaction with the phosphoinositides PtdIns(3,4,5)P3/PtdIns(3,4)P2. Akt is then activated by 3-phosphoinositide-dependent protein kinase-1 (PDK1) which, like Akt, possesses a PtdIns(3,4,5)P3/PtdIns(3,4)P2-binding PH domain [156].

DKK1, an inhibitor of the canonical Wnt signalling pathway, is produced by fibroblasts and is particularly present in the hypopigmented and very thick palmo-plantar (PP) human epidermis [157]. In this epidermis, hypo-pigmentation is not due to a loss of melanocytes but to the inhibition of both keratinocyte control over melanogensis and melanocye activity. The expression of tyrosinase, S100α, SCF receptor (c-KIT), endothelin B receptor (ETBR), SOX10, MITF and that of SCF and EDN1 as well, are significantly reduced in melanocytes and keratinocytes of PP epidermis, respectively [158].

DKK1 appears to act through four different mechanisms [159].

(i) suppressing proliferation and melanogenesis in melanocytes via inhibition of the Wnt/β-catenin/MITF pathway;

(ii) suppressing PAR-2 expression in keratinocytes, thereby decreasing melanin transfer;

(iii) potentiating keratinocyte proliferation and contraction, mainly via increased expression of αKLEIP and keratin 9 and decreased expression of β-catenin, and

(iv) induction of keratin 9 production, via Wnt5a, and reduction of fibronectin secretion, via HoxA13, in PP fibroblasts which, together, induce and maintain the palmo-plantar phenotype.

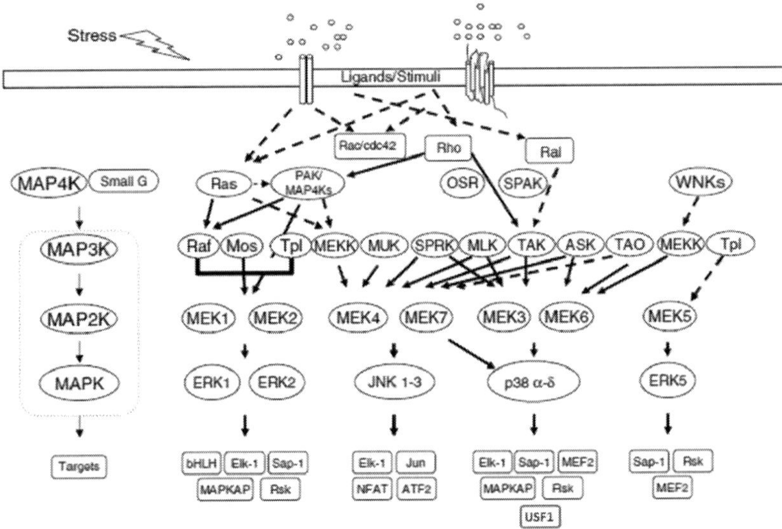


**Figure 15.3** The MAPK signalling network. The mitogen activated protein kinase (MAPK) pathway consists of four main arms, namely ERK1/2 (extracellular signal-regulated kinase), JNK (c-Jun N-terminal kinase) p38 and ERK5, that mediate functional responses to stimuli through multiple receptors such as tyrosine kinase (RTKs), G-protein coupled receptors (GPCRs) and cytokine receptors as well as ion channels. Activated MAPKs enter the nucleus to trigger transcription factor and immediate early gene activation for cellular responses such as cytokine production, apoptosis and migration. The existence of a three-tiered structure is probably essential for the amplification and tight regulation of the transmitted signal [19]. Some 18 MAPK genes, encompassing four subfamilies, have been identified in mammalian cells [1,3,9]. All MAPKs, except the larger ERKs [17], are activated by dual phosphorylation of threonine and tyrosine residues within a conserved "TXY" kinase domain motif. Upon ligand binding, RTKs and GPCRs transmit the signal to MAP3Ks [22] which then transfer the signal to MAP2Ks to induce MAPK activation [21]. Thus, MAP3Ks, create independent signalling modules that may provide stimulus specificity, whereas the MAPKs carry out the effector functions of each cascade, either through transcription factors or activation of subordinate kinases (MAPKAPKs). Multiple dual-specificity phosphatases (DUSPs) specifically dephosphorylate MAPKs, rendering them inactive either in the cytoplasm or nucleus. DUSPs also assist in shuttling or anchoring MAPKs to control their activity (modified from [7]).

Many of the above signalling pathways cross-communicate and modulate each other, involving the activation of the MAPK cascades. Thus, these pathways cannot be viewed as vertical modular entities, but rather as horizontal layers of interactive nodes (Fig. 15.3).

Furthermore, the cross-talks between RTK and GPCR-mediated signalling as well as the effective levels of MAPK/ERK signalling are governed by scaffold proteins.

## 15.3.5 The Role of Scaffold Proteins in Directing Transduction Pathways and Modulating Signalling Cross-Talks

At the plasma membrane, activated RTKs promote Ras activation through the recruitment of Grb2/Sos complexes. Here, KSR is an ERK scaffold that facilitates Ras-dependent ERK cascade activation at the plasma membrane, whereas paxillin directs ERK activation at focal adhesion structures. Furthermore, active signalling complexes containing internalized receptors together with Grb2/Sos and Ras are also found on endosomes. Here, MP1 is a MEK1/ERK1-specific scaffold that localizes to late endosomes through an interaction with the adaptor protein p14, allowing late endosomes to act as signalling loci. Activated RTKs can also direct the activation of Golgi-associated Ras through a signalling route involving RTK-associated Src and PLCγ and the Golgi-associated Ras-GRP1 complex. Here, Sef is a Golgi-localized scaffold that recruits activated MEK and promotes ERK activation. Active ERK is retained on the Sef/MEK complex and confined to cytosolic substrates. The tyrosine phosphatase Shp-2 is another effector of RTKs that positively regulates Ras signalling by antagonizing the ability of negative regulators, such as CSK, Ras GAP and Sprouty, to access and down-regulate critical enzymes involved in Ras activation [132,160,201].

Furthermore, the level of MAPK/ERK activation depends upon the activity of 14-3-3 protein family members which are implicated in the control of Raf & KSR recruitment to the plasma membrane. 14-3-3 dimers bind and retain B-Raf, C-Raf and KSR proteins in an inactive state in the cytosol. The inactive KSR1 scaffold constitutively interacts with MEK, CK2 and the catalytic subunits of PP2A, and is further sequestered from the plasma membrane by interactions with 14-3-3 proteins and IMP. This effectively prevents Ras-mediated signalling. However, PP1 or PP2A-mediated dephosphorylation of N-terminal 14-3-3-binding sites results in the recruitment of C-Raf and B-Raf to the plasma membrane as a result of Ras GTP binding. At the membrane, Raf proteins are then activated through a process involving phosphorylations and protein/lipid interactions. Heterodimerization with B-Raf also contributes to C-Raf activation and requires the binding of a 14-3-3 protein to the C-terminal Raf sites. Ras activation also mediates the translocation of the KSR1 scaffold to the plasma membrane. Here, Ras activation induces binding of the PP2A regulatory B subunit to the KSR1-associated PP2A catalytic core complex. Regulatory B subunit binding stimulates dephosphorylation and release of 14-3-3 proteins from one of the KSR1 sites, thereby unmasking the C1 domain required for membrane targeting as well as the ERK docking site. Concurrently, Ras GTP disrupts the IMP-KSR1 interaction by recruiting the inhibitory protein IMP to the cell surface and promoting its auto-ubiquitination [42,215].

Scaffold proteins also link signalling from RTKs and GPCRs to the ERK modules. Here, KSR is specifically involved in linking GPCRs to ERK1/2 module while the MP1-p14 complex interacts with MEK and ERK or with MORG 1 to direct RTK or GCPR signalling to the MEK1-ERK1 modules, respectively. The scaffolding roles of paxillin and β-arrestin appear to be involved in directing the signalling outputs from ERK-modules to specific cytosolic compartments. In particular, β-arrestin provides a spatiotemporal signalling conduit for GPCR mediated, G protein-independent ERK signalling [161,162,243].

However, stress conditions (UVR exposure) lead to significant changes in signalling cross-talk mechanisms mediated by scaffold-proteins. Four distinct JNK-scaffold proteins, namely JIP 1 and 2, JSAP1 (JIP3) and JLP (JNK-associated leucine zipper protein/JIP4) provide scaffolding functions for the JNK and p38MAPK signalling modules. These scaffold proteins play anchoring as well as catalytic role in JNK- and p38MAPK-mediated signalling pathways. In addition to their role in assembling the three-tier kinase modules, these proteins also interact with upstream signalling components, such as cell surface receptors, receptor-like proteins, upstream G proteins and/or GEFs that can then activate the corresponding kinase modules. In particular, the JLP scaffold links Hedgehog (Shh) receptor signalling (modulator of Wnt & Kit signalling) and GPCR signalling to the JNK and p38 modules [46,161,178].

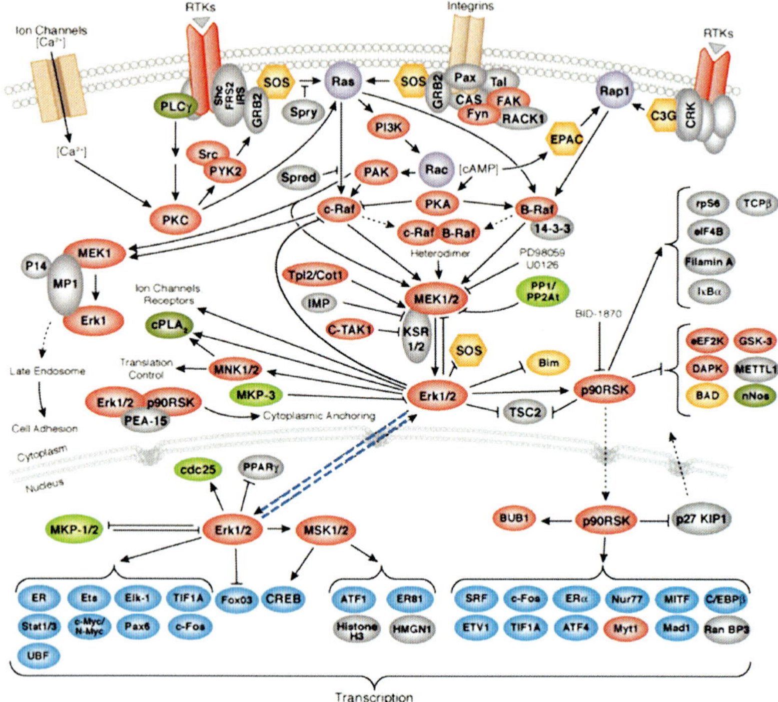


**Figure 15.4** The ERK1/2 signalling network in the epidermis represents only one arm of the MAPK signalling machinery. The RTKs involved include cKit (SCF receptor), TrkA/TrkB (NGF receptors), cMET (HGF receptor) and FGFR2b and FGFR2c (KGF and FGF2 receptors, respectively) [5]. All the components in pink ovals are subject to functional modulation through GPCRs signalling which, here, include (1) EDNRB (EDN1 receptor), which signals through Gα12/13 subunits and strongly stimulates JNK activity. However, whereas Gα12 inhibits p38MAPKs at the levels of MKKs and ERK1/2 at the level of Raf, Gα13 stimulates p38MAPKs including p38γ/ERK6 via MKK3/6 [6]. (2) EP1/EP3 and FP (PGE-2 and PGF2α receptors, respectively). EP1, a relatively low affinity PGE2 receptor, couples with Gαq/11, but not Gαi, to mediate TRP5 (receptor-activated Ca²⁺ channel) gating [8]. EP3, a high affinity PGE2 receptor, is unique in its ability to couple with multiple G proteins. The major EP3 signalling pathways are involved in inhibition of adenylyl cyclase via Gαi, and in Ca²⁺-mobilization through Gβγ from Gαi. However, along with Gαi activation, the EP3 receptor can stimulate cAMP production (via Gαs activation). FP couples with Gαq and PLA2 [10]

> leading to MAPK activation via PLC and PKC [11] and can also synergize with FGFR signalling through Mek activation while concurrently inducing the PKC-calcium-calcineurin-NFAT signalling pathways [12]. (3) MC1R (a-MSH receptor) signals through $G\alpha s$, coupling with both cAMP and $Ca^{2+}$ signalling systems [13,14], thus activating the B-Raf-ERK and MAP3K-p38 pathways while inhibiting Mekk2/3-ERK5 and C-Raf-ERK signalling. This can also synergize with c-Kit signalling to maintain C-Raf-ERK-mediated transduction [16].

Hence, as demonstrated by the ERK1/2-mediated transduction system alone (Fig. 15.4 below), the signalling intricacies are such that, without detailed proteome dynamics data, it is practically impossible to define which transcriptional mechanisms will be affected by a given signalling event, let alone reconstruct the signalling events associated with the activation/inhibition of any given transcription factor. From a very general standpoint, it is only possible to confidently state that

- Mitogens (growth factors, GPCRs, etc.) will primarily induce ERK1/2 signalling, whereas
- Stress and inflammatory cytokines will primarily induce p38 and SAPK/JNK concurrently with ERK5/BMK1 signalling.

Yet, any model of epidermal homeostasis will necessarily need to incorporate the integrated effects of multiple, highly dynamic signalling networks upon, at the very least, keratinocytes dynamics, melanocytes activity and DEJ structural evolution. The situation described above clearly demonstrates that a classical systems approach, based mainly upon interaction networks, is unlikely to succeed.

## 15.4 Approaching Dermatological Problems through Systems Biology Principles?

Given the many serious difficulties exposed in the necessarily limited overview above, the question may be asked.

However, rather than adamantly adhering to the established principles attached to the most frequently used approaches to systems biology, attempts could be made to reconsider the problem under a different light.

What characterizes the usual approaches to systems biology? It is

(1) their dependence upon relevant quantitative data arising from multiple targeted experimental interrogations in an iterative interplay between experimentation and modelling, with

(2) the aim of elucidating how the molecular components of a living system determine its phenotype by exploring their dynamic interplays as well as their interactions with the environment.

Thus, this approach interprets biological phenomena as dynamic processes, the mechanisms and consequences of which depend on the behaviour of components that constitute the living entity studied.

While this requirement may be reasonably fulfilled in the context of well-defined mechanisms (e.g. the Rab5-Rab7 toggle and cut-out switches in the conversion of early endosomes into late endosomes; [163]), it can hardly be contemplated when addressing the vast number of processes involved in tissues having the structural and functional complexity coupled to the anatomical heterogeneity of human epidermis.

Hence, given that, when dealing with issues addressing human epidermis, data on relevant molecular and cellular dynamics is seldom available to an extent and a range likely to sustain classical modelling approaches [164], one could attempt to proceed using the tremendous amount of information contained in the published scientific literature (at least 578,000 relevant publications referenced in PubMed alone).

In other words, an alternative approach to systems analysis could be based on the exploitation of existing, highly heterogeneous publicly available data rather than on homogeneous datasets arising from specifically targeted investigations.

However, the matter is much more arduous than could be anticipated.

### 15.4.1 Problem of Relevance Attached to Available Data

Most of the published data available was obtained from various animal models [129,165,166], in vitro reconstructed epidermis [167–169], cell lines [170] and, in some instances, biopsies [171–173].

Whereas data from animal models may be partly relevant to mechanisms such as epidermal stratification [174–241], it is not so to mechanisms governing epidermal pigmentation. In these models, data primarily addresses fur colour [175].

In vitro reconstructed epidermis systems are entirely bereft of key components, such as vasculature, resident immune cells, nerve termini, eccrine glands, etc., which play critical roles in epidermal physiology. Data obtained from such systems must therefore be carefully evaluated regarding their relevance to homeostatic mechanisms [176, 246].

Data from biopsies are physiologically much more relevant than most of the above. However, such data really represents "windows" open upon various time-points and snapshots on processes that remain largely obscure. This data provides what could be described as insights into "static mechanisms" separated by very substantial black boxes [171,177].

This takes particular meaning when considering that "homeostasis" of a structure such as the epidermis, even if restricted to its most basic constituents and to a given context, implicates an amazing variety of intra and extracellular mechanisms, spanning several orders of magnitude in both time and space.

Hence, irrespective of the domain being addressed, the data available is necessarily always incomplete, to an unknown extent, biased, in unknown manners and to an unknown extent, and partly erroneous, to an unknown extent.

It follows that, using this data as such, on the sole basis of positive selection (i.e. on the principle that the information is correct, relevant and can be assigned a nominal positive or negative value), will inevitably lead to an accumulation of analytically crippling inconsistencies.

Indeed, the "true" will be mixed with the "uncertain", without possibility to eliminate the "false" and even less to determine in which contexts the "true" may suddenly become "false". Furthermore, the greater the complexity addressed, the worse the negative effects these inconsistencies will have upon the analytical processes implemented.

However, the above very real difficulties certainly do not mean that the scientific literature cannot be used for the implementation of systems-based analyses.

These difficulties highlight the fact that to coherently utilize the highly heterogeneous information available, different analytical approaches become necessary.

## 15.4.2 Changing the Analytical Paradigm

By focusing mainly on chemical and physical processes with the expectation that living systems can be fully explained from this engineer's perspective, the classical approach to systems biology assumes bottom-up causation, from molecular dynamics to cellular/tissue behaviour.

However, the stability of a living system lies in its homeostatic capacity to re-establish itself.

In a living system, the outcome does not crucially depend on strictly predefined operations of the parts. Rather, the structure of the whole determines the operation of the parts. Indeed, almost all homeostatic processes are complex context-dependent entities to which genes make a necessary, but only partial, contribution. This is particularly evident in highly dynamic tissues such as the epidermis, which is continuously exposed to a wide variety of internal and external environmental conditions that can simultaneously undergo very rapid changes.

In such a system, homeostasis proceeds on the basis of functional loops wherein on-going events tell contexts how to evolve, contexts tell components how to behave and components tell future events how to arise, and so on. In other words, specific biological events do not occur because they are fated to. They occur because other events could not arise.

It follows that analyses in terms of biological components and functions now become irrelevant. What become necessary are event-driven analytical approaches.

In addition to this, the intrinsic value of any "information" is only relative. It can be profoundly modified by other, indirectly linked information as well as by the contexts it can be attached to.

Thus, both the available information and the biological processes to be considered are characterized by heavily context-dependent attributes.

Therefore, whatever event-driven analytical approach is implemented, it must also be "relativistic". That is, all available information must be treated on the basis of a negative selection procedure. In other words, what can be identified as false can be used to discover what could be true, provided that a heuristic and event-driven analytical procedure is implemented.

Heuristics can be characterized as a problem solving approach evaluating each step in a process, searching for satisfactory solutions rather than for optimal solutions, using all available qualitative information. Thus, heuristic modelling starts from accumulated knowledge to produce a model capable of describing the biological events and the mechanisms that generated the observed biological phenomenon and predict the modifications they will sustain in association with a different outcome.

The above considerations constitute the functional basis on which the CADI (computer-assisted deductive integration) analytical procedure was developed.

This alternative model-building approach, which associates algorithmics and heuristics, has repeatedly proven its efficacy in the discovery of (i) hitherto unsuspected biological mechanisms, pathways and interactions directly associated with phenotypic transitions in vivo (be they pathological or developmental) [178, 179], (ii) patent protected novel therapeutic approaches in fields ranging from oncology to neurodegenerative and infectious diseases [179–182], and (iii) the development of novel and patent protected technologies [183]. Furthermore, when applied to neurodegenerative disorders, this approach was selected by the EU's DG Research as one of 3 examples of "state-of-the-art" in systems biology that benefit to medicine [184] and was granted an industrial "Best Practice Award" by The Cambridge Health Tech Institute (USA) [185].

The logic behind this model-building approach (Fig. 15.5) does not assume functional linearity and the components of a model do not incorporate solely what is known. Indeed, since this approach relies upon strict and systematic implementation of negative selection of hypotheses, models arising from this procedure contain elements that have never been described but cannot be refuted by current knowledge and/or available biological data (Fig. 15.6).

Here, heuristic and mathematical modelling, far from being antagonistic, become complementary. Heuristic modelling plays the role of an architect (defines the nature, the structure, the functionalities and the contextual constraints of the system under study) whereas mathematical modelling, to be implemented at a later stage, plays the role of an engineer (reveals the dynamics and robustness of the structures while defining the set of parameters sufficient to give rise to similar or very different phenotypes).

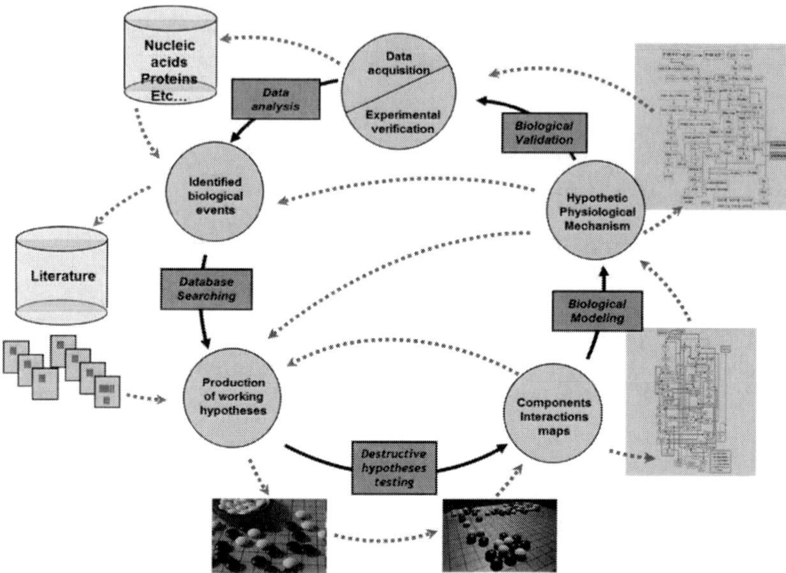


**Figure 15.5** The CADI heuristic modelling strategy. Working hypotheses, directly generated from datasets and the literature, that have resisted all destruction attempts (go boards) are merged to produce interaction maps describing the pathways that have become functional and those that have become forbidden in response to local conditions imposed by the activation of defined biological mechanisms. These maps are in turn merged to produce hypothetical physiological mechanisms. During each phase, "undetected" biological events are revealed while novel working hypotheses are being generated (dotted arrows). These are, in turn, subjected to the iterative negative (destructive) selection procedure. Hence, this model building process involves multiple levels of internal cross check procedures designed to eliminate any hypothesis that is not directly or indirectly supported by multiple data intersects. The results of experiments designed to directly challenge/ validate the model thus obtained can then be, in turn, injected into this iterative analytical process.

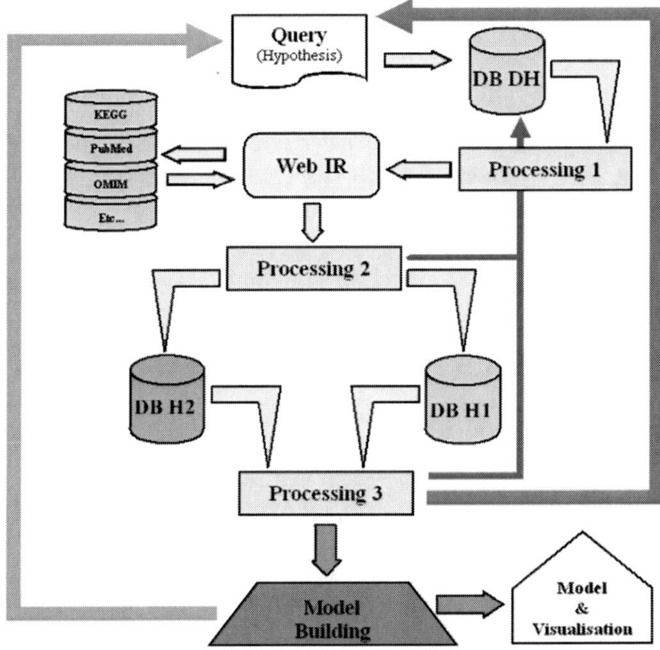


**Figure 15.6** The CADI modelling process. The procedure is initiated from a query-building interface linked to an initially empty database (DB DH) the purpose of which is threefold. First, to record all queries sent to external databases. Second, to harbour both the queries and retrieved information attached to working hypotheses demonstrated as incorrect (narrow magenta arrow). Third, to avoid unnecessary redundancies by filtering all new queries (pink and blue arrows). Following this filtration step, the queries are then dispatched (Processing Module 1) to small machines linked to public databases via a web information retrieval interface (Web IR). The information retrieved in answer to a query, largely under the form of published literature and images, is then processed (Processing Module 2) to determine whether this information could support the hypothesis attached to the query, or disagree with, or neither support nor invalidate the hypothesis but provide material for a new formulation of this hypothesis. If the information supports the working hypothesis, it is, together with the query, directed to a dedicated database (DB H1). The fact that a working hypothesis finds support in the published literature does not mean that the hypothesis is correct. It merely means that it does not contradict publicly accessible information. If data from the literature is at variance with the

hypothesis, the retrieved information and the query are directed to the DB DH database. If the hypothesis is neither invalidated nor supported, the retrieved information and the query are directed to the DB H2 database. This complex procedure is carried out by specialized biologists assisted by proprietary software. This first level of iterative query procedures is ended when most new queries lead to material directed to DB H2, the contents of this database growing over five times faster than that of any of the other two databases. At this stage, it can be considered that most available "medium-sized" pieces of the puzzle have been obtained and the model building process itself (Fig. 15.5 above) can now be implemented. The indices of the databases DB H1 and H2 are visualized to generate "meta-hypotheses" (Processing Module 3) from the merging of either already supported hypotheses (DB H1) or of supported hypotheses associated with neither supported nor ruled out hypotheses (DB H1 + DB H2). Meta-hypotheses are in turn subjected to the testing mechanism described above. Meta-hypotheses finding support in the literature enter the Model Building module, while those proved incorrect enter the DB DH database and those neither supported nor ruled out enter a new sector in DB H2. Once again, the process is ended when the contents of the new sector in DB DH2 grows much faster than those of either DB DH or of the Model Building module. At this stage, most of the "large pieces" of the puzzle that can be reconstructed using published information have been obtained. But numerous gaps and uncertainties still remain. Thus, during the model building phase, numerous questions do arise (dotted arrows in Fig. 15.5) and these are in turn processed to the query interface in order to find supported solutions or propose possible answers (not in contradiction with publicly accessible information). Model building ends when the query process mostly generates uncertainties.

Although the models arising from this analytical approach cannot, by any means, be regarded as biologically true in the absolute, they do represent a "least biased" and detailed view of the mechanisms potentially associated with a given physiological state and/or governed by the biological components under consideration, together with precise indications of the means whereby these could be manipulated. In other words, these models clearly indicate what should be biologically observed in a given experimental context, where, when, how and why. The newly gathered experimental data can then be re-injected in the model-building procedure, allowing rapid and efficient correction of the model which, thereby, now provides an exploitable representation of the biological reality addressed.

The new data arising from subsequent experimental verifications can then be re-injected into the model, rapidly leading to a clear and factual understanding of the biological processes under investigation. A concrete example, directly applying to epidermal homeostasis, will illustrate the fact.

## 15.5 The Mechanisms Whereby OA1 Differentially Affects Melanosome Biogenesis and Motility

As stated in Section 15.3.3.1, the mechanisms whereby loss-of-function mutations in OA1 lead to severe eye and hair depigmentation while having no effects at all upon skin pigmentation remain a mystery. OA1 is a G-protein coupled receptor (GPR 143) implicated in numerous steps of melanosome biogenesis and trafficking [186].

Analyses aiming to uncover the mechanisms associated with the differential effects of OA1 upon skin versus eye and hair pigmentation must necessarily take into consideration the homeostatic continuum attached to pigmentation.

Melanosome biogenesis involves vesicular traffic of proteins from the trans Golgi network (TGN) to pre-melanosomal membrane, controlling both the protein constituents and the size of melanosome. Just as melanosome motility, these mechanisms involve cytoskeletal and motor dynamics. Furthermore, the transport mechanisms associated with vesicle trafficking differ substantially from those associated with organelle motility. Since OA1 activity affects both, this also will have to be taken into account. In addition, since OA1 is a GPCR coupled to a $G\alpha$i and $G\alpha$q transducers, the effects of presence and absence of adenylyl cyclase activity (cAMP production and PKA activity) upon the signalling-dependent mechanisms that govern cytoskeleton dynamics will have to be distinguished.

### 15.5.1 The Observed Facts

Unlike other GPCRs, OA1 is not localized to the cell surface, but is exclusively found on the membranes of intracellular organelles, namely late endosomes/lysosomes and melanosomes. In stage II melanosomal membrane, OA1 is inserted the receptor side facing the melanosome lumen and the signal transducing domain facing the melanocyte cytoplasm [187]. In mice, OA1 expression parallels temporally and spatially that of TYR during development, is regulated by the transcription factor Mitf, is up-regulated by α-MSH and is inhibited by its antagonist ASP.

From a genetic standpoint, the OA1 gene is highly conserved amongst mammalian species and, in contrast to the genes for other melanosomal proteins and MC1R, no coding polymorphisms have been associated so far to OA1, underlining the critical role that this receptor plays in the development of the retina, where MC1R is not expressed [188].

OA1 is a selective L-DOPA (an early intermediate in melanin biosynthesis) receptor which signals through Gαi3 and Gαq (cytoplasmic side) [189,190] whose downstream effects (inhibition of cAMP synthesis, influx of intracellular $Ca^{2+}$ and recruitment of β-arrestin) govern spatial patterning of the developing retina. Dopamine competes with L-DOPA for the single OA1 binding site, and could function as an OA1 antagonist. The vacuolar distribution of OA1 is dependent upon intracellular tyrosine concentration. A fall in tyrosine contents leads to redistribution of OA1 to the cytoplasmic membrane [191].

OA1 is also involved in the regulation of melanosome maturation at steps II and IV, controlling the abundance of melanosomes in retinal pigment epithelial (RPE) cells and, at later stages, has a function in the maintenance of a correct melanosomal size and melanosome motility [192]. OA1 loss of function leads to decreased pigmentation and causes the formation of enlarged aberrant melanosomes harbouring disorganized fibrillar structures and displaying proteins of both mature melanosomes and lysosomes at their membrane. This strongly suggests a role for OA1 in the control of cargo vesicles import [186].

OA1 interacts biochemically with the pre-melanosomal protein MART-1 (Melan-A) which also plays a vital role in the expression, stability, trafficking, and processing of Pmel17, critical to the formation of stage II melanosomes. MART-1 acts as an escort protein for OA1 and inactivation of MART-1 leads to decreased OA1 stability accompanied by defects in melanosome biogenesis and composition similar to those arising from OA1 deficiency alone [186].

In the absence of OA1 function, melanosomes move less efficiently and especially less frequently on the tubulin cytoskeleton. However, this kinetic deficiency is not intrinsic to the microtubule (MT)-based transport system but manifests itself exclusively in the presence of intact actin-based transport [192]. This strongly suggests that the defect implicates mis-function of Rab proteins required for association with actin-based transport.

RPE and skin melanocytes of OA1-defficient mice consistently present a displacement of the organelles from the central cytoplasm towards the cell periphery. Despite their depletion from the microtubule (MT)-enriched perinuclear region, OA1-defficient melanosomes are able to aggregate at the centrosome upon disruption of the actin cytoskeleton or expression of a dominant-negative construct of myosin Va. In living cells, OA1-defficient melanosomes display a severe reduction in MT-based motility; however, this defect is rescued to normal following inhibition of actin-dependent capture at the cell periphery. Hence, there is defective regulation of organelle transport in the absence of OA1 which does not function through diffuse cytosolic signalling, but rather in an organelle autonomous fashion, implying that the cytoskeleton represent a downstream effector of this receptor [192].

## 15.5.2 Event-Driven Data Integration and Negative Selection of Working Hypotheses

### 15.5.2.1 The OA1-mediated mechanisms in melanosome biogenesis

According to the above observations, OA1 could act at either the level of

  (i)  cargo vesicle transport to pre-melanosomes, or

  (ii)  docking and fusion of cargo vesicles to pre-melanosomes.

Sorting of proteins for delivery to melanosomes depends upon the BLOC1, 2 and 3 complexes as well as upon the AP-3 adaptor complex, [193] while directionality and efficacy of vesicle delivery are in part mediated by actin filaments (AF) and microtubules (MT), which facilitate local and long-range vesicle transport, respectively.

Higher eukaryotes contain various motor proteins that are capable of powering directional vesicle transport along such molecular cables. This necessitates high specificity in the attachment of motors to vesicles, and Rab GTPases and their effectors proofread these types of interactions. In particular, actin motors of the myosin V family associate with cargo vesicles in a Rab-dependent manner [102].

Intracellular transport (Fig. 15.7) is mediated by opposite polarity MT motors or actin-dependent motors of the myosin family. AF-dependent motors, myosins, generally move the cargo to the plus ("barbed") ends of AFs [194]. MT-dependent motors include kinesins, which generally support transport to the MT plus ends [195], and dyneins, which are exclusively minus-end directed [196].

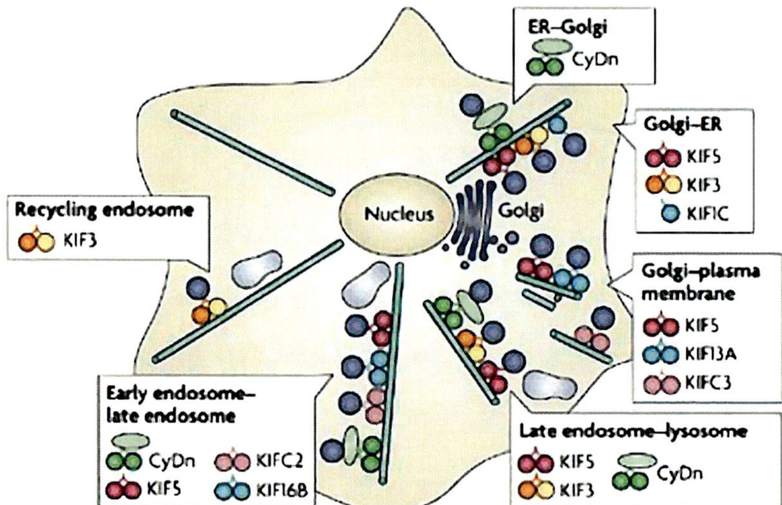


**Figure 15.7** Intracellular transport by molecular motors. In non-neuronal cells, microtubules are usually directed from the microtubule organizing centre to the periphery of the cells. Plus end-directed motors, such as the KIF5 and KIF3 and the kinesin 3 family motors KIF1C, KIF13A and KIF16B, tug against the minus end-directed motors, such as cytoplasmic dynein (CyDn), KIFC2 and KIFC3 (members of the kinesin 14B family). This might help to distribute the cargos appropriately. How these motors are differentially involved in the dynamics of intracellular membrane organelles remains largely unclear. Nevertheless, in melanocytes, it appears that this process requires PKA activity, the inhibition of which causes melanosomes aggregation at the cell's centre (retrograde transport) (Modified from [2]).

The correct delivery of organelles to their different destinations involves a precise coordination of the two transport systems. Such coordination occurs through PKA/cAMP-mediated regulation of the activities of the cytoskeletal motors [197]. Plus end-directed motor, kinesin-II, and the minus end-directed motor, cytoplasmic dynein, are tightly membrane-associated in highly purified melanosomes of Xenopus. Here, pigment aggregation (MT minus-end-directed movement) involves successive activation of PP2A and casein kinase 1ε (CK1ε). CK1ε-dependent phosphorylation of dynein intermediate chain stimulates dynein motor activity and increases minus-end-directed transport (aggregation) of pigment granules [198].

Early melanosomes must remain in the perinuclear area to receive sorting vesicles containing critical melanosomal proteins needed for their maturation and eventually for pigment biosynthesis. The movement of early melanosomes in the perinuclear area depends primarily on microtubules but not on actin filaments. In contrast, the trafficking of TYR and Pmel17 depends on cytoplasmic dynein and its interaction with the spectrin/ankyrin system involved with the sorting of cargo from the plasma membrane [199].

However, MTs represent a downstream effector of OA1 and melanosomes kinetic deficiency resulting from the absence of OA1 function manifests itself exclusively in the presence of intact actin-based transport [192].

This strongly suggests that the defect in melanosome biogenesis (giant aberrant melanosomes) is likely to implicate vesicle fusion mechanisms much more than transport mechanisms.

Besides the effects of transport mechanisms, melanosome biogenesis involves the fusion of a variety of endosomal vesicles. These complex mechanisms involve the activities of $Ca^{2+}$ channels as well as the participation of tethering proteins, the function and distribution of which are highly sensitive the nature of their phosphoinositide environment.

Rab27a and Rab27b have a key role in mediating vesicle–motor attachment and promoting targeting, transport and docking of cargo vesicles to pre-melanosome plasma membrane. However, Rab27a and Rab27b appear to perform different and non-redundant tasks in the exosomal pathway. Rab27a preferentially interacts with Slp4 (granuphilin) while Rab27b interacts preferentially with Slac2b (exophilin 5). Nevertheless, in epidermal melonosomes, Rab27b can supplement deficient Rab27a and compensate for its functional loss [200].

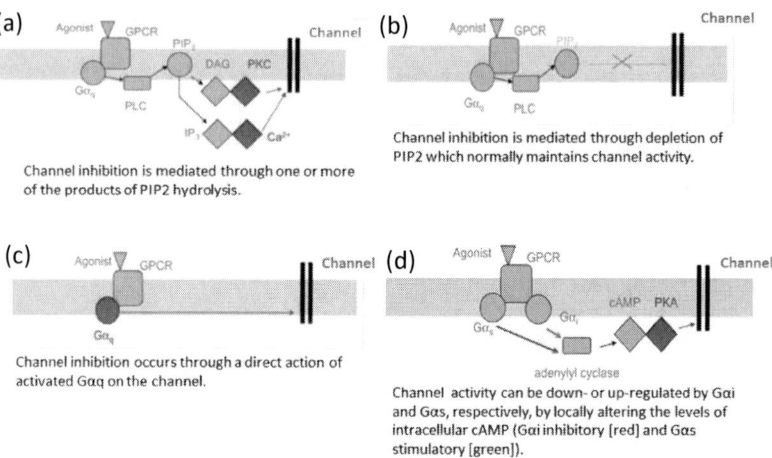



**Figure 15.8** Mechanisms whereby OA1 could inhibit tethering and fusion of cargo vesicles originating from the TGN with pre-melanosomal membrane. Activation of OA1 by intra-melanosomal L-DOPA activates *G*αq or *G*αi on the cytoplasmic side. This could lead, through 3 alternative mechanisms (a, b or c) associated with one modulatory mechanism (d) to inhibition of calcium efflux from melanosomal channels such as NCKX5, thereby impeding tethering of cargo vesicles and inhibiting fusion with the melanosomal membrane. Failure of these mechanisms through loss of OA1 function would lead to inappropriate vesicle fusion, resulting in giant, misshapen melanosomes aberrantly containing non-melanosomal proteins.

Recruitment/exchange of Rab proteins to endosomal membranes is mediated by Rab guanine nucleotide triphosphatase activating proteins (GAPs) concurrently with adaptor proteins that may be specified by golgi-stack origin (e.g. Rabaptin 5) or endosomal maturation state (e.g. EEA), the trafficking of which (shedding/recruitment) is dependent upon the phosphorylation status of phosphoinositides in membrane domains mediated by PI kinases and phosphatases. While membrane domains respond to pH (demixing under acidic conditions), the phosphoinositide-specific phosphatases/kinases respond to local ionic strengths

[201]. Member of the receptor family to which OA1 belongs are known to regulate voltage gated $Ca^{2+}$ channels (NCKX5, TPCN2), the functions of which are highly sensitive to their immediate PI(4,5) P2 environments [202].

Hence, it would appear that OA1 could be a negative regulator of vesicle fusion (melanosome biogenesis) through the control of local phosphoinosides, and subsequently $Ca^{2+}$ channels and vesicle tethering inhibition. Three hypothetical *G*αq-dependent mechanisms could lead to channels inhibition while channel activity could be down-regulated by *G*αi, through one mechanism leading to local decrease in the levels of intra-melanocyte cAMP (Fig. 15.8).

While the above mechanisms can adequately explain the effects of dysfunctional OA1 upon melanosome maturation, they do not provide satisfactory arguments for its differential effects upon melanosomal transport in RPE cells as compared to the epidermis.

Further analysis, in particular with respect to Gαq/Gαi-coupled signalling, becomes necessary.

### 15.5.2.2 The OA1-mediated mechanisms in melanosome motility

Activation of cAMP-dependent PKA or $Ca^{2+}$-dependent PKC is known to cause melanosome dispersion (activates plus end transport). Also, PKC and NO (EDN1-3 pathway) have been shown to regulate the MEK-ERK pathway where PKC, MEK and NOS inhibition each blocks bidirectional melanosome transport along microtubules, while activation of ERK stimulates transport. These effects are specific because perturbation of ERK signalling has no effect on the movement of lysosomes, organelles related to melanosomes [203]. Furthermore, stimulation of the cAMP pathway induces a rapid centrifugal transport of melanosomes, leading to their accumulation at the dendrite tips of melanocytes.

Melanosomes are transported within the melanocytes on both microtubule and actin networks [99]. The microtubule dependent transport is bi-directional and mediated through kinesin and dynein molecular motors. The actin network allows the transport of melanosomes in the dendrite outgrowths and their docking at the dendrite tips. At least three proteins, myosin-Va, Rab27a, and melanophilin/Slac2-a, play a pivotal role in the actin-dependent transport and docking of melanosomes [199,204].

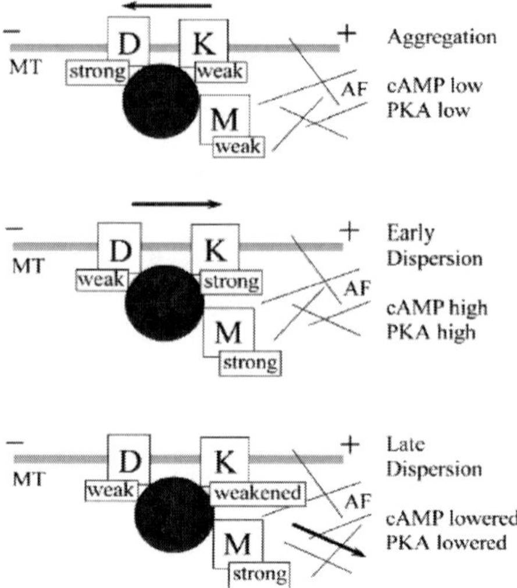



**Figure 15.9** Model for melanosome transport and switching between MTs and AFs regulation by OA1 activity and cAMP. OA1 signals through Gαi3, hence inhibiting adenylyl cyclase and decreasing the local cAMP levels of PKA signalling. (1) During aggregation (top), DOPA-mediated OA1 activation leads to locally low cAMP levels, resulting in down-regulation of kinesin and myosin Va concurrently with activation of dynein. Myosin Va and kinesin are down-regulated sufficiently that whenever there is a tug of-war between the motors, dynein wins (melanosomes are prevented from reaching the dendrites). Residual myosin Va-dependent motion allows for the granules to move along AFs until they contact MT and engage in dynein-based motion. (2) In contrast, early during dispersion (middle), OA1 signalling decreases and the levels of cAMP increase. As a result, the activity of dynein is significantly reduced, whereas kinesin and myosin Va become very active. Pigment granules thus move toward MT plus ends. Because switching onto AFs occurs during minus end runs or following kinesin-cargo dissociation, the probability for the granules to leave the MTs is low at this time. (3) At late stages of dispersion (bottom), the inputs from melanocyte-membrane-associated signalling pathways which inhibit cAMP production probably start playing a role dominant over that of OA1. At this stage, the activity of myosin Va remains high, whereas the cAMP levels and the activity of kinesin decrease. This decreases plus end-directed motion while promoting the dissociation of kinesins from melanosomes. Therefore, the number of opportunities for tripartite complex Rab27a-Mlph-myosin Va activation and transfer from MTs onto AFs is increased at this stage, resulting in increased AF-based transport. K: kinesin; M: myosin; D: Dynein. Pigment granules are shown as black circles.

cAMP stimulates the expression of Rab27a and rapidly increases the interaction of the melanophilin/Slac2-a complex with actin, allowing the rapid accumulation of melanosomes in the actin-rich region of the dendrite extremities after the action of melanocyte-differentiating agent such as α-MSH. Mlph directly activates the actin-dependent ATPase activity of myosin Va and thus its motor activity [98].

Furthermore, signalling mediated by the PI3K pathway, such as that resulting from Gαq/Gαi-mediated transduction, activates actin polymerization [205].

Cumulatively, the above considerations lead to an overall cAMP-dependent scheme of intracellular melanosome motility in which OA1 could play a central role.

Thus, OA1 might act by tethering melanosomes to tubulin filaments, thereby stabilizing the productive association between cargo and cytoskeletal route. Alternatively, OA1 could counteract the capture of melanosomes by actin filaments and as a consequence enhance the frequency by which the organelles move along MTs, while in the absence of OA1 melanosome entrapment by the actin network at the cell periphery would prevail.

This scheme could explain why in human, OA1 deficiency has the expected depigmenting effects in structures with low keratinocytes contents (retina) but is without apparent effects upon pigmentation in tissues rich in keratinocytes (epidermis). In the latter case, the OA1 activity-dependent, highly localized effects of cAMP levels upon the modulation of melanosome motility are largely supplanted by the manifold paracrine signalling pathways induced by factors concurrently originating from multiple keratinocytes in the immediate neighbourhood of each melanocyte.

As a result, in the epidermis, while the effects of OA1dysfunction upon melanosome biogenesis are partly conserved (resulting in the generation of giant aberrant melanosomes), those addressing melanosome trafficking are swamped out by keratinocytes signalling that promotes melanosome transfer.

## 15.6  Conclusion

It must be admitted that, whatever the systems-based analytical approach one could implement, current publicly accessible data alone shall certainly not allow to obtain a working understanding of epidermal homeostasis sufficiently detailed and precise to globally enable "informed interventions", be they medical or cosmetic. The major impediment lies in the signalling intricacies that govern and maintain the anatomical and functional heterogeneity of this large and deceptively "simple" organ. To be coherently approached, these difficulties will require highly contextualized differential proteomics turnover data.

However, what can most certainly be achieved, using the approach detailed above, are models of epidermal sub-domains sufficiently detailed to propose well defined

- physiological and molecular activities for components of unknown functions (e.g. SLC45A2/MATP; OCA2/p-protein; OA1/GPR143, etc.);
- mechanisms differentially governing and modulating constitutive and acquired pigmentation as well as pigmentation disorders;
- mechanisms regulating basal keratinocytes turnover and epidermal maturation (psoriasis, etc.);
- mechanisms leading to de-novo irritant or allergic contact dermatitis as well as chronic inflammatory dermatoses; etc., together with potential modes of interventions.

The latter two points are of particular importance to the use of reconstructed skin systems for safety evaluation of novel dermatologic drugs and preparations.

Nevertheless, it must be born in mind that no matter how detailed, a model can only be regarded an approximation of biological reality. The more complex this reality, the coarser the model will be. Hence, a systems model can never be more than an assistance to thoughts, and certainly not a replacement for thoughts.

## References


1. Caffrey DR, O'Neill LA, and Shields DC (1999). The evolution of the MAP kinase pathways: coduplication of interacting proteins leads to new signaling cascades, *J Mol Evol*, **49**, 567–582.

2. Hirokawa N, Noda Y, Tanaka Y, and Niwa S (2009). Kinesin superfamily motor proteins and intracellular transport, *Nat Rev Mol Cell Biol*, **10**, 682–696.

3. Roux PP and Blenis J (2004). ERK and p38 MAPK-activated protein kinases: a family of protein kinases with diverse biological functions, *Microbiol Mol Biol Rev*, **68**, 320–344.

4. Simpson CL, Patel DM, and Green KJ (2011). Deconstructing the skin: cytoarchitectural determinants of epidermal morphogenesis, *Nat Rev Mol Cell Biol*, **12**, 565–580.

5. Johnson DE and Williams LT (1993). Structural and functional diversity in the FGF receptor multigene family, *Adv Cancer Res*, **60**, 1–41.

6. Dermott JM, Ha JH, Lee CH, and Dhanasekaran N (2004). Differential regulation of Jun N-terminal kinase and p38MAP kinase by Galpha12, *Oncogene*, **23**, 226–232.

7. Jeffrey KL, Camps M, Rommel C, and Mackay CR (2007). Targeting dual-specificity phosphatases: manipulating MAP kinase signalling and immune responses, *Nat Rev Drug Discov*, **6**, 391–403.

8. Tabata H, Tanaka S, Sugimoto Y, Kanki H, Kaneko S, and Ichikawa A (2002). Possible coupling of prostaglandin E receptor EP(1) to TRP5 expressed in Xenopus laevis oocytes, *Biochem Biophys Res Commun*, **298**, 398–402.

9. Bogoyevitch MA and Court NW (2004). Counting on mitogen-activated protein kinases–ERKs 3, 4, 5, 6, 7 and 8, *Cell Signal*, **16**, 1345–1354.

10. Konger RL, Billings SD, Thompson AB, Morimiya A, Ladenson JH, Landt Y, Pentland AP, and Badve S (2005). Immunolocalization of low-affinity prostaglandin E receptors, EP and EP, in adult human epidermis, *J Invest Dermatol*, **124**, 965–970.

11. Bos CL, Richel DJ, Ritsema T, Peppelenbosch MP, and Versteeg HH (2004). Prostanoids and prostanoid receptors in signal transduction, *Int J Biochem Cell Biol*, **36**, 1187–1205.

12. Wallace AE, Catalano RD, Anderson RA, and Jabbour HN (2011). Chemokine (C-C) motif ligand 20 is regulated by PGF(2alpha)-F-prostanoid receptor signalling in endometrial adenocarcinoma and promotes cell proliferation, *Mol Cell Endocrinol*, **331**, 129–135.

13. Kim CS, Lee SH, Kim RY, Kim BJ, Li SZ, Lee IH, Lee EJ, Lim SK, Bae YS, Lee W, and Baik JH (2002). Identification of domains directing specificity of coupling to G-proteins for the melanocortin MC3 and MC4 receptors, *J Biol Chem*, **277**, 31310–31317.

14. Wachira SJ, Hughes-Darden CA, Taylor CV, Ochillo R, and Robinson TJ (2003). Evidence for the interaction of protein kinase C and melano-cortin 3-receptor signaling pathways, *Neuropeptides*, **37**, 201–210.

15. Benitah SA and Frye M (2012). Stem cells in ectodermal development, *J Mol Med (Berl)*, **90**, 783–790.

16. Newton RA, Roberts DW, Leonard JH, and Sturm RA (2007). Human melanocytes expressing MC1R variant alleles show impaired activation of multiple signaling pathways, *Peptides*, **28**, 2387–2396.

17. Yoon S and Seger R (2006). The extracellular signal-regulated kinase: multiple substrates regulate diverse cellular functions, *Growth Factors*, **24**, 21–44.

18. Chan LS (1997). Human skin basement membrane in health and in autoimmune diseases, *Front Biosci*, **2**, d343–d352.

19. Robinson MJ and Cobb MH (1997). Mitogen-activated protein kinase pathways, *Curr Opin Cell Biol*, **9**, 180–186.

20. Koster MI and Roop DR (2007). Mechanisms regulating epithelial stratification, *Annu Rev Cell Dev Biol*, **23**, 93–113.

21. Pearson G, Robinson F, Beers Gibson T, Xu BE, Karandikar M, Berman K, and Cobb MH (2001). Mitogen-activated protein (MAP) kinase pathways: regulation and physiological functions, *Endocr Rev*, **22**, 153–183.

22. Kazama T, Oguro K, and Sato Y (1989). Effect of enzyme digestion on anionic sites and charge-selective permeability of dermo-epidermal junction, *J Invest Dermatol*, **93**, 814–817.

23. Menon GK (2002). New insights into skin structure: scratching the surface, *Adv Drug Deliv Rev*, **54 Suppl 1**, S3–S17.

24. Valdes-Rodriguez R, Torres-Alvarez B, Gonzalez-Muro J, and Almeda-Valdes P (2012). The skin and the endocrine system, *Gac Med Mex*, **148**, 162–168.

25. Park JH, Park GT, Cho IH, Sim SM, Yang JM, and Lee DY (2011). An antimicrobial protein, lactoferrin exists in the sweat: proteomic analysis of sweat, *Exp Dermatol*, **20**, 369–371.

26. Rittie L, Sachs DL, Orringer JS, Voorhees JJ, and Fisher GJ (2012). Eccrine sweat glands are major contributors to reepithelialization of human wounds, *Am J Pathol*, **182**(1), 163–171.

27. Komatsu N, Saijoh K, Toyama T, Ohka R, Otsuki N, Hussack G, Takehara K, and Diamandis EP (2005). Multiple tissue kallikrein mRNA and protein expression in normal skin and skin diseases, *Br J Dermatol*, **153**, 274–281.

28. Wollina U, Abdel-Naser MB, Ganceviciene R, and Zouboulis CC (2007). Receptors of eccrine, apocrine, and holocrine skin glands, *Dermatol Clin*, **25**, 577–588.

29. Beier K, Ginez I, and Schaller H (2005). Localization of steroid hormone receptors in the apocrine sweat glands of the human axilla, *Histochem Cell Biol*, **123**, 61–65.

30. Bangert C, Brunner PM, and Stingl G (2011). Immune functions of the skin, *Clin Dermatol*, **29**, 360–376.

31. Persson AK, Black JA, Gasser A, Cheng X, Fischer TZ, and Waxman SG (2010). Sodium-calcium exchanger and multiple sodium channel isoforms in intra-epidermal nerve terminals, *Mol Pain*, **6**, 84, 1–13.

32. Boulais N and Misery L (2008). The epidermis: a sensory tissue, *Eur J Dermatol*, **18**, 119–127.

33. Paus R, Theoharides TC, and Arck PC (2006). Neuroimmunoendocrine circuitry of the "brain-skin connection", *Trends Immunol*, **27**, 32–39.

34. Slominski AT, Zmijewski MA, Skobowiat C, Zbytek B, Slominski RM, and Steketee JD (2012). Sensing the environment: regulation of local and global homeostasis by the skin's neuroendocrine system, *Adv Anat Embryol Cell Biol*, **212**, v, vii, 1–115.

35. Wang W (2005). Oxygen partial pressure in outer layers of skin: simulation using three-dimensional multilayered models, *Microcirculation*, **12**, 195–207.

36. Dao H Jr, and Kazin RA (2007). Gender differences in skin: a review of the literature, *Gend Med*, **4**, 308–328.

37. Makrantonaki E and Zouboulis CC (2010). Dermatoendocrinology. Skin aging, *Hautarzt*, **61**, 505–510.

38. de Rigal J, Des Mazis I, Diridollou S, Querleux B, Yang G, Leroy F, and Barbosa VH (2010). The effect of age on skin color and color heterogeneity in four ethnic groups, *Skin Res Technol*, **16**, 168–178.

39. Diridollou S, de Rigal J, Querleux B, Leroy F, and Holloway Barbosa V (2007). Comparative study of the hydration of the *stratum corneum* between four ethnic groups: influence of age, *Int J Dermatol*, **46 Suppl 1**, 11–14.

40. Kobayashi H and Tagami H (2004). Distinct locational differences observable in biophysical functions of the facial skin: with special emphasis on the poor functional properties of the *stratum corneum* of the perioral region, *Int J Cosmet Sci*, **26**, 91–101.

41. Querleux B, Baldeweck T, Diridollou S, de Rigal J, Huguet E, Leroy F, and Holloway Barbosa V (2009). Skin from various ethnic origins and aging: an in vivo cross-sectional multimodality imaging study, *Skin Res Technol*, **15**, 306–313.

42. Rawlings AV (2006). Ethnic skin types: are there differences in skin structure and function? *Int J Cosmet Sci*, **28**, 79–93.

43. Tagami, H. (2008). Location-related differences in structure and function of the *stratum corneum* with special emphasis on those of the facial skin. *Int J Cosmet Sci*, **30**, 413–434.

44. Amano S (2009). Possible involvement of basement membrane damage in skin photoaging, *J Invest Dermatol Symp Proc*, **14**, 2–7.

45. Hachiya A, Sriwiriyanont P, Fujimura T, Ohuchi A, Kitahara T, Takema Y, Kitzmiller WJ, Visscher MO, Tsuboi R, and Boissy RE (2009). Mechanistic effects of long-term ultraviolet B irradiation induce epidermal and dermal changes in human skin xenografts, *Am J Pathol*, **174**, 401–413.

46. Breitkreutz D, Mirancea N, and Nischt R (2009). Basement membranes in skin: unique matrix structures with diverse functions? *Histochem Cell Biol*, **132**, 1–10.

47. Mokkapati S, Baranowsky A, Mirancea N, Smyth N, Breitkreutz D, and Nischt R (2008). Basement membranes in skin are differently affected by lack of nidogen 1 and 2, *J Invest Dermatol*, **128**, 2259–2267.

48. Lai-Cheong JE, McGrath JA, and Uitto J (2011). Revertant mosaicism in skin: natural gene therapy, *Trends Mol Med*, **17**, 140–148.

49. Raghavan S, Bauer C, Mundschau G, Li Q, and Fuchs E (2000). Conditional ablation of beta1 integrin in skin. Severe defects in epidermal proliferation, basement membrane formation, and hair follicle invagination, *J Cell Biol*, **150**, 1149–1160.

50. Kwiatkowska D and Kwiatkowska-Korczak J (1999). Adhesive glycoproteins of the extracellular matrix, *Postepy Hig Med Dosw*, **53**, 55–74.

51. Gu H, Huang L, Wong YP, and Burd A (2010). HA modulation of epidermal morphogenesis in an organotypic keratinocyte-fibroblast co-culture model, *Exp Dermatol*, **19**, e336–e339.

52. Judah D, Rudkouskaya A, Wilson R, Carter DE, and Dagnino L (2012). Multiple roles of integrin-linked kinase in epidermal development, maturation and pigmentation revealed by molecular profiling, *PLoS One*, **7**, e36704.

53. Staquet MJ, Piccardi N, Msika P, and Schmitt D (2002). Langerhans cell migration. An essential step in the induction of contact hypersensitivity, *Ann Dermatol Venereol*, **129**, 1071–1077.

54. Velez-Delvalle C, Marsch-Moreno M, Castro-Munozledo F, Bolivar-Flores YJ, and Kuri-Harcuch W (2008). Fibromodulin gene is expressed in human epidermal keratinocytes in culture and in human epidermis in vivo, *Biochem Biophys Res Commun*, **371**, 420–424.

55. Iriyama S, Matsunaga Y, Takahashi K, Matsuzaki K, Kumagai N, and Amano S (2011). Activation of heparanase by ultraviolet B irradiation leads to functional loss of basement membrane at the dermal–epidermal junction in human skin, *Arch Dermatol Res*, **303**, 253–261.

56. Iriyama S, Matsunaga Y, and Amano S (2010). Heparanase activation induces epidermal hyperplasia, angiogenesis, lymphangiogenesis and wrinkles, *Exp Dermatol*, **19**, 965–972.

57. Iriyama S, Hiruma T, Tsunenaga M, and Amano S (2011). Influence of heparan sulfate chains in proteoglycan at the dermal–epidermal junction on epidermal homeostasis, *Exp Dermatol*, **20**, 810–814.

58. Iriyama S, Ono T, Aoki H, and Amano S (2011). Hyperpigmentation in human solar lentigo is promoted by heparanase-induced loss of heparan sulfate chains at the dermal–epidermal junction, *J Dermatol Sci*, **64**, 223–228.

59. Ogura Y, Matsunaga Y, Nishiyama T, and Amano S (2008). Plasmin induces degradation and dysfunction of laminin 332 (laminin 5) and impaired assembly of basement membrane at the dermal–epidermal junction, *Br J Dermatol*, **159**, 49–60.

60. Kirschner N, Rosenthal R, Gunzel D, Moll I, and Brandner JM (2012). Tight junctions and differentiation—a chicken or the egg question? *Exp Dermatol*, **21**, 171–175.

61. Uitto J, Richard G, and McGrath JA (2007). Diseases of epidermal keratins and their linker proteins, *Exp Cell Res*, **313**, 1995–2009.

62. Margadant C, Charafeddine RA, and Sonnenberg A (2010). Unique and redundant functions of integrins in the epidermis, *FASEB J*, **24**, 4133–4152.

63. De Potter IY, Poumay Y, Squillace KA, and Pittelkow MR (2001). Human EGF receptor (HER) family and heregulin members are differentially expressed in epidermal keratinocytes and modulate differentiation, *Exp Cell Res*, **271**, 315–328.

64. Muller EJ, Williamson L, Kolly C, and Suter MM (2008). Outside-in signaling through integrins and cadherins: a central mechanism to control epidermal growth and differentiation? *J Invest Dermatol*, **128**, 501–516.

65. Zeeuwen PL (2004). Epidermal differentiation: the role of proteases and their inhibitors, *Eur J Cell Biol*, **83**, 761–773.

66. Ohman H and Vahlquist A (1994). In vivo studies concerning a pH gradient in human *stratum corneum* and upper epidermis, *Acta Derm Venereol*, **74**, 375–379.

67. Fluhr JW, Kao J, Jain M, Ahn SK, Feingold KR, and Elias PM (2001). Generation of free fatty acids from phospholipids regulates *stratum corneum* acidification and integrity, *J Invest Dermatol*, **117**, 44–51.

68. Behne MJ, Meyer JW, Hanson KM, Barry NP, Murata S, Crumrine D, Clegg RW, Gratton E, Holleran WM, Elias PM, and Mauro TM (2002). NHE1 regulates the *stratum corneum* permeability barrier homeostasis. Microenvironment acidification assessed with fluorescence lifetime imaging, *J Biol Chem*, **277**, 47399–47406.

69. Hachem JP, Behne M, Aronchik I, Demerjian M, Feingold KR, Elias PM, and Mauro TM (2005). Extracellular pH Controls NHE1 expression in epidermis and keratinocytes: implications for barrier repair, *J Invest Dermatol*, **125**, 790–797.

70. Krien PM and Kermici M (2000). Evidence for the existence of a self-regulated enzymatic process within the human *stratum corneum*— an unexpected role for urocanic acid, *J Invest Dermatol*, **115**, 414–420.

71. Korting HC, Kober M, Mueller M, and Braun-Falco O (1987). Influence of repeated washings with soap and synthetic detergents on pH and resident flora of the skin of forehead and forearm. Results of a cross-over trial in health probationers, *Acta Derm Venereol*, **67**, 41–47.

72. Hachem JP, Man MQ, Crumrine D, Uchida Y, Brown BE, Rogiers V, Roseeuw D, Feingold KR, and Elias PM (2005). Sustained serine proteases activity by prolonged increase in pH leads to degradation of lipid processing enzymes and profound alterations of barrier function and *stratum corneum* integrity, *J Invest Dermatol*, **125**, 510–520.

73. Brattsand M, Stefansson K, Lundh C, Haasum Y, and Egelrud T (2005). A proteolytic cascade of kallikreins in the *stratum corneum*, *J Invest Dermatol*, **124**, 198–203.

74. Nylander-Lundqvist E and Egelrud T (1997). Formation of active IL-1 beta from pro-IL-1 beta catalyzed by *stratum corneum* chymotryptic enzyme in vitro, *Acta Derm Venereol*, **77**, 203–206.

75. Hachem JP, Houben E, Crumrine D, Man MQ, Schurer N, Roelandt T, Choi EH, Uchida Y, Brown BE, Feingold KR, and Elias PM (2006). Serine protease signaling of epidermal permeability barrier homeostasis, *J Invest Dermatol*, **126**, 2074–2086.

76. Fukunaga-Kalabis M, Santiago-Walker A, and Herlyn M (2008). Matricellular proteins produced by melanocytes and melanomas: in search for functions, *Cancer Microenviron*, **1**, 93–102.

77. Haass NK and Herlyn M (2005). Normal human melanocyte homeostasis as a paradigm for understanding melanoma, *J Investig Dermatol Symp Proc*, **10**, 153–163.

78. Pinon P and Wehrle-Haller B (2011). Integrins: versatile receptors controlling melanocyte adhesion, migration and proliferation, *Pigment Cell Melanoma Res*, **24**, 282–294.

79. Moskvina V, Smith M, Ivanov D, Blackwood D, Stclair D, Hultman C, Toncheva D, Gill M, Corvin A, O'Dushlaine C, Morris DW, Wray NR, Sullivan P, Pato C, Pato MT, Sklar P, Purcell S, Holmans P, O'Donovan MC, Owen MJ, and Kirov G (2010). Genetic Differences between Five European Populations, *Hum Hered*, **70**, 141–149.

80. Sturm RA (2009). Molecular genetics of human pigmentation diversity, *Hum Mol Genet*, **18**, R9–R17.

81. Alaluf S, Atkins D, Barrett K, Blount M, Carter N, and Heath A (2002). Ethnic variation in melanin content and composition in photoexposed and photoprotected human skin, *Pigment Cell Res*, **15**, 112–118.

82. Ito S and Wakamatsu K (2003). Quantitative analysis of eumelanin and pheomelanin in humans, mice, and other animals: a comparative review, *Pigment Cell Res*, **16**, 523–531.

83. Garcia-Molina F, Munoz-Munoz JL, Garcia-Molina M, Garcia-Ruiz PA, Tudela J, Garcia-Canovas F, and Rodriguez-Lopez JN (2010). Melanogenesis inhibition due to NADH, *Biosci Biotechnol Biochem*, **74**, 1777–1787.

84. Munoz-Munoz JL, Acosta-Motos JR, Garcia-Molina F, Varon R, Garcia-Ruiz PA, Tudela J, Garcia-Canovas F, and Rodriguez-Lopez JN (2010). Tyrosinase inactivation in its action on dopa, *Biochim Biophys Acta*, **1804**, 1467–1475.

85. Alaluf S, Barrett K, Blount M, and Carter N (2003). Ethnic variation in tyrosinase and TYRP1 expression in photoexposed and photoprotected human skin, *Pigment Cell Res*, **16**, 35–42.

86. Raposo G, Tenza D, Murphy DM, Berson JF, and Marks MS (2001). Distinct protein sorting and localization to premelanosomes, melanosomes, and lysosomes in pigmented melanocytic cells, *J Cell Biol*, **152**, 809–824.

87. Theos AC, Truschel ST, Raposo G, and Marks MS (2005). The Silver locus product Pmel17/gp100/Silv/ME20: controversial in name and in function, *Pigment Cell Res*, **18**, 322–336.

88. Kawakami A, Sakane F, Imai S, Yasuda S, Kai M, Kanoh H, Jin HY, Hirosaki K, Yamashita T, Fisher DE, and Jimbow K. (2008). Rab7

regulates maturation of melanosomal matrix protein gp100/Pmel17/ Silv, *J Invest Dermatol*, **128**, 143–150.

89. Hurbain I, Geerts WJ, Boudier T, Marco S, Verkleij AJ, Marks MS, and Raposo G (2008). Electron tomography of early melanosomes: implications for melanogenesis and the generation of fibrillar amyloid sheets, *Proc Natl Acad Sci USA*, **105**, 19726–19731.

90. Berson JF, Theos AC, Harper DC, Tenza D, Raposo G, and Marks MS (2003). Proprotein convertase cleavage liberates a fibrillogenic fragment of a resident glycoprotein to initiate melanosome biogenesis, *J Cell Biol*, **161**, 521–533.

91. Clague MJ (2002). Membrane transport: a coat for ubiquitin, *Curr Biol*, **12**, R529–R531.

92. Gautam R, Novak EK, Tan J, Wakamatsu K, Ito S, and Swank RT (2006). Interaction of Hermansky-Pudlak Syndrome genes in the regulation of lysosome-related organelles, *Traffic*, **7**, 779–792.

93. Theos AC, Tenza D, Martina JA, Hurbain I, Peden AA, Sviderskaya EV, Stewart A, Robinson MS, Bennett DC, Cutler DF, Bonifacino JS, Marks MS, and Raposo G (2005). Functions of adaptor protein (AP)-3 and AP-1 in tyrosinase sorting from endosomes to melanosomes, *Mol Biol Cell*, **16**, 5356–5372.

94. Setty SR, Tenza D, Truschel ST, Chou E, Sviderskaya EV, Theos AC, Lamoreux ML, Di Pietro SM, Starcevic M, Bennett DC, Dell'Angelica EC, Raposo G, and Marks MS (2007). BLOC-1 is required for cargo-specific sorting from vacuolar early endosomes toward lysosome-related organelles, *Mol Biol Cell*, **18**, 768–780.

95. Hearing VJ (2005). Biogenesis of pigment granules: a sensitive way to regulate melanocyte function, *J Dermatol Sci*, **37**, 3–14.

96. Wasmeier C, Hume AN, Bolasco G, and Seabra MC (2008). Melanosomes at a glance, *J Cell Sci*, **121**, 3995–3999.

97. De Matteis MA and Morrow JS (2000). Spectrin tethers and mesh in the biosynthetic pathway, *J Cell Sci*, **113 (Pt 13)**, 2331–2343.

98. Passeron T, Bahadoran P, Bertolotto C, Chiaverini C, Busca R, Valony G, Bille K, Ortonne JP, and Ballotti R (2004). Cyclic AMP promotes a peripheral distribution of melanosomes and stimulates melanophilin/ Slac2-a and actin association, *FASEB J*, **18**, 989–991.

99. Wu X, Bowers B, Rao K, Wei Q, and Hammer JA, 3rd. (1998). Visualization of melanosome dynamics within wild-type and dilute melanocytes suggests a paradigm for myosin V function in vivo, *J Cell Biol*, **143**, 1899–1918.

100. Jordens I, Fernandez-Borja M, Marsman M, Dusseljee S, Janssen L, Calafat J, Janssen H, Wubbolts R, and Neefjes J (2001). The Rab7 effector protein RILP controls lysosomal transport by inducing the recruitment of dynein-dynactin motors. *Curr Biol*, **11**, 1680–1685.

101. Jordens I, Westbroek W, Marsman M, Rocha N, Mommaas M, Huizing M, Lambert J, Naeyaert JM, and Neefjes J (2006). Rab7 and Rab27a control two motor protein activities involved in melanosomal transport, *Pigment Cell Res*, **19**, 412–423.

102. Seabra MC and Coudrier E (2004). Rab GTPases and myosin motors in organelle motility, *Traffic*, **5**, 393–399.

103. Kuroda TS and Fukuda M (2004). Rab27A-binding protein Slp2-a is required for peripheral melanosome distribution and elongated cell shape in melanocytes, *Nat Cell Biol*, **6**, 1195–1203.

104. Trichet L, Sykes C, and Plastino J (2008). Relaxing the actin cytoskeleton for adhesion and movement with Ena/VASP, *J Cell Biol*, **181**, 19–25.

105. Yonezawa S, Yoshizaki N, Sano M, Hanai A, Masaki S, Takizawa T, Kageyama T, and Moriyama A (2003). Possible involvement of myosin-X in intercellular adhesion: importance of serial pleckstrin homology regions for intracellular localization, *Dev Growth Differ*, **45**, 175–185.

106. Tokuo H, Mabuchi K, and Ikebe M (2007). The motor activity of myosin-X promotes actin fiber convergence at the cell periphery to initiate filopodia formation, *J Cell Biol*, **179**, 229–238.

107. Lin CB, Chen N, Scarpa R, Guan F, Babiarz-Magee L, Liebel F, Li WH, Kizoulis M, Shapiro S, and Seiberg M (2008). LIGR, a protease-activated receptor-2-derived peptide, enhances skin pigmentation without inducing inflammatory processes, *Pigment Cell Melanoma Res*, **21**, 172–183.

108. Seiberg M, Paine C, Sharlow E, Andrade-Gordon P, Costanzo M, Eisinger M, and Shapiro SS (2000). The protease-activated receptor 2 regulates pigmentation via keratinocyte-melanocyte interactions, *Exp Cell Res*, **254**, 25–32.

109. Nagataki M, Moriyuki K, Sekiguchi F, and Kawabata A (2008). Evidence that PAR2-triggered prostaglandin E2 (PGE2) formation involves the ERK-cytosolic phospholipase A2-COX-1-microsomal PGE synthase-1 cascade in human lung epithelial cells, *Cell Biochem Funct*, **26**, 279–282.

110. Hume AN and Seabra MC (2011). Melanosomes on the move: a model to understand organelle dynamics, *Biochem Soc Trans*, **39**, 1191–1196.

111. Hirobe T, Furuya R, Ifuku O, Osawa M, and Nishikawa S (2004). Granulocyte-macrophage colony-stimulating factor is a keratinocyte-derived factor involved in regulating the proliferation and differentiation of neonatal mouse epidermal melanocytes in culture, *Exp Cell Res*, **297**, 593–606.

112. mokawa G (2004). Autocrine and paracrine regulation of melanocytes in human skin and in pigmentary disorders, *Pigment Cell Res*, **17**, 96–110.

113. Corre S, Mekideche K, Adamski H, Mosser J, Watier E, and Galibert MD (2006). In vivo and ex vivo UV-induced analysis of pigmentation gene expressions, *J Invest Dermatol*, **126**, 916–918.

114. Herlyn M, Mancianti ML, Jambrosic J, Bolen JB, and Koprowski H (1988). Regulatory factors that determine growth and phenotype of normal human melanocytes, *Exp Cell Res*, **179**, 322–331.

115. Scott G, Deng A, Rodriguez-Burford C, Seiberg M, Han R, Babiarz L, Grizzle W, Bell W, and Pentland A (2001). Protease-activated receptor 2, a receptor involved in melanosome transfer, is upregulated in human skin by ultraviolet irradiation, *J Invest Dermatol*, **117**, 1412–1420.

116. Scott G, Leopardi S, Parker L, Babiarz L, Seiberg M, and Han R (2003). The proteinase-activated receptor-2 mediates phagocytosis in a Rho-dependent manner in human keratinocytes, *J Invest Dermatol*, **121**, 529–541.

117. Thong HY, Jee SH, Sun CC, and Boissy RE (2003). The patterns of melanosome distribution in keratinocytes of human skin as one determining factor of skin colour, *Br J Dermatol*, **149**, 498–505.

118. Yoshida Y, Hachiya A, Sriwiriyanont P, Ohuchi A, Kitahara T, Takema Y, Visscher MO, and Boissy RE (2007). Functional analysis of keratinocytes in skin color using a human skin substitute model composed of cells derived from different skin pigmentation types, *FASEB J*, **21**, 2829–2839.

119. Ebanks JP, Koshoffer A, Wickett RR, Schwemberger S, Babcock G, Hakozaki T, and Boissy RE. (2011). Epidermal keratinocytes from light vs. dark skin exhibit differential degradation of melanosomes, *J Invest Dermatol*, **131**, 1226–1233.

120. Chakraborty AK, Funasaka Y, Slominski A, Ermak G, Hwang J, Pawelek JM, and Ichihashi M (1996). Production and release of proopiomelanocortin (POMC) derived peptides by human melanocytes and keratinocytes in culture: regulation by ultraviolet B, *Biochim Biophys Acta*, **1313**, 130–138.

121. Van Raamsdonk CD, Barsh GS, Wakamatsu K, and Ito S (2009). Independent regulation of hair and skin color by two G protein-coupled pathways, *Pigment Cell Melanoma Res*, **22**, 819–826.

122. Commo S, Gaillard O, Thibaut S, and Bernard BA (2004). Absence of TRP-2 in melanogenic melanocytes of human hair, *Pigment Cell Res*, **17**, 488–497.

123. Abdel-Malek Z, Scott MC, Suzuki I, Tada A, Im S, Lamoreux L, Ito S, Barsh G, and Hearing VJ (2000). The melanocortin-1 receptor is a key regulator of human cutaneous pigmentation, *Pigment Cell Res*, **13 Suppl 8**, 156–162.

124. Slominski A, Szczesniewski A, and Wortsman J (2000). Liquid chromatography-mass spectrometry detection of corticotropin-releasing hormone and proopiomelanocortin-derived peptides in human skin, *J Clin Endocrinol Metab*, **85**, 3582–3588.

125. Cone RD, Lu D, Koppula S, Vage DI, Klungland H, Boston B, Chen W, Orth DN, Pouton C, and Kesterson RA (1996). The melanocortin receptors: agonists, antagonists, and the hormonal control of pigmentation, *Recent Prog Horm Res*, **51**, 287–317; discussion 318.

126. Im S, Moro O, Peng F, Medrano EE, Cornelius J, Babcock G, Nordlund JJ, and Abdel-Malek ZA (1998). Activation of the cyclic AMP pathway by alpha-melanotropin mediates the response of human melanocytes to ultraviolet B radiation, *Cancer Res*, **58**, 47–54.

127. Insel PA, Bourne HR, Coffino P, and Tomkins GM (1975). Cyclic AMP-dependent protein kinase: pivotal role in regulation of enzyme induction and growth, *Science*, **190**, 896–898.

128. Busca R and Ballotti R (2000). Cyclic AMP a key messenger in the regulation of skin pigmentation, *Pigment Cell Res*, **13**, 60–69.

129. Tachibana M (2000). MITF: a stream flowing for pigment cells, *Pigment Cell Res*, **13**, 230–240.

130. Peacocke M, Yaar M, Mansur CP, Chao MV, and Gilchrest BA (1988). Induction of nerve growth factor receptors on cultured human melanocytes, *Proc Natl Acad Sci USA*, **85**, 5282–5286.

131. Yaar M, Grossman K, Eller M, and Gilchrest BA (1991). Evidence for nerve growth factor-mediated paracrine effects in human epidermis, *J Cell Biol*, **115**, 821–828.

132. Imokawa G, Kobayashi T, Miyagishi M, Higashi K, and Yada Y (1997). The role of endothelin-1 in epidermal hyperpigmentation and signaling mechanisms of mitogenesis and melanogenesis, *Pigment Cell Res*, **10**, 218–228.

133. Hara M, Yaar M, and Gilchrest BA (1995). Endothelin-1 of keratinocyte origin is a mediator of melanocyte dendricity, *J Invest Dermatol*, **105**, 744–748.

134. Scott MC, Suzuki I, and Abdel-Malek ZA (2002). Regulation of the human melanocortin 1 receptor expression in epidermal melanocytes by paracrine and endocrine factors and by ultraviolet radiation, *Pigment Cell Res*, **15**, 433–439.

135. Imokawa G, Yada Y, and Kimura M (1996). Signalling mechanisms of endothelin-induced mitogenesis and melanogenesis in human melanocytes, *Biochem J*, **314 (Pt 1)**, 305–312.

136. Imokawa G, Miyagishi M, and Yada Y (1995). Endothelin-1 as a new melanogen: coordinated expression of its gene and the tyrosinase gene in UVB-exposed human epidermis, *J Invest Dermatol*, **105**, 32–37.

137. Scott G, Leopardi S, Printup S, Malhi N, Seiberg M, and Lapoint R (2004). Proteinase-activated receptor-2 stimulates prostaglandin production in keratinocytes: analysis of prostaglandin receptors on human melanocytes and effects of PGE2 and PGF2alpha on melanocyte dendricity, *J Invest Dermatol*, **122**, 1214–1224.

138. Chun KS, Lao HC, and Langenbach R (2010). The prostaglandin E2 receptor, EP2, stimulates keratinocyte proliferation in mouse skin by G protein-dependent and {beta}-arrestin1-dependent signaling pathways, *J Biol Chem*, **285**, 39672–39681.

139. Halaban R, Langdon R, Birchall N, Cuono C, Baird A, Scott G, Moellmann G, and McGuire J (1988). Basic fibroblast growth factor from human keratinocytes is a natural mitogen for melanocytes, *J Cell Biol*, **107**, 1611–1619.

140. Hachiya A, Kobayashi A, Ohuchi A, Takema Y, and Imokawa G (2001). The paracrine role of stem cell factor/c-kit signaling in the activation of human melanocytes in ultraviolet-B-induced pigmentation, *J Invest Dermatol*, **116**, 578–586.

141. Chiba S, Shibuya K, Miyazono K, Tojo A, Oka Y, Miyagawa K, and Takaku F (1990). Affinity purification of human granulocyte macrophage colony-stimulating factor receptor alpha-chain. Demonstration of binding by photoaffinity labeling, *J Biol Chem*, **265**, 19777–19781.

142. Okuda K, Sanghera JS, Pelech SL, Kanakura Y, Hallek M, Griffin JD, and Druker BJ (1992). Granulocyte-macrophage colony-stimulating factor, interleukin-3, and steel factor induce rapid tyrosine phosphorylation of p42 and p44 MAP kinase, *Blood*, **79**, 2880–2887.

143. Mui AL, Wakao H, O'Farrell AM, Harada N, and Miyajima A (1995). Interleukin-3, granulocyte-macrophage colony stimulating factor and interleukin-5 transduce signals through two STAT5 homologs, *EMBO J*, **14**, 1166–1175.

144. Wang Y, Morella KK, Ripperger J, Lai CF, Gearing DP, Fey GH, Campos SP, and Baumann H (1995). Receptors for interleukin-3 (IL-3) and growth hormone mediate an IL-6-type transcriptional induction in the presence of JAK2 or STAT3, *Blood*, **86**, 1671–1679.

145. Kimura T, Sekido M, Chimura N, Shibata S, Kondo N, Kamishina H, Kamishina H, and Maeda S (2012). Production of GM-CSF mediated by cysteine protease of Der f in canine keratinocytes, *J Vet Med Sci*, **74**, 1033–1036.

146. Li G, Schaider H, Satyamoorthy K, Hanakawa Y, Hashimoto K, and Herlyn M (2001). Downregulation of E-cadherin and Desmoglein 1 by autocrine hepatocyte growth factor during melanoma development, *Oncogene*, **20**, 8125–8135.

147. Hinitt CA, Wood J, Lee SS, Williams AC, Howarth JL, Glover CP, Uney JB, and Hague A (2010). BAG-1 enhances cell-cell adhesion, reduces proliferation and induces chaperone-independent suppression of hepatocyte growth factor-induced epidermal keratinocyte migration, *Exp Cell Res*, **316**, 2042–2060.

148. O'Brien LE, Tang K, Kats ES, Schutz-Geschwender A, Lipschutz JH, and Mostov KE (2004). ERK and MMPs sequentially regulate distinct stages of epithelial tubule development, *Dev Cell*, **7**, 21–32.

149. Matsumoto K, Tajima H, and Nakamura T (1991). Hepatocyte growth factor is a potent stimulator of human melanocyte DNA synthesis and growth, *Biochem Biophys Res Commun*, **176**, 45–51.

150. Boccaccio C, Ando M, Tamagnone L, Bardelli A, Michieli P, Battistini C, and Comoglio PM (1998). Induction of epithelial tubules by growth factor HGF depends on the STAT pathway, *Nature*, **391**, 285–288.

151. Graziani A, Gramaglia D, Cantley LC, and Comoglio PM (1991). The tyrosine-phosphorylated hepatocyte growth factor/scatter factor receptor associates with phosphatidylinositol 3-kinase, *J Biol Chem*, **266**, 22087–22090.

152. Gentile A, Trusolino L, and Comoglio PM (2008). The Met tyrosine kinase receptor in development and cancer, *Cancer Metastasis Rev*, **27**, 85–94.

153. Monga SP, Mars WM, Pediaditakis P, Bell A, Mule K, Bowen WC, Wang X, Zarnegar R, and Michalopoulos GK (2002). Hepatocyte growth factor induces Wnt-independent nuclear translocation of beta-catenin after Met-beta-catenin dissociation in hepatocytes, *Cancer Res*, **62**, 2064–2071.

154. Guo Y, Xie J, Rubin E, Tang YX, Lin F, Zi X, and Hoang BH (2008). Frzb, a secreted Wnt antagonist, decreases growth and invasiveness of fibrosarcoma cells associated with inhibition of Met signaling, *Cancer Res*, **68**, 3350–3360.

155. Abounader R, Reznik T, Colantuoni C, Martinez-Murillo F, Rosen EM, and Laterra J (2004). Regulation of c-Met-dependent gene expression by PTEN, *Oncogene*, **23**, 9173–9182.

156. Thomas CC, Deak M, Alessi DR, and van Aalten DM (2002). High-resolution structure of the pleckstrin homology domain of protein kinase b/akt bound to phosphatidylinositol (3,4,5)-trisphosphate, *Curr Biol*, **12**, 1256–1262.

157. Yamaguchi Y, Itami S, Watabe H, Yasumoto K, Abdel-Malek ZA, Kubo T, Rouzaud F, Tanemura A, Yoshikawa K, and Hearing VJ (2004). Mesenchymal-epithelial interactions in the skin: increased expression of dickkopf1 by palmoplantar fibroblasts inhibits melanocyte growth and differentiation, *J Cell Biol*, **165**, 275–285.

158. Hasegawa J, Goto Y, Murata H, Takata M, Saida T, and Imokawa G (2008). Downregulated melanogenic paracrine cytokine linkages in hypopigmented palmoplantar skin, *Pigment Cell Melanoma Res*, **21**, 687–699.

159. Yamaguchi Y, Morita A, Maeda A, and Hearing VJ (2009). Regulation of skin pigmentation and thickness by Dickkopf 1 (DKK1), *J Invest Dermatol Symp Proc*, **14**, 73–75.

160. McKay MM and Morrison DK (2007). Integrating signals from RTKs to ERK/MAPK, *Oncogene*, **26**, 3113–3121.

161. Dhanasekaran DN, Kashef K, Lee CM, Xu H, and Reddy EP (2007). Scaffold proteins of MAP-kinase modules, *Oncogene*, **26**, 3185–3202.

162. Vanhaesebroeck B, Guillermet-Guibert J, Graupera M, and Bilanges B (2010). The emerging mechanisms of isoform-specific PI3K signalling, *Nat Rev Mol Cell Biol*, **11**, 329–341.

163. Del Conte-Zerial P, Brusch L, Rink JC, Collinet C, Kalaidzidis Y, Zerial M, and Deutsch A (2008). Membrane identity and GTPase cascades regulated by toggle and cut-out switches, *Mol Syst Biol*, **4**, 206, 1–9.

164. Herrmann F, Gross A, Zhou D, Kestler HA, and Kuhl M (2012). A Boolean model of the cardiac gene regulatory network determining first and second heart field identity, *PLoS One*, **7**, e46798.

165. Charruyer A, Barland CO, Yue L, Wessendorf HB, Lu Y, Lawrence HJ, Mancianti ML, and Ghadially R (2009). Transit-amplifying cell frequency and cell cycle kinetics are altered in aged epidermis, *J Invest Dermatol*, **129**, 2574–2583.

166. Pucci M, Pirazzi V, Pasquariello N, and Maccarrone M (2011). Endocannabinoid signaling and epidermal differentiation, *Eur J Dermatol*, **21**(Suppl 2), 29–34.

167. Driskell RR, Juneja VR, Connelly JT, Kretzschmar K, Tan DW, and Watt FM (2012). Clonal growth of dermal papilla cells in hydrogels reveals intrinsic differences between Sox2-positive and -negative cells in vitro and in vivo, *J Invest Dermatol*, **132**, 1084–1093.

168. Enomoto A, Yoshihisa Y, Yamakoshi T, Ur Rehman M, Norisugi O, Hara H, Matsunaga K, Makino T, Nishihira J, and Shimizu T (2011). UV-B radiation induces macrophage migration inhibitory factor-mediated melanogenesis through activation of protease-activated receptor-2 and stem cell factor in keratinocytes, *Am J Pathol*, **178**, 679–687.

169. Tang L, Li J, Lin X, Wu W, Kang K, and Fu W (2012). Oxidation levels differentially impact melanocytes: low versus high concentration of hydrogen peroxide promotes melanin synthesis and melanosome transfer, *Dermatology*, **224**, 145–153.

170. Yoo H, Kim SJ, Kim Y, Lee H, and Kim TY (2007). Insulin-like growth factor-II regulates the 12-lipoxygenase gene expression and promotes cell proliferation in human keratinocytes via the extracellular regulatory kinase and phosphatidylinositol 3-kinase pathways, *Int J Biochem Cell Biol*, **39**, 1248–1259.

171. Elder JT, Bruce AT, Gudjonsson JE, Johnston A, Stuart PE, Tejasvi T, Voorhees JJ, Abecasis GR, and Nair RP (2010). Molecular dissection of psoriasis: integrating genetics and biology, *J Invest Dermatol*, **130**, 1213–1226.

172. Li Y, Sawalha AH, and Lu Q (2009). Aberrant DNA methylation in skin diseases, *J Dermatol Sci*, **54**, 143–149.

173. O'Regan GM, Sandilands A, McLean WH, and Irvine AD (2009). Filaggrin in atopic dermatitis, *J Allergy Clin Immunol*, **124**, R2–R6.

174. Zhang Y, Andl T, Yang SH, Teta M, Liu F, Seykora JT, Tobias JW, Piccolo S, Schmidt-Ullrich R, Nagy A, Taketo MM, Dlugosz AA, and Millar SE (2008). Activation of beta-catenin signaling programs embryonic epidermis to hair follicle fate, *Development*, **135**, 2161–2172.

175. Enshell-Seijffers D, Lindon C, Wu E, Taketo MM, and Morgan BA (2010). Beta-catenin activity in the dermal papilla of the hair follicle

regulates pigment-type switching, *Proc Natl Acad Sci USA*, **107**, 21564–21569.

176. Yoon TJ, Lei TC, Yamaguchi Y, Batzer J, Wolber R, and Hearing VJ (2003). Reconstituted 3-dimensional human skin of various ethnic origins as an in vitro model for studies of pigmentation, *Anal Biochem*, **318**, 260–269.

177. Ultto U, Richard G, and McGarth JA (2007). Diseases of epidermal keratins and their linker proteins, *Exp Cell Res*, **313**, 1995–2009.

178. Iris F, Gea M, Lampe PH, and Santamaria P (2009). Production and implementation of predictive biological models, *Med Sci (Paris)*, **25**, 608–616.

179. Iris F (2012). Psychiatric systems medicine: closer at hand than anticipated but not with the expected portrait, *Pharmacopsychiatry*, **45**(Suppl 1), S12–S21.

180. Gadal F, Bozic C, Pillot-Brochet C, Malinge S, Wagner S, Le Cam A, Buffat L, Crepin M, and Iris F (2003). Integrated transcriptome analysis of the cellular mechanisms associated with Ha-ras-dependent malignant transformation of the human breast epithelial MCF7 cell line, *Nucleic Acids Res*, **31**, 5789–5804.

181. Gadal F, Starzec A, Bozic C, Pillot-Brochet C, Malinge S, Ozanne V, Vicenzi J, Buffat L, Perret G, Iris F, and Crépin M (2005). Integrative analysis of gene expression patterns predicts specific modulations of defined cell functions by estrogen and tamoxifen in MCF7 breast cancer cells, *J Mol Endocrinol*, **34**, 61–75.

182. Turck CW and Iris F (2011). Proteome-based pathway modelling of psychiatric disorders, *Pharmacopsychiatry*, **44 Suppl 1**, S54–S61.

183. Pouillot F, Blois H, and Iris F (2010). Genetically engineered virulent phage banks in the detection and control of emergent pathogenic bacteria, *Biosecur Bioterror*, **8**, 155–169.

184. European Commission, DG Research, Directorate of Health.(2010). From Systems Biology to Systems Medicine; pp. 5–6. ftp://ftp.cordis.europa.eu/pub/fp7/health/docs/final-report-systems-medicine-workshop_en.pdf.

185. Cambridge Healthtech Institute. (2009). Bio-IT Best Practice Awards 2009 http://www.bio-itworld.com/BioIT_Article.aspx?id = 93536.

186. Giordano F, Bonetti C, Surace EM, Marigo V, and Raposo G (2009). The ocular albinism type 1 (OA1) G-protein-coupled receptor functions with MART-1 at early stages of melanogenesis to control melanosome identity and composition. *Hum Mol Genet*, **18**, 4530–4545.

187. Schiaffino MV and Tacchetti C (2005). The ocular albinism type 1 (OA1) protein and the evidence for an intracellular signal transduction system involved in melanosome biogenesis, *Pigment Cell Res*, **18**, 227–233.

188. Schiaffino MV (2010). Signaling pathways in melanosome biogenesis and pathology, *Int J Biochem Cell Biol*, **42**, 1094–1104.

189. Young A, Jiang M, Wang Y, Ahmedli NB, Ramirez J, Reese BE, Birnbaumer L, and Farber DB (2011). Specific interaction of Galphai3 with the OA1 G-protein coupled receptor controls the size and density of melanosomes in retinal pigment epithelium, *PLoS One*, **6**, e24376.

190. Goldsmith ZG and Dhanasekaran DN (2007). G protein regulation of MAPK networks, *Oncogene*, **26**, 3122–3142.

191. Lopez VM, Decatur CL, Stamer WD, Lynch RM, and McKay BS (2008). L-DOPA is an endogenous ligand for OA1, *PLoS Biol*, **6**, e236.

192. Palmisano I, Bagnato P, Palmigiano A, Innamorati G, Rotondo G, Altimare D, Venturi C, Sviderskaya EV, Piccirillo R, Coppola M, Marigo V, Incerti B, Ballabio A, Surace EM, Tacchetti C, Bennett DC, and Schiaffino MV (2008). The ocular albinism type 1 protein, an intracellular G protein-coupled receptor, regulates melanosome transport in pigment cells, *Hum Mol Genet*, **17**, 3487–3501.

193. Rachel RA, Nagashima K, O'Sullivan TN, Frost LS, Stefano FP, Marigo V, and Boesze-Battaglia K (2012). Melanoregulin, product of the dsu locus, links the BLOC-pathway and OA1 in organelle biogenesis, *PLoS One*, **7**, e42446.

194. Wu X, Jung G, and Hammer JA, 3rd. (2000). Functions of unconventional myosins, *Curr Opin Cell Biol*, **12**, 42–51.

195. Woehlke G and Schliwa M (2000). Directional motility of kinesin motor proteins, *Biochim Biophys Acta*, **1496**, 117–127.

196. Sakato M and King SM (2004). Design and regulation of the AAA+ microtubule motor dynein, *J Struct Biol*, **146**, 58–71.

197. Rodionov V, Yi J, Kashina A, Oladipo A, and Gross SP (2003). Switching between microtubule- and actin-based transport systems in melanophores is controlled by cAMP levels, *Curr Biol*, **13**, 1837–1847.

198. Ikeda K, Zhapparova O, Brodsky I, Semenova I, Tirnauer JS, Zaliapin I, and Rodionov V (2011). CK1 activates minus-end-directed transport of membrane organelles along microtubules, *Mol Biol Cell*, **22**, 1321–1329.

199. Watabe H, Valencia JC, Le Pape E, Yamaguchi Y, Nakamura M, Rouzaud F, Hoashi T, Kawa Y, Mizoguchi M, and Hearing VJ (2008). Involvement

of dynein and spectrin with early melanosome transport and melanosomal protein trafficking, *J Invest Dermatol*, **128**, 162–174.

200. Westbroek W, Lambert J, De Schepper S, Kleta R, Van Den Bossche K, Seabra MC, Huizing M, Mommaas M, and Naeyaert JM (2004). Rab27b is up-regulated in human Griscelli syndrome type II melanocytes and linked to the actin cytoskeleton via exon F-Myosin Va transcripts, *Pigment Cell Res*, **17**, 498–505.

201. Nielsen DK, Jensen AK, Harbak H, Christensen SC, and Simonsen LO (2007). Cell content of phosphatidylinositol (4,5)bisphosphate in Ehrlich mouse ascites tumour cells in response to cell volume perturbations in anisotonic and in isosmotic media, *J Physiol*, **582**, 1027–1036.

202. Breitwieser GE (2006). Calcium sensing receptors and calcium oscillations: calcium as a first messenger, *Curr Top Dev Biol*, **73**, 85–114.

203. Deacon SW, Nascimento A, Serpinskaya AS, and Gelfand VI (2005). Regulation of bidirectional melanosome transport by organelle bound MAP kinase, *Curr Biol*, **15**, 459–463.

204. Fukuda M (2005). Versatile role of Rab27 in membrane trafficking: focus on the Rab27 effector families, *J Biochem*, **137**, 9–16.

205. Stephens L, Milne L, and Hawkins P (2008). Moving towards a better understanding of chemotaxis, *Curr Biol*, **18**, R485–R494.

# Index

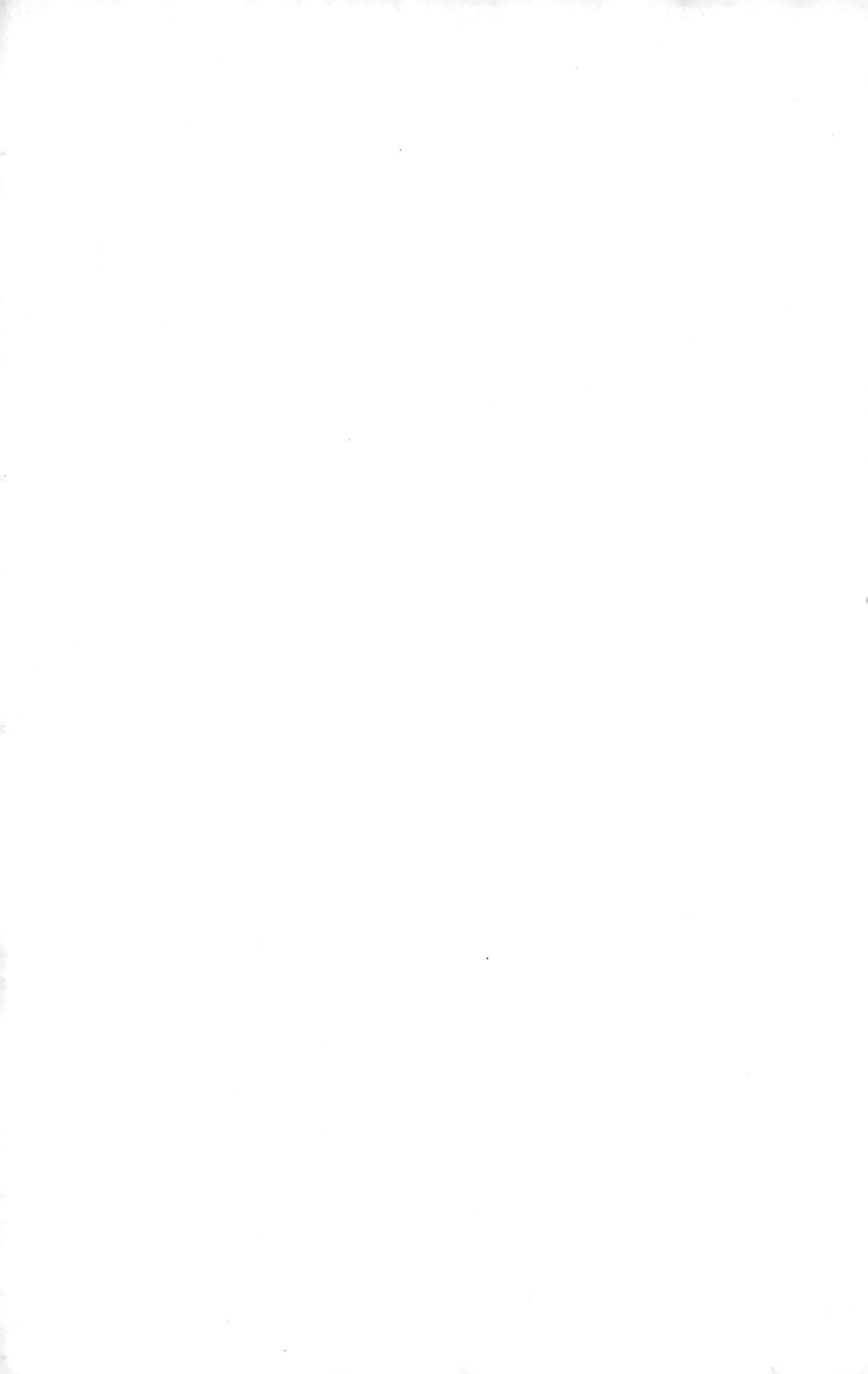